FIRE YOUR DOCTOR

Superhealth & Fitness for Lawyers and
Desk Professionals

HIRE YOURSELF!

GARY W. PITTS

Wholesale discounts for book orders are available through Ingram or Spring Arbor Distributors.

Published in Canada.

978-1-987985-23-8 (softcover)

978-1-987985-21-4 (hardcover)

978-1-987985-22-1 (ebook)

First Edition

Table of Contents

CHAPTER ELEVEN

CHAPTER TWELVE

APPENDIX A – REFERENCES AND SCIENTIFIC STUDIES

APPENDIX B – DR. INTERNET'S 10 RECOMMENDED WEBSITES 539

"FIRE YOUR DOCTOR- HIRE YOURSELF!"
SUPERHEALTH & FITNESS –

(For Lawyers & Desk Professionals)

Do it Yourself!

**"OUR FOOD SHOULD BE OUR MEDICINE;
OUR MEDICINE SHOULD BE OUR FOOD."**

— Hippocrates M.D. The Father of Medicine (425 B.C.)

**"ANYTHING THE MEDICAL PROFESSION SAYS, DO THE
OPPOSITE 99 PERCENT OF THE TIME AND YOU'LL BE RIGHT."**

—Aajonus Vonderplanitz

AUTHOR'S NOTE

This book does not contain "footnotes" in the traditional format.

For reader convenience and cohesiveness of thought, references and/or sources of information/and/or authorities are immediately referenced.

An extensive list of references, clinical studies, and recommended websites are reproduced as APPENDIX A and B respectively.

DISCLAIMER

THIS IS A <u>WARNING</u> TO THE READER. PLEASE READ!

The information and material contained in the present Book is for EDUCATIONAL PURPOSES ONLY. The statements made in this book have not been evaluated by the Food and Drug Administration and represent the PROFESSIONAL OPINIONS of the author. These opinions are based upon the research and personal and professional experiences of the author.

The information provided this book is not meant to directly, nor indirectly DIAGNOSE, TREAT, or PRESCRIBE for any MEDICAL CONDITION or DISEASE.

This book is not designed to replace medical advice of a licenced medical professional. If you know or suspect that you have a HEALTH problem, you should consult a competent appropriate health professional.

The PUBLISHER and AUTHOR specifically disclaim any liability, loss, or risk, personal or of any nature whatsoever, that may be incurred as a consequence, directly or indirectly of the use and application of ANY of the CONTENTS of this book.

This AUTHOR does not accept any responsibility for your HEALTH or how you choose o use the information contained in this book.

The reader expressly ASSUMES ANY AND ALL RESPONSIBILITY for any and ALL injuries which may be sustained; directly or indirectly, caused by and/or resulting from the reader's application of any information contained in this book.

THE OPINIONS, NUTRITIONAL ADVICE AND LIFESTYLE STRATEGIES expressed in this book are the SOLE OPINION of the author—and no one else.

The author has received no compensation, financial or otherwise, from any person, and/or corporation and/or organization mentioned and/or recommended in this book.

<u>AUTHOR'S WARNING</u>-This book is intended for an adult audience.

DEDICATION AND ACKNOWLEDGEMENTS

This book is dedicated to my 87 year-old mother; Eileen Eisenhauer, a breast cancer survivor who had the courage and wisdom to fire her conventional doctors. I love you- Mom. This book is for you.

I would also like to dedicate this book to my late stepfather Albert "Bert" Heavyside. Bert- thanks for your love and your support and for treating me as your son. In life, I have been extremely fortunate. I have had TWO phenomenal fathers; my biological father- Frank Pitts and my stepfather- Bert Heavyside. Happily for me, my Dad and Bert became great friends. I was the glue in that relationship.

My first book "The Personal Trainer's Legal Bible" was dedicated to my late father.

Mom and Bert- this book is dedicated to you.

This book is also dedicated to the great joys of my life my daughter, Tracy and my grandson- Bryan as well as all my other wonderful family members; you know who you are.

Finally- I would like to express my heartfelt special thanks to Maureen Rodrigues. Maureen- Thank you for your encouragement and your moral support. Thank you for your advice regarding this book. I am confident this book will help a lot of people become healthy- and happy.

INTRODUCTION

<u>WHY</u> I am writing this health book?

There are <u>MANY</u> reasons.

<u>YOU DESERVE TO KNOW THE TRUTH ABOUT YOUR HEALTH.</u>

<u>YOU DESERVE TO KNOW THE TRUTH ABOUT YOUR HEALTH CARE SYSTEM.</u>

<u>YOU DESERVE TO KNOW THE TRUTH ABOUT THE PHARMACEUTICAL INDUSTRY AND THE MEDICAL ESTABLISHMENT.</u>

<u>YOU DESERVE TO KNOW THAT YOU NO LONGER NEED TO BE PART OF THIS FLAWED SYSTEM!</u>

<u>YOU DESERVE TO KNOW THAT YOU HAVE THE POWER TO TAKE CONTROL OF YOUR HEATH AND THE HEALTH OF YOUR LOVED ONES.</u>

<u>YOU SHOULD FIRE YOUR DOCTOR—AND—HIRE YOURSELF!</u>

<u>YOU ARE FAR MORE POWERFUL THAN YOU THINK!</u>

<u>YOU DESERVE TO KNOW THAT THERE ARE 9 DOCTORS WHO WILL PROVIDE YOU WITH SUPERHEALTH</u>. These doctors are:

- Dr. HAPPY -☺
- Dr. PURE WATER
- Dr. EARTH
- Dr. KETOGENIC DIET
- Dr. EXERCISE
- Dr. SUNSHINE
- Dr. FRESH AIR

- Dr. SLEEP

- Dr. INTERNET

YOUR EMOTIONAL HEALTH IS YOUR PLATINUM KEY TO SUPERHEALTH. YOUR EMOTIONAL HEALTH (DR. HAPPY) IS INTIMATELY LINKED TO THE PLATINUM KEY TO SUPERHEALTH.

LOW STABLE BLOOD SUGAR/INSULIN LEVELS –(i.e. HAVING NO INSULIN RESISTANCE) IS YOUR PLATINUM KEY TO SUPERHEALTH!

What is SUPERHEALTH?

"SUPERHEALTH" IS FREEDOM FROM DISEASE AND THE ABILITY OF AN INDIVIDUAL TO FUNCTION PHYSICALLY AND MENTALLY AT HIS/ HER BEST.

UN HAPPINESS, FEAR AND STRESS ARE THE ROOT CAUSES OF MOST DISEASES. STRESS ALONE LIKELY CAUSES 85 PERCENT OF DISEASES.

We participate and are responsible for a lot of things that happen to us. If you _HATE_ your job—you are much more likely to get _SICK_ and _DIE_— i.e. at a younger age than someone who is _HAPPY_ at work and has a loving family and is EMOTIONALLY well adjusted.

YOU NEED TO REALIZE THERE IS A WAY OF TURNING AROUND JUST ABOUT ANY "HOPELESS" SITUATION.

I AM WRITING THIS BOOK TO INSPIRE YOU AND TO ENCOURAGE YOU TO TAKE CHARGE OF YOUR HEALTH!

I WANT YOU TO TAKE CHARGE OF YOUR DESTINY!

WHAT ARE YOU REALLY PASSIONATE ABOUT?

HAVE YOU DISCOVERED YOUR MISSION ON PLANET EARTH?

WHEN YOU ARE INSPIRED AND PASSIONATE—YOU ENTER A TRANCE-LIKE STATE AND YOU CAN ACCOMPLISH THINGS THAT YOU MAY NEVER HAVE FELT CAPABLE OF OR EVEN DREAMED OF!

THOUGHTS BECOME THINGS. SCIENCE TELLS US THAT WE CAN CHANGE OUR DNA IN 2 MINUTES! OMG!

I AM WRITING THIS BOOK TO PROVIDE YOU WITH A HEALTH BLUEPRINT SO THAT YOU CAN ATTAIN SUPERHEALTH BE HAPPY AND ENJOY YOUR LIFE!

I AM WRITING THIS BOOK TO PROVIDE YOU WITH THE HEALTH TOOLS AND HEALTHCARE STRATEGIES SO THAT YOU CAN TAKE CONTROL OF YOUR HEALTH—SO THAT YOU CAN BE YOUR OWN DOCTOR!

YOU DESERVE TO KNOW THE UNPLEASANT TRUTH ABOUT THE REAL HEALTH PROBLEMS EXISTING TODAY IN WESTERN SOCIETY.

I AM WRITING THIS BOOK TO EXPOSE A CORRUPT, FAILED WESTERN PARADIGM OF MEDICINE.

I AM WRITING THIS BOOK TO UN-BRAINWASH YOU AND TO AWAKEN YOU!

I AM WRITING THIS BOOK TO EXPOSE THE HEALTH PROBLEMS—BUT—

MORE IMPORTANTLY—I AM WRITING THIS BOOK TO PROVIDE YOU WITH CONCRETE—PRACTICAL SOLUTIONS THAT YOU CAN USE IMMEDIATELY!

I AM WRITING THIS BOOK TO EDUCATE YOU ABOUT YOUR HEALTH.

I AM WRITING THIS BOOK TO PROVIDE YOU WITH A PRACTICAL DO-IT-YOURSELF HEALTH SOLUTION.

I AM WRITING THIS BOOK TO INSPIRE YOU TO SEIZE CONTROL OF YOUR HEALTH TODAY!

CARPE DIEM!

YOU CANNOT OBTAIN THE NUTRITIONAL INFORMATION YOU NEED TO HEAL YOURSELF AND PREVENT ILLNESS FROM THE MEDICAL ESTABLISHMENT.

YOUR DOCTOR SIMPLY CANNOT PROVIDE YOU WITH HEALTH INFORMATION THAT YOU NEED TO KNOW.

YOUR DOCTOR DOES NOT KNOW HOW TO TAKE CARE OF HIS OWN HEALTH.

THE SAD TRUTH IS- "Your doctor does not know his arse from his elbow-☺

YOUR DOCTOR DOESN'T WANT TO KNOW THIS INFORMATION.

YOUR DOCTOR HAS BEEN BRAINWASHED BY THE BIG PHARMACEUTICAL COMPANIES (aka BIG PHARMA).

I COULD NOT SIT BY IDLY WHILE MILLIONS OF HUMAN BEINGS ARE HARMED BY AN OUT-OF-CONTROL PHARMACEUTICAL AND MEDICAL ESTABLISHMENT.

I AM WRITING THIS BOOK TO EXPOSE THE TRUTH ABOUT THE GIGANTIC HEALTH FRAUD THAT HAS BEEN UNLEASHED UPON AN ILL-INFORMED NAÏVE NORTH AMERICAN POPULATION!

YOU DESERVE TO KNOW THE TRUTH!

I'VE BEEN TRAINED AS A LAWYER TO EXPOSE THE TRUTH.

I'M AN OFFICER OF THE COURT—AS A LAWYER I TOOK AN OATH TELL THE TRUTH—THE WHOLE TRUTH AND NOTHING BUT THE TRUTH.

I COULD NOT SIT BY AND WATCH WHILE EVIL CORRUPT PHARMACEUTICAL COMPANIES HELP AN IMPOTENT MEDICAL ESTABLISHMENT KILL AND INJURE MILLIONS OF PEOPLE.

FOR THE LAST 100 YEARS—BIG PHARMA AND CONVENTIONAL DOCTORS HAVE GROWN RICHER AND BIGGER WHILE SPREADING DISEASE AND DEATH.

MEDICAL DOCTORS AND BIG-PHARMA- HAVE BRAINWASHED HUNDREDS OF MILLIONS OF PEOPLE!

DOCTORS ARE BRAINWASHED THEMSELVES FROM THE FIRST DAY THEY STEP FOOT INTO MEDICAL SCHOOL. MOST DOCTORS REMAIN BRAINWASHED UNTIL THEY DIE –(at an average age of 56 years old).

"MEDICATIONS" or "DRUGS ARE MISNAMED "MEDICINE".

MEDICATIONS SHOULD BE CALLED WHAT THEY REALLY ARE— POISONOUS DRUGS!

DOCTORS CAUSE THE DISEASES THAT THEY CLAIM TO CURE.

What is a "MEDICATION? "

100 years ago, famous biologist Sir Arthur Thompson defined "medication" as the "natural non-built external environment." He maintained that the HEALING POWER OF NATURE is also with mindful contact with the animate and inanimate natural portions of the outdoor environment.

DRUGS DO NOT PROMOTE HEALTH. IN RARE CASES—DRUGS TEMPORARILY PROLONG LIFE BUT MOSTLY—DRUGS PROMOTE DEATH AND DISEASE!

YOUR DOCTOR IS LITERALLY KILLING YOU WITH HIS POISONOUS DRUGS!

JUST SAY NO TO DRUGS! SAY YES TO HEALTHY FOOD!

THE TRUTH IS—PEOPLE HAVE BEEN SCAMMED FOR THE LAST 100 YEARS!

MAINSTREAM MEDIA, THE CHEMICAL INDUSTRY AND THE FOOD INDUSTRY HAVE CONSPIRED WITH BIG PHARMA AND THE MEDICAL ESTABLISHMENT TO SELL YOU POISONOUS CHEMICALS FOR PROFIT. PERIOD.

I AM WRITING THIS BOOK TO: "UN-BRAINWASH YOU!!"

YOU DESERVE TO KNOW THE TRUTH!

YOU DESERVE TO KNOW THE APPALLING TRUTH—THE WHOLE TRUTH—AND NOTHING BUT THE TRUTH.

AM I AN "ALARMIST"?

ABSOLUTELY! I'M A HEALTH ALARMIST! I'M RINGING THE HEALTH ALARM!

I AM WRITING THIS BOOK TO TELL YOU THAT YOU'VE BEEN LIED TO BY BIG PHARMA, BIG MEDICINE, BIG FOOD AND BIG AGRICULTURE— AND— BIG GOVERNMENT FOR MORE THAN 100 YEARS!

I AM WRITING TO INFORM THAT YOU'VE BEEN LIED TO ABOUT THE THERAPEUTIC HEALING POWERS OF NUTRITION.

I AM WRITING THIS BOOK TO TELL YOU THE TRUTH ABOUT NUTRITION.

YOU CAN USE NUTRITION TO DOCTOR YOURSELF!

YOU CAN— AND –YOU SHOULD ADOPT THE APPROACH TAKEN BY THE FATHER OF MEDICINE-Dr. Hippocrates- MORE THAN 2,500 YEARS AGO.

I AM WRITING THIS BOOK TO TELL YOU THAT YOU CAN BY-PASS EVIL BIG-PHARMA AND A CORRUPT GREEDY MEDICAL ESTABLISHMENT.

I'M EXCITED TO INFORM YOU THAT YOU CAN ABANDON THE FRAUDULENT "PILL-POPPER" APPROACH PUSHED BY WESTERN DOCTORS FOR 100 YEARS.

I AM DELIGHTED TO PROVIDE YOU WITH THE VITAL NUTRITIONAL INFORMATION YOU NEED TO ATTAIN SUPERHEALTH.

YOU CAN SAY 'ADIOS' TO CRIMINAL BIG PHARMA AND THEIR GREEDY LACKEYS.

YOU CAN TAKE YOUR FIRST STEP AND TAKE CONTROL OF YOUR HEALTH.

YOU CAN—"FIRE YOUR DOCTOR AND HIRE YOURSELF"!

IN SHORT –I'M WRITING THIS BOOK TO EMPOWER YOU- THE READER!

KNOWLEDGE IS POWER!!

I'M WRITING THIS BOOK TO EMPOWER YOU WITH A NUTRITIONAL—HEALING APPROACH TO YOUR HEALTH.

I AM WRITING THIS BOOK FOR LAYPERSONS AND HEALTH SCIENTISTS!

I USE A NEW STYLE OF UNCONVENTIONAL WRITING.

Much of this book is written in CAPS and UNDERLINED. This is my personal "Coles Notes" writing approach-☺ Hopefully, this NEW format will permit you to read my book FASTER with easier COMPREHENSION. YOU may even be able to read this book without using your EYEGLASSES-☺

"FOOD AS MEDICINE" MEDICINE AS FOOD"— IS THE ONLY AUTHENTIC MEDICAL APPROACH TO HEALTH AND WELL-BEING—PERIOD.

THIS FOOD-BASED/NUTRITIONAL APPROACH TO ACHIEVE SUPERHEALTH IS THE EXACT OPPOSITE to the modern "medical" paradigm of western medicine.

The modern-day medical profession or the "ALLOPATHIC" approach to medicine is ULTRA-SIMPLISTIC.

This model simply says "for every ill— there is a pill."

Western conventionally trained doctors are little more than legal DRUG-PUSHERS.

They simply "prescribe" (sell) drugs manufactured in a laboratory by a chemist employed by Big Pharma.

THAT'S IT— THAT'S ALL.

Conventionally trained doctors also do SURGERY- TOO. They've been taught to SLICE away superfluous body parts deemed unhealthy or unnecessary to a person's body.

THIS BARBARIC PRACTICE WAS INVENTED BY ALLOPATHIC MEDICINE TO CUT AWAY PERCEIVED HEALTH PROBLEMS. SLICING-OFF BODY TISSUE/PARTS IS A VERY BAD IDEA AND IS RARELY JUSTIFIED.

99 PERCENT OF THE TIME THIS BUTCHERY CREATES EVEN MORE PROBLEMS. THE CUTTER BENEFITS FINANCIALLY BUT THE "CUTTEE" LOSES ALMOST ALL OF THE TIME.

ALLOPATHIC MEDICINE TREATS CANCER WITH A "CUT-BURN-POISON APPROACH" (surgery, radiation and chemotherapy.)

Conventionally trained allopathic doctors (even today) are taught in medical school to "diagnose" and to "treat" symptoms of disease- and to prescribe "medications"- more accurately known as "DRUGS." Dear readers— please understand that DRUGS are NOT true "medications". The allopathic industry has literally written THEIR PERVERTED book on "medications". Allopathic "medications" are synthetic CHEMICAL-concoctions hatched up by some chemist or other white-coated individual from the Pharmaceutical Industry. Allopathic drug-oriented doctors use experimental chemicals to make money. Almost all drugs have never been PROPERLY tested to determine long-term effects on humans. Most drugs are tested on lab rats. 95 % the studies testing drugs are FRAUDULENT.

The VAST majority of scientific studies are based on "JUNK SCIENCE" and 'FABRICATED TEST RESULTS".

ALL TOXIC DRUGS HAVE HORRIFIC 'DIRECT EFFECTS". THIS INCLUDES 'MIRACLE DRUGS' SUCH AS PENICILLIN AND OTHER ANTIBIOTICS!

"Anti" means "against" health; so, it's not hard to figure out.

YOU need to understand that the medical "profession" has been transformed into a fraudulent, greed-oriented, corrupt BUSINESS!

CONVENTIONALLY TRAINED DOCTORS—AND WESTERN HEALTHCARE SYSTEMS DO MORE HARM THAN GOOD!

THEY WANT YOU to stay SICK unhealthy or diseased AND DEPENDENT ON DRUGS- so they can sell you MORE EXPENSIVE DRUGS until you DIE!

The drug-based allopathic health model has been doing this for ONE HUNDRED YEARS!

YOU ARE HUMAN LAB RATS FOR THE PHARMACEUTICAL INDUSTRY.

YOU ARE THE "CASH –COW" OF MODERN WESTERN MEDICINE!

I RECOMMEND THAT YOU ABANDON THE DRUG INDUSTRY AND THE DRUG-BASED ALLOPATHIC MODEL OF MEDICINE.

TO START- JUST- "FIRE YOUR DOCTOR AND HIRE YOURSELF!"

YOUR GUIDING HEALTH PRINCIPLE IS:

"ANYTHING THE MEDICAL PROFESSION SAYS, —DO THE EXACT OPPOSITE— 99 PERCENT OF THE TIME YOU 'LL BE RIGHT!!

Sooner or later, <u>YOU</u> will be required to make an important decision regarding your <u>HEALTH AND/OR YOUR HEALTHCARE</u>.

<u>MY TWO FUNDAMENTAL HEALTH RECOMMENDATIONS ARE</u>:

1. <u>ANYTHING THE MEDICAL PROFESSION SAYS, DO THE OP-POSITE 99 PERCENT OF THE TIME, AND YOU'LL BE RIGHT!</u>

2. <u>ADOPT THE "HEALING KETOGENIC DIET" AND YOU WILL BE RIGHT 100 PERCENT OF THE TIME!</u>

<u>THE ALLOPATHIC PRACTICE OF MEDICINE IS AN UNJUST, IMMORAL "BUSINESS".</u>

<u>YOU DESERVE TO KNOW THE TRUTH ABOUT OUR CORRUPT MEDICAL SYSTEM, ALLOPATHIC DOCTORS AND THE CORRUPT FOOD INDUSTRY.</u>

<u>YOU DESERVE TO KNOW HOW TO TAKE CONTROL OF YOUR OWN HEALTH.</u>

<u>YOU DESERVE TO KNOW WHAT YOU CAN DO ABOUT YOUR HEALTH— AND HOW TO DO IT.</u>

<u>YOU DESERVE TO KNOW THE "PRACTICAL" STEPS YOU MUST TAKE</u>

<u>TO IMPLEMENT A DO-IT-YOURSELF (DIY) APPROACH TO YOUR HEALTH.</u>

<u>YOU DESERVE TO BE INFORMED ABOUT ALTERNATIVE REMEDIES WHICH ARE FAR MORE EFFECTIVE—FAR SAFER- FASTER—AND FAR CHEAPER!!</u>

<u>I WILL PROVIDE YOU WITH THE NUTRITIONAL INFORMATION YOU REQUIRE TO "BY-PASS" THE MEDICAL ESTABLISHMENT.</u>

<u>I WILL PROVIDE YOU WITH ESSENTIAL- PRACTICAL TOOLS THAT YOU NEED.</u>

<u>I WILL PROVIDE YOU WITH THE ESSENTIAL INFORMATION YOU REQUIRE TO EMPLOY A DO-IT-YOURSELF (DIY) APPROACH TO ATTAIN SUPERHEALTH FOR YOURSELF- AND YOUR LOVED ONES.</u>

<u>YOU WILL LEARN "HOW" TO BE YOUR OWN DOCTOR!</u>

<u>YOU CAN SAY GOOD-BYE TO WASTING HOURS OF YOUR VALUABLE TIME IN YOUR DOCTOR'S WAITING ROOM. YOU CAN SAVE THOUSANDS OF DOLLARS OF YOUR HARD-EARNED CASH.</u>

<u>YOU CAN TAKE THAT MONEY AND BUY SOME HEALTHY FOOD. IT'S THAT SIMPLE! YOU MUST DO IT!</u>

<u>YOU CANNOT RELY ON YOUR SPOUSE, YOUR PARENTS OR ANY PERSON WEARING A WHITE COAT TO TAKE CONTROL OF YOUR HEALTH!</u>

<u>YOU ARE THE ONLY PERSON IN THE WORLD WHO CAN TAKE CONTROL OF YOUR HEALTH. NO ONE ELSE CAN DO IT FOR YOU.</u>

<u>YOU CAN- INDEED- YOU MUST— TAKE A DO-IT YOURSELF TO YOUR HEALTH!</u>

Dr. Hippocrates' <u>MEDICAL ADVICE</u>, 2,500 years old, <u>SHOULD HAVE</u> constituted the backbone of our modern Western Medicine. Instead, it has been <u>SUPPRESSED</u>, and <u>IGNORED</u> by Big Pharma and the medical establishment

<u>DON'T BE 'SUCKERED" BY BIG PHARMA AND THE CONVENTIONAL MEDICAL ESTABLISHMENT. YOU DO NOT NEED THEIR "DISEASE MANAGEMENT PILL-BASED APPROACH".</u>

<u>YOUR MODERN 'NUTRITIONAL APPROACH IS:</u>

<u>"LET YOUR FAT BE YOUR MEDICINE— LET YOUR MEDICINE BE YOUR FAT"</u>

<u>THE HEALING PROPERTIES OF FOOD</u> have been reported by cultures worldwide throughout history. The past decade has evidenced an <u>EXPLOSION</u> of clinical research regarding <u>THE HEALTH BENEFITS PROVIDED BY NUTRITIOUS FOODS.</u>

<u>RESEARCH HAS IDENTIFIED A BOATLOAD OF HEALTH BENEFITS PROVIDED BY NUTRIENT –DENSE WHOLE FOODS.</u>

Fruits, vegetables, and unprocessed foods have <u>PHENOMENAL HEALTH BENEFITS</u>. Studies in the past decade have taken nutritional research beyond protein, carbohydrates, fats, vitamins and minerals. Chemicals in plants called "phytochemicals" have been researched extensively. These phytochemicals offer a <u>BOATLOAD</u> of health benefits such as cancer prevention, cholesterol reduction, hormone regulation, etc.

Three decades ago,(circa 1986), the first Nutrition and Health Report by the US Surgeon-General, C. Everett Koop concluded that 8 out of 10 chronic diseases were caused by poor diet and nutrition. This report was based on hundreds of scientific studies and was co-authored by dozens of "smart" medical people.

THAT 80 PERCENT HAS NOW INCREASED TO A WHOPPING 95 PERCENT!

Has the medical establishment followed this advice? Nope. Doctors detest reading anything that they can't understand.

Today, more than 95 % of all chronic diseases are caused by food choice, toxic food ingredients, nutritional deficiencies and lack of physical exercise.

Everyone knows that we are getting fatter and sicker every year because of bad dietary information and toxic food sold by the Food companies (aka Big Food) and the pharmaceutical companies (aka as "Big Pharma") Unless you've had your head buried in the sand, you're aware that there is a GLOBAL OBESITY EPIDEMIC!

69 percent of Americans over 20 are overweight; Diabetes numbers are going through the roof!

EVERY 7 SECONDS SOMEONE IN THE WORLD DIES FROM THE COMPLICATIONS OF DIABETES!

1 in 2 men will be diagnosed with cancer and 1 in 3 women will be diagnosed with cancer. To complicate matters further, there's a new disease added to the obesity collection. It's called 'Type 3- Diabetes" or more commonly called "ALZHEIMER'S DISEASE.

This form of dementia affects an estimated 5.4 million Americans, according to 2013 statistics. About 7.2 million new cases of dementia are identified every year. With one new case of Alzheimer's diagnosed every 4 seconds— Alzheimer's has now become the FOURTH leading cause of death in the United States.

The western healthcare systems are BROKEN. They are "Ponzi-schemes" which manage disease. They use the "CUT (surgery), BURN (chemotherapy), POISON (drug) approach to medicine. This "illness" approach to medicine is deeply flawed because it only treats the SYMPTOMS of disease. It does not address the root CAUSES of disease.

WHAT IS THE NUMBER ONE CAUSE OF DEATH IN THE UNITED STATES?

Is it HEART DISEASE? Is it CANCER? Nope.

THE NUMBER ONE CAUSE OF DEATH IN THE USA IS— CONVENTIONAL MEDICINE! OMG! It's TRUE!

CONVENTIONAL (Allopathic) **DOCTORS KILL MORE THAN ONE MILLION PEOPLE EACH YEAR!** The specific number in 2013 was pegged at 1,087,000 dead people- **ANNUALLY!**

A 2003 study entitled "Death by Medicine," penned by 6 authors, Carolyn Dean MD, ND ET AL. estimated the number of people killed annually by doctors/conventional medicine at the number of 783, 936 people.

These "iatrogenic deaths" (meaning deaths resulting from the activity of physicians) include everything from adverse drug reactions to medical errors.

SHOCKINGLY—the authors specified that as few as 5 **PERCENT** and no more than 20 **PERCENT** of "iatrogenic" i.e. **DOCTOR- CAUSED DEATHS ARE EVER REPORTED!**

The estimated figure of 783,936 **WAS FAR TOO LOW**—because as the researchers intimated:

"Dead men tell no tales".

A previous Harvard Study in 1991 revealed a 4 % iatrogenic injury rate and a 14 % death rate. In 1994, Dr. Lucian L. Leope published a study in allopathic doctors' favourite journal- **THE JOURNAL OF THE AMERICAN MEDICAL ASSOCIATION (JAMA)** which authenticated 20 to 25 % **DEATH RATES.**

PUBLISHED STUDIES AND THE TRUTH ABOUT DOCTORS' DEATHS BEING THE NUMBER ONE KILLER HAVE BEEN SUPPRESSED AND "BURIED".

You will not learn **THAT TRUTH** from the mainstream media!

YOU WON'T SEE THAT STORY ON T.V. OR IN YOUR LOCAL NEWSPAPER!

Mainstream media is in bed with Big Pharma and the medical establishment.

I want to provide you with **MANY TRUTHS** in this book.

THE TRUTH ABOUT MEDICAL ATROCITIES COMMITTED BY BIG PHARMA AND THE MEDICAL ESTABLISHMENT HAVE BEEN SYSTEMATICALLY SUPPRESSED SINCE 1920.

YOU HAVE BEEN VICTIMS OF "MEDICAL McCARTHYISM".

DUE TO THE FDA, (Federal Drug Administration) <u>NO ONE</u> is legally allowed to make a health claim that a <u>FOOD, VITAMIN, MINERAL OR SUPPLEMENT CAN TREAT OR CURE ANY DISEASE/CONDITION</u>. Big Pharma and the medical establishment retain <u>THE LEGAL MONOPOLY</u> on the use of the words "diagnose" "treatment" and "cure". The medical establish employs an iron-fisted approach to prevent any alternative health care provider from using these legally protected words.

<u>IT IS WELL-KNOWN – OUTSIDE OF NORTH AMERICA— THAT THOUSANDS OF NATURAL REMEDIES</u> (e.g. Ayrudvedic and Asian) <u>HAVE BEEN SUCCESSFULLY USED FOR THOUSANDS OF YEARS</u>.

Empirical evidence and irrefutable proof for more than 5, 000 years is found in Traditional Chinese Medicine (TCM) and Ayurvedic medicine. There is no documented evidence that even <u>ONE</u> person has <u>EVER</u> died from natural remedies.

<u>THERE HAS NOT BEEN EVEN ONE REPORTED DEATH FROM SUPPLEMENTS</u>!

Big Pharma and the medical establishment argue that supplements are dangerous but— in fact the <u>EXACT OPPOSITE IS TRUE</u>! Supplements are <u>SAFE</u>, natural compounds; sometimes legally referred to as "Nutraceuticals."

<u>WHOLESOME NUTRITIOUS FOODS DO NOT KILL OR HURT PEOPLE. NUTRIENT— DENSE (KETOGENIC) FOODS HEAL PEOPLE</u>.

<u>YOU SHOULD STOP BELIEVING/TRUSTING THE MEDICAL NONSENSE THAT IS PROPAGATED BY BIG PHARMA AND THE MEDICAL ESTABLISHMENT</u>!

<u>YOU ARE VERY POWERFUL</u>!

<u>;AND THE FOOD INDUSTRY</u>.

<u>YOU CAN FIX YOUR HEALTH AND YOU CAN PROMOTE YOUR HEALTH AND THE HEALTH OF YOUR NEIGHBOURS BY SPENDING YOUR FOOD MONEY WISELY. YOU HAVE TO SPEND MONEY ON FOOD ANYWAY-SO-</u>

<u>WHY NOT BUY GOOD NUTRITIOUS FOOD AND SAVE ON HEALTHCARE EXPENSES</u>?

<u>STOP SHOPPING AT THE LOCAL DRUGSTORE</u>!

<u>STOP EATING DRUG- LACED FOOD FROM YOUR LOCAL GROCERY STORE</u>!

STOP EATING DRUGS AND PROCESSED FOODS LACED WITH ANTIBIOTIC DRUGS, POISONOUS CHEMICALS AND PESTICIDES.

STOP DRINKING HITLER'S MEDICINE! aka Fluoridated Water.

JOIN THE THOUSANDS OF CONSUMERS WHO HAVE DECIDED TO SHOP AT MOTHER NATURE'S FARMACY!

MOTHER NATURE'S FOOD IS MEDICINE.

HER FOOD will make you heal- thy, strong, and dis-ease free!

Conventional "drug-based medicine" is prescribed by doctors who went to school for 8 years or more to learn how to scribble the name of a new drug on a pad of paper. Allopathic doctors are provided LUCRATIVE incentives to sell as many drugs as possible to unsuspecting naïve patients. The truth is that simple. Most allopathic doctors make their patients wait for an hour. Then they talk at their patients 5 minutes. That's just enough time to stick their finger up a patient's butt and to scribble an illegible drug prescription on a scrap of paper. Allopathic medicine is assembly-line drug sales.

COLUMBIAN DRUG-LORDS AND ALLOPATHIC DOCTORS BOTH SELL DRUGS IN ORDER TO MAKE A LOT OF MONEY! Both are drug-pushers; WITH ONE HUGE DIFFERENCE. Doctors sell drugs legally.

ALLOPATHIC DOCTORS ALSO SUPPORT FORCED MEDICATION. (Please see infra- "Mass Murder by Water".)

ALL drug-pushers kill people with their poisonous lab-created chemical pills. Allopathic doctors kill over a MILLION people per year. No-one REALLY KNOWS how many die from eating DRUGS each year.

> "Modern medicine is a negation of health. It isn't organized to serve human health, but only to serve itself as an institution. It makes more people sick than it heals"
>
> — Ivan Illich, author, Medical Nemesis

Most enlightened consumers are aware of what stands in the way of change;—powerful Big Pharma and medical technology companies; along with other powerful corporate groups with vested interests in the BUSINESS OF BIG MEDICINE. These corporations fund medical research, support medical schools and hospitals, and advertise in medical journals. With deep pockets, they entice scientists and scientists and academics to support their efforts. Such funding can sway the balance of opinion from professional caution to uncritical acceptance of new therapies and drugs.

You have only have to look at the people who make up the hospital, medical and government health advisory boards to see rampant conflicts of interests.

A brilliant Canadian physician Sir William Osler, 100 years ago stated:

> "Drug companies are not here to bring health to the population but to scam them on one level for vast amounts of money, by treating the symptoms and not addressing the cause."

> — Sir William Osler, MD (1849-1919)

ONE CENTURY LATER—THIS SUPPRESSED TRUTH REMAINS A SHAMEFUL PILLAR OF THE MEDICAL ESTABLISHMENT.

An ill-informed North American public continues to be DUPED by an out of control allopathic medical establishment. Most allopathic doctors are brain washed by Big Pharma. Many doctors act like priests and ARE VERY ARROGANT.

Some doctors act like GODS towards their patients. Some doctors are terrified to use anything but DRUGS on their patients. Some doctors are terrified to lose their medical licence. Many doctors just cower in silence. Some doctors fear for their own lives. There are many horror stories out there whereby doctors' offices have been raided. Some doctors have had their lives and reputations destroyed by evil corporations...

BUT WAIT!

THERE ARE NEW- GREAT— EXCITING— HEALTH DISCOVERIES!

I have the GREAT pleasure to share these discoveries with YOU in this book.

A NEW HEALTH-CARE RENAISSANCE HAS BEEN STARTED!

A NEW HEALTH-CARE REVOLUTION HAS BEEN STARTED BY DR. INTERNET!

A NEW HEALTH-CARE REVOLUTION is taking place at your local farmer's market and in back-yard gardens everywhere!

Research shows that more natural health care providers, naturopathic, functional medicine doctors and functional health coaches are SPRINGING UP AND EDUCATING people about A HOLISTIC NATURAL APPROACH TO HEALTH AND WELLNESS.

THE KNOWLEDGE AND INFORMATION IN THIS BOOK WILL HELP YOU TAKE CONTROL OF YOUR HEALTH AND YOUR DESTINY!

I WILL SHOW YOU HOW TO TAKE CONTROL OF YOUR HEALTH, YOUR WELL-BEING—AND YOUR HAPPINESS!

I WILL EDUCATE AND EMPOWER YOU TO UNDERSTAND THAT— HEALTH IS WEALTH.

As Ghandi said:

> **"Real Wealth is Health- not pieces of gold and silver."**

People are discovering the food and lifestyle habits of our **ANCESTORS** and forebears.

What foods did they eat? They had no need to count calories—or even understand that a calorie meant a unit of heat. When our ancestors were hungry or wanted to feel good— they got their food/medicine from Mother Nature's "**FARMACY**'— not the local greasy spoon.

This **NATURAL/HOLISTIC APPROACH** advocates the natural healing of both mind and body through a proper food diet of plants and animals— as our Creator intended. Our body cannot be understood and healed by treating individual body parts with toxic drugs.

OUR BODY IS ONE INTEGRATED AMAZING SELF-HEALING MACHINE!

OUR BODY CAN HEAL ITSELF WHEN IT IS GIVEN NUTRITIOUS FOOD!

SUPERHEALTH IS NOT AN ABSENCE OF DRUGS!

To make matters more challenging; we are now living in a heavily **POLLUTED** environment—a virtual toxic soup. Our air, our water, our soil and our especially our **FOOD** are contaminated with toxic chemicals. We've got fossil fuels from coal-mines in China, "**CHEM-TRAILS**", glyphosate, and thousands of toxic chemicals in and around our bodies. Dozens of **NEUROTOXINS** are killing our brain and our bodies.

Much of the tap water supply of North America is poisoned with **FLUORIDE**. Tap water also contains a cocktail of heavy metals; and a cocktail of **PHARMACEUTICAL DRUGS** which damage our bodies— especially our brains.

One of the most **EVIL** effects of fluoride is its **BRAIN** damaging effects. There is **IRREFUTABLE PROOF** that this industrial toxic waste lowers human IQ and damages our brains. Chlorine and cocktails of **TOXIC** heavy metals and other chemicals compose our water supply. No one knows the full combined or 'synergistic" effect of these toxic substances. One thing we do know for sure—<u>THESE POISONS</u> are taking a <u>TERRIBLE TOLL ON GLOBAL HUMAN HEALTH</u>.

<u>I STRONGLY RECOMMEND</u> that you refrain from drinking <u>FLUORIDATED WATER</u>.

<u>I RECOMMEND THAT YOU ADDRESS YOUR BRAIN HEALTH FIRST</u>

<u>AND FOREMOST</u>!

<u>YOUR HEALTH BEGINS AND ENDS WITH YOUR BRAIN HEALTH</u>.

<u>WHEN YOU EAT SUGAR, PROCESSED FOODS AND WHEN YOU DRINK TAP WATER—YOU ARE LITERALLY EATING HOLES IN BOTH OF YOUR BRAINS- THE ONE IN YOUR BELLY AND THE ONE IN YOUR HEAD!</u>

Rather than lobotomizing your brain—<u>YOU MUST PROTECT</u> your brain and nourish your body with Mother Nature's <u>BEST ELIXIR— CLEAN, PURE WATER</u>.

The latest research suggests that <u>MOST</u> northern pristine lakes (where no human has ever all set foot) are contaminated by pharmaceutical run-offs; pesticides and herbicides. Male fish are now becoming female and/or bi-sexual as a result of endocrine disrupting chemicals such as <u>BISPHENOL</u> (BPA) aka <u>PLASTIC</u>.

These gender-bending chemicals can change your sex. I'm pretty sure that you do not want a sex change operation!-☺ Men are becoming "less male". These gender-benders are transforming men. More and more male babies are now born with an increasing number of birth defects such as smaller sexual organs, lower sperm production etc. The general male population now produces much less testosterone than their grandfathers. Male fertility has significantly decreased in the last few decades.

<u>PLASTIC IS UBIQUITOUS</u> in our modern North American society.

<u>ALL PLASTIC</u> compounds or <u>"PHTHLATES"</u> pronounced "fal-ates" which enter our bodies are actually <u>TOTALLY FOREIGN TO OUR GENETICS</u>.

The human body is <u>NOT</u> designed or programmed to <u>INGEST PLASTIC</u>. Margarine, for example, is only <u>ONE</u> molecule away from plastic! Our bodies do not know what to do with plastic; (we don't seem to be able to excrete it in our stool-☺) -so the body does what it thinks is best. Our body appears to store <u>BPA</u> in women's breasts, and ovaries. For men, the preferred storage areas appear to be the testicles and the prostate gland. The research here is just beginning; <u>BUT</u>— all of the evidence points to the toxicity of plastics and chemicals doing untold damage to our bodies. The world's oceans are awash in a sea of <u>PLASTIC</u>. All kinds of birds, fish and aquatic life is being killed by eating plastics contaminating our oceans.

The good news is that <u>YOU GET TO CHOOSE</u>!

<u>WILL YOU CHOOSE TO EDUCATE YOURSELF</u>?

<u>I recommend that you choose to educate yourself and do your due health diligence.</u>

<u>I recommend that you ditch the drugs and processed foods.</u>

<u>I recommend that you eat most nutrient-dense RAW foods.</u>

<u>THE NORTH AMERICAN FOOD SUPPLY IS HEAVILY CONTAMINATED WITH ANTIBIOTICS, PESTICIDES AND CHEMICAL FOOD ADDITIVES!</u>

To describe the Standard American Diet (SAD) …AS "<u>FOOD</u>" <u>IS A GROSS MISREPRESENTATION!</u>

<u>COMMERCIAL PROCESSED FOOD IS NOT FOOD.</u>

<u>PROCESSED FOOD IS POISONOUS GARBAGE PACKAGED & CALLED "FOOD".</u>

Some of us call it "<u>FRANKEN-FOOD</u>"…to remind us of the famous horror hero "Frankenstein"!

The choice is <u>YOURS</u>! You can choose health or you can choose sickness and dis-ease.

Are you going to choose food made from chemicals in a lab? Do you really want to be a guinea pig for fake chemical "Franken-foods?"

<u>I STRONGLY RECOMMEND THAT YOU AVOID ALL PROCESSED FOOD!</u>

You have a choice. You can eat processed junk foods that poison or— You can eat the World's Healthiest- Tastiest <u>PIZZA</u>!- and the World's Healthiest Dessert- <u>KETOGENIC BLUEBERRY GRUNT</u>! — and other <u>MOUTH-WATERING LIP-SMACKING KETOGENIC RECEIPES-</u>

Moreover, essential <u>NUTRIENTS</u> in today's food sources <u>ARE VERY LIMITED</u>. The <u>depletion</u> of minerals from food- growing soils has reached epidemic proportions. Except for some "organic" farming operations, these nutrients and essential trace minerals are not being added back to the soil. One solution is to add mineral and vitamin supplementation.

THE REAL SOLUTION IS TO GROW AS MUCH OF YOUR FOOD AS POSSIBLE. (e.g. check out Quadroponics; Sprouting using a simple bag **OR** fermenting your own veggies).

THE SECOND BEST SOLUTION IS TO SHOP AT YOUR LOCAL HEALTH FOOD STORE. But please be careful, just because it is called a health food store—does not mean that **ALL** of the food sold is **HEALTHY**!

Once our mineral/vitamin depleted food gets to the food industry-the few minerals, and nutrients it contained in the first place are then **REMOVED BY PROCESSING** and **HEATING.** The junk food industry creates "Franken- foods" filled with chemicals **NOT** listed on any label. The "legal labelling requirements" are a fraud.

I recommend that you become a "**FOOD DETECTIVE**". As a general rule, if food comes in a bag, box or can— you **SHOULD** avoid it. There are some notable exceptions, such as some canned coconut milk, for example.

Have you ever wondered **WHY** Big Food **VIOLENTLY** opposes the labelling of **GENETICALLY –MODIFIED-FOODS-aka GMO's.**? If GMO's are healthy and nutritious, why would you want people **NOT TO KNOW**? Why is there a growing trend to ban GMO's in many parts of the world? (Vermont has recently passed GMO labelling laws). Do you think humans are designed to eat food that has plant genes spliced with animal genes? If GMO food is safe—where are the scientific studies for a few months that prove it? GMO foods are another classic example of the **FOOD FRAUD** being perpetrated upon a naïve, ill-informed population.

AS A GENERAL RULE OF THUMB— IF MOTHER NATURE DID NOT MAKE IT- I recommend—

YOU SHOULD NOT EAT IT— PERIOD!

IF IT COMES IN A BOX, BAG OR CAN—DON'T EAT IT!

As an example- the cardboard portion of your cereal box likely contains more nutrition than the contents of the box.☺ There's even a good chance that your cereal contains shards of metal that you can lift with a magnet. This may be interesting for a physics student— but upsetting if you give a darn about what you eat.

LABELLING LAWS do not require legal mention of ALL of the ingredient chemicals that the "food" contains. If foods were properly labelled, the labels would be too large for the product. There are CHEMICALS in processed foods that are PROPRIETARY SECRETS that are not mentioned.

YOU SHOULD ALWAYS READ LABELS—AND EXPIRY DATES—EVEN ON ORGANIC FOODS! YOU NEED TO BECOME A FOOD LABEL DETECTIVE!

MY RECOMMENDATION IS: SHOP AT MOTHER NATURE'S FARMACY!

Natural healing, including using mankind's oldest solution seeks to use the medicine provided by Mother Nature. The natural, holistic or functional medicine approach seeks—

TO PREVENT AND HEAL HEALTH PROBLEMS before they begin.

The pill-popper approach taken by the medical establishment treats and tries to manage **SYMPTOMS** of health problems. Conventional doctors are not taught how to find the root cause of **ANY** health problem. Medical doctors' education is **GROSSLY INADEQUATE**.

ALWAYS REMEMBER—DISEASE IS NOT A DEFICIENCY OF DRUGS!

In the words of Nobel Prize Laureate, Dr. Linus Pauling:

"All disease is caused by a mineral deficiency."

DR. INTERNET HAS CAUSED A HUGE AWAKENING IN CONSUMER INTEREST TO DISCOVER THE BENEFITS OF EATING HEALTHY NUTRITIOUS FOODS.

INDEED- CONSUMER AWARENESS IS THE BIGGEST PART OF THE HEALTHCARE RENAISSANCE TAKING PLACE!

YOU ARE A BIG PART OF THAT AWARENESS!

Big Pharma, its partners, the big petrochemical companies are invested in discouraging the idea that lifestyle choices can have a **PROFOUND** effect on our Health and Wellness.

These people say that organic food and supplements, including vitamins and minerals are a waste of money.

AN INFORMED PUBLIC EATING HEALTHY FOOD COULD BANKRUPT BIG PHARMA! WHEN YOU TAKE CONTROL OF YOUR HEALTH AND TAKE A DIY APPROACH TO YOUR HEALTH—

YOU COULD PUT YOUR DOCTOR OUT OF BUSINESS!

I've written this book for **YOU**— lawyers—**AND ALL DESK PROFESSIONALS WHO WANT TO KNOW HOW TO TAKE CARE OF THEIR HEALTH.**

Whether you're a professional or ordinary folk— **YOU** definitely have the smarts to figure out what you need to eat.

<u>YOU HAVE THE ABILITY TO ATTAIN SUPERHEALTH, AND FITNESS</u>!

<u>NO DOCTOR REQUIRED</u>!

In this book—I provide <u>YOU WITH A CLEAR DETAILED DIETARY/ LIFESTYLE BLUEPRINT SO THAT YOU CAN ATTAIN SUPERHEALTH & FITNESS</u>.

I provide you with the <u>NECESSARY INFORMATION ABOUT NUTRITION; THE BIOCHEMISTRY OF NUTRITION AND HUMAN PHYSIOLOGY THAT YOU REQUIRE. THIS INFORMATION WILL ALLOW YOU TO TAKE CARE OF YOUR HEALTH. YOU WILL LEARN ABOUT THE BIOCHEMISTRY OF HUMAN METABOLISM. YOU WILL LEARN HOW OUR BODY DIGESTS FOOD</u>.

<u>YOU WILL LEARN YOU CAN APPLY THE INFORMATION IN THIS BOOK TO BY-PASS THE MEDICAL ESTABLISHMENT—AND BECOME YOUR OWN DOCTOR</u>!

<u>THE KETOGENIC DIET) AND THE KETOGENIC LIFESTYLE DETAILED IN THIS BOOK WILL TRANSFORM YOU</u>!

<u>PREPARE YOURSELF TO BE DAZZLED BY WHAT YOU LEARN</u> -☺

I will reveal to you some breath-taking <u>NEW SCIENTIFIC INFORMATION</u> that will delight and surprise you. Often I quote <u>VERBATIM</u> from the scientific study or author so that you can read the science directly from the study.

I explain the <u>SCIENCE</u> in easy-to-understand, <u>USER-FRIENDLY LANGUAGE</u>.

<u>THIS LEADING-EDGE SCIENCE WILL PUT YOU LIGHT-YEARS AHEAD OF THE WHITE-COATED CROWD</u>!

Most conventional physicians are <u>LITERALLY SO BUSY</u> pushing pills <u>AND SHUFFLING PAPERS</u> that they have no time to read medical studies or scientific literature. Moreover, doctors detest reading studies that they can't understand. Doctors are not taught to read medical literature. Big Pharma doesn't want them to learn about <u>NUTRITION AND THE BIOCHEMISTRY OF NUTRITION</u>. That's why it is not taught in medical school.

<u>THE ESSENTIAL NUTRITIONAL HEALTH INFORMATION YOU NEED HAS BEEN HIDING IN PLAIN SIGHT</u>! Who knew?

<u>A PHENOMENAL NEW HEALTH RESOURCE WEBSITE, www. GreenMedInfo.com</u> was founded in 2008 by a young genius named

Sayer Ji This site contains more than <u>23 MILLION STUDY REFERENCES WITH LINKS TO PUB.MED AND OTHER SITES.</u>

<u>AND BEST OF ALL—IT'S FREE!</u>

<u>NO DOCTOR REQUIRED!</u>

<u>YOU CAN FIND THE ANSWERS TO YOUR HEALTH QUESTIONS AT THE CLICK OF A BUTTON!</u> How cool is that?

I have provided you with <u>THE NUTRITIONAL HEALTH SCIENCE THAT YOU REQUIRE.</u> Should you require more information regarding a specific health issue—all you need to do is <u>EDUCATE YOURSELF FROM THIS OR OTHER REPUTABLE SITES</u>-but <u>NOT</u> those sites recommended by your doctor!

<u>By directly accessing the scientific literature</u>, you can read and study the literature yourself. I invite you to do some research in a particular health area that interests you.

There's no need to listen to Big Pharma's trolls and the dumb-downed corporate media talking heads. These talking heads are paid to provide the public with a distorted opinion and junk-science. The media is paid by Big Pharma and told <u>WHAT TO SAY.</u>

<u>JUST IMAGINE—</u> DOCTOR'S APPOINTMENTS, PILLS AND SURGERY WILL BECOME A THING OF THE PAST!

I will show you how to <u>BY-PASS THE CORRUPT MEDICAL ESTABLISHMENT.</u>

<u>YOU CAN TAKE A (DIY) APPROACH TO HEALTH FOR THE FIRST TIME IN HISTORY! ALL OF THIS IS POSSIBLE BECAUSE OF THE INTERNET!</u>

Back in the 1970's when garages and mechanics began charging monstrous fees for car repairs- a whole new <u>DIY PARADIGM WAS BORN.</u> People were fed up being ripped off for car repairs. People began buying used car parts and doing their <u>OWN</u> car repairs.

<u>21ST CENTURY TECHNOLOGY NOW MEANS A NEW PARADIGM OF KNOWLEDGE .THE CLICK OF A BUTTON HAS REVOLUTIONIZED THE WORLD!</u>

Need to know something? Just ask Dr. Google. All of the information you require about anything is available on-line.

<u>WHO</u> knows your body better than <u>YOU DO?</u>

<u>YOU</u> will learn to view your body in a whole new light. Your body is an <u>AMAZING SELF-HEALING MACHINE.</u> You will learn to "think outside of

the pill". When you provide your body with the <u>PROPER NUTRITION THAT IT NEEDS—</u>

<u>YOUR BODY WILL REPAIR AND HEAL ITSELF.</u>

<u>YOU HAVE FAR GREATER CONTROL OVER YOUR HEALTH AND YOUR WELL-BEING THAN YOU THINK!</u>

<u>YOU CAN REPAIR YOUR OWN BODY. YOU CAN HEAL YOURSELF WITHOUT RELYING ON SOME PILL-PUSHING DOCTOR WHO KNOWS NOTHING ABOUT HOW TO HEAL YOUR BODY.</u>

<u>THE NEW DO-IT-YOURSELF (DIY) APPROACH IS SWEEPING THE WORLD!</u>

<u>VIVA LA REVOLUTIONE!</u>

Which is more productive-<u>ONE HOUR</u> reading Time magazine in your doctor's waiting room <u>OR- RESEARCHING HEALTH LITERATURE ON LINE</u> at GreenMedInfo and/or pubmed.gov?

I promise you that you will you feel more confident about taking your own health in your OWN hands by educating yourself and reading scientific literature—rather than spending thousands of dollars on useless tests and poisonous pills.

Which will cost you less? Which will help you more? Does your doctor ever really tell you <u>ANYTHING</u> about your health issues?

<u>YOUR DOCTOR DOES NOT HAVE THE KNOWLEDGE AND EXPERTISE TO ADDRESS OR TREAT THE ROOT CAUSE OF YOUR HEALTH PROBLEMS.</u>

<u>THE TRUTH IS:</u>

<u>YOU ARE ALWAYS ON YOUR OWN WHEN IT COMES TO FIXING YOUR OWN HEALTH.</u>

<u>YOU NEED TO LEARN HOW YOU CAN HEAL YOURSELF USING NUTRITIONAL TOOLS SUPPLIED BY MOTHER NATURE.</u>

Here is the <u>MODUS OPERANDI</u> that I use in my book.

The first part of my book shall focus on the "Bad Stuff." This is all of the stuff that you need to <u>ELIMINATE FROM YOUR BODIES AND FROM YOUR LIVES.</u>

These things I call the "<u>NEUROTOXINS IN AIR, WATER, FOOD</u> and <u>OUR ENVIRONMENT.</u>

<u>THESE NEUROTOXINS ARE BRAIN-KILLERS!</u>

THESE NEUROTOXINS ARE LITERALLY KILLING PEOPLE AND DESTROYING OUR HEALTH. You need to eliminate the <u>TOXIC PEOPLE</u> and <u>TOXIC RELATIONSHIPS IN YOUR LIVES TOO</u>! A pearl of wisdom says:

<u>'A NEGATIVE THOUGHT CAN KILL YOU FASTER THAN A BAD GERM!</u>

After I've exposed the truth about the bad stuff—I'll proceed ☺

I'm convinced that <u>WE ALL NEED TO ADOPT A KETOGENIC DIET AND A KETOGENIC LIFESTYLE! THIS IS NOT JUST A DIET"</u>. KETOGENESIS(Ketogenic Nutritional approach IS A NUTRITIONAL "LIFESTYLE". We need to return to eating and living our life as we did ancestrally. The word "ketogenesis" is <u>BRAND-NEW WORD!</u>

<u>A KETOGENIC DIET IS NOT A "PALEO" DIET.</u>

<u>A KETOGENIC DIET IS PALEO ON STEROIDS!</u>

<u>THE KETOGENIC DIET IS" BRAND-NEW".</u>

<u>IT HAS ONLY EXISTED FOR 3 MILLION YEARS!</u> —☺

<u>YOU WILL RECEIVE ESSENTIAL EXERCISE INFORMATION AND KETOGENIC LIFESTYLE INFORMATION THAT YOU REQUIRE TO BE HEALTHY AND SUPERFIT.</u>

<u>MOST OF THE EXERCISE INFORMATION PROVIDED TO THE PUBLIC IS FALSE!</u>

You will learn the truth about exercise. I have been fortunate to learn my exercise knowledge from world renowned coaches such as Michael Boyle (The Godfather of Strength & Conditioning,) Mr.Gray Cook; and Mr. Al Vermeil- (the only strength coach who has coached two world championships in <u>TWO DIFFERENT SPORTS</u>! Mr. Vermeil has coached a <u>SUPERBOWL</u> football winner and a <u>NBA BASKETBALL</u> championship team. Al Vermeil has spent a half a century in the gym. He has two world-championship rings for his accomplishments. I've also had the good fortune to be educated by Dr. Tom House, Janet Alexander and several other leading fitness professionals from the Titleist Performance Institute.

It is my privilege and honour to briefly explain <u>THE SIMPLE FUNCTIONAL APPROACH</u> to exercise that you need to adopt to be strong and healthy.

<u>ESSENTIAL EXERCISE IS NOT POUNDING A TREADMILL 3 days a week!</u>

45 MINUTES OF EXERCISE PER WEEK IS SUFFICIENT—PROVIDED THAT ARE DOING THE PROPER EXERCISE!

EVERYONE KNOWS THAT GOOD HEALTH REQUIRES DOING SOME EXERCISE, UNFORTUNATELY—YOUR DOCTOR KNOWS 'SQUAT" ABOUT EXERCISE!-☺ YOUR DOCTOR DID NOT LEARN ABOUT EXERCISE IN MEDICAL SCHOOL. DRUGS AND EXERCISE DO NOT MIX WELL.

ONLY YOU CAN TAKE CONTROL OF YOUR HEALTH.

NO ONE ELSE CAN DO IT FOR YOU.

IT IS YOUR DECISION— YOURS ALONE.

YOU MUST EDUCATE YOURSELF ABOUT NUTRITION- OTHERWISE—

YOU COULD BE ON THE FAST TRACK TO CHRONIC DISEASE AND WORSE YET—YOU COULD BECOME A CASH COW FOR YOUR DOCTOR!

FOOD IS MOTHER NATURE'S SUPER-POWERFUL DRUG!

THE 'DIRECT EFFECT" OF FOOD IS TO HEAL YOU AND MAKE YOU HEAL...THY.

Hippocrates was right!

Let your Food be your Medicine and let your Medicine be your Food.

MOTHER NATURE IS FAR SMARTER THAN ANY PHYSICIAN, FOOD CHEMIST, DRUG- MAKER—or ANY PERSON WEARING A WHITE SMOCK.

YOU WILL LEARN NEW HEALTH STRATEGIES. You will learn to **FIX YOUR FOOD SO YOU CAN FIX YOUR HEALTH!**

YOU should **NOT WAIT** until you have a health problem- **YOU MUST ACT TODAY!**

SURPRISINGLY— it's much **QUICKER, SAFER, EASIER AND FAR CHEAPER** than you think!

Who doesn't want to save a fistful of cash on medical expenses and drugs? Trust me—I highly recommend eating organic food. I do not recommend that you take chemical cocktails. Better health means that **YOU WILL BE MORE PRODUCTIVE IN ALL OF YOUR PERSONAL AND PROFESSIONAL ENDEAVOURS.**

YOU WILL BE BECOME MORE OPTIMISTIC ABOUT YOUR LIFE AND YOUR FUTURE! (When you eat happy food- I guarantee that it will literally put a smile on your face!-☺

Research shows that the more <u>POSITIVE</u> that corporations or businesses are- the more <u>SUCCESSFUL</u> they are; <u>AND</u>- <u>THE MORE MONEY THEY MAKE</u>!

<u>MY FIRST RECOMMENDATION IS:</u>

<u>TO FIRE YOUR DOCTOR—AND HIRE YOURSELF!</u>

<u>YOU</u> should rely on Mother Nature and her time-honoured nutritional remedies from her <u>FARMACY</u>. This means that— <u>YOU WILL BECOME YOUR OWN CHIEF PHYSICIAN</u>. "Doctor" actually means "teacher"— <u>SO YOU WILL EDUCATE AND TEACH YOURSELF!</u>

Our Creator put everything we need on this planet for us to be strong and healthy. Pharmaceuticals made by man only separate you from your hard-earned cash. Drugs are no more than poisonous chemicals.

<u>YOU</u> can teach yourself (with the help of this book) to <u>TAKE OUT THE NEGATIVE</u>, <u>TOXIC</u> foods, emotions, (and people) from your life and— <u>REPLACE</u> them with <u>HEALTHY</u> foods and <u>POSTIVE</u> lifestyles in your life.

I recommend that you follow a <u>KETOGENIC DIET AND KETOGENIC LIFESTYLE</u>—

You will then be able to then help your spouse, family and loved ones to do the same.

Most importantly- YOU will avoid degenerative illnesses and poor health by <u>ELIMINATING ALL</u> of the bad stuff in your life; (especially the <u>SAD</u> or <u>STANDARD AMERICAN DIET</u>) Then you can add in all of the good stuff to transform your life and health.

<u>BY THE WAY- YOU WILL LIKELY SAVE YOURSELF A COUPLE OF HUNDRED DOLLARS IN FOOD BILLS AND LIKELY MANY THOUSANDS OF DOLLARS ON MEDICAL BILLS</u>! How cool is that ?

You will be able to avoid the <u>DANGERS OF THE MEDICAL DISEASE-MANAGEMENT SYSTEM(S)</u>. Research shows that the biggest cause of <u>BANKRUPTCY IN THE U.S. ...IS MEDICAL BILLS!</u>

<u>YOU WILL HAVE A MUCH BETTER QUALITY OF LIFE. WHEN YOU HAVE ADAPTED TO THE KETOGENIC DIET. YOU WILL ALSO FIND THAT YOUR ENERGY LEVELS WILL GO THROUGH THE ROOF!</u>

Does this sound too good to be true? Stay tuned and keep reading.

Everyone knows that money cannot buy happiness. Your mother was <u>RIGHT WHEN SHE TOLD YOU THE BEST THINGS IN LIFE ARE FREE!</u>

THREE of the best things to enhance your health and happiness are FREE. They are SLEEP, EXERCISE AND SUNSHINE. YOU will discover how IMPORTANT THESE STRATEGIES ARE TO YOUR SUPERHEALTH. YOU will be provided scientific proof from recent scientific literature. I'm confident that when you read about some of the scientific literature, YOU WILL BE INSPIRED to change your less than healthy habits.

If you are a salaried professional- you are likely under great pressure to increase your number of billable hours. If you are an employer or a senior partner- you will find that you and the other members of your firm will be FAR more productive when you embrace the KETOGENIC DIETARY recommendations and LIFESTYLE strategies that are detailed in this book. If you are the lady of your castle- you will have MORE energy for your career outside of your castle as well as the lion's share of the household motherly functions that are assumed by most mothers. It's very difficult for members of the distaff to juggle career obligations and motherly household obligations. It's more difficult for modern women to wear two hats than for most men- who usually delegate most of the childrearing to the mother. This may be more biological, rather than misogyny on the part of men.

If you are among the 5 percent of lawyers who do litigation- You will win more cases!

Why? How? It's SIMPLE.

YOU will eat the proper FOODS to feed, fuel and SUPERCHARGE YOUR BRAIN!

YOU will follow a BRAIN SMART DIET to get leaner AND GET SMARTER!

YOU WILL LEARN TO EAT A BRAIN –HEALTHY DIET. The same holds true if you are a non-litigious lawyer or a DESK PROFESSIONAL.

YOU MUST FEED AND NOURISH YOUR BRAIN—FIRST and FOREMOST!

WITH THAT GOOD NUTRITION—YOU WILL HAVE THE ENERGY TO DO THE RIGHT KIND OF EXERCISE FOR YOUR BODY TO REPAIR DAMAGED BRAIN CELLS AND TO BUILD NEW BRAIN CELLS (NEURONS)!

EXERCISE AND VIBRANT HEALTH IS MOSTLY ABOUT IMPROVING YOUR COGNITIVE ABILITIES AND GROWING YOUR BRAIN.

> "The chief function of the body is to carry the brain around."
>
> — Thomas A. Edison

FOOD IS EITHER MEDICINE – OR IT IS POISON— YOU GET TO CHOOSE.

Almost everyone understands the adage that "you are what you eat." The right diet helps you feel good and the wrong diet makes you feel bad.

How would you answer this question?

"What fits your busy schedule better- exercising one hour a day or being dead 24 hours a day? (Randy Glasbergen- Cartoonist)

In this book YOU will learn exactly what you need to know about EXERCISE. YOU will learn that from a World-class Strength-coach who understands how NUTRITION and our metabolism is our primary driver of health.

YOU WILL LEARN HOW EXERCISE (and sex too-☺) BUILDS BRAIN CELLS!

You can never have too many brain cells-☺ You will also learn about the MINIMUM AMOUNT that you need to be healthy and strong; (hint: it's a lot less than you think!)

YOU will also learn strategies and practical tips to counter the evils of endless hours of SITTING. Did you know that EXERCISE builds neurons (brain cells)? It also activates a protein called BDNF (Brain-Derived Neurotropic Factor)?

THIS IS A VERY POWERFUL PROTEIN TO DEVELOP A POWERFUL BRAIN!

YOU will learn how BDNF is also activated by a variety of lifestyle habits, including exercise, caloric reduction, intermittent fasting, following a KETOGENIC DIET;

By ingesting certain nutrients such as turmeric (curcumin) and Omega- 3 fat (DHA).

YOU probably know that exercise has a PLETHORA OF HEALTH BENEFITS.

YOU will learn that EXERCISE IS INDISPENSABLE IF YOU WISH TO BE AND REMAIN HEALTHY! Unknown by most conventional doctors, & most of the medical world; among ALL of the numerous physiological benefits of exercise—TWO PHENOMENAL BENEFITS stand out above the rest.

- EXERCISE re-builds the mitochondria (the little power engines of your muscle cells). Who doesn't want bigger more muscle cells?

- EXERCISE GROWS NEW BRAIN CELLS AND RE-BUILDS YOUR BRAIN!

An amazing side-effect of exercise also causes your brain to pump out all kinds of pleasure chemicals called neuro-transmitters. These" feel-good chemicals" include dopamine, serotonin, epinephrine, norepinephrine, oxytoxin, etc.) These are the kind of chemicals that your body pumps out during sex and during other physical and/or FUN-FILLED/PLEASURE FILLED ACTIVITIES.

N.B. YOU'LL BE PLEASED TO KNOW THAT SEX BUILDS BRAIN CELLS!

Who knew?

YOU will also learn about Healthcare Screening, FMS (Functional Movement Screening) that few Kinesiologists or doctors have even heard about!

Am I saying that bodily aches and pains can be fixed with EXERCISE?

YES. YES AND YES!

YOU will learn how functional movement coaches fix PAIN WITH CORRECTIVE EXERCISE.

YOU CAN THROW YOUR POISONOUS PAIN KILLER MEDS IN THE GARBAGE!

YOU CAN FIRE YOUR DOCTOR- FIX PAIN WITH CORRECTIVE EXERCISE.

YOU CAN SAVE HUNDREDS OF DOLLARS ON DRUGS THAT ONLY HELPS BIG PHARMA AND YOUR DOCTOR MAKE MONEY.

YOU CAN HEAL YOURSELF WITH MOTHER NATURE'S PAINKILLER-HEALTHY FOOD.

YOU HAVE TO EAT ANYWAY SO WHY NOT EAT YOUR MEDICINE!

THE MOST EXHILARATING SCIENTIFIC NEWS COMES FROM NEW SCIENCE CALLED "EPIGENETICS"! The naysayers who have been telling us that we are the victims of our GENETIC DNA- are wrong!

They are " DEAD"-WRONG! The medical establishment with their quackery have been wrong for more than one century!

THE JURY IS IN!

OUR FATE AND OUR HEALTH DESTINY IS LARGELY IN OUR OWN HANDS!

This includes everything from the attainment of our level of education (e.g. high-school or college degree). Everything from human health and intellectual capacity and more are caused <u>PRIMARILY BY OUR ENVIRONMENT</u>- <u>NOT OUR GENES AND OUR DNA</u>!

Recently studies, (<u>SUPPRESSED</u> by mainstream media and government) offer us <u>TREMENDOUS AMOUNTS OF HOPE FOR EVERY SINGLE ONE OF US</u>!

Recent epigenetic studies prove that we are <u>not</u> victims of our own heredity (genes).

<u>WE ARE MASTERS OF OUR OWN HEALTH AND WELL-BEING</u>!

A recent study found that 98 PERCENT of all educational attainment (i.e. whether you complete high-school or college) <u>IS ACCOUNTED FOR BY FACTORS OTHER THAN YOUR GENETIC MAKE-UP!</u> (source: <u>www.independentsciencenews.org</u>

This study did not make the headlines. The authors failed to mention the 98 percent in the title or in the summary, nor was anything mentioned in the at all by mainstream media.

<u>WHY was this study suppressed?</u>

The answer is very simple. Big Government and Big corporations have a vested interest in <u>GENETICS</u>. <u>IF</u>— the scientific evidence suggested by their genetics shows <u>GENE VARIATION</u>—it does a couple of important things.

It removes <u>ALL RESPONSIBILITY</u> from their shoulders. In essence, it's a like a get out-of-jail free card. It's also a <u>HIDDEN</u> form of social control where the opinion of the masses is steered by industry- and/ or government forces.

<u>IF</u> people can be made to believe that <u>THEIR GENES ARE THE PRIMARY DRIVERS OF DISEASE AND POOR MENTAL HEALTH</u> and even educational achievement, then, those in control do not have to change anything. Toxins need not be removed from their products and the social control mechanism that is in the American educational system can remain unaddressed.

<u>There's one little problem.</u>

<u>THE SCIENCE SAYS THE EXACT OPPOSITE!</u>

Harvard Geneticist Geneticist Richard Lewontin, summed it up in his 1992 book: "The Doctrine of DNA: Biology as Idealogy" where he said:

> <u>"The notion that the lower classes are biologically infe-</u>
> <u>rior to the upper classes... is meant to legitimate the</u>

structures of inequality in our society by putting a bio-logical gloss on them."

Authors, Hall, Mathews and Morley (2010) wrote:

"Geneticists have not identified major susceptibility alleles (gene variants) for most common diseases."

Even the findings that have been claimed (which are modest) have consistently not stood up to retrospective replication. (Ioannidis and Panagiotou 2011) The absence of evidence is now so clear that even leaders in the field of human genetics sometimes find an acknowl-edgement is necessary (though only in the context for more funding. (Manolio et. Al 2009)

As the evidence for genetic causations has continuously and stub-bornly refused to appear—critics have grown bolder.

Authors Chaufan and Joseph in 2013 felt confident enough to write:

"These variants have not been found because they do not exist."

-author's underline

To be fair and scientifically accurate, while it is true, there have been a few exceptions- such as a specific breast cancer gene BRCA I, cystic fibrosis, and Huntington's disease.

BUT— for common physical and mental health conditions such as heart disease, cancer, autism and schizophrenia the situation has proven DIFFERENT.

The epidemiological and genetic evidence suggests that GENETIC RISK IS AT MOST A MINOR contributing factor.

Latham author of the above study expressed it very well:

"The same political logic applies to any human disease- or disorder, or even any social complaint. If the disorder (e.g. autism) can be shown to have a partial generic origin- then the barn door is open for any accused vaccine maker, or polluter or policy-maker to evade the blame- both legally and in the perception of the public." (author's underline)

IN SUM —YOUR GENES WILL EXPRESS GENETIC DATA depending upon the environment in which it finds itself- meaning the presence or absence of proper nutrients, toxins, even YOUR THOUGHTS, YOUR

FEELINGS AND YOUR EMOTIONS. For example, when you are afraid, your body pumps out CORTISOL and other hormones and chemicals into your body. Research into the health of our ancestors also indicates that CANCER – for example, is a MAN-MADE DISEASE.- in large part caused by drugs, chemicals, sugars, grains, obesity, stress, poor-sleeping habits; etc.

We now understand that FOOD IS INFORMATION!

We recently learned that FOOD IS A "POWERFUL EPIGENETIC MODULATOR"- or in simple language- FOOD CAN CHANGE OUR GENETIC DNA!

FOOD ACTUALLY REGULATES (for good or bad) THE EXPRESSION OF MANY OF OUR GENES!

How cool is that!

According to recent research, only about 10 PERCENT OF LONGEVITY or how long you will live is determined by your genetics. The other 90 PERCENT IS UP TO YOU! So you take heart if you did not make a wise choice when you chose your parents.- ☺

YOUR HABITS AND LIFESTYLE mostly determines how LONG you will live and how WELL you live. Most genes get turned "on" or get turned "off" based on your behaviour. This is called "GENE EXPRESSION."

SO- YOU CAN CELEBRATE! YOU ARE NOT THE VICTIM OF POOR GENES!

You can no longer claim that you are unlucky because you chose your parents poorly! -☺

THE VAST MAJORITY OF YOUR GENES ARE UNDER YOUR CONTROL- YOU ARE LARGELY THE MASTER OF YOUR OWN HEATH!

YOU ARE LARGELY THE AUTHOR OF YOUR OWN DESTINY ON PLANET EARTH!

It is the QUALITY of the decisions YOU MAKE that helps you LIVE a long healthy life as a human being—OR—KILLS YOU PREMATURELY!

YOU can choose to be the BOSS of your life, instead of allowing food cravings or the big food companies to kill you early. A little planning and a little forethought are all that is required. When confronted by a choice between a double cheese-burger; a spinach salad, or between an all-night booze fest and a good night's sleep- ASK YOURSELF—

Which choice is in **MY** best interest? Will your choice make you smarter, stronger, healthier, better or more passionate for life? Or will it **ROB** you of something **PRECIOUS**?

Each and every day of your life—

YOU CAN CHOOSE TO BE THE BOSS OF YOUR LIFE. **YOU CAN TO CHOOSE A LONG, HEALTHY, VIBRANT LIFE**! **OR**— you can do nothing and take the unfortunate consequences.

YOU no longer have any excuses. **YOU** can no longer blame your lack of success and/or lack of happiness or whatever on being "unlucky" in Mother Nature's gene lottery.

YOU should also know that it helps to associate with like-"health-minded POSITIVE supportive individuals. If you do not make wise decisions that affect your health—will you be around to enjoy your grandchildren? Or will be suffering from Alzheimer's because you stuffed your body with carbohydrates, sugary and processed junk **FOODS**.

Recent research even suggests that **YOUR DIET WILL EVEN AFFECT FUTURE GENERATIONS TO COME**! **OMG**!

How amazing is that!

This means that, unless you take control of your health— **NOW**— it can directly affect your children, your grandchildren, and even your great-grandchildren. An alarming bad example is that research now shows that the umbilical cords of some babies **CONTAIN 2000 TOXINS**! Yuk!

The **OPPOSITE** is also true. When you take care of your health you are increasing the likelihood that your children and grand-children **WILL HAVE BETTER HEALTH**.

Scientists, researchers and even psychiatrists are finding that **EVERYTHING** we do has ripple effects on the **EMOTIONAL AND PHYSICAL HEALTH OF OUR FAMILIES**.

We are electrically-charged bacterial human beings; with our bodies surrounded by an energy force of about 12 feet. All of our 10 **TRILLION CELLS** are talking to each other and to other people's cells! Who knew?

Actually, we are composed of **99.9999 PERCENT WATER AT THE MOLECULAR LEVEL**. It's **TRUE**!

<u>EVEN MORE AMAZING</u> — <u>WE ARE MORE CREATURES OF BACTERIA</u> than anything else! We have more than <u>100 TRILLION BACTERIA</u> in and on our bodies!!

Our bodies are truly remarkable. There are many different ways of <u>HEALING</u> our bodies that science is only just beginning to understand.

Do you believe that we can <u>REGENERATE</u> (grow) <u>A NEW IMMUNE SYSTEM IN ONLY 72</u> HOURS? <u>YES</u> -WE <u>CAN</u>.

<u>IT'S ABSOLUTELY TRUE! AND</u>— IT'S FREE!

<u>PLUS</u>- <u>YOU CAN DO IT YOURSELF!</u> It's called "<u>FASTING</u>" and has been used for <u>THOUSANDS OF YEARS TO HEAL HUMANS!</u> Later, you will learn about the science and the protocol and how to use this amazing <u>HEALING TOOL</u>.

<u>CLINICAL STUDIES</u> <u>PROVE THAT IT HAS BEEN USED BREAST CANCER PATIENTS TO REVERSE CANCER!</u>

Even more amazing- <u>FASTING</u> has proved effective even when used by breast cancer patients undergoing horrific chemotherapy cancer treatment!

<u>TAKING CARE OF OUR HEALTH IS ALL ABOUT EDUCATION, EDUCATION, EDUCATION AND</u> <u>MORE EDUCATION!</u>

Everyone knows that "<u>KNOWLEDGE IS POWER</u>". This is especially important when it comes to our HEALTH.

Your allopathic (conventionally-trained) physician <u>DOES NOT POSSESS</u> the nutritional tools and knowledge of lifestyle strategies to help you take control of your health. But that's okay. Your doctor will need to take the same health journey as you do. Your doctor only knows how to treat symptoms of "dis-ease" by prescribing toxic drugs-which do the <u>EXACT OPPOSITE!</u>

<u>SUPERHEALTH IS NOT ATTAINED BY EATING DRUGS</u>.

Vibrant health is accomplished by using <u>FOOD AS YOUR MEDICINE</u>.

Humans have done this for the last 2.9 million years. Unfortunately- your doctor was not taught this in medical school. Only <u>YOU</u> can take responsibility for your own health. It begins with <u>YOUR</u> decision to stop relying on <u>SOME</u> white-coated pill pusher.

<u>ALL YOU REALLY NEED IS</u>-

<u>THE DESIRE AND THE COURAGE TO ADOPT THE "KETOGENIC" NUTRITIONAL AND LIFESTYLE STRATEGIES DETAILED IN THIS BOOK</u>.

This book is your "COMPREHENSIVE HEALTHCARE BIBLE". It was written to educate YOU; it provides YOU with the necessary information that YOU need so that YOU can take control of your health- and attain SUPERHEALTH AND FITNESS.

FOLLOWING THE HEALING KETOGENIC NUTRITIONAL APPROACH IS THE HEALTH SOLUTION THAT YOU REQUIRE. (For science-oriented readers—dozens of the most recent clinical studies are listed in the REFERENCE SECTION at the end of this book.)

Switching health gears—

Did you know that THOUGHTS BECOME THINGS?

YES—IT'S TRUE!

WE ARE MORE POWERFUL AS HUMAN BEINGS THAN ANYONE EVER IMAGINED!

ENERGY HEALING IS A HUGE NEW FIELD OF MODERN MEDICINE!

YOU can buy all kinds of books recently written about ENERGY MEDICINE- aka— ENERGY HEALING.

There are energy healers; it's even possible TO HEAL AND TO FIX all kinds of health problems by ENERGY HEALING- EVEN FROM A

DISTANCE!

THIS NEW SCIENCE IS CALLED "QUANTUM PHYSICS".

How cool is that?

THE SCIENCE OF GENETICS is nicely summed up by Bruce Lipton, PhD. Follows:

> "The implication is that this basic idea we have that we are controlled by our genes is false. It's an idea that turns us into victims. I'm saying that we are the creators of our situation. The genes are merely the blueprints. We are the contractors; and we can adjust these blueprints; and we can even rewrite them."

SCIENCE PROVES THAT:

YOU ARE MASTER OF YOUR OWN HEALTH—AND YOUR OWN DESTINY!

THERE ARE MANY WAYS TO CHANGE YOUR GENOME (aka GENETICS) AND

SWITCH ON YOUR HEALTHY GENES.

YOU CAN FLIP YOUR GENETIC SWITCH. THIS WILL HELP YOU TO BUILD NEW BRAIN CELLS. SWITCHING ON YOUR "HEALTHY" GENES WILL ALLOW YOU TO LIVE A LONG, HEALTHY, HAPPY LIFE.

BUT— SUPERHEALTH ALL STARTS WITH EATING A NUTRIENT-RICH DIET.

Which diet you ask? —There are dozens of "so-called healthy" diets out there. THE BEST THERAPEUTIC (HEALING) DIET IS MORE THAN A "DIET." IT IS A COMPLETE NUTRITIONAL APPROACH COUPLED WITH KEY LIFESTYLE CHANGES.

THIS NUTRITIONAL APPROACH— IS KNOWN AS "THE KETOGENIC DIET".

This diet is prescribed by most knowledgeable nutritionists and healthcare/functional medicine doctors to PREVENT AND REVERSE A BOATLOAD OF DISEASES/ADVERSE HEALTH CONDITIONS- FROM A TO Z!

SUPERHEALTH BEGINS AND ENDS WITH A DIET WHICH NOURISHES AND GROWS OUR BRAIN! This is the real magic behind the keto-genic diet.

Dr. Ketogenic Diet is a "BRAIN DIET". This diet and Ketogenic Foods will make you smart; lean, fit, and best of all- HEALTHY AND HAPPY!

YOU could describe the Ketogenic Diet as "PALEO –ON- STEROIDS" -☺

THIS "DIET" IS A BRAND- NEW NUTRITIONAL APPROACH. This dietary approach is virtually unknown by conventional doctors and die-ticians. The Ketogenic diet has ONLY existed for more than 2.9 million years; i.e. since humans have roamed around here on planet Earth.-☺!!

VERY FEW PEOPLE HAVE EVEN HEARD ABOUT THE KETOGENIC DIET.

It's not taught in medical/die-tician schools. Registered Dieticians are taught medical therapy rather than Nutrition. Indeed, the word "Nutrition" has only become commonplace in the last decade- even in fitness circles. Most of the Western World is totally ignorant about the KETOGENIC DIET. Even the athletic community is ignorant about the importance of a ketogenic diet.

THIS EVIDENCE —BASED SCIENTIFIC SUPPORTING LITERATURE HAS BEEN HIDING in plain sight for many years. Actually, Dr.Ketogenic Diet has been suppressed for almost 50 years!

<u>YOU WILL ADORE THE DELICIOUS BRAIN-SMART- "SCRUMPTIOUS" KETOGENIC RECIPES</u> provided in this book.

How do the following foods sound...almond fudge bars or cancer-fighting comfort coconut cake?

<u>Does the WORLD'S HEALTHIEST BEST TASTING PIZZA sound appealing to you?</u>

Before reading further you might want to jump to my recipe section at the end of chapter 7 (Dr. Ketogenic Diet...

Our ancestors had the hunter-gatherer's <u>GENOME</u> (our genetic-make-up); which means that we are— (and always have been) hard-wired to consume a <u>KETOGENIC DIET</u>.

<u>A KETOGENIC DIET BASICALLY CONSISTS OF:</u>

> <u>75-80 % FAT- 15-20 % PROTEIN- and 5 % CARBOHYDRATES</u>
>
> <u>A KETOGENIC DIET IS VERY HIGH FAT (healthy fats); MODERATE PROTEIN, and VERY –LOW CARBOHYDRATE DIET.</u> Extensive CLINICAL studies are analyzed and references are provided in the Appendix A.

The vast majority of people living in the western world are "carboholics." Carboholics are people that have a carbohydrate addiction. Basically, the entire Western world is <u>ADDICTED TO PROCESSED FOOD</u>-i.e. the Standard American Diet (SAD) diet. Processed, refined foods are more accurately described as "Frankenfoods"; this type of food is often laced with toxic chemicals and additives; often comes from drug-laced, antibiotic foods sources and is almost always <u>NUTRIENT-DEFICIENT</u>, and loaded with <u>REFINED POISONS; SUGARS AND HIGH-FRUCTOSE CORN SYRUP, (HFCS)</u>.

<u>"CARBOHYDRATE ADDICTION" IS THE LEADING CAUSE OF GLOBAL OBESITY.</u>

The United States has exported their Standard American Diet (<u>SAD</u>) to most parts of the globe. The disease called "carbohydrate addiction has been rapidly spread to most parts of the planet. Even more importantly, this carbohydrate addiction is not only limited to "refined" or "processed" carbohydrates.

Carbohydrate addiction is caused by <u>UNHEALTHY CARBOHYDRATES!</u>

Humans have only subsisted on a <u>CARBOHYDRATE DIET</u> for about the <u>LAST 10,000 YEARS</u> (i.e. <u>SINCE THE DAWN OF AGRICULTURE</u>). Prior to that, almost all humans on planet earth ate a healthy, healing Ketogenic Diet.

OUR HUMAN GENOME AND ESPECIALLY OUR BRAINS— ARE HARD-WIRED TO EAT THIS KIND OF DIET—PERIOD!

IF MOTHER NATURE DOESN'T SUPPLY IT—WE'RE NOT GENETICALLY DESIGNED/PROGRAMMED TO EAT IT!

This meant that our ancestors ate what they killed as wild game, fish, nuts, seeds, and some plants that would grow wild. As for fruits- our ancestors might have been lucky enough to eat some seasonal wild berries. The only "sugary food" was honey- which was scarce and hard to find. Honey is actually food for bees. We are hard-wired to know that if a food is sweet that it is good for us. Most animals and humans know instinctively that food that is rotten and or foul-smelling often tastes that way for a reason.

Some populations still eat in this ancestral way. The Massai warriors and Inuit (aka Eskimo peoples) are good examples. The Massai used to eat about 3 pounds of animals, blood, & milk each day. Now they eat less meat because they have lost most of their herds, so they are sometimes forced to eat more veggies and plant food. For the Inuit, whales, and seals (98 % good fats) and fish/ animal fats were the mainstay of their diets. There are not many fruits and veggies that grow on the arctic tundra.-☺ Inuit native peoples were quite healthy until they adopted the standard North American diet and unhealthy lifestyles.

WHEN MODERN AGRICULTURE CAME ALONG—THAT'S WHEN OUR HEALTH PROBLEMS BEGAN. For example, we are **NOT GENETICALLY DESIGNED TO EAT BREAD AND GRAINS**. Some of that **JUNK FOOD** pizza that you ate last week may be still rotting in your colon. Many people are literally walking around with several pounds of undigested fecal matter in their colons. Yuk!

THE HUMAN BODY AND HUMAN METABOLISM WERE NOT DESIGNED— OR ENGINEERED TO EAT AND DIGEST ALMOST ALL CARBOHYDRATES.

HUMANS HAVE VIRTUALLY A "ZERO" REQUIREMENT FOR CARBOHYDRATES!

AS SURPRISING as this seems, **CARBOHYDRATES** should **NOT** even be considered as a **MACRONUTRIENT**. Think of carbohydrates as an ingredient found in small amounts in most plants. If Mother Nature does not provide the food from **HER FARMACY—YOU WERE NOT INTENDED TO EAT IT!** This is a good starting point to look at nutrition. Humans are supposed to eat to live—not live to eat.

In this book YOU WILL LEARN:

1. <u>FAT IS THE PREFERRED FUEL OF HUMAN METABOLISM!</u>

2. <u>FAT (especially SATURATED FAT) IS YOUR BEST FRIEND;</u>

3. <u>FAT IS THE PREFERRED SUPERFUEL FOR YOUR BRAIN & YOUR HEART!</u>

<u>HOW AMAZING AND REVOLUTIONARY IS THAT?</u>

<u>Who knew?</u>

<u>Sidebar-</u>

In this book— there are <u>NO FOOTNOTES</u>. Instead, there are immediate citations and/or references which will permit you to verify the accuracy of the information discussed.

Footnotes are cumbersome; they are old school; they are awkward; time- consuming and thought-breaking. Who wants to see little numbers in the text and explanations at the bottom of a page or at the end of each chapter? Footnotes are frustrating; (time consuming too) to flip to an index of footnotes and read these during the text.

The modern way is to provide the source of the article, study; scientific or other. In this way, <u>YOU</u> the reader, if you so desire, you can verify the veracity for yourself.

Here are a few brief comments about how I have structured my book.

The first chapter "The Evolution of Modern Western Medicine" traces the origin of our modern day "healthcare" systems; with analysis of the why's, how's, and wherefores of the <u>FRAUDULENT</u>, <u>BARBARIC</u>, <u>DYSFUNCTIONAL ALLOPATHIC MEDICAL</u> <u>APPROACH TO MEDICINE.</u>

My first chapter provides <u>DOZENS OF REASONS TO FIRE YOUR DOCTOR!</u>

My second or "flagship" chapter provides the <u>THREE TOP REASONS WHY FIRING YOUR DOCTOR IS YOUR FIRST CRUCIAL STEP TO TAKE CONTROL OF YOUR HEALTH. I WILL ALSO PROVIDE YOU WITH REASONS WHY YOU SHOULD HIRE YOURSELF AS YOUR OWN DOCTOR.</u>

<u>I WILL ALSO PROVIDE YOU WITH THE PRACTICAL STUFF THAT YOU "NEED-TO-KNOW SUCH AS THE IMPORTANT HEALTH TESTS AND HOW TO GET THEM.</u>

<u>KNOWLEDGE OF THESE TESTS- WHAT THEY MEAN AND HOW TO USE THEM WILL EMPOWER YOU!</u>

THIS INFORMATION IS WHAT YOU NEED TO BY-PASS THE MEDICAL ESTABLISHMENT AND ESCAPE THE CLUTCHES OF BIG PHARMA.

YOU WILL BE PROVIDED THE KNOWLEDGE, NEED-TO-KNOW INFORMATION, AND ESSENTIAL TOOLS YOU NEED TO PERMIT YOU TO SEIZE CONTROL OF YOUR OWN HEALTH. NO DOCTOR IS REQUIRED!

I provide you with my personal recommendations regarding the information that you require to take control of your health.

YOU MUST TAKE A "DO –IT- YOURSELF" (DIY) APPROACH TO YOUR HEALTH!

INDEED- YOU MUST LEARN TO BE YOUR OWN DOCTOR!

In chapter two, you will learn about the IMPORTANT HEALTH TESTS THAT ARE NOT USED BY 98 percent of conventionally- trained doctors. Some tests that your doctor gives you are the WRONG TESTS. ALMOST ALL HEALTH ADVICE provided by your doctor IS COMPLETELY ERRONEOUS.

THE SAD TRUTH IS THAT 99 percent of what your doctor tells you is WRONG!

This book will reveal to YOU the SUPPRESSED TRUTHS ABOUT FUNCTIONAL HEALTH AND FUNCTIONAL MEDICINE.

Your doctor was taught "DYSFUNCTIONAL MEDICINE";(aka how to prescribe a pill for any symptoms" that he might guess.

YOU WILL LEARN MORE ABOUT "FUNCTIONAL MEDICINE" THAN CONVENTIONAL DOCTORS LEARN IN A LIFETIME!

YOU WILL BE LIGHT-YEARS AHEAD OF YOUR (FORMER) DOCTOR!

YOU WILL LEARN ABOUT NUTRITION/ BIOCHEMISTRY OF NUTRITION.

CONVENTIONAL PHYSICIANS ARE CLUELESS ABOUT HUMAN PHYSIOLOGY AND HUMAN BIOCHEMISTRY- BECAUSE THEY HAVE NOT BEEN TRAINED IN NUTRITION OR IN THE BIOCHEMISTRY OF NUTRITION!

THIS BOOK WILL PROVIDE YOU WITH THE NECESSARY BIOCHEMISTRY OF NUTRITION, /CUTTING-EDGE NUTRITIONAL INFORMATION THAT YOU NEED TO APPLY SO THAT YOU CAN BE STRONG, HEALTHY AND DIS-EASE FREE.

(Please check out the world's "Healthiest best- tastingPizza Recipe and other DELICIOUS HEALTHY Ketogenic Recipes which will blow you away! -☺)

Chapter Eleven is a special chapter entitled: "Diseases that your Doctor cannot Diagnose", This chapter explains and analyzes the importance of Digestive Health and how so much illness is linked to poor GUT HEALTH.

YOU WILL LEARN HOW YOUR GUT IS YOUR FIRST BRAIN!

YOU will learn cutting-edge scientific information about the complex interactions between our gut microbes and our "traditional brain".

YOU WILL LEARN THE FIRST NUTRITIONAL STEP THAT YOU NEED TO TAKE TO RESTORE YOUR OVERALL HEALTH. YOU WILL LEARN HOW TO:

   " TO RESTORE YOUR GUT HEALTH-

   AND HOW TO " HEAL AND SEAL" YOUR GUT"

Probably 90 percent of people in modern Western society suffer from" leaky gut". Once your GUT is healed; vital nutrients can then be properly absorbed by your body.

More importantly, PATHOGENS can be prevented from entering your gut. Think of healing a leaky gut as healing a leaky brain too- -☺) literally! You need to strengthen the fortress walls of your intestinal lining from invading armies of pathogens!

ONCE YOUR GUT LINING/GUT HEALTH IS RESTORED—THEN YOU CAN RE-POPULATE YOUR GUT WITH " THE GOOD IMMUNE (FOOD) SOLDIERS."

YOU MUST LEARN HOW TO DO THIS NUTRITIONAL HEALING PROCESS FOR YOURSELF. YOU WILL LEARN THAT THE KEY TO YOUR HEALTH IS THE PROPER COMPOSITION OF MICROBIAL GUT BACTERIA.

NO DOCTOR KNOWS YOUR BODY. ONLY YOU KNOW YOUR OWN BODY.

YOU MUST LEARN TO HEAL YOURSELF. NO ONE ELSE CAN DO IT FOR YOU!

In chapter four —NEUROTOXINS are analyzed; chapter 5 analyses the "Queen of Neurotoxins"; and the "Sugar Factory" in chapter 6, (with an in depth analysis of Diabetes). Chapter 7- is my "core" chapter- "THE HEALING KETOGENIC DIET"

The remaining chapters analyze other important doctors such as Dr. Sunshine; Dr. Exercise and Dr. Sleep, and Dr. Water etc.

My final chapter, "Listen with your Ketogenic Heart"(Dr. Happy-☺ deals with EMOTIONAL HEALTH, OUR HAPPINESS AND WELL-BEING.

OUR EMOTIONAL HEALTH IS THE MOST IMPORTANT ASPECT OF OUR HEALTH.

85 PERCENT OF ALL DISEASES ARE TRIGGERED AND/OR CAUSED BY STRESS- SO A SUPERHEALTH PROGRAM MUST ADDRESS EMOTIONAL HEALTH.

EATING A BRAIN- HEALTHY- KETOGENIC DIET WILL SUPERCHARGE YOUR BRAIN AND YOUR LIFE. YOU WILL LEARN HOW TO RE-BUILD YOUR BODY AT A CELLULAR LEVEL!

ALMOST ALL HEALTH ISSUES— CAN BE SUCCESSFULLY RESOLVED BY FOLLOWING A WELL-CONSTRUCTED KETOGENIC DIET.

We are all unique human beings; with unique genes, unique bio-chemistry; unique health histories, and unique metabolisms. There is NO one-size that fits all. We must each determine our "Goldilocks Health Zone".

GENERALLY SPEAKING— A KETOGENIC NUTRITIONAL APPROACH WHICH LIMITS CARBS AND EMPHASIZES HEALTHY FATS IS THE BEST APPROACH FOR ALL HUMANS.

THE GOLDEN KEY TO GOOD HEALTH IS TO MAINTAIN STABLE- LOW BLOOD SUGAR AND GREAT INSULIN SENSITIVITY.

To conclude this introduction:

WHEN YOU ADOPT A KETOGENIC DIET AND LIFESTYLE— YOU WILL SUPERCHARGE YOUR BRAIN AND YOUR ENTIRE BODY.

WHEN YOU FOLLOW DR. "KETO'S" PRESCRIPTION YOU WILL ENTER 'NUTRITIONAL KETOSIS".

YOU WILL LEARN TO ENJOY EATING GREAT TASTING- DELICIOUS –LIP-SMACKING FOODS. THESE KETOGENIC FOODS WILL SATISFY YOU LIKE NO OTHER FOODS THAT YOU HAVE EVER EATEN!

KETOGENIC FOODS ARE HIGH-FAT/LOW CARBOHYDRATE FOODS THAT WE ARE BIOLOGICALLY PROGRAMMED AND DESIGNED TO EAT.

KETOGENIC FOODS ARE THE MOST SATISFYING FOODS THAT YOU WILL EVER EAT!

ONCE YOU ENTER 'NUTRITIONAL KETOSIS" YOU WILL LIKELY WANT TO STAY THERE FOR THE REST OF YOUR LIFE!

DR. HIPPOCRATES WAS RIGHT!

"Let your Food be your Medicine; let your Medicine be your food." His medical philosophy was right 2,500 years ago. It continues to be right today.

I'm convinced that—

DR. KETOGENIC DIET WILL TRANSFORM YOU AND YOUR HEALTH—FOREVER.

A KETOGENIC DIET WILL SUPERCHARGE YOUR BRAIN, YOUR HEALTH, AND EVERY ASPECT OF YOUR LIFE!

Enjoy your Ketogenic Journey.

Nutritional Ketogenesis has transformed my life. I know it can transform your life too.

Ketogenic Love, Strength and Honour.

January 12th, 2016

Gary W. Pitts

CHAPTER ONE

THE EVOLUTION OF WESTERN (ALLOPATHIC) MEDICINE

"Modern medicine is a negation of health. It isn't orga-
nized to serve human health, but only to serve itself
as an institution. It makes more people sick than it
heals" – Ivan Illich, author of "Medical Nemesis"

A. ALLOPATHIC MEDICINE

The American Medical Association (AMA) refers to MD medical
students as "allopathic" medical students. This term describes
the conventional Western medical system of practice. The word
"Allopathic" comes from the Greek word "allos," which means other
or apposite—and "pathos" which means suffering or disease.
Stedman's Medical Dictionary refers to allopathic medicine as "a
therapeutic system in which a disease is treated by producing a
second condition which is incompatible with or antagonistic to
the first". Conventional allopathic medicine is the kind of medicine
practiced by most health care providers in western healthcare
systems. It is a "disease management" approach; rather than a
"preventative health care" approach.

Allopathic medicine is very warlike; it uses razor-sharp knives
called scalpels and poisons. It removes tumors, masses, infections,
and other unwanted tissues by surgery. Bacteria, cancer cells, and
undesirable tissues are killed with <u>POISONS</u> called <u>DRUGS</u>; and
burnt with chemicals aka-chemotherapy. The general idea is to kill
the bad unwanted tissue or organ or whatever— without killing
the patient. Unwanted tissue and body parts can be radiated

(burned up) while obliterating the unwanted body part or tissue- without in theory— damaging healthy skin/tissue, cells and/ or healthy body organs.

The allopathic approach can be summed up as the "CUT, POISON, BURN" paradigm. In medical school, allopathic physicians are taught essentially how to prescribe DRUGS and DO SURGERY. Allopathic doctors are taught to TREAT SYMPTOMS.

ALLOPATHIC CONVENTIONALLY- TRAINED PHYSICIANS NOT TAUGHT TO IDENTIFY OR TO TREAT THE ROOT CAUSE OF ANY MEDICAL PROBLEM OR OTHER ADVERSE HEALTH SYMPTOM.

Allopathic medicine works best to fix gunshot wounds; slap on casts for broken bones and employ similar emergency medicine for acute injuries—PROVIDED that you are lucky enough to escape from the hospital without contracting a deadly virus, C-DIFFICILE or other deadly bacterial infection spread by the widespread use of antibi- otics. In Latin "hospital" means "a place to die.". Hospitals were very aptly named.

HOSPITALS ARE NOW RANKED AS THE NUMBER 3 KILLER IN THE USA!

One out of every 25 patients that quest for treatment will lead to a hospital-related infection. According to the Center for Disease Control (CDC) and estimated 722,000 patients will fall prey to infec- tion attributed to the care they receive in US hospitals. Of those, 75,000 will lose their lives. But hospital- borne infections is only one part of the story.

An estimated 440,000 Americans each year are DYING from pre- ventative hospital errors—including injury, illness and infection! According to research by The Leapfrog Group, research reveals the LACK OF PROGRESS WITHIN MODERN MEDICINE.

In a Senate Subcommittee hearing in 2014, expert testimony con- cluded that this "medical care" cost an estimated ONE TRILLION DOLLARS ANNUALLY! Testimony indicated that 1,000 patients die EVERY DAY from medical errors; and another 10,000 patients experi- ence serious complications.

The take-home message is to AVOID HOSPITALS. There are innumera- ble natural alternative remedies; life-style modifications, which have been proven time and time again to minimize the effects of disease. Foods and supplements that are high in antioxidants are effective in safeguarding against CELLULAR damage that can lead to disease. There are 3 primary ingredients such as Vitamin C, Beta-Carotene and Vitamin E and a boatload of nutrients found in coloured fruits and vegetables

If a <u>MEDICAL EMERGENCY</u> arises and/or other medical procedure arises—e.g. surgery—I <u>STRONGLY RECOMMEND THAT YOU</u>:

<u>MAKE SURE THAT THE PATIENT RECEIVING CARE HAS A PATIENT ADVOCATE!</u>

<u>THE PATIENT ADVOCATE</u> should be prepared to ask questions- interrogate doctors if necessary and monitor the administration of care to help reduce the risk of injury and infection. This patient advocate may even consider bringing some nutritious food to the patient. Chances are high that hospital food will be sub-par nutrition.

Even <u>EMERGENCY</u> medicine as practiced by "allopaths" is now being eroded with techniques such as <u>AED's</u> (automated external defibrillators) to treat SCA's (sudden heart attacks). Moreover, some hospitals are starting to use natural substances such as honey to treat wounds. During World War 1- honey was often successfully used on the battlefield to treat wounded soldiers. After 100 years, allopathic emergency medicine is slowly starting to change. Some enlightened allopathic doctors are starting to wake up-but it's a slow process.

In practice, emergency first responders i.e. (paramedics) likely save more lives than do most emergency- room physicians. Most allopathic doctors do not even know how to use these talking <u>AED BOXES</u>; many do not even have them in their offices. These devices can be safely used by a schoolchild. Many people, (including cardiologists) do not even know of their existence outside of the ambulance/emergency room.

<u>If you have a SCA (sudden heart attack) if an AED is NOT administered WITHIN FIVE (5) MINUTES of your SCA—your chances of survival are SLIM AND NONE</u>.

<u>AED</u>'s are mandatory in most American states. In Canada, Manitoba is the <u>only</u> province that has enacted this legislation that literally saves lives every day. This law came into force on January 1st, 2014. Most American Appellate Court judges know and understand the importance of <u>AED</u> and <u>CPR</u> (cardio-pulmonary resuscitation). In Canada, it appears that due to the lack of legislation, the importance of <u>AED</u> and <u>CPR</u> has not been yet been judicially recognized by the Canadian Judicial system. But then, even the medical industry in Canada has turned a blind eye to the importance of <u>AED</u> and <u>CPR</u>. As a general rule, Canadian cardiologists are still pushing drugs, and heart surgery— such as stents, by-passes etc. <u>AED</u>'s probably save more lives after SCA's than does the medical establishment. If a talking

box can be used by a 10-year old to <u>SAVE A LIFE</u> after a sudden heart attack- Shouldn't you buy one? It could be the best $ 1,500.00 that you will ever spend. You may even save a loved one's or neighbours life.

$ 1, 500 to save your life in 5 minutes is more valuable than any "life-saving surgery "or heart procedure. But this would make your cardiologist unhappy. He would not be able to pay for his new Mercedes. (See infra: Cardiologists or Criminals)

<u>How did allopathic medicine begin?</u>

<u>How has Big Oil conquered the world?</u>

Transformation of the Practice of Medicine went into full force in 1901-with the establishment of the Rockefeller Institute for Medical Research.

Before that, naturopathic based herbal medicine had been the norm.

Rockefeller- an <u>OIL KING- PIN SET OUT TO SHIFT THE MEDICAL INDUSTRY TOWARD OIL-DERIVED PHARMACEUTICALS INSTEAD.</u> The Institute was headed up by Simon Flexner, whose brother Abraham was contracted by the Carnegie Foundation to author a report on the current state of the medical education. (the "Flexner Report of 1910". The effectiveness of therapies being taught by medical colleges and institutions was evaluated. Any remedy that could not be patented was vigorously dismissed as "<u>QUACKERY</u>".

New partnerships with people like Andrew Carnegie and J.P. Morgan began to convince state and federal legislators to create laws (regulations and licensing "red-tape") that strictly promoted <u>DRUG MEDICINE</u>. The idea was to build a new medical profession— <u>while snuffing out and shutting down alternative, inexpensive, natural remedies.</u>

These "natural remedies" were called "quackery". Medical colleges and institutions that did <u>NOT</u> conform to this "new "approach" were simply eliminated.

<u>THE SOLE FOCUS OF MEDICINE SHIFTED TO THE USE OF SYNTHETIC DRUGS AND SURGERY.</u>

<u>THIS MEDICAL PARADIGM QUICKLY RESULTED IN A "MASSIVE MEDICAL ECONOMY!</u>

<u>THE TRUTH OF THE MATTER IS:</u>

<u>THE ALLOPATHIC MEDICAL DOCTORS ARE THE REAL "QUACKS"!</u>

MODERN MEDICINE IS A PROFIT-DRIVEN BUSINESS DIVORCED FROM HEALING.

The Flexner Report was conveniently titled "Medical Education in the United States and States were <u>halved</u> as a result of the Flexner Report. In less than 15 years the number of medical schools was reduced from 160 to 80. By World War II the number of medical schools was reduced further below 70.

THE CONCENTRATED CONTROL OF MEDICAL EDUCATION AND THE WESTERN ALLOPATHIC MODEL OF MEDICINE HAD BEEN CREATED.

This new "profession" began a massive categorization of "new diseases" which are used to describe a huge array health of health issues today in our western civilization. The government and Big Pharma both control our "healthcare" <u>more accurately described as "our disease- management care".</u>

In 1910 —at the time of the Flexner report— <u>HEART ATTACKS WERE ALMOST NON-EXISTENT. PEOPLE WERE BRAINWASHED TO FORGET ABOUT THE PREVENTION OF DISEASE BASED ON THE PREMISE THAT FOOD IS MEDICINE.</u>

THE TRUTH IS THAT THERE IS NOT A SINGLE RECORDED CASE OF HEART DISEASE WHICH IS MORE THAN 100 YEARS OLD!

TODAY IN 2015— HEART FAILURE/AND/OR CARDIOVASCULAR DISEASE IS THE SECOND LEADING CAUSE OF DEATH in Western countries.

HEART DIS- EASE HAS EXPLODED PARTLY DUE TO A BROKEN HEALTH CARE SYSTEM AND INCOMPETENT ALLOPATHIC DOCTORS.

The average drug use for children up to 18 years old is 4 prescriptions per capita.

The average drug use for seniors 65 years old is 28 prescriptions per capita.

ALLOPATHIC DOCTORS RECEIVE NO NUTRITIONAL EDUCATION IN MEDICAL SCHOOL. THEY ARE CLUELESS ABOUT THE BIOCHEMISTRY OF NUTRITION.

This ignorance has not stopped the medical establishment from verbally "prescribing" <u>HORRIFIC- TOTALLY- FLAWED NUTRITIONAL ADVICE FOR THE LAST 75 YEARS.</u> Did you know that allopathic doctors used to advertise that CIGARETTES were healthy and good for you? OMG! How horrific is that? How many people were killed and/or suffered serious injuries by following such horrific advice?

DOCTORS AND DIE-TICIANS HAVE PROVIDED THE WORST POSSIBLE NUTRITIONAL ADVICE. THEIR INSANE ADVICE HAS ADVOCATED THAT PEOPLE EAT A HIGH-CARBOHYDRATE AND LOW-FAT DIET.

No one will ever know how many people have been killed or seriously injured by this flawed dietary advice.

HERE ARE SOME RESULTS OF THIS HORRIFIC DIETARY ADVICE.

In **1910, only 1 in 100,000 PEOPLE HAD DIABETES.**

In **1910, ALZHEIMER'S DISEASE,** (aka "all-timer's disease" was not even heard of! Forty years ago, Alzheimer's did not exist. Most people (especially baby-boomers) have naively listened to their allopathic physicians' "sick advice" (pun intended).

Consumers been told for **SEVEN DECADES** by allopathic doctors and their die-itician colleagues to eat a high carbohydrate /low-fat diet. Most have followed that awful advice and have gone to an early grave as a result.

Following this flawed advice North Americans are now **FATTER** and **SICKER** than ever. People are now being diagnosed in ever-increasing numbers with **DIABETES** and a **PLETHORA** of related diseases. Doctors tell their patients that obesity, diabetes and chronic diseases are a natural result of old age, drinking and smoking and/or bad genes. Allopathic doctors have no use for vitamins, herbs or other nutrients.

IT HAS NOW BEEN SCIENTIFICALLY PROVEN THAT HIGH CARBOHYDRATE DIETS CAUSE Alzheimer's disease in two ways.

1. **THE BRAIN IS STARVED BY NOT RECEIV-ING ENOUGH GOOD DIETARY FAT and**

2. **CARBOHYDRATES LITERALLY EAT AWAY YOUR BRAIN.**

In 2010, in the United States, according to the CDC, there were **18.8 MILLION** people diagnosed with **DIABETES**; plus another **7 MILLION people** who went **UNDETECTED.** You can add to those numbers another **80 MILLION people** who are **PRE-DIABETICS.**

ALZHEIMER'S DISEASE now has about **5.4 MILLION** sufferers; (source: www.diabetes.org) Alzheimer's Disease has now been dubbed "Type 3 Diabetes".

From having **NO** heart disease in 1910, a mere 20 years later— in 1930, heart disease was causing 4,000 deaths per year. By 1950 heart disease was the **LEADING** cause of death in the United States.

CANCER –another man-made disease is discussed below. It's esti-mated that <u>every other man will get cancer</u> in his lifetime- <u>every third woman will get cancer</u> in her lifetime.

B.   WESTERN MEDICINE'S SUPPRESSION OF KNOWLEDGE

It's only been 100 years since the discovery of some of the most vital nutrients humans (and animals) need to maintain health and prevent sickness—but mainstream allopathic doctors will not recom-mend them. At the turn of the twentieth century, US medicine wasn't PROFITABLE. People were eating organic foods from farms where the soil had no pesticides. The soil was full of nutrients. Heart disease, cancer, diabetes, Alzheimer's, arthritis, etc. was unheard of.

<u>THERE WERE ALMOST NO PHARMACEUTICAL DEATHS EITHER!</u>

In 1905, Dr. William Fletcher was researching "Beriberi", when he discovered that if special things called "vitamins" were removed or absent from food—<u>DISEASE OCCURRED.</u>

<u>By 1912, DEFICIENCY DISEASE WAS DISCOVERED.</u> The general public began to believe that a lack of vitamins could make you sick; and eventually could <u>KILL</u> you.

Vitamin B12 was discovered by accident in an effort to cure perni-cious anemia. Numerous scientists helped to isolate Vitamin B12 as they realized that the disease was directly caused by its deficiency. Elmer McCollum discovered Vitamin A in 1912. At the same time, sci-entists determined nutritional levels that kept cattle healthy. They discovered that the <u>ABSENCE OF VITAMINS</u> had detrimental effects.

By 1916, experiments showed that fat-soluble Vitamin-A was nec-essary for normal growth. By 1919, Edward Mellanby proved that <u>RICKETS WAS CAUSED BY DEFICIENCIES OF VITAMIN D AND CALCIUM.</u>

But shortly thereafter, the Flexner Report came about. The American Medical Association (AMA) and the allopathic founders quickly real-ized the <u>THREAT</u> that this "nutritional information presented to their newly created allopathic profession. The AMA began to label natural doctors "quacks" because the latter used vitamins and minerals to prevent disease. Soon Americans began believing that there were "magic pills" and <u>VACCINES THAT CURED ALL SERIOUS HEALTH ISSUES.</u>

Thus began "<u>THE SUPPRESSION OF TRUTHFUL INFORMATION</u>" e.g. <u>ABOUT THE VALUE OF VITAMINS AND MINERALS.</u> Ironically the earli-est medical textbooks advocated using Nutritional Therapy (High Fat

Ketogenic Diets) to treat Diabetes and other diseases. As you might expect the new allopathic establishment made sure that medical students were shielded from reading this "quackery."

The allopathic approach says: just eat ANY food; take our pills and vaccines and "your health will be just fine". People who tout nutrition as important have been shouted down; ridiculed and discredited as "quacks". The American public has been <u>VERY BADLY BRAIN-WASHED</u>!

Allopathic doctors have been brain-washed with a deficient education. To make matters worse, most allopathic doctors sleep quietly in their ignorance about nutrition. Allopathic doctors have been disciplined by the iron-fisted approach of the AMA and the medical licensing authorities.

Since its formation, the American Medical Association (AMA), which represents Western Medicine, has waged a relentless attack on <u>ALL</u> forms of natural and indigenous medicine.

The Western medical system has systematically sought to <u>SUPPRESS NEARLY ALL TRUTHFUL INFORMATION</u> about the disease prevention and treatment potential of <u>FOODS, MEDICINAL HERBS, NUTRITIONAL THERAPIES, HEALING ARTS TREATMENTS</u>; etc. The AMA, Big Pharma and governments are all in collusion or "in cahoots". Each group has vested interests in the "<u>disease-care management</u>" system that is erroneously called "health-care". These vested interests have managed to <u>INTIMIDATE</u> and <u>ELIMINATE</u> competition from <u>ALTERNATIVE/NATURAL HEALTH CARE SOURCES AND HEALTH CARE PROVIDERS</u>. Here is a newsflash!

<u>THE TRUTH ABOUT HEALTH CARE AND ALTERNATIVE REMEDIES CAN NO LONGER BE SUPPRESSED</u>!

<u>THE DAYS OF MEDICAL McCARTHYISM ARE GONE</u>!

<u>THE TRUTH IS NOW ACCESSIBLE TO EVERYONE</u>!

Governments, Big Pharma, the medical establishment and the talking heads of mainstream media can no longer suppress the truth. Most consumers living in industrialized countries now have access to a little thing called the <u>INTERNET</u>.

The jig is up for Big Pharma.

<u>PEOPLE ARE FED UP WITH THE LIES AND FRAUDULENT PRACTICES OF MAINSTREAM MEDICINE</u>.

WITH THE PRESS OF A BUTTON AND IN THE BLINK OF AN EYELASH —ALL KNOWN HUMAN HEALTH INFORMATION IS NOW AVAILABLE- 24/7!

YOU no longer need to listen to the talking heads in mainstream media who are paid to spout medical junk science. NOW- YOU can take control of your own health by educating yourself WITH THE HELP OF THIS BOOK- AND DR. INTERNET.

YOU no longer need to be an ill-informed victim to mainstream allopathic medicine controlled by Big Pharma. YOU can easily and quickly educate yourself. YOU must do your own due diligence; investigate and search out the truth about health for YOURSELF.

YOU CAN CONSULT HEALTH SOURCES SUCH AS: www.Gopher.com ; www.natural news.com, www.Mercola.com and www.GreenMedInfo. com

YOU CAN GET INSTANT HEALTH ADVICE; YOU can use your Smartphone, Ipad, or computer to Google Up- Functional Medicine- Functional doctors, alternative medicine, Naturopathic doctors; alternative medicine, natural remedies- ETC. ETC. Trips to the local pharmacy will be a thing of the past. Trips to your local health food store, your well-stocked kitchen and/or pantry will be YOUR MEDICAL ARSENAL.

GOVERNMENTS, BIG PHARMA, ALLOPATHIC DOCTORS AND MAINSTREAM MEDIA CAN NO LONGER SUPPRESS HEALTH INFORMATION!

YOU NOW HAVE INSTANT ACCESS TO TRUTHFUL INFORMATION ABOUT YOUR HEALTH!

YOU DO NOT NEED TO LISTEN TO TALKING MEDIA HEADS DECEIVE YOU ABOUT A HALF-BAKED SUMMARY OF A FRAUDULENT CLINIC STUDY.

YOU ONLY NEED TO GO READ A STUDY OR ARTICLE YOURSELF.

THIS BOOK WILL PROVIDE YOU WITH THE SOLID SCIENCE THAT YOU NEED TO TAKE CARE OF YOUR HEALTH.

For the last 100 years Big Government, Big Pharma, The Medical Establishment and Mainstream Media have waged a war on natural medicine.. Big Pharma pays thousands of dollars to SUPRESS THE TRUTH ABOUT ITS HORRIFIC DRUGS. Big Pharma's biggest con job was is 1986 when VACCINE MANUFACTURERS convinced American legislators to grant them immunity from lawsuit. (See infra).

Since 1986, Big Pharma, Big Government and Big media <u>HAS SUCCESSFULLY SUPPRESSED THE TRUTH ABOUT THE HORRIFIC DANGERS OF VACCINES THEIR INSANE "COMPENSATION SCHEME" AND OTHER FRAUDS.</u>

But- the jig is up!

The big evil corporations who have profited from human misery for the last 100 years are now being exposed. People are waking up. <u>PEOPLE ARE WAKING UP TO REALIZE THAT—"DRUGS" ARE NOT "MEDICATIONS"!</u>

The word "MEDICATION" is a "BASTARDIZATION OF THE <u>ENGLISH LANGUAGE!</u>

<u>DRUGS ARE TOXIC CHEMICALS SOLD TO MAKE MONEY—PERIOD.</u> Drugs cure nothing. They never have and they never will.

<u>DRUGS MAKE YOU FATTER, SICKER AND DEPENDENT ON BIG PHARMA—FOR THE REST OF YOUR LIFE!</u> Do you really want to be a drug addict for the rest of your life?

<u>TRUTH CAN NO LONGER BE HIDDEN OR SUPPRESSED BY EVIL FORCES!</u>

<u>THERE ARE NOW 100 MILLION NATURAL HEALTH CONSUMERS OUT THERE WHO ARE TAKING CONTROL OF THEIR HEALTH!</u>

<u>THERE IS A NEW HEALTHCARE REVOLUTION TAKING PLACE. YOU NOW HAVE A CHOICE. YOU CAN USE THE INFORMATION IN THIS BOOK AND DR. INTERNET TO CREATE A NEW HEALTHCARE SYSTEM—STARTING WITH ONE PERSON—YOU!</u>

<u>YOU CAN ABANDON THE FAILED DISEASE MANAGEMENT SYSTEM INVENTED BY BIG PHARMA.</u>

<u>YOU SHOULD NOT TRUST BIG PHARMA. YOU SHOULD NOT TRUST YOUR DOCTOR!</u>

<u>WE HAVE NOW (Thanks to Dr. Internet) ENTERED THE AGE OF DO-IT-YOURSELF MEDICINE-aka (a new (DIY) APPROACH TO HEALTHCARE!</u>

<u>YOU SHOULD TRUST YOURSELF- FIRST AND FOREMOST!</u>

For more than 100 years conventionally trained doctors have treated non-allopathic, natural and/or alternative naturopathic doctors as "quacks" who should not be allowed to practice medicine. The <u>TRUTH IS</u> allopathic doctors are doing <u>MORE HARM THAN GOOD!</u>

The real "medical quacks" are the <u>ALLOPATHIC DOCTORS!</u> The <u>"COMPETENT DOCTORS"</u> are the ones who use an all-natural "<u>_ – HOLISTIC FULL BODY APPROACH</u>" to healing our bodies.

<u>COMPETENT DOCTORS USE A NUTRITIONAL APPROACH TO HEAL PEOPLE.</u>

Medical quacks use poisonous chemicals to treat symptoms—<u>ONLY NOT TO HEAL ANYONE.</u>

Dr. Hippocrates was <u>100 PERCENT RIGHT</u>. He advised us that:

<u>"All disease begins in the gut".</u>

Recent research—("<u>THE HUMAN GENOME PROJECT</u>") <u>HAS UNEQUIVOCALLY PROVEN THAT THESE 6 WORDS MAY BE THE 6 MOST IMPORTANT HEALTH WORDS IN THE ENGLISH LANGUAGE!</u>"

Indigenous, traditional healing is an ancient, deeply- rooted practice <u>WORLDWIDE.</u>

Our self-healing body and its complex systems are best <u>NURTURED BY MOTHER NATURE HERSELF</u>. Humans have the best <u>SELF-HEALING</u> bodies on the planet.

The jury is in.

Synthetic chemicals and sloppy, ill-advised surgery pollutes the body with toxins and leaves the body to repair damage caused by injured body parts. Allopathic doctors cannot think outside of the pill. Why? Because their medical education is <u>DEFICIENT</u>. It is a drug-based medical education. Allopathic doctors are taught <u>ONLY TO DIAGNOSE SYMPTOMS</u>. They are taught to match a symptom to a drug.

<u>ALLOPATHIC QUACKS ARE TAUGHT NOTHING ABOUT FINDING THE ROOT CAUSE OF A DISEASE OR ANY OTHER MEDICAL PROBLEM.</u>

<u>DOCTORS SPEND (WASTE) HUNDREDS OF THOUSANDS OF DOLLARS ON THEIR MEDICAL EDUCATION</u>- They only learn how to sell drugs to an ill-informed population- who erroneously believe that the letters M.D mean that doctors have the medical expertise to help patients get healthy.

<u>IN AMERICA TODAY</u> —<u>AT LEAST 400 PEOPLE DIE EVERY SINGLE DAY FROM TAKING DRUGS!</u>

<u>IT'S TIME TO STOP THIS INSANITY!</u>

THE "PILL FOR AN ILL APPROACH" IS A RECIPE FOR A HEALTH DISASTER!

THE ALLOPATHIC MODEL OF MEDICINE HAS NOT ONLY FAILED TO HELP PEOPLE—IT HAS DONE MORE HARM THAN GOOD!

Conventionally trained doctors do not deserve the title of "doctors". Doctor means 'TEACHER'. Conventional doctors have taught us one important lesson.

What has the ALLOPATHIC profession taught North American consumers?

They have taught us **TO APPLY THE 99 PERCENT HEALTH RULE**.

What is the 99 percent rule?

THE 99 PERCENT HEALTH RULE IS VERY SIMPLE. IT SAYS:

> **"ANYTHING THE MEDICAL PROFESSION SAYS, DO THE OPPOSITE and 99 PERCENT OF THE TIME AND YOU'LL BE RIGHT!!"**

YOU SHOULD LET MY 99 PERCENT HEALTH RULE GUIDE YOU IN YOUR QUEST FOR SUPERHEALTH & FITNESS!

YOU will observe the **ACCURACY** of this rule throughout the rest of this book.

Often I will refer to the 99 Percent Health rule. The information and scientific knowledge you gain from this book **WILL CONVINCE YOU TO ADOPT MY** 99 PERCENT HEALTH RULE.

Indigenous medicine comes directly from **MOTHER NATURES' FARMACY**—**NOT** from some laboratory where scientists need masks and gloves to concoct **A TOXIC CHEMICAL POISON PILL THAT MIGHT** make you feel better **TEMPORARILY**. Almost always this chemical either makes you sicker, or worsens the condition that was supposed to treat. If you're unlucky—this chemical **KILLS YOU**.

SUPERHEALTH IS NOT FOUND IN A PILL.

SUPERHEALTH IS OBTAINED BY EATING NUTRITIOUS FOOD.

WHY have **NUTRIENTS** (such as Vitamin C and D) been deliberately suppressed?

WHY has the truth about natural herbs and substances such as colloidal silver been suppressed?

WHY HAVE ALL NUTRITIONAL THERAPIES BEEN SUPPRESSED?

WHY HAVE MANY DOCTORS WHO HAVE TRIED TO USE NUTRITIONAL, AND/OR ALTERNATIVE MEDICINE BEEN VICIOUSLY ATTACKED, AND VILIFIED BY MODERN MEDICINE?

WHY HAVE MANY ALTERNATIVE DOCTORS BEEN PERSECUTED, ARRESTED and/or HAD THEIR MEDICAL LICENSES STRIPPED?

The answer is very simple.

IF PEOPLE KNEW THE TRUTH ABOUT HEALING YOUR BODY BY EATING HEALTHY FOOD-

Do you think Big Pharma would sell any DRUGS?

NUTRITIONAL INTERVENTION WILL SOON KILL BIG PHARMA!

Within the last year, there has been a spate of mysterious deaths of out-spoken HOLISTIC AMERICAN DOCTORS DYING UNDER SUSPICIOUS CIRCUMSTANCES!

Are you naïve enough to believe that these are just coincidences?

THE AMA HAS RECENTLY ISSUED A NEW THREAT TO OUTSPOKEN DOCTORS.

The AMA recently re-drafted its "Ethical Guidelines for Physicians in the Media". This was done allegedly to "defend the integrity of the profession." The new guidelines will target unorthodox medical information that the AMA deems dubious and unsubstantiated. The guidelines create disciplinary guidelines for medical doctors who make claims that do not align with the best available science".

What this means is that allopathic drug-pushers who do not toe the company line will be disciplined. This is not controlling "ethics "of doctors; this is a blatant attempt to silence drug doctors who publicly speak out about alternative health remedies.

THIS IS A DELIBERATE ATTEMPT TO SUPPRESS KNOWLEDGE OF HEALING OUR BODIES WITH NUTRITIONAL THERAPIES AND NATURAL, SAFE REMEDIES!

THIS IS A DIRECT ATTACK ON HONEST DOCTORS WHO SPEAK THE TRUTH ABOUT HEALTH. THIS IS DONE TO INTIMIDATE AND SCARE DOCTORS TO KEEP SILENT AND TO ONLY TALK ABOUT DRUGS!

MAINSTREAM MEDIA IS VERY HAPPY TO REPORT THIS INFORMATION BECAUSE MAINSTREAM MEDIA IS PAID ALSO TO KEEP THE PUBLIC IGNORANT.

Here's an example of the 99 percent health rule in practice in everyday life.

As a matter of fact- the <u>AMA</u> is <u>NOT</u> a legal body. It is a trade association whose roots go <u>DEEP</u> in American medicine. It has a powerful influence on the way state licensing boards oversee and discipline doctors in USA and Canada. The AMA is a trade group that seeks to control allopathic doctors who have the temerity to speak the truth about non-drug medicine. People who discover the truth about drugs may decide to buy some good nutritious food- or take some vitamin supplements <u>INSTEAD</u> of filling their prescription for toxic drugs.

The <u>AMA</u> allegedly managed to scrounge up <u>20 MILLION DOLLARS FOR LOBBYING IN</u> 2014-.—not too shabby for a trade association during difficult economic times.

Btw: Did you hear that the beloved TV doctor- Dr. OZ had to defend his reputation before Congress? Imagine—T.V's beloved heart doctor having to justify his actions when he publicly tells people to eat good nutritious food- (and implicitly says to ditch the drugs.)

Why do you suppose the medical establishment has always suppressed the <u>TRUTH</u> about alternative and natural remedies? Well, the main reason is that:

<u>YOU CANNOT GET A PATENT ON A PLANT or A NATURAL SUBSTANCE.</u>

<u>IT COSTS ABOUT 1 BILLION DOLLARS TO GET A DRUG APPROVED BY THE FDA!</u> That's a lot of money to get permission to sell a chemical pill to the public. That's why Big Pharma has come up with a new plan. Big Pharma can sell a vaccine (which is actually a drug cocktail.

<u>BEST of all for Big Pharma, since 1986—</u>

There's a law that says that <u>VACCINE MANUFACTURERS CANNOT BE SUED!</u>

("See below-"Medical Crimes Against Humanity".

Can you imagine what would happen if everyone ate an avocado every day?

<u>BIG PHARMA AND ALLOPATHIC DOCTORS MAKE "BEEEG" MONEY FROM SELLING DRUGS!</u> If Big Pharma doesn't sell drugs- they would go bankrupt. And their drug pushing medical doctors <u>WOULD GO OUT OF BUSINESS!</u>

To discover how many lives would be saved if the allopathic doctors' business were shut down- please read the next section.

In what other job do you get paid without regard to the quality of your work or for poisoning people?

BIG PHARMA HAS TRANSFORMED THE PRACTICE OF WESTERN (ALLOPATHIC) MEDICINE INTO A FRAUDULENT, PROFIT-ORIENTED BUSINESS.

THE TAKEOVER OF EDUCATION, OF MEDICINE, OF THE MONETARY SYSTEM, AND THE FOOD SUPPLY ITSELF SHOWS THAT THE AIM OF THE OIL INDUSTRY IS TO MONOPOLIZE ALL ASPECTS OF OUR LIVES!

THESE PEOPLE HAVE MIND-BOGGLING AMOUNTS OF MONEY TO SPEND TO ACCOMPLISH THEIR MONOPOLIZATION OF OUR LIVES.

DEMOCRATIC SOCIETY IS AT RISK. THE OIL OLIGARCHS WISH TO MONOPOLIZE EVERY ASPECT OF OUR LIVES!

THE VAST MAJORITY OF THE WORLD'S POPULATION IS STILL PLAYING THE SHELL GAME THAT THE OIL OLIGARCHS PERFECTED DECADES AGO.

ALL CITIZENS MUST BAND TOGETHER TO STOP THIS OPPRESSION.

C.   DEATH BY MEDICINE

Here's a trivia question for you.

What's the NUMBER ONE KILLER IN THE UNITED STATES? (Hint: it's NOT heart disease; OR cancer.

In 2003, a very powerful article, entitled "Death by Medicine" authored by Dr. Caroline Dean and Gary Null Ph.D. found that "iatrogenic" DEATHS accounted for more than ONE MILLION PEOPLE IN THE UNITED STATES!

Are you shocked? I was too when I learned about this several years ago!

The author's estimated figure of 784,000 being was too low). "Iatrogenic" means doctor-caused. The authors' specified that this number was between 5 to 15 percent was TOO LOW! Remember that dead men tell no tales. -☺

This study also found that the second leading cause of death in the US was heart disease with about 600, 000 deaths; the third leading cause of death was cancer which caused more 200

SOME MORE SHOCKING FACTS: (source: deathclock.com)

- Since Jan 1st, 2000- <u>CHEMOTHERAPY DRUGS HAVE KILLED 16,086, 202 PEOPLE!</u>

- Yes- more than <u>TWO MILLION PEOPLE ARE KILLED BY DOCTORS AND CHEMO EACH YEAR IN THE USA!</u>

- Since Jan. 1st, 2000, <u>SUPERBUGS HAVE KILLED 11,260,362 PEOPLE WORLDWIDE!</u>

- <u>STATIN DRUGS HAVE KILLED HUNDREDS OF MIL-LIONS OF PEOPLE-WORLDWIDE!!</u>

- The number of people having in hospital, adverse drug re-actions (ADR) to a prescribed medicine is 2.2 MILLION.

- Dr. Richard Besser of the CDC in 1995 said the num-ber of unnecessary antibiotics prescribed annu-ally for viral infections was 20 MILLION...

- The number of unnecessary medical and surgical pro-cedures performed annually is 7.5 MILLION.

- The number of people exposed to unneces-sary hospitalization annually is 8.9 MILLION.

In 2010, a mere 7 years later, two more studies have shown that things have not changed in the medical "business". One report in the New England Journal of Medicine and another in the Journal of Internal Medicine- showed for example:

- out of <u>62 MILLION DEATH CERTIFICATES</u> dated between 1976 to 2006, <u>ALMOST A QUARTER-MILLION DEATHS</u> were specified as having occurred in a hospital setting <u>DUE TO MEDICATION ERRORS"</u>

- an estimated 450,000 preventable medication-relat-ed adverse events occur <u>EVERY YEAR</u> in the USA;

- The costs of adverse drug reactions to society are 136 BILLION ANNUALLY- greater than the to-tal cost of cardiovascular or diabetic care.

<u>More facts you should know:</u>

- According to the 2011 Health Grades Hos-pital Quality in America Study-

  The incidence of medical harm occurring in the United States is "estimated" to be over 40,000 harm-ful and/or lethal errors each and every day.

- In 2011, an estimated 722, 000 patients contracted an infection during a stay in an acute care hospital in the U.S, and about 75,000 patients died as a result of it.

MORE DISTURBING DRUG FACTS:

More than a decade ago, Professor Bruce Pomerance of the University of Toronto concluded that properly pre-scribed (and correctly taken) pharmaceutical DRUGS were the 4th leading cause of death in the United States.

- In 2010, there were 38,329 pharmaceutical drug overdose deaths reported in the U.S. of which 74.3 % were unintentional.

- Did you know that every 19 minutes someone dies in the USA from an accidental over prescription of drugs?

- From 2006 to 2010 there have been 270,827 deaths from FDA approved drugs!!

- Most of you have likely heard that the drug VIOXX killed 60,000 people before it was yanked from the market. (It seems that the case was settled out of court for about 250 million dollars). How much are our lives worth?

What was the penalty for creating this this bad medicine? It was a wee fine... a few million dollars and a slap on the wrist. It's treated by Big pharmaceutical companies just the cost of doing business. Killing 60,000 people was not serious enough to justify putting anyone in prison.

HOW MANY PEOPLE WENT TO PRISON? NONE.-ZERO!

- In reports between 2006 and 2010, there have been a to-tal of 1,702,973 cases documented as "serious." "Serious" means that one or more of these outcomes were stated in the report: death, hospitalization, life threatening, disabil-ity, congenial anomaly, and/or other serious outcome.

(Source of drug facts: www.DrugWar.Facts.org)

- NARCOTIC OVERDOSE DEATHS HAVE QUA-DRUPLED IN THE LAST 10 YEARS.

- Finally—IT APPEARS THAT BETA-BLOCKERS (drugs given to prevent heart attacks) HAVE ACTUALLY KILLED MORE THAN ONE MILLION PEOPLE IN EUROPE! (Google it up)

D. CARDIOLOGISTS— OR CRIMINALS?

Cardiovascular disease is the leading cause of death around the world. It claims the lives of over <u>17 MILLION PEOPLE PER YEAR</u>. According to WHO (World Health Organization)' "cardiovascular disease can be prevented".

Probably no one has corrupted modern medicine more than cardiologists. Cardiologists in the USA are making millions of dollars—not from saving lives or curing diseases. They're <u>AMASSING</u> their fortunes by manipulating their patients by <u>demanding</u> that they submit to needless surgeries and drugs. You should not be surprised. This is allopathic medicine at its money— making best.

There are shocking details from the U.S. Justice Department that reveal that many cardiologists are likely causing more harm by <u>CAUSING</u> heart disease in otherwise healthy patients. They are doing this by pushing drugs on patients and twisting patients' arms to submit to <u>SURGERIES THAT PATIENTS DO NOT NEED!</u>

Cardiologists make their money by using heart drugs, technology and surgery. For the most part they are <u>OPPOSED</u> to the general concept of analyzing your health and/or finding/exploring ways to improve it.

It's a true, sad state of affairs that most cardiologists <u>CAN'T</u> tell you more about how to improve the health of your heart—<u>THAN THE AVERAGE PERSON</u> you meet on the street!

After a triple or quadruple by-pass, cardiologists typically tell their patients <u>"GO HOME- TAKE YOUR MEDS AND DO NOT DO ANYTHING;— AND BY ALL MEANS- DON'T GO NEAR A TREADMILL!"</u>

The reality is that these ill-treated patients need to do exactly the opposite. These patients need HIIT (High Intensity Interval Training); (see Exercise, infra). The reality is these heart patients <u>SHOULD</u> be weaned off of their poisonous drugs; to get some exercise so that their hearts can become strong and healthy.

Cardiologists, (poor devils), really know very little about how to make your heart strong and healthy. All they know is how to push drugs and slice holes in your heart.

<u>ONE SMALL PROBLEM</u> with heart drugs is: <u>THEY DO NOT ENHANCE YOUR HEART HEALTH!</u> IT'S THE 99 Percent Rule—<u>AGAIN!</u>

Heart drugs only make your doctor's wallet fatter.

The worst heart drugs of all appear to be— <u>BETA-BLOCKERS</u>. Before these drugs <u>KILL</u> you, over time they will typically turn your heart into a fat, lazy water balloon.

If you had high blood pressure to begin with, you will end up with an even weaker heart.

According to the CDC, the total number of surgeries performed in the U.S. is 51.4 million, of which 4.7 million are cardiac-related. Using this statistic, the number of Americans potentially affected by dangerous beta-blockers is 46.7 million.

<u>THAT MEANS THAT THERE COULD BE AS MANY AS 11 MILLION DEATHS EACH YEAR CAUSED BY BETA-BLOCKER DRUGS! OMG!</u>

Do these deaths show up in deaths caused by drugs? Some do- but most do not. Few deaths are followed by an autopsy; and few death certificates are likely to say- patient died from his beta-blocker/heart drugs. As you might imagine, no one can know for sure how many people really are <u>KILLED BY MEDICINE</u>!

It appears that <u>ONE MILLION EUROPEANS </u>with little or no heart problems were <u>KILLED NEEDLESSLY</u>! Google Up the horrors of <u>BETA— BLOCKERS</u> before you decide to take them.

<u>BLOOD THINNERS</u> (such as <u>WARFARIN</u>- aka <u>RAT POISON</u>) <u>ARE THE LEADING CAUSES OF DEATH IN EMERGENCY ROOMS</u>! (source: Duke University).

Anti-coagulants also known as "blood thinners" have been used for many decades. Since blood-thinners are considered a "preventative medication", many conventional doctors prescribe these. These doctors erroneously believing the benefits outweigh the risks.

Actually drinking water and walking barefoot on the grass are <u>FAR MORE EFFECTIVE</u> <u>NATURAL WAYS TO THIN YOUR BLOOD</u>-see Grounding/Earthing, infra.

<u>BY 2018- IT'S PREDICTED THAT BLOOD THINNERS WILL BE THE BIGGEST CASH –COW</u> ($$$$ maker) <u>FOR BIG PHARMA</u>!

<u>WALKING BAREFOOT ON THE GRASS OR BEACH</u> (see "Grounding" or "Earthing" infra) <u>IS FAR BETTER AND A HECK OF A LOT SAFER THAN RAT POISON</u>!

A word of caution—if you take blood thinners and walk outside on bare grass or beach- you might make your blood too thin!

<u>The take-home message is:</u>

DITCH BIG PHARMA'S HEART DRUG POISONS!

JUST SAY NO TO DRUGS!

JUST SAY NO TO ALL DRUGS- PRESCRIPTION, OTC AND RECREATIONAL DRUGS!

Do you want to die from ingesting rat poison or would you rather take use some natural remedies provided by MOTHER NATURE'S FARMACY?

One of the most profitable SCAMS used by cardiologists is the STENT. A stent is a small medical tube inserted into a blocked artery to keep it open.

Yes, sometimes, stents can be helpful. However, if you do some research, you will find that cardiologists pushing stents on patients who have little or NO SIGNS OF HEART DISEASE.

For the patient/victims, it means injury, amputations, permanent disability and death.

Health care economists have stated that with 110 BILLION DOLLARS generated from STENTS over the last decade, the rush for big money can lead to corrupted practices...

According to the U.S. Justice Department lawsuits filed by "whistle-blowers" are sealed by federal judges. No one can talk about these cases. This corruption is placed under lock and key. That is the reason you will likely never hear about these cases in the mainstream media. Court records show that the hospitals that employ these corrupt cardiologists help cover-up their tricks hide them from prosecution and continue to employ them.

FOLKS- THIS IS JUST ANOTHER CASE OF THE TRUTH BEING SUPPRESSED SO THAT YOU ARE SCAMMED BY BIG PHARMA AND BIG MEDICAL.

Who cares whether these cardiologists are injuring or killing patients? Hey- it's just the cost of doing medical business! Here's a typical scenario—

Patient to his doctor: "Hey Doc—how do my X-rays look?"

> Doctor's reply: "Well, I've just spoken to my Accountant and it looks like you're going to need surgery." -☺

DON'T LET YOUR DOCTOR CUT A HOLE IN YOUR HEART TO GET TO YOUR WALLET!

<u>What causes heart attacks</u>?

The spectrum of heart disease, which includes angina, unstable angina, and myocardial infarction, (heart attack) is better understood from the perspective of events happening in the myocardium (heart)—<u>AS OPPOSED</u> to events happening in the coronary arteries; (the arteries that supply the heart).

The conventional-medical view claims that the central event of heart disease occurs in the <u>ARTERIES WITH A BUILD-UP OF A BLOCKAGE CALLED " PLAQUE"</u>.

Conventional "medical theory" says that most MI's (heart attacks) are caused by the progressive blockage caused by plaque build-up in the <u>FOUR MAJOR ARTERIES</u> leading to the heart. These plaques were thought to be composed of <u>CHOLESTEROL</u> that built up in the arterial lumen (inside of the vessel), which eventually cut off the blood supply to certain area of the heart, resulting in <u>OXYGEN DEFICIENCY</u> in that area, causing first <u>PAIN</u> (<u>ANGINA</u>) and then progressing to <u>ISCHEMIA</u> (aka <u>HEART ATTACK</u>).

The simple solution say allopathic doctors is to unblock the "<u>STENOSIS</u>" (aka <u>THE BLOCKAGE(S)</u> with either <u>ANGIPLASTY OR A STENT; OR—IF THIS IS IMPOSSIBLE— BY BYPASSING THIS AREA WITH CORONARY BYPASS GRAFTING</u> (CABG).

It's a simple problem- simple solution- right? <u>NOT SO FAST</u>!

<u>THIS "CORONARY ARTERY THEORY" IS COMPLETELY BOGUS!</u>

<u>THIS MEDICAL THEORY- LIKE 99 PERCENT OF ALLOPATHIC THEORY IS UTTERLY FALSE!</u>

During the last <u>50 YEARS</u> this flawed theory has cost North Americans <u>BILLIONS OF DOLLARS IN UNNECESSARY SURGERY COSTS!</u>

<u>THIS FLAWED THEORY HAS ALSO PROMOTED DRUGS THAT CAUSE MORE HARM THAN POSITIVE BENEFITS- AND HAVE COST BILLIONS OF DOLLARS!</u>

It gets worse.

After surgery— which is most times unnecessary; most cardiologists <u>COMPOUND THE DAMAGE BY GIVING THEIR PATIENTS THE WORST DIETARY ADVICE IN THE WORLD</u>! Most cardiologists then worsen unnecessary injury (surgery).

Il-informed cardiologists (the vast majority) advise heart patient <u>TO FOLLOW A LOW-FAT LOW-CHOLESTEROL DIET</u>! <u>OMG</u>!

THIS IS LIKE POURING GASOLINE ON A FIRE!

THIS FLAWED NUTRITIONAL ADVICE DEPRIVES THE HEART OF ITS PREFERRED AND MOST EFFICIENT MOST VITAL FUEL SOURCES;- FAT ! FAT! & FAT! —in the form of fat bodies called **KETONES**— **AND FATTY ACIDS!**

THE PREFERRED, MOST EFFICIENT FUEL SOURCES FOR OUR HEART (and our brain too) ARE(FATS) KETONES AND FATTY ACIDS.

Ketones are "fat-bodies" manufactured by our bodies. Later herein, you will learn that ketones (fat) is the preferred fuel of the brain, the heart and of the human body. Have you ever seen how much fat covers our hearts? Heart surgeons forget to tell their clients this little fact. Gee- does this mean that **HEALTHY FAT IS CRUCIAL TO OUR HEART HEALTH? ABSOLUTELY!**

A heart cutter (surgeon) who gives a heart patient- low-fat/ high carb dietary advice should be prosecuted and jailed for **CRIMINAL NEGLIGENCE!**

Studies show that most heart surgery is **USELESS**. For example, a 2003 study at the Mayo Clinic on the efficacy of bypass surgeries, stents and angioplasty concluded that these surgeries did very little- except relieve the **SYMPTOMS OF CHEST PAIN**. The study proved that surgery **DOES NOT PREVENT FURTHER HEART ATTACKS;**

AND THAT ONLY VERY-HIGH RISK PATIENTS CAN BENEFIT FROM BY PASS SURGERY WITH A BETTER CHANCE FOR SURVIVAL.

So- what REALLY causes heart attacks?

First of all, I invite you to go to the website of Dr. Knut Sroka- namely: www.heartattacknew.com and read his entire website, and watch the heart video.

The video shows how the collateral circulation nourishes the heart even with severe **BLOCKAGE OF A CORONARY ARTERY**. On his website, you should read at least 2 articles entitled: G. Baroldi " The Etiopathologies of Coronary Heart Disease: a Heritical theory based on Mophology," and K. Sroka-"On the Genesis of Myocardial Ischemia."

You will see that if and when a **BLOCKAGE** occurs in one of our 4 major coronary arteries, our bodies are **AMAZING!** Our bodies **DO NOT WAIT** for some cutter wielding a scalpel to begin repair work. Our bodies do their **OWN NATURAL BY-PASSES!**

These are called **COLLATERAL CIRCULATIONS!**

THESE ARE OUR OWN NATURAL HEART BYPASSES THAT OUR BODY MAKES AUTOMATICALLY IF THERE IS A BLOCKAGE IN AN ARTERY!

Starting soon after birth, the normal heart develops and extensive network of small blood vessels develop called <u>COLLATERAL VESSELS</u>. Eventually, these vessels compensate for the interruption of flow in <u>ANY ONE OR MORE OF THE MAJOR BLOOD VESSELS</u>.

As Dr. Sroka points out—coronary angiograms fail to show the collateral circulation.—i.e. (our bodies' natural by-passes). Most heart surgeries are done on <u>MINIMALLY SYMPTOMATIC PATIENTS WITH 90% in ONE OR MORE ARTERIES</u>. These arteries are almost always <u>COLLATERALIZED</u>.

<u>IT IS NOT THE SURGERY THAT RESTORES BLOOD FLOW BECAUSE THE BODY HAS ALREADY DONE ITS OWN BY-PASS!</u>

In addition to the <u>BOGUS</u>-possibly "<u>FRAUDULENT</u>") blocked artery explanation is the "unstable" or "friable" plaque theory. Acute thrombosis does happen in patients having heart attacks but it is a <u>CONSEQUENCE NOT THE CAUSE OF THE MI</u>. While thrombosis associated with <u>MI</u> is a real phenomenon; it does not occur in more than <u>50 PERCENT</u> of cases. In sum, this is another flawed theory of what causes heart attacks.

<u>THE MAJORITY OF HEART ATTACKS ARE CAUSED BY A MALFUNCTION OF YOUR CENTRAL NERVOUS SYSTEM. (CNS)</u>.

<u>SPECIFICALLY- MOST HEART ATTACKS ARE CAUSED BY AN IMBALANCE BETWEEN YOUR SYMPATHETIC AND PARASYMPATHETIC BRANCHES/SYSTEMS</u>.

<u>THE MAJORITY OF HEART ATTACKS ARE NOT CAUSED BY CLOGGED ARTERIES AND COMPROMISED BLOOD FLOW</u>. This is medical nonsense!

In essence, when arteries are more than 90 percent blocked, in almost all cases, our bodies compensate for that blockage by forming a collateral blood supply. Who knew? We have such an amazing clever body! In other words, your body naturally performs its own natural by-pass. This explains why the majority of angioplasty and by-pass surgeries provide only <u>MINIMAL</u> benefit.

According to Dr. Cowan, most heart attacks occur as a result of the following <u>MECHANISM</u>—

If a person experiences decreased healing activity of his or her parasympathetic nervous system over time—typically— from <u>CHRONIC STRESS</u>- then a strong <u>EMOTIONAL</u> stressor activates a sympathetic response to compensate. This causes an uncontrolled release of adrenalin, which breaks down the myocardial cells.

THIS is a classic example of "BUSTED CELLS"(a technical term-☺ Chronic stress interferes with cells and their metabolism—and causes "BUSTED METABOLISM"(another technical term-☺

THE TERMS "BUSTED CELLS" AND "BUSTED METABOLISM" ARE USED THROUGHOUT THIS BOOK to explain the concept of cellular damage and damage to our entire metabolism.

When our heart is deprived of its normal (best) fuel sources; this in turn impairs the heart's ability to contract and a HEART ATTACK OCCURS.

According to Dr. Cowan, heart attacks typically occur without any disruption in blood flow—so it's the HEART MUSCLE ITSELF THAT EXPERIENCES THE PROBLEM —NOT YOUR ARTERIES!

The implications are ENORMOUS with respect to the effects of UNMANAGED STRESS ON YOUR HEART!

Is STRESS making you a heart attack waiting to happen?

NOT ONLY DOES STRESS INCREASE INFLAMMATION— BUT—

IT ACTIVATES YOUR SYMPATHETIC NERVOUS SYSTEM; ("Fight or flight response").

STRESS ALSO SUPPRESSES YOUR PARASYMPATHETIC NERVOUS SYSTEM.

HEART ATTACKS RESULT FROM A SUPPRESSED PARASYMPATHETIC NERVOUS SYSTEM.

TO PREVENT HEART ATTACKS— YOU NEED TO NURTURE AND PROTECT THIS PART OF YOUR CENTRAL NERVOUS SYSTEM.

THIS MEANS KEEPING YOUR STRESS LEVELS UNDER CONTROL!

THIS MEANS KEEPING YOUR CORTISOL LEVELS UNDER CONTROL!

THE LATEST RESEARCH SHOWS THAT STRESS IS A "BIG" CAUSE OF OBESITY AND WEIGHT GAIN!

DRUGS USED IN CARDIOLOGY ATTEMPT TO UP-REGULATE THE PARASYMPATHETIC NERVOUS SYSTEM—(Nitrates stimulate NO (nitric oxide) production; aspirin and statins also stimulate the pro-duction of NO etc...

THESE DRUGS ONLY WORK— <u>TEMPORARILY</u> —UNTIL-

<u>THEY CAUSE A REBOUND DECREASE IN THESE SUBSTANCES THAT MAKES THE PARASYMPATHETIC SYSTEM FAIL!</u>

-EVEN WORSE—

The most consistent <u>RISK FACTORS</u> for a person having <u>HEART DISEASE ARE</u>:

- Male sex, diabetes, cigarette use and psycho-logical and/or or <u>EMOTIONAL STRESS</u>.

<u>The bottom line:</u>

<u>THE TWO BEST STRATEGIES TO AVOID HEART DISEASE ARE:</u>

1. <u>ELIMINATE AND/OR MANAGE THE EMOTION-AL AND OTHER STRESS IN YOUR LIFE</u> and—

2. <u>EAT A LOW-CARB HIGH-FAT KETOGENIC DIET.</u>

E.   VACCINATIONS = MEDICAL CRIMES AGAINST HUMANITY

I've been a Quebec- licenced attorney since 1974. I took an oath to uphold the <u>LAW</u> and the integrity of the Canadian Judicial System. As an officer of the Court, I also took an oath to protect the most vulnerable, downtrodden, and oppressed members of our society. I've been trained to be an exposer of facts. I am also a <u>TRUTH –TELLER</u>.

I could not stand by and watch the <u>DAMAGE</u> being wreaked upon society by villainous, greedy pharmaceutical companies getting richer and richer by selling their poisonous products to a naïve- ill-informed population.

<u>DRUG COMPANIES AND DOCTORS CAUSE MORE THAN 2 TWO MILLION DEATHS EVERY YEAR IN THE USA!</u>

<u>VACCINES ARE THE MOST EVIL DRUGS EVER CREATED!</u>

<u>WORSE YET— IN THE U.S.A. VACCINE MANUFACTURERS CANNOT BE SUED IN COURT BY INJURED VICTIMS!</u> In 1986, the Pharmaceutical companies and big corporations convinced American legislators to enact legislation that shields vaccine manufacturers from lawsuits. <u>CANADIAN LAW IS DIFFERENT.</u>

Vaccinations are routinely administered by ill-informed allopathic doctors under the erroneous belief that <u>VACCINES SAFE AND EFFECTIVE</u>.

<u>THIS IS A BIG-FAT LIE!</u>

<u>THE TRUTH OF IS VACCINES ARE EXTREMELY DANGEROUS AND VACCINES ARE NOT EFFECTIVE!</u>

<u>VACCINES CAUSE MORE HARM THAN GOOD!</u>

<u>VACCINES ARE MORE THAN "TREATMENT."</u>

<u>VACCINES ARE INVASIVE. VACCINES ARE SURGERY!</u>

Has your doctor explained that to <u>YOU</u>?

<u>MOST DOCTORS ARE TOTALLY IGNORANT ABOUT THE DANGERS OF VACCINES</u>. (Remember- the 99 percent rule and doctors don't know their arse from their elbow.)

They are also <u>CLUELESS</u> about VACCINES. Most doctors' knowledge of these horrific <u>DRUGS</u> comes from the local Big Pharma representative. Many doctors likely have never even taken the time to read the insert packaged with <u>VACCINE DRUGS</u>.

<u>THESE WRITTEN "INSERTS" CONTAIN A SHOPPING LIST OF HORRIFIC "DIRECT" EFFECTS OF VACCINES!</u>

Has your doctor shown you <u>THAT</u> list? Has your doctor advised you about the dangers and side-effects of vaccine drugs? Has your doctor ever discussed vaccine drugs with you? Has your doctor told you that he requires your "informed consent" before <u>ANY TREATMENT</u>? Has your doctor obtained your "informed consent"? Has your doctor lied to you about the legalities of vaccinations?

<u>MY DEAR READERS- UNDER MEDICAL LAW- YOU HAVE A HUGE CHOICE!</u>

<u>MEDICAL LAW IMPOSES VERY STRICT LEGAL OBLIGATIONS ON DOCTORS</u>.

<u>BEFORE DOCTORS CAN EVEN TOUCH YOU- THEY REQUIRE YOUR CONSENT!</u>

<u>IF YOU DO NOT GIVE YOUR CONSENT- FREELY AND VOLUNTARILY— YOUR DOCTOR CAN BE ACCUSED OF CRIMINAL ASSAULT AND BATTERY!</u>

<u>DOCTORS HAVE THE LEGAL OBLIGATION TO OBTAIN A CLIENT'S</u>

INFORMED CONSENT—BEFORE DOING ANY MEDICAL TREATMENTS OR BEFORE PERFORMING MEDICAL PROCEDURES OF ANY KIND.

YOUR DOCTOR MUST OBTAIN YOUR INFORMED CONSENT BEFORE HE/SHE PERFORMS VACCINATION OR ANY OTHER KIND OF SURGERY ON YOUR BODY!!

Many doctors tell their patients "sit down; shut up; and roll-up your sleeve" or get your kid to roll-up his sleeve. Frequently they say: "Your kids can't go to school without the vaccines". They say:

"IT'S THE LAW"… "YOU MUST BE VACCINATED!"

UNDER CANADIAN LAW- THIS IS A BIG-FAT FRAUDULENT LIE!

This is unadulterated "medical excreta". Canadian doctors who tell their Canadian patients vaccinations are mandatory ARE MEDICAL LIARS! Ignorance of the law is no excuse.

Canadian doctors who ignorantly MISINFORM or DO NOT INFORM their patients regarding VACCINATION LAW are guilty of MEDICAL MALPRACTICE.

Canadian doctors who knowingly NO NOT RESPECT THE VACCINATION LEGAL REQUIREMENTS WHICH REQUIRE DOCTORS TO OBTAIN YOUR INFORMED CONSENT— SHOULD BE JAILED!

IN THE UNITED STATES, VACCINE LAWS ARE DIFFERENT.

American doctors who say that vaccination is mandatory are most often telling a HALF-TRUTH. A half-truth is of course a disguised LIE.

There ARE a FEW American states where vaccinations are LEGALLY MANDATORY- e.g. California). HOWEVER- for most American states there are VARIOUS KINDS OF LEGAL EXEMPTIONS- e.g. religious, philosophical, "medical" for VACCINATIONS.

IF YOU LIVE IN THE UNITED STATES IT I STRONGLY RECOMMEND THAT YOU purchase a book entitled "Vaccine Exemptions" written by Alan Phillips, J.D—

This VACCINE EXEMPTIONS BOOK will provide YOU with essential legal information that YOU NEED TO PROTECT YOURSELF FROM HORRIFIC VACCINE

i.CANADIAN VACCINE LAW IS CRYSTAL CLEAR.

1. THERE ARE NO MANDATORY VACCINATIONS IN CANADA.

Health Canada echoes this by saying:

"Immunization is not mandatory in Canada".

There <u>ARE TWO</u> Canadian provinces that have legislation requiring Vaccination of school children is as a <u>pre-condition</u> to attending school ; (Ontario and New Brunswick)-

<u>BUT— THESE VACCINATIONS ARE NOT MANDATORY!</u>

<u>CANADIANS- YOU CAN CHOOSE NOT TO BE VACCINATED BY SIMPLY FILLING OUT A SIMPLE FORM!</u>

<u>YOU ONLY NEED TO FILL OUT A VERY- VERY- SIMPLE EXEMPTION FORM.</u> This is a simple <u>sworn</u> statement of conscience or religious belief.

<u>YOU CAN OBTAIN THIS FORM on line at</u> www.VaccinechoiceCanada.com. or from local government websites/offices.

In Canada, the web is rife with calls to create a <u>NO-FAULT COMPENSATION SCHEME</u> to compensate victims for vaccine-related injuries. An impotent UNICEF (United Nations Children's Fund) is tracking the rise of on-line anti-vaccination sentiments in Eastern and Central Europe.

In 1985 Quebec legislators were shamed into creating a <u>NO-FAULT COMPENSATION</u> SCHEME. Vran.org says that only 109 cases have been evaluated with only 27 successful applicants in the last 30 years.

And <u>why</u> is that?

That's because "<u>ALMOST NO ONE KNOWS OF THE EXISTENCE OF THIS PROGRAMME.</u>" On top of that- <u>THREE CONVENTIONALLY-TRAINED DOCTORS</u> decide whether vaccine-compensation is awarded!

<u>DO YOU REALLY EXPECT THAT CONVENTIONAL VACCINE-PUSHING DOCTORS ARE LIKELY TO COMPENSATE VACCINE-INJURED VICTIMS??</u>

The "legal foxes" that are supposed to be <u>GUARDING</u> the chicken-coop are <u>IN THE CHICKEN COOP! OMG!</u> Big Pharma and the medical establishment control the legal mechanism that indemnifies vaccine victims!

<u>WHERE'S THE JUSTICE IN THAT?</u>

Fortunately- Canadian law does offer <u>LEGAL PROTECTION AGAINST VACCINES.</u>

    <u>i.CANADIAN MEDICAL LAW IS CRYSTAL CLEAR</u>

<u>Every individual in Canada has the legal right to make a voluntary and informed decision about medical procedures, including surgery that carry a risk of injury or death.</u>

<u>CANADIAN MEDICAL LAW UPHOLDS YOUR RIGHT TO "INFORMED CONSENT".</u>

<u>CANADIAN MEDICAL LAW ALSO UPHOLDS FREEDOM OF CONSCIENCE AND RELIGION AND SECURITY OF THE PERSON.</u>

<u>UNDER THE CANADIAN CHARTER OF RIGHTS AND FREEDOMS— THE MEDICAL PRINCIPLE OF INFORMED CONSENT IS SOLIDLY ENTRENCHED.</u>

<u>YOU ARE PROTECTED FROM MEDICAL ASSAULT AND BATTERY!</u>

In 1980 in a famous Supreme Court decision in <u>Reibl</u> vs. <u>Hughes</u>, Mr. Justice Laskin speaking for a unanimous bench:

<u>POSTULATED THE DOCTRINE OF INFORMED CONSENT INTO CANADIAN LAW</u> with these immortal words:

> <u>"In summary, the decided cases appear to indicate that, in obtaining the consent of a patient for the performance upon him of a surgical operation, a surgeon, generally should answer any specific questions posed by the patients as to the risks involved, and should without being questioned, disclose to him the nature of the proposed operation, its gravity, and material risks, and any special or unusual risks."</u>

Mr. Justice Laskin emphasized that the relationship between a doctor and a patient gives rise <u>TO THE DUTY OF THE DOCTOR TO DISCLOSE MATERIAL RISKS ASSOCIATED WITH A PROCEDURE- WITHOUT HAVING TO BE QUESTIONED BY THE PATIENT.</u>

<u>YOUR DOCTOR MUST PROPERLY INFORM YOU ALL THAT YOU NEED TO KNOW- AND THIS WITHOUT THE NECESSITY OF YOU HAVING TO ASK QUESTIONS.</u>

Several Appellate Court Judgments since the <u>Riebl</u> decision have <u>BROADENED AND CLARIFIED THE MEDICAL LAW OF " INFORMED CONSENT".</u>

One Alberta Appellate case confirmed that the <u>DUTY OF DISCLOSURE IS NOT JUST CONFINED TO RISKS; but extends to other material information- such as any ALTERNATIVES to the treatment being proposed and the risks associated therewith- which a reasonable patient would want to have.</u>

In another recent Alberta case, <u>Rhine</u> vs. <u>Millan</u>, Judge Ritter, in the context of a medical malpractice action involving an allegedly inappropriate prescription of corticosteroids, reviewed the law in relation to <u>INFORMED CONSENT</u>. The learned judge stated:

> <u>"The doctor/patient relationship requires the doctor to disclose to a patient all the material risks of procedures or treatments being recommended. In determining whether this has been accomplished, the Court should adopt a patient-centered approach to defining these material risks. The test includes consideration of what the patient would have found relevant—as well as what the medical profession deems material.</u>
>
> <u>In determining whether facts are material necessitating disclosure- the test is what the patient would have wanted to know.</u> (Author's underline)

<u>DOCTORS HAVE A LEGAL DUTY TO PROVIDE MATERIAL INFORMATION THAT A REASONABLE PATIENT WOULD WANT TO KNOW.</u>

The Court will determine whether there has been a <u>MATERIAL NON-DISCLOSURE OF FACTS OR RISKS</u>, having regard to the expert evidence and the evidence as a whole.

<u>THE DUTY TO DISCLOSE AVAILABLE ALTERNATIVES IS ESPECIALLY IMPORTANT WHERE THESE ARE MORE CONSERVATIVE, AND INVOLVE FEWER RISKS THAN THE TREATMENT BEING PROPOSED.</u>

<u>Bottom line:</u>

<u>IF A PHYSICIAN FAILS TO OBTAIN AN INFORMED CONSENT—</u>

<u>LIABILITY (RESPONSIBILITY) WILL ONLY ATTACH WHERE IT CAN BE ESTABLISHED—</u>

<u>THAT A REASONABLE PERSON IN THE PATIENT'S POSITION WOULD HAVE DECIDED TO FORGO THE SURGICAL PROCEDURE HAD HE OR SHE BEEN PROPERLY INFORMED.</u>

When our Supreme Court of Canada speaks—<u>EVERYONE SHOULD LISTEN!</u>

<u>VACCINES ARE HORRIBLE DRUGS WHICH KILL AND INJURE THOUSANDS OF PEOPLE.</u> Toxic threats engendered by prescription drugs and <u>medical VACCINES</u> have been around for decades.

THE MEDICAL TRUTH ABOUT HOW DANGEROUS VACCINES REALLY ARE HAS BEEN SUPPRESSED AND HIDDEN FROM A BRAINWASHED POPULATION.

Vaccine TRUTH number one:

1. **VACCINES ARE MEDICAL CRIMES AGAINST HUMANITY.**

Vaccines are dangerous, **TOXIC CHEMICALS/DRUGS** that do more **HARM** than good. Vaccines and vaccinations should be outlawed! Vaccine pushers should be stopped!

YOU must do **your own due diligence.** Liars figure but figures don't lie. The scientific literature is **CLEAR**. Sadly, most conventional doctors are clueless about **VACCINES**. Most conventional doctors simply listen to the local drug representative explain the latest vaccine promotion. Most allopathic doctors either are too brainwashed by Big Pharma to read the scientific literature about vaccines.

YOU MUST BE YOUR OWN DOCTOR!

YOU MUST RESEARCH AND LEARN THE COLD HARD TRUTH ABOUT VACCINES!

Some sources are provided below. **YOU** need to fire your doctor-Hire yourself!

YOU CAN SELF-DIAGNOSE USING THE INTERNET.

If you have a health concern- your family doctor cannot help you. **YOU** must consult **DR. INTERNET**. In this book I have provided YOU with some great sources of health information.

THE SELF-HELP & SELF-MANAGEMENT TOOLS AND EDUCATIONAL MATERIALS ARE OUT THERE!

CONSULT A TRUSTWORTHY SITE; (hint—not the ones your doctor might suggest). Some trustworthy websites are suggested throughout this book.

YOU can discover the truth about **VACCINES** for yourself!

Vaccine truth number two:

2. **VACCINES ARE A FRAUD!**

Vaccines have been foisted upon an ill-informed human population by a greedy, corrupt pharmaceutical industry whose sole goal is to sell drugs. Allopathic doctors, trained as drug-pushers are obviously strong proponents of vaccines. The unpopular truth is that vaccines are <u>FRAUDULENT DRUGS</u> that have been introduced to mankind with the "alleged" goal of preventing diseases from polio, measles, mumps, and various kinds of <u>FLU</u>. Here's an example of this truth-

<u>THE FASTEST WAY TO GET THE FLU IS TO GET A VACCINE FLU SHOT!</u>

OMG! IT'S TRUE!

<u>Vaccine truth number three:</u>

3. <u>TAKE HEART! YOU CAN AVOID VACCINES AND</u>
<u>THEIR HORRIFIC HEALTH CONSEQUENCES!</u>

<u>THERE EXISTS A SAFE-NON-TOXIC-NON –INVASIVE, MORE EFFECTIVE ALTERNATIVE TO VACCINES!</u>

<u>YOU CAN IMMUNIZE YOURSELF EFFECTIVELY—AND SAFELY— WITHOUT USING VACCINES!</u>

<u>THIS NATURAL HOMEOPATHIC REMEDY IS CALLED HOMEOPROPHYLAXIS!</u>

<u>HOMEOPROPHYLAXIS WILL SAFELY IMMUNIZE YOU AGAINST A BOATLOAD OF DISEASES!</u>

<u>HOMEOPROPHYLAXIS IS BACKED BY SCIENTIFIC STUDIES DONE IN CUBA!</u>

i.AMERICAN VACCINATION LAW

In 2011, the United States Supreme Court stated:

"<u>VACCINES ARE UNAVOIDABLY UNSAFE</u>"-

Governments, Big Pharma, Mainstream Medical Authorities and Mainstream Media for <u>DECADES</u> have told people that Vaccines are <u>SAFE</u>.

<u>THIS IS A BIG-FAT LIE! IT'S ALSO A FRAUDULENT BIG-FAT LIE!</u>

<u>VACCINES ARE MEDICAL CRIMES AGAINST HUMANITY!!</u>

<u>FOR DECADES THESE MEDICAL CRIMES HAVE BEEN COMMITTED.</u>

How has this happened?

The answer is very simple—<u>THE TRUTH HAS SUPPRESSED. CRITICS OF THE VACCINATION CRIMES AND TRUTH-TELLERS HAVE BEEN UNJUSTLY DEMONIZED.</u>

<u>HERE ARE SOME SOURCES OF "TRUTHFUL" INFORMATION:</u>

1. "THERE IS NO EVIDENCE THAT VACCINES CAN PREVENT DEATHS OR PREVENT DEATHS OR PERSON-TO-PERSON- INFECTION" (source: Thomas Jefferson, researcher with Cochrane Collaboration, Northwestern EDU, January 13th, 2013;

2. THE NATIONAL VACCINE INFORMATION CENTRE (NVIC) Website at www.NVIC.org

3. Here are 6 MORE WEBSITES THAT PROVIDE TRUTHFUL INFORMATION AND ACCURATE STATISTICS- These are: www.GreenMedInfo.com , www.Mothering.com, www.vran.org (Vaccine Risk Awareness Network). www.naturalnews.com , www.mercola.com and www.TruthVac.com

VACCINATION IS ONE OF THE BIGGEST HEALTH CARE SCAMS EVER!

IT IS YOUR MORAL DUTY TO EDUCATE YOURSELF ABOUT VACCINES. YOU MUST AVOID THESE HORRIFIC LITTLE PRICKS.

YOU NEED TO DISCOVER THE TRUTH ABOUT THE HORRORS OF VACCINES.

YOU NEED TO PROTECT YOUR HEALTH.

THE HEALTH OF YOUR FAMILY AND LOVED ONES AND THE HEALTH OF FUTURE GENERATIONS DEPENDS ON YOUR DECISION TO TAKE CONTROL OF YOUR OWN HEALTH.

YOU MUST LEAD BY YOUR OWN EXAMPLE.

Vaccines (like most drugs) are routinely fast-tracked for approval by the FDA without little or no testing or any scientific evidence that they are effective.

If Vaccines are "SAFE"- why have the United States, and some countries s established a COMPENSATION SCHEME to indemnify VICTIMS HURT BY VACCINES?

Canada and Russia are the only G8 nations without a national No-Fault Compensation Scheme. In the United States, The Vaccine Act provides IMMUNITY to vaccine manufacturers for vaccine-related injuries.

The US Vaccine Injury Compensation Program, better known as "Vaccine court" has paid out over 3 BILLION DOLLARS to vaccine victims. It recently awarded millions of dollars to two children suffering autism from vaccine-injury.

THE GOVERNMENT DOES NOT ADMIT THAT VACCINES CAUSE AUTISM.

All files are sealed; hushed up, unpublished, and/or access to medical records and "court" documents and exhibits is blocked. (See www. huffingtonpost.com . In "vaccine court," the U.S. Department of Health and Human Services acts as the defendant and the Justice Department attorneys act as counsel. The US Supreme Court has acknowledged that it is powerless to overrule the "Vaccine Court".

The late senator, John Kennedy Jr. published an excellent article in which he publicized the VACCINE HORROR STORY and how vaccines were linked to autism in children. He was immediately discredited by mainstream media. This story emphasizes how big government, big Pharma and Big Medicine have been able to SUPPRESS THE TRUTH ABOUT THE DANGERS OF VACCINES. (Please see article July 2009, Kennedy 2005 in www.globalresearch.org)

A few weeks ago, a MASSIVE FRAUD was uncovered in the Centre of Disease Control (CDC.) A Dr. Thompson came forward and announced to the world (virtual world) that for the last 12 years he took part in a giant cover-up of information. Apparently, the CDC deliberately fudged their research numbers regarding the number of young American black boys who had allegedly became autistic and/ or suffered autistic injuries caused by vaccines aka "those horrific little pricks."

Please Google up the story of Dr. Andrew Wakefield, a British doctor who was vilified for having told the truth about his clients suffering the effects of autism attributed to injuries from vaccines.

THE LATEST VACCINE BOMBSHELL DROPPED ON SEPTEMBER 8, 2014!

As reported by Global Research, (supra)—A study published September 8th, 2014 in the Journal of Public Health and Epidemiology reveals a significant correlation between Autism and 3 specific vaccines:

- MMR (measles, mumps, and rubella)

- Varicella (chicken pox)

- Hepatitis- A- vaccines

Using statistical analysis from the US Government, UK, Denmark, and Australia; scientists at Sound Choice Pharmaceutical Institute (SCPI) found that increases in autistic disorder correspond with the introduction of vaccines using human fetal cell lines and retroviral contaminants.

Even more alarming, Dr. Theresa Deisher, lead scientist, SCPI founder stated plainly:

"Not only are the human fetal contaminated vaccines associated with autistic disorder throughout the world, but also with epidemic leukemia and lymphomas."

The clincher was the introduction of vaccines manufactured with human fetal cell lines containing fetal and retroviral contaminants. The cell line in question is known as "WI-38".

According to the authors—autism rates rose sharply each time another one of those vaccines were released.

In the US, autism rates jumped in 1980-1981 following the approval of MerovaxII an MMR II both of which are made of the human fetal cell line WI-38.

Another jump in autism prevalence occurred in 1988; corresponding to three factors:

- The addition of a second dose of MMRII;

- A highly successful measles vaccination campaign that raised compliance from 50 to 82 percent between the years 1987-1989;

- The introduction of Poliomax in 1987;

In 1995, autism rates jumped again in response to the introduction of the VARICELLA VACCINE VARIVAX. The authors conclude:

"Rising autistic disorder prevalence is directly related to vaccines manufactured utilizing human fetal cells."

At press time for this book, it appears that Canadian and American authorities are gearing up to fast track ANOTHER VACCINE to jab us with. Allegedly it will be used to help inoculate people against the Ebola virus.

GOD knows what HORRIFIC DAMAGE THIS VACCINE WILL DO TO HUMANITY!

Dr. David Brownstein, a Holistic Practitioner describes the CDC horrific little pricks latest debacle in the following words:

"What is happening is a media blackout on THE BIGGEST SCANDAL TO HIT MEDICINE in recent times" (author's caps)

He adds:

"What needs to be publicized is that all of our children, and especially African-American, may be harmed when they receive a commonly prescribed vaccine—the MMR vaccine—before 35 months of age. The decline of our children's health should be a national priority that should be addressed at the highest levels of our Government."

ON TOP OF ALL THIS- IT APPEARS THAT ABOUT 200 NEW VACCINES ARE IN THE PIPELINE! God help us.

A PREMIER PREVENTATIVE HEALTH RECOMMENDATION IS:

- AVOID BECOMING A VACCINE VICTIM!

- PROTECT YOUR CHILDREN AND LOVED ONES FROM SUFERING HORRIFIC VACCINE INJURY OR DEATH.

- JUST SAY NO TO ALL DRUGS!

- PLEASE HELP STOP THESE CRIMES AGAINST HUMANITY—PLEASE!

F.   THE TRUTH ABOUT CANCER

"To sell chemotherapy as a "therapy" is most likely the biggest deceit in the history of medicine.

Whoever masterminded this chemo-torture deserves a monument in hell.

Dr. Ryke Geerd Hamer, M.D.

CANCER IS A RECENT MAN-MADE DISEASE.

Science Daily in 2008 projected CANCER to be the NUMBER ONE KILLER IN THE WORLD by 2015. That's not exactly true. Iatrogenic doctor deaths and chemotherapy drugs are the number two and number one causes of DEATH RESPECTIVELY.

According to the news report, the burden of cancer doubled globally between 1975 and 2000. It is estimated that it will double again by 2020; and nearly triple by 2030.

This translates to far greater numbers of people living with-and dying from- the disease. The report estimates that there were 12 million new cancer diagnoses worldwide this year.

More than 7 million people will die from the disease.

The projected numbers for the year <u>2030 are 20 to 26 million new diagnoses—and between 13-17 million deaths</u>!

<u>BUT YOU SHOULD NOT BE ALARMED!</u>

<u>WHEN YOU ADOPT THE "KETOGENIC DIET" AND THE "KETOGENIC LIFESTYLE"—YOU WILL MAKE YOUR IMMUNE SYSTEM BULLETPROOF!</u>

<u>YOU WILL SHIELD YOURSELF FROM DISEASES SUCH AS CANCER AND OTHER CHRONIC DISORDERS.</u>

This means no more doctors' visits-; no more expensive drugs; you will become leaner, healthier, and happier. You will also likely save a couple of hundred dollars a month in grocery bills! How cool is that!

<u>HOW AND WHY IS CANCER INCREASING?</u>

What about the "War on Cancer" declared by former President Richard Nixon? What about all of the big ads, commercials and "pink-ribbon" campaigns?

These campaigns have raised more than <u>TWO TRILLION DOLLARS</u> in the last 25 years!

Have you figured out who has pocketed all of this cash? How can the rates of cancer be skyrocketing when <u>TRILLIONS OF DOLLARS ARE SPENT ON CANCER "RESEARCH"</u>? Who really benefits from <u>ALL OF THIS MONEY</u>?

The answer is <u>SIMPLE</u>.

<u>ALL YOUR HARD-EARNED CASH (DONATIONS)</u> is being used to fund research to "create new cancer drugs" and to line the pockets of the Cancer Industry.

My advice is to forget the "pink ribbons". Spend your hard-earned cash to buy some healthy nutritious food. Stop giving your money to the cancer industry. The only people they help are part of the cancer industry. The color pink has been chosen to sucker you into contributing to helping the cancer industry. What have the cancer people done with the trillions of dollars sucked from the public? They have feathered their own nest. There are dozens of other charities which actually help people. Spend your health dollars wisely. The best way to spend your health dollars is to purchase nutritious food. Nutritious healthy organic food is <u>YOUR BEST MEDICINE</u>. You need to get your <u>NATURAL MEDICINE</u> from Mother Nature's <u>FARMACY</u>.

<u>YOU CAN DEFEAT CANCER BY EATING A CANCER-BUSTING KETOGENIC DIET!</u>

Does Big Pharma know this? <u>OF COURSE THEY DO!</u>

Why is information about the therapeutic value of <u>VITAMINS,</u> <u>MINERALS AND NUTRIENTS IN FOOD AND SUPPLEMENTS</u> <u>SUPPRESSED BY MAINSTREAM MEDIA; BIG PHARMA, AND</u> <u>ALLOPATHIC DOCTORS</u>?

Conventional cancer treatments- i.e." <u>cut, poison</u> and <u>burn</u>" (aka "surgery "chemotherapy" and "radiation") <u>especially POISONOUS</u> <u>DRUGS CAUSE MORE HARM THAN THEY DO GOOD</u>. The "side-effects" caused by these drugs are legendary.

To find about the "effects" of <u>ANY</u> drug—<u>OR THE BENEFITS OF</u> <u>ANY</u> natural health issue- just <u>GOOGLE UP such</u> websites as <u>www.</u> <u>GreenMedInfo.com; www.mercola.com,</u> www.pubmed.gov.com <u>ETC</u>.

<u>THE TRUTH IS:" SIDE-EFFECTS" ARE "DIRECT" EFFECTS!</u>

The words "side effects" are 'MARKETING WORDS"— <u>CHOSEN TO</u> <u>CON YOU INTO USING DRUGS</u>. Have you ever heard of any drug that <u>CURED ANYTHING?</u>

<u>THE ALLOPATHIC INDUSTRY AND THEIR MENTORS- BIG PHARMA</u> <u>HAVE NO REASONS TO BE PROUD</u>.

<u>EVERYONE CONNECTED TO THE PHARMACEUTICAL INDUSTRY AND</u> <u>ENTIRE MEDICAL ESTABLISHMENT SHOULD BE ASHAMED OF THEIR</u> <u>BEHAVIOUR</u>.

<u>THESE PEOPLE AND THEIR SUPPORTERS SHOULD BE ASHAMED OF</u> <u>THE HARM THAT THEY HAVE CAUSED TO THE WORLD'S POPULATION</u>.

<u>IT IS TIME TO STOP THIS HUMAN SUFFERING AND MISERY ALL IN THE</u> <u>NAME OF PROFIT!</u>

<u>THE FAILURE OF ALLOPATHIC MEDICINE AND THE HORRIFIC DAMAGE</u> <u>IT HAS CAUSED (AND CONTINUES TO CAUSE) IS A BIG REASON THAT</u> <u>INSPIRED ME TO WRITE THIS BOOK</u>.

<u>YOU NEED TO TAKE RESPONSIBILITY FOR YOUR OWN HEALTH!</u>

<u>YOU CANNOT RELY ON BIG PHARMA AND THEIR HENCHMEN—THE</u> <u>ALLOPATHIC CROWD TO LOOK AFTER YOUR HEALTH</u>.

<u>THE PUBLIC IS FINALLY WAKING UP TO THE HORRORS OF</u> <u>CONVENTIONAL WESTERN (ALLOPATHIC) MEDICINE</u>.

<u>VIBRANT HEALTH CANNOT BE FOUND IN A SYNTHETIC PILL OR</u> <u>CHEMICAL COCKTAIL</u>

JUST SAY NO TO BIG PHARMA'S POISONOUS "MEDS"!

IF MOTHER NATURE DOESN'T MAKE IT—YOU DON'T NEED IT!

THE TRUTH ABOUT PENICILLIN-

About 75 years ago, the world's first "miracle drug" came to market. It could "cure" severe and potentially fatal diseases. It was a landmark event that kicked off modern medicine as we know it.

Penicillin is touted as the single greatest medical discovery in history. One medical historian even calls it a "turning point" in human history.

ONE BIG PROBLEM WITH THIS DISCOVERY; it accidently spun off a handful of ALL-POWERFUL DRUG COMPANIES! This elite group was able to piggyback on the original invention of penicillin- without— it appears, funding any of the research. These companies altered and patented various strains.

Using clever marketing, they grabbed 1.2 **TRILLION DOLLARS OUT OF THE PUBLIC PURSE—WITHOUT CURING ANYTHING!**

THE CONSEQUENCES FOR OUR HEALTH HAVE BEEN DISASTROUS!

BIG PHARMA DEVELOPS DRUGS TO PROFITABLY MANAGE THE SYMPTOMS OF DISEASE. IT'S NOT IN THEIR FINANCIAL INTERESTS TO FIND "CURES"!

CURES WOULD CUT OFF THEIR PROFITS AND KILL THE DRUG INDUSTRY.

Dr. Rath, a leading health researcher comments:

"Throughout the 20th Century, the pharmaceutical industry has been constructed by investors, the goal being to replace effective but non-patentable natural remedies with mostly ineffective but patentable and highly profitable pharmaceutical drugs. The very nature of the pharmaceutical industry is to make money from ongoing diseases. Like other industries, the pharmaceutical industry tries to expand their market- that is to maintain ongoing diseases and to find new diseases for their drugs."

Prevention and cure of diseases damages the pharmaceutical business. The eradication of common diseases threatens its very existence. Therefore, Big Pharma fights the eradication of disease at all costs. The pharmaceutical industry itself is the main obstacle. This is the real reason why widespread diseases are further expanding- including heart attacks, strokes, cancer, high blood pressure, diabetes, osteoporosis, etc. etc.

PHARMACEUTICAL DRUGS ARE NOT INTENDED TO CURE DISEASES.

According to health insurers, over 24,000 pharmaceutical drugs are currently marketed and prescribed- without any proven therapeutical value; (source: AOK Magazine 4/98) According to medical doctor's associations, the known dangerous "side-effects" of pharmaceutical drugs have become the 4TH LEADING CAUSE OF DEATH (after heart attacks, cancer and strokes) (source: Journal of the American Medical Association (JAMA) April 15th, 1998). (**N.B. Allopathic doctors are number one cause of death. See: death of medicine infra.)

WHEN PEOPLE STOP USING POISONOUS DRUGS, PEOPLE CAN BANKRUPT THE PHARMACEUTICAL INDUSTRY. Doing this will also put a nail in the coffin of their partners- THE ALLOPATHIC INDUSTRY.

CANCER ALONE IS A $ 125 BILLION A YEAR MARKET (source: National Cancer Institute). The cancer industry is projected to grow to $ 173 BILLION BY 2020- a 39 PERCENT INCREASE!

THE DRUG INDUSTRY NOW IS A $ 1.2 TRILLION DOLLAR ANNUAL MARKET!

IT SPENDS $ 180 MILLION ANNUALLY ON LOBBYISTS TO PUSH LEGISLATION ON ITS BEHALF.

A 2008 British study reported by ABC news in November 2008 found that:

"1 IN EVERY 4 CANCER DEATHS HAD EITHER BEEN SPED UP OR EVEN BEEN CAUSED BY CHEMOTHERAPY."

The study's findings also included the discovery that 2 out of every 5 of the patients had suffered significant poisoning from the treatment. Pink ribbons are a pink scam.

A team of researchers from Washington State had a giant "OOPS!' moment recently!

They accidently uncovered the DEADLY TRUTH about chemotherapy while investigating WHY PROSTATE CANCER CELLS ARE SO DIFFICULT TO KILL USING CONVENTIONAL METHODS.

CHEMOTHERAPY IS THE NUMBER ONE KILLER OF ADULTS IN THE USA!

CHEMOTHERAPY DOES NOT "TREAT" OR "CURE" CANCER AT ALL!

It's a fraudulent scheme to make money by using "treatments" that do the EXACT OPPOSITE of what they are advertised to do! A recent study published in the New York Times Academy of Sciences proves that:

CHEMO KILLS CANCER PATIENTS 4X FASTER THAN NO TREATMENT AT ALL!

What chemotherapy actually does is: IT FUELS THE GROWTH AND PROLIFERATION OF CANCER CELLS! This is what is referred to as "METASTASIS OF CANCER". MOST OFTEN— DEATH RESULTS NOT FROM THE CANCER.

DEATH RESULTS FROM THE HORRIFIC EFFECTS OF THE "CUT, BURN, & POISON" CANCER APPROACH USED BY ALLOPATHIC DOCTORS.

You will not see any death certificates that indicate the cause of death was chemotherapy, radiation or poisoning of the patient. For example, once chemotherapy has been initiated, it usually suppresses the immune system and spreads the cancer. Most times, when surgeons (oncologists), "cut out" breast cancer tissue with the goal of cutting out cancerous cells—this actually severs lymph nodes; an integral part the LYMPHATIC SYSTEM— resulting in a swollen arm— possibly for the rest of the patient's life.

Sidebar-

My 87 year-old mother, Eileen, a breast-cancer survivor personally experienced this. Fortunately— I PERSONALLY FIRED MY MOM'S ONCOLOGIST- BEFORE THE LATTER COULD DO ANY FURTHER DAMAGE!

My mom's oncologist had also prescribed some poisonous chemo drugs. My mom (with my persuasion) never took ANY drugs.

Seven years later, my mom remains HEALTHY AND DRUG FREE – at age 87 years young!

Conventional doctors are taught very little about the LYMPHATIC SYSTEM infra- (Oops—another reason to fire your doctor-☺

Oncologists never explain (perhaps because they are ignorant or do not care) that cancer is a METABOLIC DISEASE.

Cancer exists and spreads throughout the body. It does not exist ONLY in the cancerous tumour and/or tissues. Cancer is said to "metastasize " or spread throughout the body.

ALLOPATHIC DOCTORS DO NOT TREAT THE CAUSES OF ANY DISEASES.

THEY ONLY TREAT THE SYMPTOMS OF DISEASES.

CONVENTIONALLY TRAINED ONCOLOGISTS ONLY TREAT THE SYMPTOMS OF CANCER—NOT THE ROOT CAUSES OF CANCER!

They just e.g. cut out malignant tumours; then apply the old one, two, three, standardized cookie-cutter approach…one size fits all —CUT, BURN, POISON APPROACH.

In her book, "Outsmart Your Cancer", Tanya Pierce, outlines 6 main ways in which CANCER STATISTICS ARE FUDGED AND/OR MANIPULATED to make them look better than they actually are. She obtains these findings principally from the outstanding work of Lorraine Day, M.D and Ralph W. Moss, Ph.D.

"CURE" is defined as being alive for 5 years after diagnosis. This means a person could be very sick with cancer for 5 years and ONE day later—he or she dies—but still is declared

"CURED" BY CHEMOTHERAPY!

IN THE HEALTHCARE INDUSTRY—THE WORD 'CURE' IS A 4 LETTER WORD!

What is the solution? It's very simple.

In order to avoid losing their medical licenses and/or being raided by the medical mafia, enlightened "healers" are careful about using the "CURE" WORD or the "C" word for short.

A POPULAR ALTERNATIVE METHOD OF DESCRIBING "TREATMENTS" THAT ACTUALLY WORK AND/OR "CURE" DISEASES HAS NOW EVOLVED.

INSTEAD OF THE FOUR-LETTER WORD "CURE";

SMART KNOWLEDGEABLE PEOPLE USE THE WORDS:

" REVERSE AND PREVENT THE DISEASE"

Saying that nutrition and healthy lifestyle changes "reverse and prevent" disease does TWO IMPORTANT THINGS:

Firstly, it does not unduly offend the allopathic crowd and their supporters. Using these euphemistic words helps keep the users out of harm's way and allows them to practice real healing by using NUTRITIONAL THERAPIES and other kinds of NATURAL HEALING METHODS.

The allopathic industry has a legal monopoly on the use of the words "treat, cure and prescribe" when used in the medical sense. The C word is particularly threatening to the allopathic crowd. Most health books use a disclaimer in order not to inflame the allopathic crowd.

THE ONLY DISEASE AND ILLNESS THAT ALLOPATHIC DOCTORS HAVE CURED IS:

"THEIR OWN POVERTY"

IT'S MORE ACCURATE TO SAY THAT OUR CREATOR "CURES" US- OR THAT WE "CURE" OURSELVES FROM DISEASE. No one can cure anyone of any disease.

We have the power to control what we eat and our lifestyle choices.

OUR BODY IS THE MOST AMAZING SELF-HEALING MACHINE EVER CREATED!

SICKNESS AND DISEASE CANNOT BE CURED BY ANYONE BUT THE PERSON WHO IS SICK OR DISEASED.

It is the doctor within each of us who does the healing. Dr. Hippocrates, the Father of Medicine was right 2,500 years ago. Let your Food (fat-☺) be your medicine; let your medicine be your food-fat-☺

YOU WILL LEARN HOW TO USE A KETOGENIC NUTRITIONAL APPROACH TO REVERSE AND PREVENT DISEASES AND TO BE HEALTHY.

A KETOGENIC DIET WILL REVERSE AND PREVENT CANCER, DIABETES, HEART DISEASE MANY OTHER ADVERSE HEALTH CONDITIONS.

WHO CARES ABOUT THE 4 LETTER WORD "CURE"? Let Big Pharma and the failed allopathic industry keep the word cure. Let them put the word cure wherever they like.

It is symbolic of a failed paradigm –namely Big Pharma and the allopathic industries invented 100 years ago. Isn't it paradoxical that the Hippocratic Oath has been removed from allopathic oath?

BIG PHARMA CAN'T GET A PATENT ON THE WORD CURE!-☺

Back to cancer—

Certain types of cancer and certain groups of people that exhibit poor recovery rates are simply EXCLUDED from the overall statistics. This artificially raises the average cure rate. Interesting?

HOW DECEPTIVE IS THAT!

Easily curable cancerous and even pre-cancerous conditions are included in overall statistics. For example, ductal carcinoma in situ (DCIS), which was included in and now accounts for a significant portion of breast cancer statistics. This clever deceptive tactic, artificially, increases the overall recovery rates.

Earlier detection is taken to mean— longer survival time. This means that a person may die at the exact same point of cancer development as another person, BUT the former is taken to have lived longer simply by virtue of the fact that his tumour was discovered earlier. In other words, different starting points are used.

HOW CLEVERLY DECEPTIVE IS THAT?

Patients who fail to "complete" conventional treatment protocols are excluded from overall statistics. This means that IF a patient prescribed a 10- course chemotherapy protocol DIES after 9 sessions, he is not included as a "FAILURE" rate!

How outrageous is that!

Some people will sell their grandmother to make a buck. Your oncologist might be one of them. Chances are that he/she is more interested in their bank account rather than reversing your cancer. Control cancer groups as well play by different rules and protocols (gimmicks).

AGAIN— THIS ARTIFICIALLY RAISES CURE RATES FOR CONVENTIONAL TREATMENT PROTOCOLS.

How scientific is this? Are you appalled too?

Dr. Ralph Moss adds:

> "Relative survival rates take into account the "expected mortality figures." Put simply, this means that if a person hadn't died of cancer, he might have been run over by a truck, and that must be factored into the equation."

> Once again, this artificially raises the success rates of conventional treatment."

Alan Nixon, Ph. D. Past President of the American Chemical Society, stated the TRUTH VERY BLUNTLY—

> "As a chemist trained to interpret data, it is incomprehensible to me that physicians can ignore the clear evidence that CHEMOTHERAPY DOES MUCH, MUCH MORE HARM THAN GOOD". (authors caps)

THE SHOCKING UNTOLD TRUTH IS:

CONVENTIONAL PHYSICIANS AND CHEMO-DRUGS KILL MORE THAN TWO MILLION PEOPLE EVERY YEAR!

YES—2 MILLION PEOPLE EVERY YEAR! This is a not a misprint!

YOUR ALLOPATHIC DOCTOR IS THE BIGGEST KILLER OF ALL!

More proof that: Doctors do not know their arse from their elbow. **MOST DOCTORS ARE CLUELESS ABOUT DRUG "DIRECT EFFECTS AND IATROGENIC DEATHS** (aka Doctor-caused deaths).

Where did chemotherapy drugs come from?

THE UGLY TRUTH IS:

After WWI there was a huge stockpile of **POISONOUS NERVE GAS.** After the Second World War, there still remained a **VAST SUPPLY OF POISONOUS NERVE GAS.**

Then someone from the American Defense Department got a bright idea.

Why not use this available **NERVE GAS IN THE DRUG INDUSTRY?** This was the sick perverted **GENESIS OF CHEMOTHERAPEUTIC DRUGS!** Imagine using a chemical outlawed by the Geneva Convention (rules of warfare) to kill cancer **AND BRAINWASHED PATIENTS.**

A recent survey of **ONCOLOGISTS** showed that—

86 (EIGHTY- SIX PERCENT OF PHYSICIANS would refuse chemotherapy for **THEMSELVES!**

THESE SAME DOCTORS WOULD NOT PRESCRIBE IT FOR THEIR FAMILY MEMBERS EITHER!

SO —THIS PROVES THAT MOST ONCOLOGISTS ARE NOT STUPID.

MOST ARE INVETERATE LIARS AND FRAUD ARTISTS!

THIS IS ALSO EVIDENCE THAT MANY ONCOLOGISTS SHOULD BE CHARGED WITH CRIMINAL NEGLIGENCE AND JAILED!

It's time to stop insane killing for profit.

THIS EXPLAINS HOW THE CHEMICAL- BASED CANCER INDUSTRY WORKS.

THE TIME HAS COME TO STOP THIS INSANE KILLING FOR PROFIT!

So what IS the REAL cause(s) of the cancer epidemic?

Medical historian Hans Ruesch states:

> "Despite the general recognition that 85 percent of all cancers are caused by environmental influences; less than 10 percent of the U.S. National Cancer Institute budget is given to environmental causes. And despite the recognition that the majority of environmental causes are linked to NUTRITION; less than ONE percent of the National Cancer Institute's Budget is devoted to nutrition studies."

According to the National Cancer Institute, **AN ESTIMATED 84 THOUSAND CANCER CASES ARE LINKED TO OBESITY!** So you see, the Cancer Industry **KNOWS** what causes cancer. What do they do? They solicit your hard-earned cash (donations) to "research" for a "cure" for cancer!

DO NOT SUPPORT THIS FRAUD WITH YOUR HARD-EARNED CASH!

DOZENS OF CLINICAL STUDIES IRREFUTABLY PROVE ALL TYPES OF CANCER CAN BE REVERSED BY EATING A KETOGENIC DIET.

EVEN GLIOBLASTOMA (aka BRAIN CANCER) CAN BE PREVENTED AND CAN BE REVERSED BY EATING A KETOGENIC DIET!

TELL THAT TO YOUR CHOWDER HEADED DOCTOR- WHEN YOU GIVE HIM HIS PINK SLIP-☺

I IMPLORE YOU—DEAR READERS TO TELL ALL OF YOUR FRIENDS, FAMILY AND LOVED ONES ABOUT THE KETOGENIC WAY TO DEFEAT CANCER! (I will explain the biochemistry mechanics later in this book.)

IMAGINE HOW GOOD YOU'D FEEL IF WERE TO SAVE THE LIFE OF EVEN ONE PERSON! BY USING NUTRITIOUS HEALING FOOD! Just the thought of saving lives gives me goose bumps.-☺

It is a scientific fact that **EVERYONE** develops between 1,000 to 10,000 cancer cells as a by-product of metabolic processes every day. Fortunately, we all have a **POWERFUL IMMUNE SYSTEM THAT HEALS AND DESTROYS** these abnormal cells, (This process is called cell "apoptosis;" or cell death).

THIS ENTIRE PROCESS KILLS OR REPAIRS damaged ("busted") cells and rebuilds our healthy cells—**PROVIDED THAT WE PROVIDE OUR BODIES WITH THE NECESSARY MEDICINE.**

THAT MEDICINE IS KETOGENIC HEALING KETONES MADE BY OUR BODY

90 PERCENT OF YOUR IMMUNE SYSTEM resides in your gastrointestinal tract (G.I); (aka GUT).

EITHER YOU ARE "BUILDING UP" YOUR IMMUNE SYSTEM WITH FOOD THAT YOUR BODY REQUIRES—OR

YOU ARE "TEARING IT DOWN" AND CAUSING ALL KINDS OF BAD CELLS TO GROW. There is no 3rd. option.

What are you doing to your body with the food that you eat? Are you eating wholesome nutritious cancer-fighting foods like cruciferous veggies; (e.g. broccoli & cauliflower).

OR-

Are you eating poisonous, cancerous junk food like hot-dogs, pizza and bagels?

IT IS YOUR CHOICE!

YOU CAN FEED YOUR CANCER OR ANY OTHER CHRONIC DISEASE—

OR—YOU CAN STARVE OUT YOUR CANCER!

YOU CAN REBUILD YOUR IMMUNE SYSTEM SIMPLY BY EATING THE PROPER FOOD.

FOOD =MEDICINE—&— MEDICINE=FOOD.

Everyone knows that it usually takes <u>MANY YEARS</u> for a cancerous tumour to develop.

CONVENTIONAL CANCER THERAPY IS MADNESS! IT'S ABSOLUTE INSANITY!

Conventionally trained oncologists are killing people and profiting from human suffering and misery.

Instead of by brest cancer patients paying out hundreds of thousands of dollars on chemo drugs, radiation and surgery (aka- "cut, burn & poison")—

YOU CAN REVERSE CANCER FOR A FEW HUNDRED BUCKS BY EATING A WELL-CONSTRUCTED KETOGENIC DIET!

You have to eat food <u>ANYWAY</u>; why not eat a high-fat- low-carb **KETOGENIC DIET?**

It will not cost you any more than the (SAD) junk food diet you could be eating. YOU will save thousands of dollars on poisonous drugs (aka "medications.")

IT'S ALSO LIKELY THAT YOU WILL EVEN SAVE SOME MONEY ON FOOD!

How cool is that?

How can our body heal itself if you destroy its defense (aka immune) system with poisonous drugs?

Does it make sense to undergo treatments that make you <u>VOMIT</u> buckets; <u>LOSE</u> your hair <u>AND COST THOUSANDS OF DOLLARS ONLY TO KILL YOU WITH A SLOW AGONIZING PAINFUL DEATH?</u>

<u>DO ONCOLOGISTS TELL CANCER PATIENTS THAT CHEMOTHERAPY DRUGS KILL MORE THAN ONE MILLION PATIENTS EVERY YEAR SINCE 2000?</u>

Would any sane person who knew that chemo kills you and that there are natural non-invasive cures for cancer decide to opt for chemo?

Where is the common sense in paying thousands of dollars to kill yourself? There are dozens of less painful ways to kill yourself than using chemo.

Conventional cancer treatment wants to focus on destroying the cancer from the <u>OUTSIDE</u>. (chemo, radiation etc.)

<u>THE BEST NON-INVASIVE WAY TO KILL CANCER COMES FROM MAXIMIZING OUR OWN INNATE HEALING ABILITIES AND OUR IMMUNE SYSTEM.</u>

<u>OUR BODIES ARE AMAZING SELF-HEALING MACHINES IF WE GIVE THEM THE APPROPRIATE RAW MATERIALS TO HEAL AND SELF-REPAIR.</u>

90 percent of our immune system is in our gut—so it makes sense to inoculate our immune system with good food to rebuild and repair "busted cells". (More on "busted cells" later in this book)

<u>CANCER IS NOT MYSTERIOUS! CANCER IS MAN-MADE DISEASE IN THE LAST 100 YEARS.</u>

<u>YOU DO NOT GET CANCER BY BEING UNLUCKY!</u>

Your doctor is clueless about what causes cancer or any other disease.

Your doctor has been brainwashed by Big Pharma the first day he walked into medical school.

HERE IS THE TRUTH ABOUT CANCER.

The causes of cancer were discovered by a brilliant German Physiologist/ medical doctor Dr. Otto Heinrich <u>WARBURG</u>. He discovered that <u>CANCER IS A METABOLIC DISEASE.</u> Cancer is characterized by cellular mitochondrial respiratory insufficiency.

<u>THROUGHOUT THIS BOOK I USE TERMS SUCH AS MITOCHONDRIAL DYSFUNCTION AND/OR METABOLIC DYSFUNCTION.</u>

<u>IN SIMPLE TERMS —YOU CAN THINK OF CANCER AS "BUSTED CELLS" OR "BUSTED METABOLISM."</u>

The mitochondria are the little power plants in our cells where energy is created). The entire subject of cellular energy and cellular dysfunction will be thoroughly analysed later in this book.

Dr. Otto Warburg in 1931 won the Nobel Prize in Medicine for his discovery <u>THAT THE PREFERRED FUEL FOR CANCER IS SUGAR!</u> He was also the first to discover the <u>HEALING DISEASE- CURING POWER OF THE</u> 8th element on the Periodic Table- namely: <u>OXYGEN!</u> His conclusions were downright outstanding! He said this to a prestigious gathering of Nobel Laureates:

"Cancer, above all other diseases, has countless secondary causes. But even for cancer, there is only one prime cause. Summarized in a few words, the prime cause of cancer is the replacement of the respiration of oxygen in normal body cells by a fermentation of sugar. In other words-the lack of oxygen is the <u>NUMBER ONE CAUSE OF CANCER.</u>

According to Dr. Warburg-

> <u>"It is indisputable that all cancer could be prevented if the respiration of body cells were kept intact. In short, supplying your cells with oxygen not only kills cancer cells and tumours, it blocks future cancer cells from forming. It's that simple."</u>

<u>GOOGLE UP —"OXYGEN CANCER". THERE ARE MORE THAN 39 MILLION RESULTS!</u>

<u>IN SUM- THE 8TH ELEMENT PROTOCOL (i.e. OXYGEN TREATMENT) CAN CURE ALL 213 TYPES OF CANCER!</u>

<u>IF THIS CANCER CURE WERE ALLOWED TO THRIVE— IT COULD TOPPLE THE ENTIRE $ 300 BILLION DOLLAR CANCER INDUSTRY</u>

<u>THIS CURE HAS BEEN BANNED IN NORTH AMERICA. BUT- IT APPEARS THAT</u>

49

THIS OUTLAWED NATURAL CANCER THERAPY IS USED BY FDA OFFICIALS TO CURE THEMSELVES!

How outrageous is THAT!

While the FDA has banned the 8th Element (Oxygen Therapy) in America since the 1940's, highly respectable doctors report treating FDA officials and their families with the very same treatment they banned for Americans. According to Dr. Hans Kelper, the world-famous German cancer doctor who administers the 8th Element Therapy-

> "You wouldn't believe how many FDA officials or relatives or acquaintances of FDA officials come to see me as patients in Hanover."

RESEARCH PROVES THAT OXYGEN THERAPY REDUCES CANCER CELLS GROWTH BY 38 PERCENT!

In real life practice- 15,000 credible courageous physicians have used oxygen therapy to CURE 50 DISEASES.

Here are some testimonials:

Molecular biologist Stephen A Levin, from the University of California Berkeley, concludes that: "a lack of oxygen in the tissues is the fundamental cause of all degenerative diseases".

Dr. Arthur G. Guyton, renowned author of the classic textbook on Medical Physiology, wrote-

> "All chronic pain, suffering, and diseases are caused by a lack of oxygen at a cellular level."

Dr. Perris M. Kidd, an internationally recognized cell biologist, states:

> "We can look at oxygen deficiency as the single greatest cause of all disease".

Dr. W. Spencer Way, who wrote in the Journal of the American Association of Physicians

> "The link between insufficient oxygen and disease has now been firmly   established."

LOW OXYGEN IS ONE UNIVERSAL CAUSE OF ALL DISEASE.

IMAGINE IF OXYGEN THERAPIES WENT MAINSTREAM?

THE IMPLICATIONS ARE ENORMOUS!

IT WOULD BRING THE 1.2 TRILLION DOLLAR DRUG INDUSTRY TO A GRINDING HALT!

Most ignorant oncologists simply tell their patients to go home — take their "medicine" and eat whatever they like!

THIS IS SHEER MADNESS!

TREATING WOMEN WITH BREAST CANCER WITH CONVENTIONAL THERAPY AS BEEN DUBBED –

"A CRIME AGAINST HUMANITY"!

Cancer is very often "triggered" by **A TOXIC AND/OR DEFICIENT LIFESTYLE**

CHOICES.

FOOD AS "MEDICINE" gives the body what it needs on a **CELLULAR LEVEL.**

ELIMINATION OF ALL TOXIC NEUROTOXINS AND THE REPLACEMENT WITH NUTRITIOUS FOOD WILL REVERSE AND PREVENT CANCER.

THE MEDICAL/DRUG MAFIA HAVE ALWAYS SUPPRESSED SUCCESSFUL INEXPENSIVE NATURAL NUTRITIONAL THERAPIES THAT HEAL AND PREVENT CANCER.

HERE ARE SOME OTHER NATURAL TREATMENTS WHICH HAVE BEEN SUCCESSFULLY USED TO TREAT AND HEAL CANCER—

- **Hoxsey Remedies**

- **Gaston Nassens**

- **Max Gerson**

- **Raymond "Royal" Rifle**

- **Burzynski's Antineoplastons**
  (Please watch his documentary: "Cut, Poison, Burn")- IT'S A REAL EYE-OPENER!

- **Live Cell Therapy**

- **Ozone/Oxygenation Therapy;**

- **LAETREILE THERAPY, (using Amygdalin- a natural compound (apricot seeds)**

  You can review the latest scientific study called

"Amygdalin blocks bladder cancer cell growth in vitro by diminishing cyclin A and adte 2."

This German study was published on August 19th, 2014. (Source: The Journal PLoS PuBMed no. 25136960)

A documentary film was even made on this subject!

This film reveals how the Cancer Industry FRAUDULENTLY SUPPRESSED the research of a Japanese doctor. HIS SCIENTIFIC EVIDENCE PROVING the benefits of laetrile (amygdalin) was covered up and suppressed.

Guess what?

SEVERAL OF THE DOCTORS who participated in the fraudulent suppression of laetrile—subsequently THEMSELVES DIED OF CANCER! OMG!

- RAW FOODS AND SUPERFOODS!

- EXTRA-VIRGIN OLIVE OIL HAS BEEN PROVEN TO KILL CANCER CELLS IN 30 MINUTES!! Dr. Hippocrates dubbed OLIVE OIL "THE GREAT THERAPEUTIC!"

  WOWIE! How cool is that!

LADIES AND GENTLEMEN— I'm excited to tell you about—

THE NEWEST AND BEST NUTRITIONAL THERAPY THAT YOU CAN USE TO DESTROY CANCER IS:

Drum roll please…-☺)

THE MOST EFFECTIVE NUTRITIONAL THERAPY OF ALL IS:

THE MAGICAL KETOGENIC DIET!

HALLELUJAH! AND— HALLELUJAH!

THIS NUTRITIONAL APPROACH IS THE MAGIC BULLET THAT EVERYONE HAS BEEN SEARCHING FOR!

THE KETOGENIC DIET HAS BECOME THE NEW GOLD STANDARD OF NUTRITION AND THE NEW GOLD STANDARD OF NUTRITIONAL HEALTH!

KETOGENIC DIETS ARE BECOMING VERY POPULAR BECAUSE OF DR INTERNET.

A ketogenic diet works by <u>SIMPLY STARVING CANCER CELLS FROM THEIR FAVOURITE FOOD</u>—SUGAR. The underpinning cellular bio-chemistry and metabolism will be fully explained in later chapters.

<u>THE KETOGENIC DIET- (A HIGH-FAT- LOW CARBOHYDRATE DIET) IS THE CORE PHILOSOPHY OF THIS BOOK.</u>

<u>THIS NUTRITIONAL APPROACH WILL REVERSE AND PREVENT A PROVERBIAL BOATLOAD OF CHRONIC DISEASES/CONDITIONS</u>...such as: Cancer, Alzheimer's, diabetes, obesity, Multiple Sclerosis and other diseases from A to Z – How and why this dietary approach woks will be fully explained in subsequent chapters. In sum, to be cancer-free and dis-ease-free, and <u>HEALTHY</u> –YOU should adopt <u>THE HAPPY HEALING KETOGENIC DIET.</u>

<u>WHEN YOU FOLLOW A WELL-CONSTRUCTED KETOGENIC DIET—YOU CAN KISS THAT UGLY BELLY FAT GOODBYE!</u>

<u>YOU WILL EMBRACE SPARKLING HAPPY HEALTH!</u>

<u>YOU CAN KISS YOUR DOCTOR GOODBYE!</u> (You don't have to unless you want to...he may have germs on his skin...-☺)

G. THE GREATEST HEALTH- SCAM OF THIS CENTURY!

<u>THE GREATEST HEALTH SCAM OF THIS CENTURY IS THE CHOLESTEROL SCAM!</u>

<u>HERE'S HOW THE TYPICAL MEDICAL SCAM WORKS:</u>

> "Mr. (s) Smith,—you are overweight. You need to lose some weight. Your blood sugar levels are too high. I am going to prescribe a medication to help you control them. I will need you to watch your diet closely. Limit your sugar; eat plenty of whole grains and vegetables; you must AVOID ALL FATS and fatty foods; especially avoid SATURATED FAT; you should eat low-fat or no-fat foods.

> Because diabetes runs in your family you'll probably need to take this medication for the rest of our life. In addition to this medicine, Your CHOLESTEROL is way too high. High cholesterol causes heart problems— so I'm also going to put you on a STATIN DRUG to lower your CHOLESTEROL.

<u>THIS IS: THE GREATEST MEDICAL SCAM OF THE 21st CENTURY!</u>

PRESCRIBING STATIN DRUGS (CHOLESTEROL-LOWERING DRUGS) SUCH AS "LIPITOR" IS HOW THE MEDICAL ESTABLISHMENT OPERATES THIS SCAM— (FRAUD).

"CHOLESTEROL"—HAS BEEN WRONGFULLY DEMONIZED. You're constantly told that cholesterol is EVIL! Just the mention of the word "cholesterol" strikes TERROR into the hearts and heads of most people.

MEDICAL EXPERTS AND THEIR MEDIA LACKEYS SAY THAT CHOLESTEROL IS AN EVIL SUBSTANCE THAT CLOGS OUR ARTERIES WHICH THEN CAUSES HEART ATTACKS.

Often the word 'cholesterol" is spoken in the same sentence as heart disease, diabetes, cancer, stroke and almost any medical condition known to man!

Just Google up "cholesterol" and you will get 105,000,000 results. Just the mention of this other "C" word causes some people's blood pressure to rise – especially when it is uttered by someone in a white-coat.

SHOULD YOU FEAR CHOLESTEROL? ABSOLUTELY NOT!

CHOLESTEROL IS ONE OF THE MOST IMPORTANT- ESSENTIAL SUBSTANCES REQUIRED BY YOUR BODY!

YOUR BODY NEEDS CHOLESTEROL TO SURVIVE.

YOUR BRAIN IS 50—YES- FIFTY PERCENT CHOLESTEROL!

YOUR BODY CRAVES CHOLESTEROL—AND FAT TOO!

Does it make sense to prescribe STATIN DRUGS WHICH PREVENT YOUR BODY FROM MAKING CHOLESTEROL!!!!

DEAR READERS –PLEASE DO NOT FALL FOR THE CHOLESTEROL SCAM!

BIG PHARMA AND DOCTORS HAVE 100 BILLION REASONS TO ADORE CHOLESTEROL-LOWERING STATIN DRUGS.

STATIN DRUGS EARN 100 BILLION DOLLARS PER YEAR!

Statin Drugs reached the market in 1986 when Merck received FDA approval for "Lovastatin". In the last 20 years, obesity, diabetes, heart disease and cancer rates have all skyrocketed. Is this a coincidence? ABSOLUTELY NOT!

CHOLESTEROL is just an excuse to prescribe STATIN DRUGS.

Satin drugs (such as Lipitor, Crestor, Zocor etc.), are routinely pre-scribed for life as illustrated in the abovementioned classical medical scenario. It's very sad.

IT'S SHOCKING HOW THE PUBLIC HAS BEEN BRAINWASHED—AND DUPED— BY BIG PHARMA, BIG MEDICAL AND BIG GOVERNMENT!

WHAT IS "CHOLESTEROL" ANYWAY?

CHOLESTEROL IS A FATTY, WAX-LIKE SUBSTANCE NATURALLY FOUND IN EVERY CELL AND MOST ORGANS—BRAIN, HEART, LIVER AND MOST OTHER PARTS OF YOUR BODY!

CHOLESTEROL PLAYS A CRITICAL ROLE IN OUR BODY!

Cholesterol plays a critical role within your cell membranes. Research also shows that cholesterol also interacts with proteins inside your cells;—adding MUCH MORE IMPORTANCE.

CHOLESTEROL IS SO IMPORTANT THAT —EVERY CELL IN YOUR BODY HAS A WAY TO MAKE ITS OWN SUPPLY!

Your body is literally composed of TRILLIONS of cells that need to interact with each other. Cholesterol is one of the molecules that allow for these reactions to take place. For example, cholesterol is the precursor to BILE ACIDS; so without sufficient amounts of choles-terol, your digestive system be adversely affected.

CHOLESTEROL PLAYS A CRITICAL ROLE IN OUR BRAIN.

RESEARCH SHOWS THAT FAT AND CHOLESTEROL ARE SEVERELY DEFICIENT IN DISEASED BRAINS.

RESEARCH ALSO SHOWS THAT HIGH TOTAL CHOLESTEROL LEVELS IN LATE LIFE ARE ASSOCIATED WITH INCREASED LONGEVITY!

OMG! Isn't that the exact opposite of what your doctor told you?... oops another reason to fire your doctor..-☺

YOUR BRAIN CONTAINS ABOUT 25 PERCENT OF THE TOTAL CHOLESTEROL IN YOUR BODY!

Cholesterol is critical for BRAIN synapse formation; i.e. the connec-tions between your BRAIN'S NEURONS which allow you to think; learn new things and form memories. Cholesterol is essential to grow new synapses; it also is a crucial component in the myelin coating around each neuron.

CHOLESTEROL IS A POWERFUL ANTIOXIDANT FOR OUR BRAIN!

CHOLESTEROL IS NEUROPROTECTIVE. IT PROTECTS OUR BRAIN AGAINST FREE RADICALS — (aka ROS) reactive oxygen species.

LOW LEVELS OF HDL CHOLESTEROL CAUSE MEMORY LOSS AND ALZHEIEMER'S DISEASE AND HEAVEN KNOW WHAT ELSE.

LOW LEVELS OF CHOLESTEROL ALSO INCREASES DEPRESSION, STROKE VIOLENT BEHAVIOUR AND SUICIDE.

CHOLESTEROL IS REQUIRED TO FORM CELL MEMBRANES.

CHOLESTEROL IS ABSOLUTELY ESSENTIAL TO PRODUCE IMPORTANT SEX HORMONES SUCH AS TESTOSTERONE, PROGESTERONE AND ESTROGEN!

CHOLESTEROL HELPS PRODUCE BILE ACIDS THAT HELP YOU DIGEST FAT.

BILE SALTS THAT ARE SECRETED BY THE GALLBLADDER ARE MADE OF CHOLESTEROL. Bile salts are needed to allow the body to properly digest FAT and to ABSORB FAT SOLUBLE VITAMINS A, D. AND K.

VITAMIN D IS DIRECTLY FORMED FROM CHOLESTEROL.

NO CHOLESTEROL IN YOUR BODY MEANS YOUR BODY CANNOT MAKE VITAMIN D! OMG! YOU CANNOT SURVIVE WITHOUT VITAMIN D!

HAVING A LOW LEVEL OF CHOLESTEROL IN YOUR BODY SERIOUSLY COMPROMISES THE BODY'S ABILITY TO DIGEST FAT ALSO.

THIS POINT CANNOT BE OVER EMPHASIZED.

FAT IS THE PREFERRED FUEL OF HUMAN METABOLISM!

YOUR BRAIN AND YOUR HEART MUST HAVE CHOLESTEROL AND HEALTHY FATS IN ORDER TO BE HEALTHY!

STATIN DRUGS ARE VERY EFFECT AT LOWERING CHOLESTEROL. BUT—

THE LAST THING IN THE WORLD THAT YOU WANT TO DO IS TO LOWER YOUR CHOLESTEROL!

STATIN DRUGS ARE ONE OF THE MOST EVIL HARMFUL DRUGS THAT HAVE EVER BEEN INVENTED!

99 PERCENT OF WHAT YOUR DOCTOR SAYS TO DO IS WRONG.

ONCE AGAIN—

ALL YOU HAVE TO DO IS TO APPLY MY 99 PERCENT HEALTH RULE-i.e.

DO THE EXACT OPPOSITE OF WHAT DOCTORS SAY—

AND YOU'LL BE RIGHT!

DOCTORS WHO PRESCRIBE STATIN DRUGS ARE GUILTY OF MEDICAL MALPRACTICE AND THEY SHOULD HAVE THEIR MEDICAL LICENSES REVOKED.

TAKING STATIN DRUGS IS ONE OF THE MOST HARMFUL THINGS THAT YOU CAN EVER DO TO HARM YOUR BODY!

STATIN DRUGS SHOULD BE OUTLAWED!

STATIN DRUGS DO NOT PREVENT HEART ATTACKS—STATINS CAUSE THEM!

LADIES AND GENTLEMEN—THE JURY IS IN.

DOZENS OF CLINICAL STUDIES HAVE PROVEN THE LETHAL EFFECTS OF STATIN DRUGS.

In a (2010) study, 300 patients diagnosed with heart failure were studied for an average of 3.7 years. The study found that the STATIN drug users WITH THE LOWEST LEVELS OF LDL CHOLESTEROL HAD THE HIGHEST RATES OF MORTALITY!

Conversely— patients with the HIGHEST LEVELS OF CHOLESTEROL HAD A LOWER RISK OF DEATH!

STATIN DRUGS CAUSE HEART DISEASE, CANCER AND DIABETES— AND A BOATLOAD OF HEALTH PROBLEMS!

STATIN DRUGS ARE ONE OF THE MOST POISONOUS CHEMICALS EVER DEVELOPED BY BIG PHARMA!

CHEMOTHERAPY DRUGS DESERVE THE TITLE OF THE "KING" OF POISONOUS DRUGS.

STATIN DRUGS DESERVE THE TITLE OF THE "QUEEN" OF POISONOUS DRUGS.

STATIN DRUGS DO NOT PREVENT HEART ATTACKS.

STATIN DRUGS DO THE EXACT OPPOSITE. STATIN DRUGS CAUSE HEART ATTACKS AND A BOATLOAD OF OTHER KINDS OF MEDICAL PROBLEMS.

CHOLESTEROL AND SATURATED FAT DO NOT CAUSE HEART PROBLEMS.

JUST THE OPPOSITE!

CHOLESTEROL AND SATURATED FAT PREVENT HEART PROBLEMS!

THIS IS THE EXACT OPPOSITE OF WHAT CONVENTIONAL MEDICINE SAYS!

This is another example of the 99 PERCENT RULE-supra)

Is it true that there is "good" and "bad" cholesterol?

OF COURSE NOT! Remember the 99 % rule?

THIS IS ANOTHER BIG, BIG, BIG MEDICAL FRAUD!

THIS IS THE GREATEST MEDICAL SCAM OF THE 21st CENTURY!

CONVENTIONAL MEDICINE SAYS THERE ARE 2 KINDS OF CHOLESTEROL:

The "Good" Cholesterol (HDL) and the "Bad" Cholesterol (LDL)

Guess what?

HDL AND LDL—ARE NOT EVEN CHOLESTEROL!! OMG!

THESE "CHOLESTEROLS" ARE ACTUALLY KINDS OF PROTEINS!!!

"HDL" stands for "HIGH –DENSITY- LIPOPROTEIN"!

"HDL" IS A PARTICLE IN THE BLOOD THAT CARRIES CHOLESTEROL FROM THE ARTERIES TO THE LIVER.

"LDL" stands for "LOW-DENSITY-LIPOPROTEIN"!

"LDL" IS A PARTICLE MADE BY THE LIVER THAT CARRIES CHOLESTEROL AND FAT SOLUBLE VITAMINS FROM THE LIVER TO THE CELLS. (Occasionally, LDL is referred to as the AMOUNT of cholesterol carried in these particles.)

HDL—HIGH-DENSITY LIPO—PROTEIN IS NOT ONLY GOOD—IT IS GREAT! YOU WANT TO RAISE YOUR HDL AS HIGH AS POSSIBLE.

LDL—LOW-DENSITY LIPO—PROTEIN IS ONLY BAD" OR DANGEROUS FOR YOU WHEN:

- **LDL PARTICLES** are **VERY SMALL ONES**; these tiny suckers are able to penetrate heart and other tissue and do great damage to our cardiovascular system); Research shows that when these LDL particles are **LARGE AND FLUFFY—THEY ARE NOT DANGEROUS.**

- **THESE SMALL LDL PARTICLES BECOME OXIDIZED; AND/OR**

- **THESE SMALL LDL PARTICLES BECOME VERY NUMEROUS;**

THE BIOCHEMISTRY OF LIPID (FAT) METABOLISM AND HOW OUR BODY PRODUCES AND MANUFACTURES DIFFERENT TYPES OF CHOLESTEROL IS A MYSTERY TO CONVENTIONAL DOCTORS.

FIFTY (50) PERCENT of people who suffer heart attacks have normal cholesterol levels. Doctors are taught that high cholesterol is a risk factor for heart disease. They are also taught that a high triglyceride level was also a risk factor for heart disease. It was drilled into every medical student's head that a lower cholesterol level was always better than a high one.

Medical doctors are not taught that higher cholesterol levels are pre-dictive of a longer lifespan in the elderly. Lowering cholesterol levels with cholesterol- lowering drugs (statins) **DESTROYS THE HEALTH OF 97 PERCENT OF THE PATIENTS (PEOPLE) WHO TAKE THEM!**

A recent study (2015) reported in the Journal Critical Care Medicine studied 724 hospitalized patients who suffered acute heart attacks. The study found that those with OF **RISK** when compared with patients with higher LDL-cholesterol and triglyceride levels.

In fact- lower LDL- cholesterol (less than 110 ng/dl and triglycerides less than 62.5 ng/dl were identified as optimal threshold values for predicting 30 day mortality.

The lower the LDL-cholesterol level was associated with a 65 **PERCENT INCREASED MORTALITY RISK AND THE LOWER TRIGLYCERIDE LEVEL WAS ASSOCIATED WITH A 405 PERCENT INCREASED MORTALITY RATE!**

Furthermore, as compared to patients with LDL-cholesterol levels >110 ng/dl and triglycerides > 62.5 ng/dl- those with **LOWERED LDL AND TRIGLYCERIDE LEVELS HAD A 990 PERCENT OR TEN TIMES AN INCREASED RISK FOR MORTALITY!**

Why? How can this be?

Why would lowered cholesterol levels and triglyceride levels be asso-ciated with a higher mortality rate?

The answer is simple.

FATS FROM TRIGLYCERIDES ARE A MAJOR ENERGY SOURCE AND LDL-CHOLESTEROL IS CRITICAL FOR CELL MEMBRANE SYNTHESIS AND IS NEED TO FIGHT INFECTIONS!

ADEQUATE LDL-CHOLESTEROL AND TRIGLYCERIDE LEVELS ARE CRUCIAL FOR CELL FUNCTION AND SURVIVAL IN THE CASE OF A HEART ATTACK AND TO STAY HEALTHY!

TAKING STATIN DRUGS IS A DISASTER!

MOST DOCTORS ARE CLUELESS ABOUT HOW STATINS. DOCTORS DO NOT UNDERSTAND HOW STATINS POISON THE HUMAN BIOCHEMISTRY—AND THE DIRECT EFFECTS CAUSED BY THEIR USE.

STATINS ARE POISONS—THEY SHOULD BE PULLED FROM THE MARKET NOW!

DOCTORS WHO PRESCRIBE STATINS- SHOULD BE PROSECUTED AND JAILED FOR CRIMINAL NEGLIGENCE.

IN SUM- CHOLESTEROL IS YOUR FRIEND.

WHEN YOU EAT THE RIGHT FOODS IT WILL PROTECT YOU AND MAKE YOUR BODY STRONG AND HEALTHY.

YOUR LIVER IS YOUR BODY'S MAIN FAT- BURNING ORGAN!

YOUR LIVER METABOLIZES MOST OF THE FOOD THAT YOU PUT INTO YOUR BODY.

WHEN YOU SHUT DOWN THE PRODUCTION OF CHOLESTEROL BY TAKING STATIN DRUGS- YOU COMPLETELY DESTROY LIVER FUNCTION!

WHEN YOU DESTROY PRODUCTION OF CHOLESTEROL WITH STATINS- YOU DESTROY THE LIVER'S ABILITY TO BURN FAT.

WHEN YOU SHUT DOWN YOUR LIVER- YOUR LIVER STORES FAT! Yuk!

WHEN YOU SHUT DOWN YOUR LIVER (esp.CoQ10 Enzyme)- YOU SHUT DOWN YOUR FAT- BURNING FURNACE! OMG!

CoQ10 Enzyme IS ESSENTIAL TO PRODUCE CELLULAR ENERGY (called ATP). This mechanism is more fully explained later in this book.

STATIN DRUGS SHUT DOWN THE MITOCHONDRIA (tiny power engines in cells that produce ATP).

STATIN DRUGS BUST YOUR MITOCHONDRIA—THEN YOUR BUSTED CELLS DIE OFF- THEN YOU DIE TOO!

THIS EXPLAINS WHY MOST PEOPLE WHO TAKE STATINS SUFFER MUSCLE WEAKNESS AND FATIGUE AND LOW-ENERGY.

FIRE YOUR DOCTOR—HIRE YOURSELF!

Sidebar:

<u>In chapter two- "Fire Your Doctor- Hire Yourself"- I relate my mother's story many years ago, how her doctor wanted to prescribe STATIN drugs to her. I explain how I prevented this fraud from being perpetrated on my mother.</u>

<u>ANOTHER LETHAL EFFECT OF STATIN DRUGS IS:</u>

<u>STATIN DRUGS PREVENT YOUR BODY FROM ABSORBING NUTRIENTS!</u>

<u>SO – LIKE MOST DRUGS-STATINS ARE A TERRIBLE DOUBLE HEALTH-WHAMMY!</u>

For an excellent book on how drugs rob your nutrients; I highly recommend a book called "Drug Muggers" written by Suzy Cohen, a brilliant Pharmacist.

To repeat, a carrier protein, LDL, has been given the derogatory title of "bad cholesterol." In reality, LDL is not a <u>cholesterol</u> molecule at all; good or bad.

<u>HIGH CHOLESTEROL LEVELS HAVE NOTHING TO DO WITH CORONARY OR ANY OTHER TYPE OF HEART DISEASE!</u>

<u>THIS THEORY IS MEDICAL "NONSENSE"</u>(another word comes to mind-☺)

<u>STATIN DRUGS ACTUALLY "CAUSE" HEART DISEASE!</u>

A recent study in 2012, reported in the Journal Atherosclerosis found that <u>STATIN USE IS ASSOCIATED WITH A 52 PERCENT INCREASE OF CALCIFIED CORONARY PLAQUE. CORONARY ARTERY CALCIFICATION IS "THE" HALLMARK OF HEART DISEASE!</u>

<u>How can a competent doctor prescribe a statin drug and tell patients that it will prevent heart disease?</u> This is the biggest medical scam is in this century. Doctors who participate in this medical scam as an excuse to prescribe statins should be jailed!

According to world-renown neurologist, Dr. David Perlmutter, M.D. author of "Grain Brain"

> <u>"The fundamental role of LDL in the brain, again, is to capture life-giving cholesterol and transport it to the neuron, where it performs critically important functions...</u>

And now we have the evidence in the scientific literature to prove that when cholesterol levels are low, the
brain simply doesn't work well; individuals with low
cholesterol are at a much greater risk for dementia and
other neurological problems.

We need to change our attitudes about cholesterol and
even LDL;

They are our friends, not foes."

(Authors underline.)

Science tells us that the REAL CAUSE of diabetes, heart diseases, Alzheimer's and God knows what other disease IS...— OXIDIZED LDL PARTICLES.

IT IS NOT—CHOLESTEROL!

Sally Fallon, the President of the Weston A. Price Foundation, and Mary Enig, Ph.D an expert in lipid biochemistry, says:

"HIGH CHOLESTEROL- IS AN INVENTED DISEASE"

Professor Yeon-Kyun Shin, a noted authority from Iowa University, talking about how cholesterol functions within neural networks to transmit messages, stated in 2009:

"If you deprive cholesterol from the brain, then you
directly affect the machinery that triggers the release of
neurotransmitters. Neuro-transmitters affect the data
processing and memory functions. In other words—
how smart you are and how well you remember things.
If you try to lower the cholesterol by taking medication
that is attacking the machinery of cholesterol synthesis
in the liver; that medicine goes to the brain too. And
then it reduces the synthesis of cholesterol, which is
necessary in the brain. Our study shows a direct link
between cholesterol and the neurotransmitter release,
and we know exactly the molecular mechanics of what
happens in the cells. Cholesterol changes the shape of
the proteins to stimulate thinking and memory."

Dr. David Brownstein, in his book, "Drugs that Don't work and Natural Therapies That Do" highlights the mechanics behind statin damage. He points out that statins work by poisoning an enzyme known as HMG-CoA reductase, which the body uses to produce cholesterol, adrenal hormones, sex hormones and memory proteins.

HMG-CoA reductase is also responsible for maintaining cell energy, which is needed by every system in the body.

Artificially blocking or otherwise inhibiting this vital enzyme is a receipe for a HEALTH DISASTER. He advises anyone against taking statin drugs.

Cholesterol is primarily produced in the liver and your body uses a specific enzyme- HMG-CoA reductase to produce it. Statins work by blocking this enzyme, which significantly reduces cholesterol production in the liver and lowers cholesterol levels in the blood. Statins also block the production of CoQ10 because the enzyme that statins block is also key to the production of CoQ10. CoQ10 is an enzyme with a variety of purposes. Including acting as an antioxidant and a key player in cellular energy production.

Decreased CoQ10 levels can result in muscle damage.

Dr. Brownstein also questions why any "cognizant" doctor would prescribe them, knowing that as many as 3.6 MILLION PEOPLE have reported BRAIN DYSFUNCTION as a result of their use. OMG!

THE BRAIN IS THE ORGAN THAT SUFFERS THE MOST WHEN CHOLESTEROL PRODUCTION IS BLOCKED! OMG!

Dr. Brownstein states: "You can't poison a crucial enzyme or block an important receptor for the long term and expect a good result." For me, this is another way to describe the process of killing your mitochondria, busting your cells, busting your mitochondrial health… and slowly BUSTING YOU!

Dear readers for more research and clinical information about STATIN POISONS—

YOU can consult The National Library of Medicine, (http://nlm.nih.gov/). It contains peer-reviewed published research on more than 300 known ADVERSE EFFECTS ASSOCIATED WITH THE USE OF STATINS. For a summary of these studies—please go to: www.GreenMedInfo.com.

OTHER PROBLEMS CAUSED BY STATIN DRUGS INCLUDE:

INCREASED RISK OF CERTAIN CANCERS, DIGESTIVE PROBLEMS, ASTHMA, INFLAMMATION OF THE PANCREAS AND LIVER DAMAGE.

Based on the thousands of entries published in the US Food and Drug Administration short-term memory loss, disorientation, to chronic depression and dementia. This same database reports over 100.000 adverse events.

PLEASE KEEP IN MIND THAT VERY FEW ADVERSE DRUG REACTIONS ARE EVER REPORTED TO THE FDA!

ADVERSE EVENTS ARE BASED ON A ONE –TO– TEN PERCENT REPORTING RATE!

THIS MEANS THAT MILLIONS OF PEOPLE ARE BEING HARMED BY STATINS!

WE MUST BAN STATIN DRUGS AND ELIMINATE THE ALLOPATHIC MODEL OF MEDICINE! You can help yourself and your fellow human beings. You can begin this process.

YOU CAN START TO IMPROVE YOUR HEALTH IMMEDIATELY!

JUST SAY NO TO ALL POISONOUS DRUGS!

In 2009, Dr. Stephanie Seneff, a senior researcher and **WORLD RENOWN SCIENTIST** at the Computer Science and Artificial Intelligence Laboratory at MIT wrote an ground- breaking essay explaining why **low-fat diets and statins cause Alzheimer's Disease**.

In it she details statins' side effects, discusses how the brain suffers from statins. She also synthesizes the latest science and inputs from other experts in the field.

(A sad commentary is that the statin industry advertises its products saying that they interfere with cholesterol production in the **BRAIN** as well as the liver.)

Dr. Seneff also examines how statins deplete COQ10 enzyme pro-duced by the liver. Unfortunately, as we age our bodies **MAKE LESS COQ10** which is a double whammy!

The depletion of this enzyme from our liver causes things like fatigue, depression, shortness of breath, mobility and balance problems. Deficiency in COQ10 has been linked to heart failure, hypertension, and Parkinson's disease.

STATINS DRUGS CAUSE DIABETES TOO.

So, if you're a few pounds overweight or you have slightly elevated blood pressure, you should avoid being sucked in by your doctor's recommendation to take statin drugs!

A recent study published in January (2012) carried out by The **AMERICAN MEDICAL ASSOCIATION** and published in the Archives of Internal Medicine showed conclusively that—

"THAT THERE WAS A WHOPPING 48 PERCENT INCREASED RISK OF DIABETES AMONG WOMEN TAKING STATIN MEDICATIONS!

OMG!

IMAGINE! STATIN DRUG USE INCREASES WOMEN'S RATE OF DIABETES BY A WHOPPING 48 PERCENT!

Earlier this year, The New York Times published an opinion piece in which a Harvard Medical School faculty member decried the use of statins. The article entitled "Don't give Patients More Statins," not only cited statin therapy's significant side effects and failure to mean-ingfully protect against heart disease, but also another issue: false assurances which distract patients from the true "cure" for "high cho-lesterol", poor lifestyle choices. The piece strongly cautioned patients against following any guidelines related to statins, and instead advised them to consider all of the evidence in order to determine the best course of treatment. (source: http://www.nytimes.com)

How sad is it when a doctor begs other doctors not to use statins. What would have happened if implored his fellow doctors to stop their criminal behaviour by prescribing statins? This sane doctor would likely had a visit from his local licencing board.

ONE OUT OF EVERY FOUR AMERICANS TAKES STATIN DRUGS.

BIG PHARMA AND THE MEDICAL ESTABLISHMENT WANT TO PUT STATIN DRUGS IN YOUR DRINKING WATER! OMG!

HORRIFIC NEW GUIDELINES FOR PRESCRIBING STATIN DRUGS HAVE BEEN LOWERED!

Dear readers—statin drug use is now becoming AN EVEN BIGGER HORROR STORY!

More and more young overweight young children are now "eligible" recipients. Some neuroscientists even predict that statins prescribed for pregnant overweight women might mean "kiddies born with no arms and legs in the next ten years! OMG!

How awful is that?

The old horrific drug Thalidomide given to pregnant women will look safe compared to statin drugs. In the early 1970's thalidomide was a drug prescribed by allopathic doctors to help pregnant women with nausea. It caused a vast number of babies to be born with a wide variety of birth defects. After the drug companies settled out of court with thousands of maimed victims, this horrific drug was taken off of the market.

But- Guess What?

It now appears that Thalidomide has once again re-surfaced and has become a prescribed drug for another "medical" condition! It costs at least 80 million dollars to get a drug approved for the market.

NEVER TRUST BIG PHARMA OR ALLOPATHIC DOCTORS.

BOTH ARE ENGAGING IN CRIMINAL FRAUD.

MANY DRUG COMPANIES HAVE KILLED PEOPLE AND HAVE SIMPLY PAID MILLIONS OF DOLLARS IN FINES.

BIG PHARMA IS LIKE 007 JAMES BOND.

BOTH HAVE A LICENSE TO KILL!

ALLOPATHIC DOCTORS ALSO HAVE A LICENCE TO KILL TOO!

Guess what?

NO ONE GOES TO JAIL FOR KILLING PEOPLE!

THIS "LEGALIZED KILLING" IS CONSIDERED AS JUST THE COST OF DOING BUSINESS!

You must make your own decisions. Think for yourself.

Beware of the letters M.D.

MOST PEOPLE BELIEVE THAT THESE LETTERS MEAN

"Medical Doctor".

Personally, I've come to believe THAT THE LETTERS " M.D." actually mean:" MORE DINERO"! -☺

YOU NEED TO TAKE CONTROL OF YOUR OWN HEALTH.

YOU MUST FIRE YOUR DOCTOR- AND HIRE YOURSELF!

THE CHOLESTEROL MEDICAL SCAM HAS MUSHROOMED INTO A TRILLION DOLLAR INDUSTRY! Big Pharma and conventional medicine's only goal is to MAKE MONEY.

THE BIG BUCKS ARE IN "DIS-EASE- NOT HEALTH. NEXT TO CANCER DOLLARS,—STATIN DRUGS ARE THE BIGGEST MEDICAL CASH COW.

DON'T LET BIG PHARMA AND MEDICAL DOCTORS "MILK YOU"! -☺

Dr. George Mann, a researcher with the Framington Heart Study summed up the <u>WHOLE CHOLESTEROL SCAM</u> in these immortal words:

> "The diet heart hypotheses that suggests that a high intake of fat or cholesterol causes heart disease has been repeatedly shown to be wrong, and yet, for complicated reasons of pride, profit, and prejudice, the hypothesis continues to be exploited by scientists, fund-raising enterprises, food companies, and even governmental agencies.
>
> THE PUBLIC IS BEING DECEIVED BY THE GREATEST HEALTH SCAM OF THE CENTURY."
>
> The take-home message:
>
> JUST SAY NO TO DRUGS!

H. PHAT PHOBIA—"THE LIPID HYPOTHESIS"

The Greatest Scam in Medical History concerns the statin drug connection to cholesterol.

<u>THE CHOLESTEROL SCAM IS INEXTRICABLY LINKED TO WHAT HAS BECOME KNOWN AS THE "LIPID HYPOTHESIS."</u>

<u>WHAT HAS BEEN DUBBED "THE LIPID HYPOTHESIS" HAS SPAWNED WHAT CAN BE CALLED "THE PHAT PHOBIA".</u>

"<u>THE PHAT PHOBIA</u>" is a huge myth which has been destroying the health of North Americans for the last half-century. In 2015 this myth is still pervasive in mainstream nutrition. What is the "lipid hypothesis" and how did it spawn "phat phobia?"

Here's how this flawed theory—this so-called "lipid hypothesis" got started.

Fat Phobia began about the end of the nineteenth century. It really took America by storm in the mid-twentieth century. Just around the time of the First World War, the US Department of Agriculture began to keep track of food and eating trends among Americans. Up to that point in time, most people had been eating <u>LOTS OF HEALTHY FATS</u>, including butter, eggs, and cheese. Most North Americans were cooking with lard.

About 1950 many Americans starting ditching their butter and lard for vegetable oils and margarine. About this time, conventional doctors were even advertising the health benefits of <u>SMOKING CIGARETTES</u>!

How sad that people did not know the 99 <u>PERCENT RULE</u>!

Doctors, "scientists" and food companies also started to push the <u>"THEORY" THAT "A FATTY DIET" CAUSED FATTY ARTERIES.</u>

<u>ACCORDING TO THEORY—THIS "EXCESS IVE FAT CLOGGED OUR ARTERIES WITH CHOLESTEROL. BLOCKED ARTERIES WHICH THEN CAUSED HEART ATTACKS.</u>

<u>THE RISING INCIDENCE OF CORONARY HEART DISEASE</u> (CAD) <u>WAS BLAMED ON SATURATED FATS AND CHOLESTEROL.</u>

For 200 years previously, Americans had eaten <u>HIGH-FAT DIETS</u> but heart problems had been largely unknown. To confront this "new" crisis, American health "experts" <u>DECLARED A BIG WAR ON FAT.</u>

<u>ILL-INFORMED DOCTORS AND DIE-TICIANS—AND OTHER SELF-PROCLAIMED EXPERTS LABELLED ALL FAT—ESPECIALLY SATURATED FAT AS EVIL.</u>

<u>THE WORD "FAT" BECAME A 4-LETTER WORD.</u>

<u>THE SOLUTION TO PREVENT HEART ATTACKS</u> (they said) <u>WAS TO ELIMINATE THE EVIL VILLAIN FAT—ESPECIALLY FAT AND CHOLESTEROL—ITS EVIL PARTNER!</u>

<u>"SATURATED FAT" WAS DUBBED THE KING OF EVIL FATS. FATS OF ALL KINDS WERE SAID TO BE BAD FOR EVERYONE.</u>

<u>THUS BEGAN THE FEAR OF FAT—OR— "PHAT PHOBIA"</u>

<u>THIS NEW THEORY WAS CALLED "THE LIPID HYPOTHESIS".</u> (Lipid means Fat).

<u>THE LIPID HYPOTHESIS " THEORY" CLAIMED THAT:</u>

- <u>SATURATED ANIMAL FAT" RAISES BLOOD CHOLESTEROL LEVELS.</u>

- <u>THIS LEADS TO THE DEPOSITION OF CHOLESTEROL AND OTHER FATS AS PLAQUES WHICH THEN CLOGGED ARTERIES.</u>

- <u>EVIL FAT AND EVIL CHOLESTEROL THEN CAUSES CLOGGED ARTERIES AND CAUSES HEART ATTACKS AND EVERY CARDIOVASCULAR PROBLEM UNDER THE SUN!</u>

<u>HOW</u> did this "lipid hypothesis" originate?

The "<u>FATHER</u>" of this lipid hypothesis was a man named Ancel Keys. The lipid hypothesis came out of his head. The lipid hypothesis was <u>HIS</u> brainchild; he also appears to have created K-rations for WWII. The latter actually helped to keep soldiers alive. His former flawed approach has likely caused <u>MILLIONS OF PREMATURE DEATHS</u>.

Ancel Key's <u>GOAL WAS TO PROVE A DIRECT CORRELATION BETWEEN CALORIES FROM FAT IN THE DIET AND CORRESPONDING DEATH FROM HEART DISEASE AMONG VARIOUS POPULATIONS</u>.

Mr. Keys, a physiologist from the University of Minnesota, carried out what has become known as the "Seven Countries Studies". He studied 22 countries but decided to "cherry-pick "his study results <u>TO PROVE</u> his theory. He focused on 7 countries only. He conveniently forgot about the results from the other countries. From his 7 countries Mr. Keys showed a nearly <u>direct correlation between calories from fat in the diet and deaths from heart disease</u>.

Mr. Keys ignored the countries that didn't fit his pattern.

<u>THIS INCLUDED MANY WHERE PEOPLE EAT A LOT OF FAT BUT DON'T GET HEART DISEASE—AND OTHERS WHERE THE DIETS ARE LOW IN FAT BUT THEIR POPULATIONS HAVE A HIGH INCIDENCE OF FATAL HEART ATTACKS</u>!

History also shows that Mr. Keys swiftly silenced his critics. Remember too that at that time there were newspaper ads by physicians extolling the health benefits from smoking.

<u>CONVENTIONAL DOCTORS, DIE-TICIANS, BIG PHARMA, BIG FOOD AND GOVERNMENT AUTHORITIES QUICKLY</u> <u>RUBBER-STAMPED THIS JUNK SCIENCE.</u>

<u>THIS "JUNK SCIENCE" PERSISTED FOR THE NEXT SEVERAL DECADES</u>.

<u>THIS IS YET ANOTHER CLASSIC ILLUSTRATION OF A MASSIVE FRAUD UNLEASHED ON AN UNSUSPECTING NAÏVE POPULATION</u>!

<u>MY MISSION IN THIS BOOK IS TO TEACH PEOPLE THE 99 PERCENT RULE</u>!

This rule says to do the exact opposite of what medical doctors tell you and ...

<u>YOU WILL BE RIGHT 99 PERCENT OF THE TIME</u>!

<u>HALLELUJAH</u>!

THE BEST THING YOU CAN DO FOR YOUR HEALTH IS TO SIMPLY FOLLOW THIS GOLDEN HEALTH ADVICE!

Phat phobia spawned the "low-fat theory". The low-fat theory PAVED the way for statin drugs to control cholesterol. The American Heart Association circa 1956 began pushing the "prudent diet" which advocated replacing butter, lard eggs and beef with margarine, vegetable oils, cold cereal etc. By the late 1970s the lipid hypothesis, LOW-FAT AND CHOLESTEROL SCAM had become entrenched in the hearts and minds of a naïve, gullible North American population.

MILLIONS OF PEOPLE WERE SCARED TO DEATH TO EAT FAT AND CHOLESTEROL-RICH FOOD.

WE WILL NEVER KNOW HOW MANY MILLIONS OF PEOPLE HAVE DIED OR SUFFERED NEEDLESSLY DUE TO THE LOW-FAT DIET!

FOR THE LAST 60 YEARS- DOCTORS WHO HAVE ADVOCATED LOW-FAT DIETS- AND WHO HAVE PRESCRIBED STATIN DRUGS TO LOWER CHOLESTEROL SHOULD BE ASHAMED OF THEMSELVES!

According to the Harvard School of Public Health:

> The Food Companies saw a tremendous marketing opportunity and re-engineered thousands of foods to be lower in fat or 'FAT FREE'.

HEALTH AUTHORITIES ADVISED CONSUMERS TO REPLACE THE "BAD FATS" WITH HEART-HEALTHY" FATS SUCH AS PROCESSED VEGETABLE OILS, INCLUDING SOYBEAN, CORN, COTTONSEED, CANOLA, PEANUT, SAFFLOWER AND SUNFLOWER OILS.

THIS HORRIFIC NUTRITIONAL ADVICE IS LIKE THROWING YOUR BODY FROM THE FRYING PAN INTO THE FIRE!

Decades ago when FOOD PROCESSING first began, it became regular practice to ALTER that which Mother Nature provided. Thus began the era of "FRANKENFOODS". Whole nutritious foods that came mostly from the farm to the table were replaced by OVER-PROCESSED, REFINED AND CHEMICAL-LADEN CONVENIENCE FOODS.

MORE THAN 5 DECADES OF HEALTHY SOURCES OF FATS WERE REPLACED WITH "VEGETABLE OILS".

Vegetable oils were pushed as "HEALTHIER FOR YOU".

THIS IS ANOTHER MEDICAL LIE!

DOCTORS WHO ADVISE THEIR CLIENTS TO EAT ANY OF THESE FOUR VEGETABLE OILS BELOW—SHOULD BE JAILED!

DIET-ICIANS WHO ADVISE PEOPLE TO EAT THESE BAD FOODS SHOULD NOT BE JAILED IF THEY CAN CONVINCE CROWN PROSECUTORS THAT THE FORMER ARE JUST INNOCENT VICTIMS OF A MASSIVE FRAUD PERPETRATED BY THE MEDICAL/DRUG ESTABLISHMENT.

THE TRUTH IS THESE VEGETABLE OILS HAVE DONE MUCH MORE HARM THAN GOOD.

HERE ARE 4 OF THE WORST OILS:

1. CANOLA OIL

There is no such thing as canola in nature. Canola Oil is actually a modified version of rapeseed oil. Asian and Indian cultures used rapeseed oil for centuries; but it was never family, contains cyanide-containing compounds and in nature wild animals and even insects avoid it. The refining process of deodorizing and bleaching to become canola oil involves exposing rapeseed oil to <u>HIGH</u> heat which greatly reduces the Omega-3 content; (its only original redeeming factor.) Consumption of tis "GMO oil" has been linked to muscular disorders, and fatty degeneration of the heart, kidneys, adrenals and thyroid gland. This oil is ubiquitous, so check labels carefully. Unfortunately, it's even in "so-called healthy products."

2. COTTONSEED OIL

Thousands of commercially produced foods contain cottonseed oil; everything from canned foods to chips and other packaged items. It is even in beverages such as Gatorade. However- cotton is <u>NOT</u> a food crop. Therefore, it is not treated like an edible crop but an industrial one. Virtually nothing can be sprayed on cotton plants to ward off insects and induce growth. Dangerous poisons such as trifluralin, cyanide, dicofol, propargite, and naled are used on cotton crops. These penetrate deep into the plants, literally transforming them into toxic organisms. While this may be okay for the making of pants and shirts; cottonseed oil is not really SAFE to consume. The majority of cotton plants are genetically modified- altered at the molecular level. Even though we ae not eating the cotton plant directly, the extracted oil contains the same properties as the plant. Besides a high-amount of Omega-6 fatty acids, cottonseed oil has a similar protein structure to peanuts; so people who are allergic to PEANUTS may have a serious allergic reaction to this oil, as well. However, the FDA does not require an allergy label on the oil. Peanut Oils can be toxic- even fatal to some people.

3. SAFFLOWER OIL

Studies show than an increase of too much Omega- 6 also increases the risk of death by heart disease. What is important is the ration of Omega 3: to Omega 6 in our diets. The ratio should be no more than 1:1 or 2:1 in favour of O-3's. Studies have found that by substituting animal fats with vegetable oils such as safflower; cholesterol levels would indeed drop. BUT- what these studies failed to evaluate was the <u>HIGH RATIO OF</u> <u>OMEGA 6 TO OMEGA 3 FATS</u> in these oils. The amount of Omega- 6 fatty acids in the American diet has been skyrocketing. Researchers now have evidence that it is not the CHOLESTEROL that kills, but too much Omega ^'s. When a group of individuals replaced animal fats with Omega 6-rich safflower oil, their cholesterol levels decreased; BUT- the rates of death from cardiovascular disease and coronary artery disease increased significantly as compared to those consuming animal fats/ These results prompted researchers to re-evaluate their theories on saturated fat, cholesterol and heart disease. The finger was pointed at the formerly "heart healthy Omega 6 in oils.

4. SOYBEAN OIL

The GMO hormone disrupting nightmare "health food" they keep telling you to eat is SOY. Soy is not beneficial; this is one of the <u>BIGGEST NUTRITIONAL MYTHS</u> out there. Asians eat soy regularly- but in its <u>FERMENTED STATE</u>. 93 percent of American soy is GMO. This highly-processed soy has been linked to a variety of bad health outcomes- including thyroid damage and hormone disruption due to its large quantities of estrogen-like compounds called phytoestrogens.

<u>UP TO 80 PERCENT TO THE OIL CONSUMED TODAY IS SOYBEAN OIL.</u>

<u>IT'S HIGHLY PROCESSED; HEAVILY HYDROGENATED AND FOUND IN THE VAST MAJORITY OF PRODUCTS ON SUPERMARKET SHELVES.</u>

<u>ORGANIC SOY IS NOT SAFE EITHER!</u> Some so-called "organic soy farms" have been found to be fraudulent...passing off the GMO-product for the real thing.

<u>IT'S BEST TO AVOID SOYBEAN OIL.</u>

<u>MY DEAR READERS-</u>

<u>YOU HAVE BEEN LIED TO BY THE MEDICAL ESTABLISHMENT BY THE FOOD INDUSTRY AND BY GOVERNMENT AUTHORITIES!</u>

<u>THIS MASSIVE FRAUD STILL CONTINUES TODAY.</u>

IT IS MY MORAL AND LEGAL DUTY TO ADVISE YOU TO AVOID THIS TERRIBLE HEALTH TRAP.

The adoption of the lipid- hypothesis has resulted in skyrocketing obesity rates, heart disease, cancer and every bad health condition known to man.

ONE FLAWED STUDY BY ONE MAN (Mr. Ancel Keys) HAS DECIMATED THE HEALTH OF NORTH AMERICANS FOR MORE THAN 60 YEARS.

THERE HAS NOT EVEN BEEN ONE SCIENTIFIC STUDY that demonstrates that eating a low-fat, low-cholesterol diet prevents or reduces heart attack or death.

Despite the lack of scientific evidence for the lipid hypothesis, and fat-phobia, the low-fat approach has flourished. Big Pharma has been happy to vilify **CHOLESTEROL AND FATS.**

How else can they dupe the public and sell statin drugs to lower cholesterol?

THE VILIFICATION OF FATS HAS BEEN MADE WORSE BY MAINSTREAM MEDICINE AND DIETICIANS WHO CONTINUE TO PROMOTE THIS JUNK SCIENCE.

EATING A LOW-FAT-HIGH CARBOHYDRATE DIET HAS PROVEN TO BE A PRESCRIPTION FOR HEALTH DISASTER!

WHATEVER THE MEDICAL PROFESSION SAYS TO DO—DO THE OPPOSITE AND 99 PERCENT OF THE TIME YOU'LL BE RIGHT!

YOU MUST DITCH THE LOW-FAT-HIGH CARB APPROACH TO HEALTH PUSHED BY THE WHITE-COATED CROWD.

THE LOW-FAT-HIGH-CARB APPROACH IS A PRESCRIPTION FOR A HEALTH DISASTER! (Studies references).

WE MUST STUFF OUR BODY WITH HEALTHY FATS.

WE MUST KEEP OUR CARB INTAKE AS LOW AS POSSIBLE.

This is the essence of the Ketogenic Diet. There is a **BOATLOAD** of scientific evidence that **SATURATED FATS ARE HEART HEALTHY** and **LOW-FAT DIETS PROMOTE CARDIOVASCULAR DISEASE, DIABETES, CANCER AND A BOATLOAD OF OTHER MEDICAL PROBLEMS.**

Dozens of scientific studies prove that "good" fats (especially saturated) fats are among **HEALTHIEST FOODS** that you can put in your belly **TO PROMOTE SUPERHEALTH.**

GOOD/HEALTHY FATS AND SATURATED FATS ARE VERY HEALTHY FOR YOU!

SATURATED FATS ARE YOUR BEST FRIENDS!

SATURATED FATS MAKE MAGIC KETONE BODIES WHEN EATEN AS PART OF A KETOGENIC DIET.

For many years, saturated fats have been VILIFIED as the cause of a long list of human health problems. Mainstream medical personnel, the American Government, and the media constantly remind us that eating saturated fat will clog our arteries, raise our cholesterol levels and increase our risk of atherosclerosis and death from heart disease.

However, nothing could be further from the truth.

For instance, a paper published in the Journal of the American Medical Association was based on data from the famous Framingham study and reports THAT FAT IN THE DIET PROTECTS AGAINST STROKE.

In an article titled "What if saturated fat is not the problem, Richard Feinman, a Professor of Biochemistry at the State University Medical Center in Brooklyn writes:

> " Perhaps the most compelling research was published in a 2004 issue of the American Journal of Clinical Nutrition by researchers from Harvard School of Public Health. Their study showed that in postmenopausal women with heart disease, a higher saturated fat intake was associated with less narrowing of the coronary and a reduced progression of disease. Even with similar levels of LDL cholesterol, women with lower saturated fat intake had much higher rates of disease progression. Higher saturated fat intake was also associated with higher HDL (the "good" cholesterol) and lower triglycerides." (author underlines)

Do you see how mainstream medicine and the media LIES TO YOU?

DOZENS OF STUDIES AND RESEARCH CLEARLY PROVE THAT –

"CARBOHYDRATE CONSUMPTION" IS THE TRUE VILLAIN WHEN IT COMES TO OUR HEALTH!

CARBOHYDRATES (aka CARBS) POISON OUR PANCREAS AND THEY POISON OUR BRAIN!

CARBS CAUSE OUR PANCREAS TO PRODUCE A HORMONE CALLED "INSULIN."

CONTROLLING OUR INSULIN PRODUCTION AND BLOOD SUGAR LEVELS IS THE NUMBER ONE GOAL FOR US TO BE HEALTHY AND DIS-EASE FREE.

YOU CAN TAKE CONTROL OF YOUR HEALTH BY TAKING CONTROL OF YOUR BLOOD SUGAR.

YOU WILL LEARN HOW TO REGULATE YOUR BLOOD SUGAR LEVELS.

YOU WILL UNDERSTAND WHY MAINTAINING STABLE SAFE BLOOD SUGAR LEVELS IS THE PLATINUM KEY TO OPTIMIZING YOUR HEALTH!

SATURATED FATS EATEN AS PART OF A LOW-CARB DIET HAVE A HUGE BENEFICIAL EFFECT on arterial health and blood sugar.

THE LOWER YOUR CARB INTAKE AND THE HIGHER YOUR SATURATED FAT INTAKE—the less fat, blood sugar, and insulin in the bloodstream. Blood biomarkers that indicate heart disease, insulin resistance, and the symptoms of diabetes, are IMPROVED WHEN EATING A HIGH-FAT LOW-CARB DIET.

Dr. Jeff Volek et al. have authored several studies clarifying the relationship between FAT INTAKE, CARBOHYDRATE INTAKE AND HEALTH CONDITIONS SUCH AS ATHEROSCLEROSIS AND DIABETES.

In one study, Dr. Volek and his team compared the markers for heart disease from the blood of a group of people on a VERY LOW- CARB /HIGH FAT DIET (35 grams of carbs and 100 grams of fat- with 36% percent as SATURATED FAT) with a group on a LOW-FAT DIET (l90 grams of carbs and 24 grams of FAT). Both groups ate about 1,500 calories per day.

DESPITE THE CONSUMPTION OF 3 TIMES THE AMOUNT OF ANIMAL FAT—

> THE GROUP ON THE LOWER CARB DIET HAD LOWER LEVELS OF SATURATED FAT IN THEIR BLOOD THAN THE LOW-FAT GROUP DID!

How amazing is that!

The explanation for this is that when carbohydrate intake is LOW; the body burns FAT as an energy source instead. Since the body is burning the FAT being eaten for energy, there is LESS SATURATED FAT to circulate in the blood.

The take-home message—

- THE FAT CONTENT OF YOUR DIET IS NOT AN INDICATOR OF THE

AMOUNT OF FAT CIRCULATING IN YOUR THE BLOODSTREAM.

- EATING FAT AND CHOLESTEROL HAS NOTHING TO DO WHAT-SOEVER WITH HOW "CLOGGED" YOUR ARTERIES MIGHT BE!

- MOREOVER—THE HIGHER YOUR CARB INTAKE, THE HIGHER YOUR BLOOD SUGAR AND INSULIN AND THE MORE LIKELY YOU WILL DE-VELOP HEART DISEASE—NO MATTER WHAT YOUR FAT INTAKE IS.

- FINALLY—HIGH LEVELS OF BLOOD SUGAR AND INSULIN PRO-MOTE STORAGE OF FAT, INCREASE YOUR BLOOD TRIGLYCER-IDE LEVELS AND INFLAMMATION WITHIN YOUR ARTERIES.

- THIS INFLAMMATION THEN TRIGGERS THE BODY TO BRING CHO-LESTEROL TO THE SITE OF THE INJURY AS A REPAIR MECHANISM.

In sum, you can see that the "lipid hypothesis" which spawned the "Phat Phobia" is another FRAUD.

THESE FRAUDS TOGETHER COMPOSE THE BIG CHOLESTEROL SCAM.

FAT AND CHOLESTEROL ARE YOUR BEST HEALTH FRIENDS.

BIG PHARMA AND THE MEDICAL ESTABLISHMENT ARE YOUR WORST HEALTH ENEMIES.

I. FORCED MEDICATION- MASS MURDER BY WATER

72 PERCENT OF NORTH AMERICANS ARE FORCEFULLY MEDICATED BY DRINKING FLUORIDATED WATER IN THEIR MUNICIPAL WATER SUPPLY.

FLUORIDE IS A NEUROTOXIN- i.e. POISONOUS TO OUR BRAIN!

Water has been fluoridated in North America since 1945 when his inane practice actually began in Grand Rapids Michigan. Putting fluoride in the drinking water of people has been done illegally and without THE CONSENT OF THE PUBLIC!

"Mandatory Fluoridation is medical treatment" stated Professor Aron Afek, an expert in pathology and medical administration who serves as Israel's Health Ministry's Director-General. Israel recently banned all water fluoridation as a result of the latest science confirming that sodium fluoride is poisonous and highly neurotoxic. My chapter on Neurotoxins examines the other toxic poisonous substances that must be eliminated from our diet and from our life.

Fluoride deserves the title- "THE GOD-FATHER OF NEUROTOXINS".

Think of fluoride as a tiny dose of RAT POISON in every single glass of tap water!

Forced medication by placing a neurotoxin- sodium fluoride in the drinking water of millions of consumers is ILLEGAL AND IMMORAL. It contravenes the American Constitution (& American Bill of Rights). Mandatory fluoridation also contravenes the Canadian and Quebec Charters of Rights and Freedoms. A strong legal argument could be made that it also contravenes the Hague Convention/Nuremberg rules of war! The use of poisonous gases such as mustard gas (in WW1) has long been outlawed.

France, Germany, Japan, Sweden, Holland, India, and Great Britain have all rejected its use after its health authorities confirmed its horrific effects on human health. Only a handful of countries such as Australia, Canada, Ireland, New Zealand, the UK and USA, continue this out-dated, barbaric illegal, practice of water fluoridation.

Why has sodium fluoride been put into our drinking water?

The main reason given by authorities is that fluoride is put in your drinking water "for your teeth." It is supposed to fight cavities and strengthen bones. Part of the fraud- the part about fluoride being beneficial for teeth was removed from the "American Fluoride Campaign. This language was removed because this way the masses could still be hoodwinked into believing that fluoride helps with cavities.

THE TRUTH IS- fluoride, technically known as "fluorosilic acid" DOES AFFECT YOUR TEETH. Instead of helping with tooth decay, fluoride actually causes DENTAL FLUOROSIS!

Dental fluorosis is often caused by over-exposure to fluoride when the dental enamel is mineralizing during childhood. Fluoride is extremely powerful in its ability as an acid to penetrate tissue; causing soft tissue damage and bone erosion as it leaches calcium and magnesium from the body. (source: http://tuberose.com/ Flouride.html)

But fluoride does MUCH more than damage teeth:

FLUORIDE IS PROVEN TO:

- Cause all kinds of cancers;
- Calcify the pineal gland (in your skull);
- Cause brain damage in Unborn fetus;

- Impair & lowers IQ- **(
- Damages the Stomach
- Cause heart problems
- Initiate Thyroid Tumours & impairs Thyroid functions
- Create many Reproductive problems
- Impair kidney function
- Cause various skin problems
- Cause receding gums
- Depress cell growth rate

Recent studies show that the latest Chinese fluoride has some bonus- "extras" in it. Recent analysis studies indicate that fluoride now has a wide array of toxic metals- including lead, arsenic, aluminum—and even uranium. This latest version of fluoridated water gives a new meaning "heavy water". This means that fluoride water today is far more TOXIC than it was in 1945. Today it is laced with dozens of heavy metals which are NEUROTIC BY THEMSELVES. Only heaven knows how poisonous the latest fluoridated water really is! The last thing in the world that people need is more toxic metals in their drinking water.

IS IT ANY WONDER WHY MOST OF THE WORLD HAS BANNED THE USE OF THIS DANGEROUS NEUROTOXIN CALLED FLUORIDE?

1. What is sodium fluoride anyway?

Well, it's actually one of the basic ingredients in MILITARY NERVE GAS!

SODIUM FLUORIDE IS A HAZARDOUS WASTE BY-PRODUCT THAT IS PRODUCED AS A BY-PRODUCT OF ALUMINUM.

IT IS ALSO A COMMON INGREDIENT IN ROACH AND RAT POISONS!

2. How and when did this forced mass medication start?

The short explanation is that sodium fluoride was the brainchild of Nazi scientists. History indicates that in the 1930's and 1940's both Hitler and Stalin began using sodium fluoride in the water in the prison camps. This became a great strategy. It was a convenient and very cost-effective way to keep the prisoners docile and dumb-downed. When prison camps were liberated by allied soldiers; often prisoners were found wandering around in a reduced state of awareness. Fluoridation began to cause brain damage and lowered IQ in various ways.

3. Who supplies this poisonous chemical?

Actually, the fluoride used in 90 percent of North American water systems is a lesser quality poison. Unlike that used during the Hitler era, it is Hexafluorosilcic acid —known as silicon fluoride.

China does not fluoridate their public drinking water. They produce and sell 50 percent of all the fluoride which is consumed around the world. The Chinese have now done over 80 experiments that prove fluoride interferes with brain functions that show damage to IQ, fetal damage etc.

The Chinese are laughing all the way to the bank at the stupidity of North American consumers. Apparently it should cost about $ 6,000.00 or $ 7, 000.00 a barrel to DISPOSE OF THIS TOXIC WASTE!

Would you spend billions of dollars to dispose of your toxic industrial waste when you can sell it to people who are ill informed? Would you tell these people that you are selling them toxic poison which causes cancer, brain damage and all kinds of other horrific health problems? Do you see the pattern here? Big Pharma, the medical establishment, and the suppliers of fluoride are all in the same business. They all sell poisonous chemicals FOR PROFIT.

What do you think of this public scam? Sources say that any testing done by municipal water companies, for toxic metals (required by EPA) is done UPSTREAM from where the fluoride is added. It seems that many communities have found a "mysterious residue" in their water treatment systems. The CDC says not to worry. Officials are saying that this doesn't mean that your water is "unsafe." Fluoride does not dissolve- but how can anyone really believe that fluoride causes gummed-up pipes? Some people would have the public believe that people have clogged pipes because of too much bubble gum.-☺

4. Has anyone been publicly sounding the alarm about the dangers of sodium fluoride in our drinking water?

ABSOLUTELY!

There have been DOZENS OF SCIENTIFIC STUD-IES that have shown that sodium fluoride is A NEU-ROTOXIN VERY HARMFUL TO OUR HEALTH!

As early as 1971, Dr. Dean Burke, a Ph.D. did a study of the effects of fluoride in drinking water in the United States and in 1981 he said:

"We estimate that since fluoridation was introduced in the U.S. there have been almost as many deaths associated with fluoridation as the sum total of all American military deaths since 1776 and that one-tenth of the 350,000 cancer deaths in the U.S. are linked with artificial water fluoridation." (authors underline)

Dr. Burke publicly added:

"THIS AMOUNTS TO PUBLIC MURDER ON A GRAND SCALE.

IT IS A PUBLIC CRIME TO PUT FLUORIDE INTO THE DRINKING WATER OF PEOPLE".

(Authors caps)

WATER FLUORIDATION IS MEDICATED MASS MURDER!

WATER FLUORIDATION IS A CRIME AGAINST HUMANITY!

In the last 30 years all kinds of experts have spoken out against the terrible dangers and health consequences of putting fluoride in our water system. Recently, there have been pockets of citizens who are waking up and DEMANDING that fluoride be removed from the public water system.

5. How about more current scientific proof?

There is no doubt about it. Fluoride should not be ingested. Scientists from the EPA's National Health and Environmental Effects research laboratories have classified Fluoride as:

" A chemical having substantial evidence of developmental neurotoxicity. Furthermore, according to the CDC, 41 percent of American adolescents now have dental fleurosis- unattractive discoloration and mottling of teeth that indicates over-exposure to fluoride.

Renowned medical doctor and neurosurgeon, Dr. Russell Blaylock sheds some light on the real dangers of fluoride exposure. When fluoride interacts and is COMBINED with other toxic chemicals commonly found in municipal water supplies.

In his "Why Fluoride is Toxic" report, Dr. Blaylock explains how we all are being lied to about the safety of fluoride chemicals in our water. Widespread government health claims that fluoride is completely safe at current exposure levels are false. Dr. Blaylock argues that they ignore lots of scientific evidence showing both brain and nervous system damage and elevated risk of cancer linked to fluoride exposure.

Another major concern area of research involves fluoride's role in apparently triggering brain diseases such as Alzheimer's. Also, fluoride appears to worsen brain problems in people who have already been diagnosed with dementia.

Dr. Blaylock adds:

> "One study shows that adding fluoride to water in the presence of even small amounts of aluminum caused the destruction of brain cells in the part of the brain which controls learning and memory."

There are studies which show that fluoride enhances the "bioavailability of aluminum."

In a 1998 study reported in the journal "Brain Research", the presence of fluoride and aluminum was identified as a "double whammy". Fluoride mixed with aluminum made aluminum much more toxic. The World Health Organization (WHO) suggests in a report on aluminum that aluminum (salts) coupled with fluoride chemicals resulted in increased aluminum concentrations of aluminum at many water treatment plants. Again, the heavy metal combo effect was strongly evidenced. (source: http://w3.newsmax.com)

THE MOUNTING SCIENTIFIC EVIDENCE IS CONCLUSIVE AND COMPELLING.

And people who already have compromised immune systems or with pre-existing health problems are at an even greater risk. Even at very "low doses" considered safe by government, FLUORIDE can have a dramatic impact on neurological function, brain chemistry and cardiovascular function. All of the foregoing is clearly outlined in the scientific literature—which is hiding in plain sight.

For more information, you can check out the relevant literature prepared by groups like FLUORIDE ACTION NETWORK (FAN) – www.FluorideAlert.org.

The latest study, hot off of the press— was published on September 28th, 2014 in the journal Toxicology. The article was entitled "Effect of Water Fluoridation in the development of medial vascular calcification in euremic rats."

Commenting at www.GreenMedInfo.com , its founder Sayer Ji commented as follows:

> "Now a provocative new study published in journal Toxicology not only provides some vindication for our previous interpretations, but also raises serious concern

over the cardiovascular complications associated with water fluoridation practices, showing for the first time that despite exhibiting anti-calcifying effects in vitro (cell model), fluoride exposure at levels found in people who drink fluoridated water exhibits artery-calcifying effects in the more important in vivo (animal model).

This latest study also confirmed previous science concerning fluoride, namely, according to the authors:

"More than 90 % of the ingested fluoride is absorbed through the intestine and quickly distributed between plasma/soft tissues and calcified structures, where it can be sequestered for years.(Buzalf & Whiteford 2011)."

(author underline)

You can read an excellent article concerning the evils of fluoride—an article called "Fluoride is Killing us softly" published in the above website on December 4th, 2013.

6. What other things contain fluoride?

FLUORIDE IS CONTAINED IN HUNDREDS OF DIFFERENT FOODS AND BEVERAGES.

FLUORIDE IS PRESENT IN EVERYTHING FROM PHOSPHATE FERTILIZERS TO CRACKING AGENTS FOR THE PETROLEUM INDUSTRY.

FLUORIDE IS THE FIRST NEUROTOXIN THAT YOU MUST ELIMINATE FROM YOUR WATER, FROM YOUR ENVIRONMENT AND FROM YOUR LIFE

Take-home message:

- YOU MUST AVOID FLUORIDE. IT IS "THE GOD-FATHER OF NEUROTOXINS".

- CLEAN PURE WATER IS A PRE-REQUISITE TO OPTIMUM HEALTH.

- DR. CLEAN WATER IS ONE OF YOUR BEST DOCTORS-☺

- CLEAN PURE WATER IS THE NUMBER ONE SU-PERFOOD IN THE WORLD.

- YOU MUST ELIMINATE FLUORIDE FROM YOUR DIET!

J.   THE END OF ANTIBIOTICS- 'SUPERBUGS' ARE HERE!

When you were young you were told that germs, bugs and viruses were bad things to be avoided. They were all kind of lumped together. You didn't necessarily understand what they were, but you knew that they were <u>BAD</u> for you. If you got an infected cut or caught a severe cold, you were taken to the doctor. You likely left with an antibiotic to take care of your "health problem."

Today- thanks to science- we're a lot smarter. Now we know and understand that there are <u>TWO KINDS BACTERIA</u>- the <u>GOOD</u> and the <u>BAD</u>. You will learn later in this book about the importance of our quadrillion little bacteria in and on our bodies. If you're a healthy, smart person you may even have some <u>pro-biotic yogurt</u> in your fridge.

<u>FERMENTED –PROBIOTIC FOODS SUCH AS YOGURT ARE ESSENTIAL TO GOOD HEALTH. FERMENTED FOOD PRODUCTS ARE GOOD BACTERIA THAT PROMOTE GOOD "GUT FLORA".</u>

What's happening with antibiotics?

Scientists are experimenting with viruses to battle diseases such as HIV. Antibiotics have emerged as being a double-edged sword.

<u>MANY ANTIBIOTICS PRESCRIBED FOR DECADES BY CONVENTIONAL MEDICINE ARE NO LONGER EFFECTIVE.</u>

Worse yet- now we're becoming victims of the "cure."

<u>ANTIBIOTICS HAVE SPAWNED NEW DRUG-RESISTANT "SUPERBUGS".</u>

<u>PENICILLIN</u> was discovered in 1928. At that time, <u>IT WAS A MIRACLE CURE</u>. For almost eight decades, penicillin has been the pride and joy of <u>BIG PHARMA</u> and the <u>ALLOPATHIC</u>, conventional medical community.

There is only one little problem. Mother Nature is fighting back against poisonous man-made chemicals called "antibiotics." The overuse of penicillin and other antibiotics has spawned a new bunch of drug-resistant <u>SUPERBUGS</u>. These new superbugs spawned by Mother Nature are now defeating antibiotics (chemical drugs) invented by humans.

Before the discovery of the first antibiotic, anything from syphilis to splinters could and often did lead to death. Once an infection entered the body, it spread rapidly. With the birth of antibiotics, <u>ALLOPATHIC MEDICINE</u> mistakenly believed that it had finally conquered <u>INFECTION</u>.

ALLOPATHIC MEDICINE IS WRONG ABOUT OUR HEALTH 99 PERCENT OF THE TIME!

THE END OF ANTIBIOTICS IS MORE SAD PROOF THAT ALLOPATHIC MEDICINE HAS BEEN A DISMAL FAILURE.

In 1961, the first case of what would become known as "Methicillin Resistant Staphyloccus" (MRSA) was diagnosed in the United Kingdom. MSRA, as its name suggests is a staph infection that's immune to Methicillin, a POTENT ANTIBIOTIC.

THE DANGEROUS TRUTH — MRSA IS NOT THE ONLY "SUPERBUG" WHICH HAS BEEN SPAWNED BY ANTIBIOTICS.

DO NOT "ESKAPE" TO YOUR NEAREST HOSPITAL!

"ESKAPE" is a clever acronym for ENTEROCOCCUS, STAPHYLOCCUS, KLEBSIELLA, ANCINETOBACTER, PSEUDOMONAS, and ENTEROBACTER.

THESE " SUPERBUGS" ARE NOW THE MOST COMMON ORGANISMS FOUND IN THE STANDARD HOSPITAL ENVIRONMENT. ("Hospital" literally means "a place to die.")

HOSPITAL ACQUIRED INFECTIONS KILL AT LEAST 48,000 PEOPLE EVERY YEAR. That's 3 TIMES MORE than people who die from HIV.

WITH THE PASSAGE OF TIME, AND THE OVERUSE OF ANTIBIOTICS, MANY ORGANISMS HAVE DEVELOPED "SUPERBUGS" OR BASICALLY AN IMMUNITY TO TREATMENT.

The same is true with such "old" diseases such as gonorrhea, chlamydia, and syphilis. One night's indiscretion once meant an embarrassing visit to the doctor and an injection. NOW— once again- it can mean a DEATH sentence!

BIG PHARMA'S DRUGS ADMINISTERED BY ALLOPATHIC DOCTORS HAVE UTTERLY AND COMPLETELY FAILED. ANTIBIOTICS HAVE NOW BECOME MORE DANGEROUS THAN LIFE-SAVING!

THE END OF ANTIBIOTICS SPELLS THE END OF THE VIABILITY OF DRUG- PUSHERS. TIME TO REJOICE...HALLELUJAH!

Even TUBERCULOSIS is reappearing on the medical horizon. Resistant strains are popping up in various areas of the world. Once TREATABLE—nearly 1.5 MILLION PEOPLE DIE FROM THIS ANCIENT DISEASE VERY YEAR.

More than 500,000 of those infected suffer from a strain that is <u>RESISTANT TO TREATMENT</u>. Is this a coincidence? I think not. My research suggests that this is another example of the overuse and misuse of <u>ANTIBIOTICS</u>.

<u>SOME</u> conventional doctors have realized that antibiotics are a double edged sword so they are starting to cut back on their usage. Most often, however, when someone brings in a child to a doctor's office with a runny nose—they leave with a prescription for <u>ANTIBIOTICS</u>.

If people wish to take antibiotics—all they have to do is eat commercial meat! Commercial beef and poultry is laced with <u>ANTIBIOTICS</u>.

If the meat that you are eating is <u>NOT ORGANIC; YOU ARE UNKNOWINGLY INGESTING MASS QUANTITIES OF ANTIBIOTICS!</u>

<u>TODAY</u>— <u>MORE THAN 80 PERCENT OF ANTIBIOTICS</u> in the United States are not given to humans. Instead, they are force-fed to "healthy" animals and poultry. The convoluted logic is that antibiotics promote growth and healthier food.

There are at least <u>TWO</u> small problems.

- <u>THESE ANTIBIOTICS ARE INCREASING THE CASES OF DRUG-RESISTANT E. COLI AND SALMONELLA.</u>

- <u>THE ANTIBIOTICS EATEN BY ANIMALS</u> (cows, chickens, pigs and poultry.) <u>ARE DESTROYING THE HEALTH OF THE NORTH AMERICAN POPULATION!</u>

Are you unknowingly <u>EATING ANTIBIOTICS?</u>

When Jonas Salk "cured" polio in 1955, he made the compassionate choice to give it away for the benefit of humanity as a whole. His <u>GENEROSITY</u> has improved the lives of millions. While his vaccine certainly helped, it turns out that the number of cases was actually <u>PETERING OUT</u> anyway.

<u>THE WHOLE SUBJECT OF VACCINES IS BADLY MISUNDERSTOOD BY THE ENTIRE MEDICAL ESTABLISHMENT</u>. Please see Crimes Against Humanity-(supra).

Currently, only 5 major drug companies are currently researching new antibiotics.

As at 2008, only 15 out of 167 drugs under development have the <u>POTENTIAL</u> to treat organisms with multi-drug resistance. None are marketed presently.

There are 3 reasons for the <u>END OF ANTIBIOTICS.</u>

- <u>1. BIG PHARMA CANNOT DEFEAT MOTHER NATURE'S POWER.</u>

- <u>2. BIG PHARMA DOES NOT WANT TO FIND A "CURE" WITH NEW ANTIBIOTICS.</u>

- <u>3. THERE IS NO MONEY TO BE MADE FROM A NEW ANTIBIOTIC.</u>

- Why give someone a drug that is a quick-fix? Where's the money in that? Big Pharma would much rather sell heart pills, pills for diabetics; cholesterol-lowering drugs etc. It's much more profitable to sell pills that a patient has to take for a lifetime!

  It's all about separating people from their hard-earned cash.

  <u>BIG PHARMA AND THEIR ALLOPATHIC CRONIES MAKE BIG MONEY FROM DISEASE MANAGEMENT— NOT PROVIDING HEALTH CARE.</u>

  Why research and discover new antibiotics?

<u>IT'S FAR MORE PROFITABLE TO SELL VACCINES.</u>

<u>VACCINE MANUFACTURERS ARE IMMUNE FROM LAWSUITS—</u>

That's why there are 200 <u>NEW VACCINES</u> coming down the drug pipe-line -☹

<u>SEVEN REASONS TO AVOID ANTIBIOTICS—</u>

1. <u>80 PERCENT OF THE ANTIBIOTICS USED ARE PUMPED INTO FARM ANIMALS</u> (used for meat and dairy) by the CAFA (Confined Animal Feed Animals).

2. Clostridium Difficile Infection

   One of the very common side effects of antibiotic use is infection of the colon. Toxins given off from the strain of bacteria, known as "Colstrum Difficile, ("C-Diff" Infections,) as they are known in the medical community, cause severe <u>DIARRHEA AND SEVERE DAMAGE TO THE GASTROINTESTINAL TRACT</u>—C-Diff infections are notorious for causing Leaky Gut Syndrome (see infra).

3. <u>Liver Damage</u>

   The liver is the organ that has the greatest responsibility for filtering out toxins and other unwanted substances from the body. Because of this, it is also the organ <u>MOST</u> likely to be harmed by certain medications like antibiotics. A new study from the medical Journal Gasterenterology found that antibiotics were the <u>WORST</u> group of medications to damage the liver.

4. <u>The cancer link</u>

Antibiotic use has been linked to cancer. One shocking study found that those who had taken 6 or more antibiotic prescriptions had a <u>1.5 TIMES GREATER RISK</u> for developing certain more usual types of cancer in comparison with those who had a lower antibiotic exposure.

5. <u>Chronic Fatigue Syndrome</u> (CFS)

CFS is a chronic viral illness that has been linked to antibiotic use as well. Belgian researchers believe they have uncovered a link between the onset of CFS and a build-up of hydrogen sulphite in the body.

This build-up can occur after antibiotic use, a Salmonella infection or excessive mercury exposure.

6. <u>Aids</u>

Some researchers also believe that there might be a link between overuse of antibiotics and a weakened or damaged immune system; which ironically can lead to even more problems with bacterial and other types of infections. AIDS patients are among the highest users of antibiotics in North America.

7. <u>Fungal and Bacterial Overgrowth</u>

Antibiotics do destroy bacteria but they also trigger and increase endotoxins from the body itself, which suppress the immune system. This suppression of immunity along with killing off of good bacteria can lead to bacterial or fungal overgrowths such as an infestation of Candida. That is why yeast infections are so common after a round of antibiotics.

8. <u>A weakened immune system</u>

Using antibiotics to fight off an infection is a sort of "Quick Fix". That may do the job but does not allow the body to develop its own resistance. This lack of resistance development may lead to a weakened immunity that actually makes infections more of a possibility.

<u>The take-home message:</u>

<u>BE CAREFUL</u> about taking antibiotics at the first sign of a sniffle. These pills <u>MAY</u> temporarily provide relief for the problem in the

SHORT run. BUT—they WILL also cause long-term health issues that actually make you more vulnerable to infection and disease.

ANTIBIOTICS DAMAGE YOUR IMMUNE SYSTEM- BIG TIME!

ANTIBIOTICS EAT A HOLE IN THE LINING OF YOUR GUT.

ANTIBIOTICS DECIMATE THE GOOD BACTERIA IN YOUR GUT.

ANTIBIOTICS LIKE ALL POISONOUS DRUGS CAUSE MORE HARM THAN THEY DO GOOD.

According to a landmark report entitled "Antibiotic Resistance Threat Report" published by the Center for Disease Control (CDC):

> "2 million Americans become infected with antibiotic-resistant bacteria each `year, and at least 23, 000 of them die as a direct result of those infections. Even more die from complications." (author underline)

The CDC has admitted that we are now living in a "post-antibiotics era."

Dr. Arjun Srinivasan, Associate director of the CDC stated in a PBS interview:

> "We've reached the end of antibiotics, period...we're here. We're in the post-antibiotic era. There are patients for whom we have no therapy; and we literally are in a position of having a patient in a bed who has an infection, something that five years ago even we could have treated, but now we can't. "

THE END OF ANTIBIOTIC DRUGS MEANS THE COLLAPSE OF THE ALLOPATHIC MEDICAL EMPIRE! HALLELUJAH!

We're quickly heading in that direction. Imagine hip surgery without antibiotics!

Modern medicine has shot itself in the foot. Most "allo-pathetic" doctors refuse to use natural substances to treat infections, which is why they erroneously BELIEVE that no defenses exist against SUPERBUGS. Mainstream conventional doctors have been totally and utterly BRAINWASHED BY BIG PHARMA.

Allopathic doctors cannot even CONCEIVE of the idea that an herb, a food, or something from Mother Nature's Farmacy might provide the answer to antibiotic-resistant SUPERBUGS.

Allopathic doctors are clueless about the nutritional and natural methods used by Dr. Hippocrates—he Father of Medicine. He used therapeutic— NATURAL ANTIBIOTICS supplied by Mother Nature. He used onions, garlic, honey, red wine, and many other natural antibiotics.

History reveals that the Yellow Emperor (4th Century B.C.) successfully used FMT (Fecal Microbial Transplants) to transplant good bacteria (poop) into unhealthy people.☺

This may sound gross—BUT –FMT IS NOW being successfully used by the Mayo Clinic to CURE C-DIFFICILE INFECTIONS WITH A 98 PERCENT SUCCESS RATE!

NO CHEMIST OR DRUG-MAKER CAN OUTSMART MOTHER NATURE.

What does the RESEARCH say?

Studies show that store-bought meat is OFTEN CONTAMINATED WITH SUPERBUGS! Many studies show a multitude of resistant organisms on meat and poultry products purchased in grocery stores. A recent study of meat and poultry from five U.S. cities found STAPHYLOCOCEUS AUREUS ON 47 PERCENT OF SAMPLES!

- 96 PERCENT OF THOSE SAMPLES WERE RESIS- TANT TO AT LEAST ONE ANTIBIOTIC— and

- 52 PERCENT WERE MULTI-DRUG RESISTANT!

Tests conducted by the FDA every year routinely show high levels of antibiotic bacteria on retail meat.

IN 2010, 52 PERCENT OF CHICKEN BREAST TESTED WAS CONTAMINATED WITH ANTI-BIOTIC-RESISTANT E-COLI!-☹

You'd better say good-bye to your local greasy spoon and fast food joint.

What does the farm use of antibiotics REALLY DO TO HUMANS?

When farm animals receive antibiotics in doses too low to kill all of the infectious bacteria in them, those bacteria that survive and flourish, do so because they are resistant to the drug. As they multiply and interact with other bacteria, they pass on their resistance.

Bacteria can even share the traits that make them drug resistant with other kinds of bacteria leading to widespread drug-resistance and the creation of bacterial SUPERBUGS!

How do these SUPERBUGS spread?

Antibiotic resistant bacteria generated in CAFO's (Confined Animal Feeding Operations) (aka monster agricultural farms) spread in several ways.

By food—As mentioned, testing of meat in retail stores typically finds drug-resistant bacteria on meats and poultry products. Bacteria on food carried into the kitchen where other foods can become cross-contaminated by contact with infected knives, cutting-board, surfaces, our hands etc. We then inadvertently spread these bacteria to other people.

By air and water—Drug-resistant bacteria have been found in drinking water; near hog facilities in 3 states ad have been detected in the air DOWNWIND from industrial swine facilities. (source: Natural Resources Defense Council) www.nrdc.org)

Have you ever smelled pig manure? PHEW! ☺) If you do– you may never want to eat bacon again.-☺

Low doses of antibiotics have been used since the 1950's to enhance growth.

IN THE U.S.— 80 PERCENT OF ALL ANTIBIOTICS ARE NOW USED ON FARM ANIMALS. But- LOW DOSES encourage resistance, just as Alexander Fleming (creator of penicillin—WARNED! Not only have recent studies shown that antibiotic- drug resistant bacteria been found widely in farm animals raised for meat...they have ALSO BEEN FOUND IN WILD ANIMALS; including crows, foxes and skunks.

Scientists are fighting and losing— a running battle with SUPERBUGS!

Why? It is very simple.

Chemists in labs cannot create magic potions to outsmart Mother Nature! Chemists in labs cannot outsmart bacteria-resistant bugs. Drugs have never cured or solved anything.

ANTIBIOTICS HAVE NOW LOST THEIR ABILITY TO SAVE LIVES!

Another factor is that livestock workers sometimes accidently transport drug-resistant bacteria on their clothing and bodies. Unwittingly, they sometimes pass them on to other family members, friends and communities.

Many European countries STOPPED using penicillin, streptomycin, and tetracyclines to promote faster growth in animals in the 1970's. This policy was expanded to other antibiotics in the 1990's and to all antimicrobial growth promoters across the European Union. In May 2011, NRDC filed a lawsuit against the FDA to end the use of antibiotics in animal feed. It appears that that lawsuit is now in progress.

In 1928, Alexander Fleming who discovered the first antibiotic (penicillin) won the Nobel Prize for Medicine in 1945 warned of the dangers of antibiotic resistance.

He said:

> " It is not difficult to make microbes resistant to peni-cillin in the laboratory by exposing them to concen-trations not insufficient to kill them...There is the danger that the ignorant man may easily under dose himself and by exposing his microbes to non-lethal quantities of the drug make them more resistant." (source: www.NobelPrize.org)

Fleming's predictions proved right! Penicillin- resistant bacteria arrived while the drug was still being given to only a few patients. Now each class of antibiotics since has been greeted by resistant bacteria. Beta-agonist drugs such as Zilmax belong to a class of non-hormone drugs used as a growth promoter in American livestock. As a class, beta-agonist drugs have been used in US cattle production since 2003.

Ractopamine, another beta-agonist, is yet another drug used in the USA; even though it's been **BANNED** in 160 other countries due to its potential health hazards. Beta-antagonist drugs like Ractopamine and Zilmax are fed to cattle in the weeks prior to slaughter to increase weight by as much as 30 pounds of lean meat per cow. As much as **20 PERCENT** of the drug administered may remain in the meat you buy! The horrific effects Zilmax has on cattle includes lost hooves and lameness—and a host of other terrible effects —**TOO GROSS** to even mention.

The latest scientific discovery disputes all claims that low concen-trations of pharmaceutical drugs in our environment are harm-less. In fact, their evolutionary capabilities have proven to be very **DANGEROUS**!

In a Swedish study published on October 7th, 2014 in the Journal Bio, (source: http://www.eurekalert.org) scientists discovered that heavy metals —combos like copper, silver and arsenic coupled with low levels of antibiotics help develop harmful dangerous drug-resis-tant bacteria.

"Biocides" are chemicals used to suppress organisms that are harmful to human or animal health or that cause damage to natural or manufactured materials. Examples, according to the European Commission are insect repellents, industrial chemicals and disinfectants.

According to this Swedish study:

- **About 50 % of the antibiotics used to treat humans and animals are UNCHANGED and in ACTIVE FORM ARE EXCRETED IN THE URINE!**

Professor Andersson says:

> **"These results are worrying and suggest that substances other than antibiotics that are present in very small quantities can drive development of resistance as well. The results underline the importance of reducing the use of antibiotics—but also suggests that our high use of Heavy metals and Biocides in various contexts should decrease too".**

Excrement containing pharmaceutical drugs eventually ends up in the environment, which is ALARMING because the environmental aspects of this process are WIDELY UNKNOWN. This new study sheds some light on what is happening these days and how their presence in the environment contributes to antibiotic resistance; as well as their REACTION WITH HEAVY METALS present in nature due to natural sources and human activities.

Professor Andersson continued:

> **"These antibiotics then disperse usually in very low concentrations, through sewage systems into the water and soil where they can remain active in the environment for a very long period, and so contribute to the enrichment of resistant bacteria...**

> **...in most environments there are complex mixtures of antibiotics, biocides and heavy metals that together have intensified combination effects. "**

The take-home message:

THE END OF ANTIBIOTICS HAS ARRIVED—THAT'S THE BAD NEWS.

THIS MEANS —THE END OF MODERN MEDICINE- THAT'S THE GOOD NEWS!

HALLELUJAH! IT'S TIME TO REJOICE!

THE OVERUSE OF PENICILLIN AND ANTIBIOTIC DRUGS HAS SPAWNED A NEW GENERATION OF "DRUG-RESISTANT SUPERBUGS".

THIS IS THE ULTIMATE PROOF THAT "ALL DRUGS" DO MORE HARM THAN GOOD.

MOTHER NATURE HAS TRIUMPHED ONCE AGAIN.

FOOD IS MOTHER NATURE'S SOLUTION TO HEAL US.

NO PERSON WEARING A WHITE-COAT WILL EVER TRUMP MOTHER NATURE.

TO HEAL OURSELVES—

WE MUST GET OUR MEDICINE FROM MOTHER NATURE'S FARMACY.

MOST OF THE WORLD HAS DONE THIS FOR MILLENNIA.

K. THE MOST IMPORTANT HEALTH DISCOVERY EVER! (Dr. EARTH)!

"Since the late 20th century, chronic degenerative diseases have overcome infectious disease as the major causes of death in the 21st century, so an increase in human longevity will depend on finding an intervention that inhibits the development of these diseases and slows their progress."

-De Flora et al.

"Earthing the human body influences human physiological processes, including increasing the activity of catabolic processes and may be the primary factor regulating endocrine and nervous systems"

-K. Sokal and P. Sokal

Introduction

HUMANS ARE ELECTRICAL BEINGS!

Your body is capable of generating electricity, and this ability is actually a key part of achieving health. Electricity allows your nervous system to send signals to your brain. These signals are electrical charges that are delivered from cell to cell; from synapse to synapse for almost instantaneous communication.

The messages conducted via electrical signals in your body are responsible for controlling the rhythm of your heartbeat, the circulation of blood throughout your body and much more.

Your biological clock uses electrical activity in order to help keep your circadian rhythms in order.

YOU ARE QUITE SIMPLY AN ELECTRICAL BEING.

If electrical activity stops in your body, you die.

How does this electrical activity take place?

Your body uses a complex process to generate electricity. Inside your body are atoms that are made up of positively charged protons, negatively charged electrons and neutrons-(neutral).

An atom with unbalanced charges will become either positively or negatively charged, and the switch from one charge to the other allows electrons to flow from one atom to another. This is what is referred to as "electricity".

Your cells generate electrical charges via electrolytes like sodium and potassium using a mechanism known as the "sodium-potassium gate." As Discovery Magazine explained:

"When your body needs to send a message from one point to another, it opens the gate. When the membrane gate opens, sodium and potassium ions move freely into and out of the cell.

Negatively charged potassium ions leave the cell, attracted to the positivity outside the membrane; and positively charged ions enter it, moving toward the negative charge. The result is a switch in the concentrations of the two types of ions-and rapid switch in charge.

...this flip between positive and negative generates an electrical pulse. This impulse triggers the gate on the next cell to open, creating another charge, and so on. In this way, an electrical pulse moves from nerve to nerve in your stubbed toe to the part of the brain that senses pain."

Defibrillators work because of your body's electricity; they deliver an electric shock to your heart which jump starts your heart rhythm and why receiving the wrong type of shock, like an electric shock, or lighting strike can essentially "fry" your body's electrical system.

The opposite also hold true.

YOU CAN ACTUALLY HARNESS THE ELECTRICAL CHARGE OF THE EARTH TO POSITIVELY INFLUENCE YOUR HEALTH IN NUMEROUS WAYS.

EARTHING (OR "GROUNDING") refers to the discovery of benefits-including better sleep, and reduced pain—from walking barefoot outside or sitting, working, or sleeping indoors connected to conductive systems that transfer the **EARTH'S ELECTRONS FROM THE GROUND INTO THE BODY.**

YOUR BODY CAN ABSORB A LIMITLESS NUMBER OR FREE ELECTRONS FROM MOTHER EARTH!

OUR CREATOR CREATED US AND HE CREATED DR. EARTH TO SUPPLY US WITH AN UNLIMITED SUPPLY OF FREE ELECTRONS!

The Earth carries an enormous negative charge. It's always electron-rich and serves as a powerful abundant supply of **ANTIOXIDANT AND FREE-RADICAL BUSTING ELECTRONS.**

Your body is finely tuned to "work" with the Earth in the sense that there is a constant flow of energy between your body and the Earth. When you put your feet on the ground, you absorb large amounts of negative electrons through the soles of your feet.

The effect is sufficient to maintain your body at the same negatively charged electrical potential as the Earth. This simple process is called "grounding" or "earthing".

THE GROUNDING EFFECT IS ONE OF THE MOST POWERFUL ANTIOXIDANTS WE KNOW OF!

WHEN YOU WALK BAREFOOT OUTSIDE ON GRASS OR A SANDY BEACH—YOU ARE RECEIVING THE BEST MEDICINE IN THE WORLD FROM DR. EARTH!

Throughout history, humans mostly walked barefoot or with footwear made of animal skins. They slept on the ground or on skins. Through direct contact or through perspiration-moistened animal skins used as footwear or sleeping mats, the ground's abundant free electrons were able to enter the body, which is electrically conductive.

Through this mechanism, every part of the body could equilibrate with the electrical potential of the Earth, thereby stabilizing the electrical environment of all organs, tissues, and cells.

Modern lifestyle has increasingly separated humans from the primordial flow of Earth's electrons. For example, since the 1960s, we have increasingly worn insulating rubber or plastic soled shoes, instead of the traditional leather fashioned from hides.

During recent decades, chronic illness, immune disorders, and inflammatory diseases have increased dramatically, and some researchers have cited environmental factors as the cause. However, the possibility of modern disconnection with Earth's surface as a cause has not been considered.

At the end of the last century, experiments initiated independently by Ober in the USA and K. Sokal in Poland revealed distinct physiological and health benefits with the use of conductive bed pads, mats, EKG-and TENS type electrode patches, and plates connected indoors to the Earth outside.

Ober, a retired cable television executive, found a similarity between the human body (a bioelelectrical, signal-transmitting organism) and the cable used to transmit cable television signals. When cables are "grounded" to the Earth, interference is virtually eliminated from the signal. Furthermore, all electrical systems are stabilized by grounding them to the Earth.

D. Sokal meanwhile discovered that grounding the human body represents a "universal regulating factor in Nature" that strongly influences bioelectrical, bioenergetics and biochemical processes and appears to offer a significant modulating effect on chronic illnesses encountered daily by healthcare professionals.

Environmental medicine is the wave of the future. Environmental medicine focuses on the interactions between human health and the environment, including factors such as compromised air and water and toxic chemicals, and how they cause or mediate disease. Omnipresent throughout the environment is a surprisingly beneficial, yet overlooked global resource for health maintenance, disease prevention and clinical therapy; the surface of the Earth itself. It is an established, though not widely appreciated fact, thobat the Earth's surface possesses a limitless and continuously renewed supply of free or mobile electrons. The surface of the planet is electrically conductive (except in ultra dry areas such as deserts); and its negative potential is maintained (i.e. its electron supply is replenished) by the global atmospheric electrical circuit.

Mounting evidence suggests that the Earth's negative potential can create a stable internal bioelectrical environment for the normal functioning of all body systems.

Moreover, oscillations of the intensity of the Earth's potential is important for setting the biological clocks regulating diurnal body rhythms, such as CORTISOL SECRETION.

Research has also proven that electrons from antioxidant molecules neutralize reactive oxygen species (ROS), or "free radicals" involved in the body's immune and inflammatory responses. It is assumed that the influx of free electrons absorbed into the body through direct contact with the Earth neutralize (ROS) and thereby reduce acute and chronic inflammation.

EARTHING (aka GROUNDING refers to contact with the Earth's surface electrons by walking barefoot outside or sitting, working, or sleeping indoors connected to conductive systems, some of them patented, that transfer the energy from the ground into the body.

Emerging scientific research supports the concept that the EARTH'S ELECTRONS INDUCE BETTER SLEEP, A SHIFT FROM SYMPATHETIC TO PARASYMPATHETIC TONE TO THE AUTONOMOUS NERVOUS SYSTEM (ANS), AND A BLOOD-THINNING EFFECT.

HERE ARE DR. EARTH'S MAGICAL GROUNDING EFFECTS:

1. Sleep, chronic pain, stress and cortisol

The studies show that most grounded subjects described symptomatic improvement while the control subjects did not. Many subjects reported significant relief from asthmatic and respiratory conditions, rheumatoid arthritis, PMS, sleep apnea, and hypertension while grounded. These results indicated that the effects of earthing go WAY beyond reduction of pain and improvements in sleep.

Studies focused on the cortisol levels in grounded and ungrounded subjects. Cortisol levels before and after grounding were monitored. In unstressed subjects, the normal 24-hour cortisol secretion profile follows a predictable pattern: lowest around midnight and highest around 8 a.m. The studies showed a realignment and normalization trend of patterns after 6 weeks of sleeping grounded. Subjective symptoms of sleep dysfunction, pain and stress were reported daily during the 8 week test periods. The majority of subjects with high-to out-of range night time secretion levels experienced improvements in sleeping grounded. Restoration of normal day-night cortisol secretions was observed. And—all subjects reported falling asleep more quickly—and—all subjects reported waking up fewer times during the night.

Grounding the body at night during sleep also positively affected morning fatigue levels, daytime energy, and night time pain levels.

About 30 percent of the American adult population complain of sleep disruption, and 10 percent have associated symptoms of daytime functional impairment consistent with the diagnosis of insomnia. Insomnia often correlates with major depression, general-ized anxiety, substance abuse, dementia, and a plethora of pain and physical problems.

The direct and indirect of insomnia have been estimated <u>AT TENS OF BILLIONS OF DOLLARS IN THE USA ALONE.</u>

2. Reduction in overall stress levels and shift to ANS Balance

A study investigated the effects of grounding on human physiology. Earthing was accomplished with a conductive adhesive patch placed on the sole of each foot. A biofeedback system recorded electrophys-iological and physiological parameters. Subjected were exposed to 28 minutes in the unearthed condition followed by 28 minutes with the earthing wire connected. (Controls were unearthed for 56 minutes.)

Upon earthing 50 percent of the subjects showed an <u>abrupt, almost instantaneous change in root mean square</u> (rms) values of electro-encephalograms (EFGs) from the left hemisphere, (but not from the right hemisphere) at all frequencies analyzed by the biofeedback system (beta, alpha, theta and delta)/

All grounded subjects presented an abrupt change in rms values of surface electromyograms (SEMGs) from right and left upper trape-zius muscles.

Earthing decreased blood volume pulse (BVP) in 19 of 22 subjects.

Earthing the human body showed significant effects on electrophysi-ological properties of electrophysiological recordings.

<u>Taken together, the changes in EEG, FMG, and BVP, PROVE REDUCTIONS IN OVERALL STRESS LEVELS AND TENSIONS AND A SHIFT IN ANS BALANCE UPON EARTHING.</u>

Another grounding study involved a 2-hour grounding sessions while subjects were seated in comfortable recliners.

<u>The results proved quite amazing!</u>

These results were documented:

- an immediate decrease (within a few seconds in skin conductance (SC) at grounding and an immediate in-crease at un-grounding. (no change for controls).

- Respiratory rate (RR) increased during grounding, an ef-fect that lasted after un-grounding. RR variance increased immediately after grounding and then decreased;

- Blood oxygenation (BO) variance decreased during grounding, followed by a dramatic increase after un-grounding;

- Pulse rate (PR) and perfusion index (PI) variances increased toward the end of the grounding period. And this change persisted after un-grounding.

- THIS IMMEDIATE DECREASE IN SC INDICATED A RAPID ACTIVATION OF THE PARASYMPATHETIC NERVOUS SYSTEM AND A CORRESPONDING DEACTIVATION OF THE SYMPATHETIC NERVOUS SYSTEM.

The immediate increase in SC at cessation of grounding indicates an opposite effect. Increased RR, stabilization of BO, and slight rise in heart rate suggested...

"the start of a metabolic healing response necessitating an increase in oxygen consumption".

3. Immune cell and pain responses with Delayed-Onset Muscle Soreness Induction

Pain reduction from sleeping grounded has been documented in previous studies.

Another pilot study looked for blood markers that might differentiate between grounded and ungrounded subjects who completed A SINGLE SESSION OF INTENSE

ECCENTRIC EXERCISE RESULTING IN DELAYED-ONSET-MUSCLE SORENESS (DOMS) OF THE GASTROCNEMIUS (calf muscle).

DOMS is a common complaint in the Fitness and Athletic world following excessive/extreme physical activity; and involves acute inflammation in "overtaxed" muscles. DOMS develops in 14 to 48 hours and persists for more than 96 hours. There are several known treatments that reduce the recovery period.

THESE INCLUDE MASSAGE FOAM ROLLING, HYDROTHERAPY (and CONTRASTS), AND ACUPUNCTURE.

In one study healthy young men did a toe-raise routine with a barbell equal to 1/3rd of their body weight. The grounded group placed a conductive patch on the sole of each foot during active hours and a conductive sheet at night. Complete blood counts, blood chemistry, enzyme chemistry, serum and saliva cortisol, MRI, spectroscopy, and pain levels;

A TOTAL OF 48 PARAMETERS WERE TAKEN—at 24, 48 and 72 hours afterwards).

Parameters that differed by these criteria included white blood cell counts, bilirubin, creatine kinase, phosphocreatine/organic phosphate ratios, glycerolphosphorycholine, phosphorylcholine, the visual analogue pain scale, and pressure measurements on the right gastrocnemius.

THE STUDY RESULTS WERE AMAZING!

The results showed that grounding the body to the Earth <u>alters measures of immune system activity and pain</u>.

Among the ungrounded men, there was an expected, sharp increase in white blood cells at the stage when DOMS is known to reach its peak, and a greater perception of pain.

This effect demonstrates a typical <u>inflammatory response</u>.

The grounded men had only a slight decrease in white blood cells, <u>indicating scant inflammation;</u>—

FOR THE FIRST TIME EVER OBSERVED—A SHORTER RECOVERY TIME!

The researchers commented that there were significant differences in the pain reported by the grounded men! Ungrounded men expressed the perception of greater pain and muscle soreness.

4. <u>Heart Rate Variability</u>

Studies also show that grounding improves heart rate variability (HRV).

In one study, participants were grounded with adhesive electrode patches placed on the soles of their feet and the palms of their hands. Two hour grounding sessions showed amazing results- again!

In a nutshell- during the grounding sessions, participants had statistically significant **IMPROVEMENTS IN HRV THAT WENT WAY BEYOND BASIC RELAXATION RESULTS!**

GROUNDING CALMS YOUR SYMPATHETIC NERVOUS SYSTEM.

This supports your heart rate variability.

WHEN YOU SUPPORT (HRV) THIS PROMOTES HOMEOSTASIS (OR BALANCE) OF YOUR AUTONOMIC NERVOUS SYSTEM.

ANYTIME YOU IMPROVE YOUR HEART RATE VARIABILITY (HRV)—

YOU ARE IMPROVING YOUR ENTIRE BODY AND ALL OF ITS FUNCTIONS!

5. Body vitamins and minerals and osteoporosis

In one study involving non-medicated subjects, grounding during a SINGLE NIGHT OF SLEEP:

RESULTED IN STATISTICALLY SIGNIFICANT CHANGES IN CONCENTRATIONS OF MINERALS AND ELECTROLYTES IN THE BLOOD SERUM, IRON, IONIZED CALCIUM, INORGANIC PHOSPHOROUS, SODIUM, POTASSIUM AND MAGNESIUM!

RENAL EXCRETION OF BOTH CALCIUM AND PHOSPHORUS WAS REDUCED SIGNIFICANTLY.

THE OBSERVED REDUCTIONS IN BLOOD AND URINARY CALCIUM AND PHOSPHORUS PROVES THAT:

EARTHING FOR A SINGLE NIGHT REDUCES PRIMARY INDICATORS OF OSTEOPOROSIS. Translation:

EARTHING CAN BE AN AMAZING TOOL TO PREVENT AND TREAT OSTEOPOROSIS! No poisonous drugs and no doctor required!

6. Grounding reverses diabetes mellitus

In one grounding study, diabetic patients had been prescribed the drug glibenclamide, an anti-diabetic drug for 6 months—BUT at the time of the study had UNSATISFACTORY GLYCEMIC CONTROL DESPITE DIETARY AND EXERCISE ADVICE AND GLIBENCLAMIDE DOSES OF 10 mg/day!

When these diabetic patients grounded continually during rest and physical activity over a 72- HOUR PERIOD THEY HAD DECREASED FASTING GLUCOSE!

GROUNDING (Dr. EARTH) REVERSES DIABETES FAR BETTER THAN DRUGS AND GROUNDING IS FAR SAFER AND FAR CHEAPER!

7. Grounding regulates thyroid hormones

In another study, 6 healthy males and 6 healthy females with no history of thyroid disease, grounded for a SINGLE NIGHT.

BLOOD SAMPLES SHOWED A SIGNIFICANT DECREASE OF FREE-TRI-IODOTHYRONINE AND AN INCREASE OF FREE THYROXINE AND THYOID-STIMULATING HORMONE.

THIS PROVES EARTHING HAS A PROFOUND EFFECT ON HEPATIC, HYPOTHALAMUS AND PITUITARY RELATIONSHIPS WITH THYROID FUNCTION.

Ober et al have observed that many individuals on thyroid "medications" reported symptoms of HYPERTHYROID, SUCH AS HEART PALPITATIONS AFTER STARTING GROUNDING. SUCH SYMPTOMS TYPICALLY VANISH AFTER "MEDICATION" IS ADJUSTED DOWNWARD.

THIS IS EXTREMELY IMPORTANT BECAUSE:

THROUGH A SERIES OF FEEDBACK REGULATIONS, THYROID HORMONES AFFECT ALMOST EVERY PHYSIOLOGICAL PROCESS IN THE BODY, INCLUDING GROWTH AND DEVELOPMENT, METABOLISM, BODY TEMPERATURE, AND HEART RATE!

ZOWIE!

Grounding produces many changes in many electrical properties of our bodies.

Grounding produces important changes in the electrical properties of our BLOOD.

A SUITABLE MEASURE IS THE ZETA POTENTIAL OF RED BLOOD CELLS (RBCs) AND RBC AGGREGATION.

ZETA POTENTIAL is a parameter closely related to the number of negative charges on the surface of an RBC. The higher the number is the greater the ability of the RBC to repel other RBCs.

THUS THE GREATER THE ZETA-POTENTIAL— THE LESS COAGUABLE THE BLOOD- translation— the THINNER YOUR BLOOD IS.

Grounding the body to the earth substantially increases the ZETA-POTENTIAL AND DECREASES RBC AGGREGATION, THEREBY REDUCING BLOOD VISCOSITY.

A pilot study on the electrodynamics of red blood cells (zeta-potential) has revealed that earthing significantly reduces BLOOD VISCOSITY; an important but neglected parameter in cardiovascular diseases and diabetes, and circulation in general.

THUS —THINNING THE BLOOD ALLOWS FOR MORE OXYGEN DELIVERY TO TISSUES AND FURTHER SUPPORT THE REDUCTION OF INFLAMMATION.

RESEARCH SHOWS THAT GROUNDING INCREASES ZETA-POTENTIAL BY A WHOPPING 280 PERCENT!

STRESS REDUCTION HAS BEEN CONFIRMED WITH VARIOUS MEASURES SHOWING RAPID SHIFTS IN ANS FROM SYMPATHETIC TO PARASYMPATHETIC DOMINANCE, IMPROVEMENT IN HEART RATE VARIABILITY, AND NORMALISATION OF MUSCLE TENSION.

SUBJECTS IN PAIN REPORTED REDUCTION TO ALMOST ZERO PAIN!

In 2008, Adak and colleagues DISCOVERED THE PRESENCE OF BOTH HYPERCOAGULABLE BLOOD AND POOR ZETA-POTENTIAL AMONG DIABETICS.

ZETA-POTENTIAL WAS PARTICULARLY POOR AMONG DIABETICS WITH CARDIOVASCULAR DISEASE.

More amazing research by Mess'rs Ober and K Sokal et al. in last 20 years shows that:

REGULAR EARTHING:

- improves blood pressure

- cardiovascular arrhythmias and autoimmune conditions such as lupus, multiple sclerosis, and rheumatoid arthritis.

From a practical standpoint, healthcare providers could recommend outdoor "barefoot sessions" to patients, weather and conditions permitting. Ober et al. have observed that going barefoot as little as 30 or 40 minutes daily can significantly reduce pain and stress. The studies mentioned here explain why this is the case.

Obviously, there is no cost for barefoot grounding. However, the use of conductive systems while sleeping, working, or relaxing indoors offer a more convenient and routine-friendly approach.

The big take-home warning:

DR. EARTH (Grounding) IS A PHENOMENAL HEALING DOCTOR.

YOU ARE HEREBY WARNED—if you are taking "medications" of any kind, you are strongly advised to be careful.

If you are taking medications to thin your blood (e.g. Coumadin poison), blood sugar drugs, drugs to control blood pressure, and/or drugs to regulate thyroid hormone levels—

IF YOU WALK BAREFOOT ON THE GRASS OR BEACH YOU COULD SERIOUSLY THREATEN YOUR HEALTH—UNLESS YOU ADJUST YOUR MEDICATION ACCORDINGLY!

Earthing influences thyroid function, so if you are on thyroid medication, you may begin to feel symptoms of over-medication. Similarly, if you are on Coumadin, you need to know that there could be a compounded response, and <u>TOO MUCH</u> blood thinning.

You will need to monitor your blood carefully and check with a knowledgeable healthcare advisor (not the pill pusher who put you on blood thinners – that doctor probably does not know his arse from his elbow-☺ …Your doctor has likely never heard of Dr. Earth-☺

We also know that the regulation of blood sugar improves so— if you take blood sugar pills or anti-diabetic "meds" <u>YOU</u> will have to monitor yourself.

Also, if you are taking any anti-inflammatory drugs, you will also have to monitor your response and dosage.

<u>REMEMBER</u>—

<u>YOU MUST BE YOUR OWN DOCTOR.</u>

<u>YOU MUST LISTEN TO YOUR BODY.</u>

<u>YOU MUST WEAN YOURSELF OFF POISONOUS DRUGS WHEN YOU ARE BEING HEALED BY DR. EARTH AND/OR DR. KETO OR THE OTHER NATURAL DOCTORS…</u>

<u>VERY OFTEN POISONOUS DRUGS DO NOT MIX WITH HEALTHY FOOD.</u>

<u>NO ONE KNOWS HOW DRUGS INTERACT WITH VARIOUS FOODS/SUPPLEMENTS.</u>

<u>OFTEN DRUGS HAVE HORRIFIC EFFECTS WHEN COMBINED WITH DR. EXERCISE- TOO!</u>

Whether you are barefoot on the ground outside, or grounding yourself indoors for many hours with an Earthing system, you want to have the best and safest experience possible.

If you have any doubts at all whether Earthing may be safe for you, simply go out in your backyard, or to your nearest grassy park, or sandy beach and sit/stand/walk barefoot for at least <u>30 TO 40 MINUTES.</u>

Your body is absorbing the same natural energy from the Earth.

It's a simple experiment and often a surprising one.

<u>YOU WILL FEEL BETTER AND NOTICE A DIFFERENCE IN A VERY SHORT PERIOD OF TIME!</u>

YOU CAN PURCHASE GROUNDING MATS AND GROUNDING PRODUCTS FOR INDOOR GROUNDING AT VERY REASONABLE PRICES AT WEBSITES SUCH AS EARTHING.CA.

YOU WILL BE AMAZED WITH HOW GREAT YOU FEEL AFTER A SHORT BOUT OF GROUNDING WITH DR. EARTH!

YOU WILL COME TO LOVE DR. FEEL-GOOD-☺ (aka DR. EARTH).

GROUNDING IS THE GREATEST HEALTH DISCOVERY EVER!

GROUNDING IS A HEALING ENERGY THAT OUR ANCESTORS DID.

GROUNDING WILL REGULATE YOUR BLOOD SUGAR LEVELS AND YOUR ENTIRE METABOLISM.

GROUNDING WILL REVERSE YOUR DIABETES.

GROUNDING WILL PERMIT YOU TO WEAN YOURSELF OFF ANTI-DIABETIC, BLOOD- SUGAR, BLOOD THINNING/PRESSURE PILLS AND THYROID DRUGS.

GROUNDING IS A POWERFUL "STRESS BUSTER" WHICH WILL CALM YOU AND INCREASE YOUR HEART-RATE VARIABILITY (HRV).

GROUNDING WILL FIX DOMS AND SORE MUSCLES.

GROUNDING WILL PROVIDE THE BEST SLEEP AND HEAL YOU DURING YOUR SLEEP- FOR THE REST OF YOUR LIFE!

GROUNDING WILL CHANGE YOUR BLOOD FROM THICK RED CATSUP TO THE CONSISTENCY OF RED WINE-☺

GROUNDING WILL TURN ON YOU PARASYMPATHETIC NERVOUS SYSTEM.

GROUNDING WILL RELAX AND CALM YOU AND SHUT OFF YOUR CORTISOL PUMP...

GROUNDING WILL INCREASE YOUR ZETA-POTENTIAL, DECREASE INFLAMMATION; BOLSTER YOUR IMMUNE SYSTEM, AND ALLOW YOUR BODY TO RECOVER FROM STRESSFUL EXERCISE.

DR. EARTH IS YOUR BEST SOLUTION TO STOP INFLAMMATION THAT REDUCES YOUR RISK OF HEART DISEASE AND OTHER INFLAMMATORY ILLNESSES.

DR. EARTH WILL HELP YOU TO ATTAIN SUPERHEALTH AND FITNESS.

AND BEST OF ALL...DR. EARTH (grounding) is FREE!

ENJOY!

CHAPTER TWO
FIRE YOUR DOCTOR—
HIRE YOURSELF!

"Anything the medical profession says, do the opposite-

99 percent of the time and you'll be right."

Aajonus Vonderplanitz,

A. Introduction

In chapter one, I traced the evolution of modern western allopathic medicine. We saw how Western Medicine has SUPPRESSED THE NUTRITIONAL-BASED APPROACH TO MEDICINE.

BIG PHARMA, BIG MEDICAL AND BIG MEDIA HAVE SUPPRESSED NATURAL MEDICINE. We saw how Big Government, Big Pharma, Big Medicine and their puppets—LAMESTREAM MEDIA have supressed the unpleasant truth about how drug-based Western medicine has damaged North American people. We analyzed how western medicine has evolved into a greedy corrupt BUSINESS manipulated by the pharmaceutical companies. Western health-care systems have become corrupt "Ponzi-schemes" which profit from human misery and death caused by conventional doctors and Big Pharma.

THE ALLOPATHIC MODEL OF MEDICINE HAS FAILED MISERABLY.

WE HAVE HEALTHCARE SYSTEMS AND ALLOPATHIC DOCTORS THAT COULD CARE LESS ABOUT NUTRITION. PLUS—

WE HAVE A FOOD SYSTEM THAT DOES NOT CARE ABOUT HEALTH!

ALLOPATHIC MEDICINE AND ALLOPATHIC DOCTORS ARE THE EXACT ANTITHESIS TO HEALTH!

ALLOPATHIC DOCTORS ARE PILL— PURVEYORS OF DISEASE AND DEATH!

DRUGS AND PILLS HAVE NEVER CURED ANYTHING—AND NEVER WILL!

99 PERCENT OF WHAT ALLOPATHIC DOCTORS ARE DOING AND SAYING IS COMPLETELY WRONG!

"ANYTHING THE MEDICAL PROFESSION SAYS—DO THE OPPOSITE, 99 PERCENT OF THE TIME YOU'LL BE RIGHT!"

Doctors have become the number one <u>KILLER</u> of adults in North America. In my opening chapter, other topics covered were the "Truth about cancer, Cardiologists—or Criminals". The" Great Cholesterol Scam, the "Lipid Hypothesis"- "Phat Fhobia" and "Mass Medical Murder" by water fluoridation.

I also examined the subject of <u>VACCINATIONS</u>—aka "CRIMES AGAINST HUMANITY. Sadly, we have reached the end of <u>ANTIBIOTICS</u>. Once antibiotics were the 'pride and joy" of allopathic medicine used to fight disease. The <u>OVERUSE</u> of antibiotics by Big Agriculture and ill-informed doctors has transformed antibiotics into <u>PURVEYORS OF INFECTIONS AND DISEASE.</u>

Antibiotic drugs have now become <u>DANGEROUS</u>. They have spawned <u>NEW DRUG-RESISTANT BACTERIA</u> that cause more harm than good. Moreover, the Pharmaceutical Industry has conceded defeat. They know that investing millions of dollars in research for new antibiotic <u>DRUGS</u> is a waste of time and money. Big Pharma knows that they can manufacture hundreds of other drugs and make <u>BAZILLIONS OF DOLLARS</u>. There is no financial incentive to create new antibiotics... so Big Pharma does not give a hoot...about anything but selling profitable drugs.

Chapter one finished on a very <u>POSITIVE NOTE!</u>

<u>YOU LEARNED ABOUT THE GREATEST HEALTH DISCOVERY EVER!</u>

<u>YOU NOW CAN HEAL YOURSELF. NO DOCTOR REQUIRED!</u>

<u>YOU NOW CAN HIRE YOURSELF.</u>

<u>AND DR. EARTH'S RATES ARE VERY AFFORDABLE</u>-☺ **(24/7!)**

THE DEMISE OF ANTIBIOTIC DRUGS MEAN THAT ALLOPATHIC MEDICINE NO LONGER HAS ANY DRUGS THAT CAN HELP MANAGE DISEASE SYMPTOMS.

YOUR DOCTOR WILL SOON NOT EVEN BE ABLE TO GIVE YOU A SHOT OF PENICILLIN-OR ANY OTHER INJECTION THAT WILL HELP YOU REGAIN HEALTH.

ALLOPATHIC DOCTORS HAVE LOST THE ONLY DRUG THAT HAD ANY THERAPEUTIC VALUE!

How will surgeons be able to do surgery? …they won't!

Medical doctors spend hundreds of thousands of dollars on their education. They go to medical school with noble intentions. Doctors pay thousands of dollars for the privilege to use the letters "MD"; and—AFTER THAT—THEY ARE UNLEASHED UPON AN ILL-INFORMED NAÏVE PUBLIC TO PRACTICE SELLING DRUGS FOR BIG PHARMA.

Allopathic doctors receive a VERY-FLAWED EDUCATION which teaches them ALMOST NOTHING about how to help sick people get well. Their medical education teaches them NOTHING about how to prevent illness or disease. Their pharmaceutical teachers do not want them to know about NUTRITION. Big –Pharma cannot tolerate "their doctors" learning about NATURAL, NON-PHARMACEUTICAL WAYS TO HEAL SICK PEOPLE. Medical students are taught to diagnose symptoms and to match those symptoms with poisonous drugs and/or how to use a scalpel; aka- "CUT, BURN POISON"

WHEN PEOPLE LEARN that eating nutritious food makes them healthy-

BIG PHARMA WILL GO BANKRUPT! ALLOPATHIC DOCTORS WILL GO OUT OF BUSINESS!

IF DOCTORS PRESCRIBED NUTRITIOUS FOOD AND EXERCISE-DOCTORS' WAITING ROOMS WOULD BE EMPTY.

IF DOCTORS PRESCRIBED VITAMIN D— MOST DOCTORS' WAITING ROOMS WOULD BE EMPTY! (so would their bank accounts-☺)

THE WORST THINGS ABOUT A DOCTOR'S EDUCATION ARE:

1. At the end of medical school what has been taught to doctors is OBSOLETE.

2. What doctors are taught is in any event COMPLETELY WRONG!

CAN YOU SEE HOW "MEDICALLY IMPOTENT" MOST DOCTORS ARE?

THE DECISION TO FIRE YOUR DOCTOR IS ONE OF THE MOST IMPORTANT DECISIONS THAT YOU WILL EVER MAKE.

This chapter- "Fire Your Doctor and Hire Yourself" is divided into two sections—Section B in which I explain the top three reasons you should "FIRE YOUR DOCTOR"

In Section C- I analyze many reasons why you should "HIRE YOURSELF".

Conceptually- I have separated the perceived NEGATIVE part- (Fire Your Doctor) from the VERY POSITIVE part – (Hire Yourself)-☺

THE STRUCTURE OF MY BOOK MIRRORS THIS CONCEPTUAL APPROACH.

THROUGHOUT MY BOOK I ANALYZE THE SERIOUS CHALLENGES AND APPARENT BARRIERS TO YOUR HEALTH- BUT—

THEN PROPOSE THE POSITIVE HEALTH STRATEGIES YOU CAN USE TO TAKE CONTROL OF YOUR HEALTH- BE YOUR OWN DOCTOR –SO THAT YOU CAN TAKE A DO-IT-YOURSELF (DIY) APPROACH TO YOUR HEALTH.

MY BOOK CELEBRATES THE POWER OF MOTHER NATURE AND THE POWER OF OUR CREATOR!

MY BOOK CELEBRATES THE AMAZING HEALING POWERS OF OUR BODIES USING A WELL-CONSTRUCTED KETOGENIC DIET.

MY BOOK CELEBRATES THE HEALING POWER OF NUTRITIOUS FOODS!

FOOD HAS BEEN OUR REAL MEDICINE FOR THE LAST 30 MILLION YEARS!

FOOD WILL CONTINUE TO BE OUR MEDICINE UNTIL THIS PLANET CEASES TO EXIST.

EVERYTHING THAT WE NEED TO BE HEALTHY, STRONG AND DISEASE-FREE HAS EXISTED SINCE HUMANS HAVE ROAMED THIS PLANET.

DR. HIPPOCRATES WAS RIGHT 10 MINUTES AGO- in the 5th Century B.C.-☺

AYURVEDIC AND CHINESE MEDICINE HAVE USED FOOD AS MEDICINE FOR THE LAST 5,000 YEARS!

DRUGS AND ALLOPATHIC DOCTORS WILL NEVER BE THE ANSWER!

HUMAN SOCIETY DOES NOT NEED BIG PHARMA AND ITS ALLOPATHIC DRUG DEALERS.

THE ONE HUNDRED YEAR DRUG EXPERIMENT USED BY THE ALLOPATHIC MEDICAL ESTABLISHMENT HAS NOT ONLY FAILED—IT HAS MORPHED INTO A CRIMINAL BUSINESS AND SHOULD BE OUTLAWED—PERIOD!

You do not need to wait for sleepy corrupt politicians to wake up and pass laws that change the allopathic medical model. You do not need to wait any longer to learn how to take care OF YOUR HEALTH AND WELL-BEING

I'm excited and pleased to provide you with leading-edge health knowledge and practical tools/strategies.

THE TOOLS AND HEALTH INFORMATION PROVIDED HEREIN WILL ALLOW YOU TO BY-PASS BIG PHARMA AND THE MEDICAL ESTABLISHMENT!

YOU WILL BE PROVIDED WITH THE TOOLS SO THAT YOU CAN TAKE A DO-IT-YOURSELF (DIY) APPROACH TO YOUR HEALTH AND WELL-BEING.

LET'S GET STARTED WITH YOUR ACTION HEALTH CARE PLAN!

YOUR FIRST ACTION STEP IS:

TO FIRE YOUR DOCTOR—AND HIRE YOURSELF!

B. REASONS TO FIRE YOUR DOCTOR

It is very likely have already you have already identified some good reasons to dismiss your doctor from chapter one. Here are another 99 good reasons to fire your doctor:

NINETY-NINE PERCENT OF WHAT YOUR DOCTOR SAYS TO DO—IS WRONG!

IF YOU DO THE OPPOSITE OF WHAT YOUR DOCTOR SAYS—99 PERCENT OF THE TIME YOU'LL BE RIGHT!

FROM A BOATLOAD OF REASONS TO FIRE YOUR DOCTOR— HERE ARE MY TOP 3 REASONS.

REASON NUMBER ONE—

YOUR DOCTOR DOES NOT KNOW "HIS ARSE FROM HIS ELBOW".

The expression to "not know your arse from your elbow" was apparently used from 1700 for about the two hundred years until circa

1920, when it fell into disuse in North America because it was perceived to be vulgar. This is not true. This expression is still widely used in Britain to denote someone who is very ignorant—or dumb-witted.

This expression accurately describes most allopathic doctors. The reason that your doctor does not know his arse from his elbow is due to your doctor's medical training.

In short—

YOUR DOCTOR RECEIVED A BADLY –FLAWED MEDICAL EDUCATION!

> Your doctor likely spent 7-8 years of his life and paid a quarter million dollars for his medical education. Conventionally trained doctors should ask for a refund of their medical school expenses-☺
>
> In medical school allopathic doctors are BRAINWASHED BY BIG PHARMA. Many allopathic doctors never wake up to the truth about their medical ignorance until they get sick or a family member gets sick. That's when they learn that drugs and surgery are USELESS; and only make HEALTH PROBLEMS WORSE.
>
> By then of course—it's too late for them or their patients.
>
> DOCTOR MEANS "TEACHER"-SO-
>
> YOU SHOULD FIRE YOUR "TEACHER" AND HIRE YOURSELF!
>
> YOUR TEACHER HAS RECEIVED A FLAWED EDUCATION.
>
> HAS YOUR DOCTOR TAUGHT YOU ANYTHING ABOUT YOUR HEALTH OR HOW TO TAKE CARE OF YOUR HEALTH?
>
> ALLOPATHIC DOCTORS HAVE RECEIVED AN INCOMPLETE – DRUG BASED EDUCATION; - ALLOPATHIC DOCTORS TAKE THAT MEDICAL IGNORANCE AND FOIST THEMSELVES ON A NAÏVE POPULATION.
>
> ON TOP OF THAT, MANY WESTERN DOCTORS VIEW THEMSELVES AS GODS AND THEIR PATIENTS AS THEIR SUBJECTS. YOUR DOCTOR LIKELY TREATS YOU WITH ARROGANCE AND A CONDESCENDING ATTITUDE BECAUSE HE WEARS A WHITE FROCK DECORATED WITH A RUBBER TUBE PROVIDED BY BIG PHARMA.

YOUR LOCAL BUTCHER ALSO WEARS A WHITE FROCK—TOO.

YOUR BUTCHER IS MORE ESSENTIAL TO YOUR GOOD HEALTH THAN YOUR DOCTOR IS.

YOUR DOCTOR PROVIDES POISONOUS CHEMICALS (aka "MEDICATIONS". YOUR BUTCHER KNOWS MORE ABOUT NUTRITION AND HEALTHY MEAT THAN YOUR DOCTOR.

YOUR BUTCHER DESERVES MORE RESPECT.

DOCTORS CAUSE THE DISEASES THEY CLAIM TO CURE!

DOCTORS ARE TRAINED TO TREAT DISEASE—NOT THE PATIENT.

MODERN MEDICINE IS DISEASE-CENTRED- NOT PATIENT-CENTERED.

"Diagnosis" in Greek means knowing the central under- standing of a problem".

"Differential diagnosis" means "What disease does this patient have?

ALLOPATHIC MEDICINE IS A SHAMEFUL DYSFUNCTIONAL APPROACH.

YOU NEED TO ASK ENVIRONMENTAL QUESTIONS.

YOUR DOCTOR KNOWS NOTHING ABOUT NUTRITION.

YOUR DOCTOR KNOWS LITTLE ABOUT BIOCHEMISTRY.

YOUR DOCTOR KNOWS LITTLE ABOUT HUMAN PHYSIOLOGY.

YOUR DOCTOR IS ALSO CLUELESS ABOUT ENVIRONMENTAL HEALTH.

At most, your doctor had a few hours provided in his medical curricu- lum. Your grandmother probably knows more about nutrition than your doctor.

Your doctor has never studied ANYTHING about herbs, naturopathic, homeopathic, Traditional Chinese or Ayurvedic medicine Chinese and Ayurvedic medicine use a patient-centered NON-INVASIVE – NON-TOXIC MEDICAL APPROACH.

YOUR DOCTOR IS CLUELESS ABOUT THE BIOCHEMISTRY OF NUTRITION.

YOUR DOCTOR HAS INADEQUATE KNOWLEDGE OF HUMAN PHYSIOLOGY.

YOUR DOCTOR IS CLUELESS ABOUT "ALTERNATIVE-AND/OR NATURAL" MEDICINE APPROACHES.

YOUR DOCTOR IS CLUELESS ABOUT NATUROPATHIC, HOMEOPATHIC AND OSTEOPATHIC MEDICINE.

YOUR DOCTOR IS CLUELESS ABOUT CHIROPRACTIC MEDICINE.

YOUR DOCTOR IS CLUELESS ABOUT ACUPUNCTURE, ENERGY HEALING AND A BOATLOAD OF OTHER NON-TOXIC HEALTH REMEDIES.

YOUR DOCTOR IS ALSO IGNORANT ABOUT THE IMPORTANCE OF EATING NUTRIENT-DENSE FOOD.

YOUR DOCTOR DOES NOT CARE ABOUT NUTRITION.

YOUR DOCTOR HAS BEEN TAUGHT TO SCOFF AT VITAMINS AND MINERALS AND OTHER MICRONUTRIENTS.

YOUR DOCTOR PROBABLY REFERS PATIENTS TO A DIE-TICIAN.

WHILE YOU'RE AT IT—

YOU PROBABLY SHOULD FIRE YOUR DIE-TICIAN TOO!

(My Persian cat knows more about nutrition than most die-ticians-☺}

YOUR DOCTOR IS CLUELESS ABOUT THE HEALING POWERS OF NUTRITIOUS FOODS, AND THE HUGE VARIETY OF MICRONUTRIENTS AND OTHER COMPOUNDS CONTAINED IN ORGANIC FRUITS AND VEGETABLES.

YOUR DOCTOR IS CLUELESS ABOUT MOTHER NATURE'S FARMACY!

FACT—94 percent of physicians have a financial relationship with the Pharmaceutical Industry.

<u>FACT—Only 6 percent of drug advertising material sent to doctors is supported by the scientific evidence.</u>

<u>YOUR DOCTOR TAKES HIS MARCHING ORDERS FROM BIG PHARMA.</u>

<u>YOUR DOCTOR DOES NOT KNOW WHAT TO DO—SO HE DOPES YOU UP!</u>

<u>Your doctor tries to match a drug to your symptoms. Your doctor has been taught—"a pill for every ill." So— your doctor prescribes poisonous drugs to YOU. These drugs only make you sicker. These drugs CAUSE you to come back to his office. Then your doctor prescribes even MORE drugs. More drugs make YOU even sicker!</u>

<u>YOUR DOCTOR DOES NOT KNOW HOW TO FIND THE CAUSE OF ANY MEDICAL CONDITION!</u>

<u>YOUR DOCTOR HAS NOT BEEN "TAUGHT" HOW TO DISCOVER THE ROOT CAUSE OF ANY DISEASE.</u>

<u>YOUR DOCTOR TREATS SYMPTOMS WITH DRUGS (or surgery)-PERIOD!</u>

<u>AS YOU GET SICKER AND SICKER—YOUR DOCTOR AND BIG PHARMA GET RICHER AND RICHER!</u>

<u>YOU ARE ONLY A "CASH-COW" FOR YOUR DOCTOR.</u>

<u>YOU ARE ONLY A PILL-PURCHASER TO YOUR DOCTOR.</u>

<u>WHEN YOU VISIT YOUR DOCTOR- IT'S LIKE GOING TO THE LOCAL DRUGSTORE TO BUY DRUGS. THE ONLY DIFFERENCE IS THE PILLS YOU PURCHASE WITH A SCRIBBLED NOTE FROM YOUR DOCTOR COST A LOT MORE MONEY!</u>

<u>THE PLAIN TRUTH IS-</u>

Your doctor has been conditioned to believe <u>ANYTHING BIG PHARMA SAYS.</u>

W.C Fields said "There's a sucker born every minute". Your doctor likely is a sucker who has been brainwashed by Big Pharma since his first year of medical school. Unlike lawyers- doctors bury their mistakes! Don't let your doctor brainwash you with his medical non-sense! You should fire your doctor!

Big Pharma continues to brainwash allopathic doctors post medical school by providing continuing "education" (think drug) courses.

Big Pharma makes sure that your doctor's continuing education courses DO NOT INCLUDE ANYTHING TO DO WITH NUTRITION.

BIG PHARMA HAS BEEN SUPPRESSING THE TRUTH ABOUT THE HEALING POWERS OF NUTRITION SINCE THE DAY THAT THE MEDICAL PROFESSION WAS CREATED- almost 100 years ago.

ALLOPATHIC DOCTORS AND BIG PHARMA HATE NUTRITION!

NUTRITION IS A THREAT TO THE VERY EXISTENCE OF BIG PHARMA AND THE MEDICAL ESTABLISHMENT! Big Pharma can't get a PATENT ON FOOD.

NO PATENT MEANS NO MONEY. THE PRACTICE OF ALLOPATHIC MEDICINE IS THE MEDICAL PRACTICE OF MATCHING DRUGS TO A SYMPTOM. YOUR DOCTOR HAS BEEN TAUGHT TO " Name that symptom and then to whip out a drug that "appears" to... match...or have helpful effects...

THE MAIN DIFFERENCES BETWEEN A PHARMACIST AND AN ALLOPATHIC DOCTOR ARE:

1. A pharmacist sells drugs over a counter. Your pharmacist is your doctor's BUSINESS partner. Together- your doctor and your pharmacist manage a very lucrative legalized DRUG BUSINESS. Unfortunately, ONE HORRIFIC EFFECT of this drug business is that MANY OF THESE POISONOUS DRUGS END UP IN THE HANDS OF TEEN-AGERS!

2. MANY OF PRESCRIPTION DRUGS ALSO END UP CONTAMNATING THE LOCAL WATER SUPPLY—FOREVER!

   YOUR DOCTOR WITH HIS DRUG PUSHER—THE LOCAL PHARMACIST) BOTH KILL PEOPLE LEGALLY WITH POISONOUS DRUGS.

   Doctors and pharmacists cause drug deaths by selling prescription drugs to patients. Patients either flush these drugs down the toilet (and/or pee them out); either way, these drugs end up in the local water supply. When a patient leaves a medicine cabinet open and readily accessible to any household member- very often these dangerous prescription drugs end up on the street being used by teen-agers to get HIGH AND DIE!

3. A pharmacist is a chemist who makes and sells DRUG COCKTAILS. These drug-cocktails have never been tested. Rather than buy an untested drug cocktail compounded (created)

by your local pharmacist—you'd be better off buying a <u>COCK-TAIL</u> from your local bartender. A bartender's cocktail is far safer, much cheaper and gives you an immediate <u>BUZZ</u>!-☺

4. A pharmacist does not wear a stethoscope-but doctors and pharmacists both wear white-coats to impress a naïve public. White-coats are phenomenal marketing tools.

   Your local butcher and garbage- man also like to wear them. Doctors' and pharmacists wear white-coats that do not show the excrement and bodily fluids of the people injured by their toxic poisonous pills. Meat butchers and garbage men deserve more respect than convention doctors.

   How do doctors and pharmacists get to sleep at night?

5. Your local pharmacist is not interested to probe your anus with his finger.☺

6. Unlike a doctor- a pharmacist does actually sell hundreds of <u>NON-DRUG ITEMS THAT CAN BE BENEFICIAL TO YOUR HEALTH.</u>

   <u>YOUR DOCTOR CANNOT HELP YOU TO REVERSE AND OVERCOME ANY ADVERSE HEALTH PROBLEMS.</u>

   <u>YOUR DOCTOR DOES NOT POSSESS THE NUTRITIONAL KNOWLEDGE AND HEALTH EXPERTISE WHICH YOU REQUIRE.</u>

   <u>YOUR DOCTOR IS CLUELESS ABOUT HOW TO TREAT OBESITY!</u> (Your doctor likely has a bigger belly than you do...-☺

   <u>YOUR DOCTOR IS MEDICALLY IMPOTENT WHEN IT COMES TO HELPING YOU BECOME LEAN, STRONG AND HEALTHY.</u>

   How <u>SAD</u> is that!

Your doctor is like a carpenter with only a hammer and thus all he sees are nails.

<u>IF</u> you want to reverse any health condition and/or get <u>HEALTHY</u>— rather than visiting your doctor, you should take on the job of looking after your own health.

You would be better off to attend church and pray for your health!

Several large studies of cancer patients showed that patients who attended Church had fewer and greatly reduced adverse symptoms of cancer treatment. Patients who view God as a loving, benevolent being have better than those patients who have a sense of fatalism and harbour anger towards God. Attendance at Church provides patients with strength and comfort.

Moreover when you exit the church—<u>YOU WILL DEFINITELY FEEL BETTER</u> than when you exit your doctor's office.

<u>EVERYONE KNOWS THAT EXERCISE IS ESSENTIAL FOR GOOD HEALTH.</u>

<u>WHAT YOUR DOCTOR KNOWS ABOUT EXERCISE HE PROBABLY LEARNED FROM WATCHING THE DR. OZ SHOW.</u>

<u>YOUR DOCTOR IS NOT TAUGHT ABOUT EXERCISE AND MUSCLES IN MEDICAL SCHOOL.</u>

<u>YOUR DOCTOR IS CLUELESS ABOUT EXERCISE AND THE THERAPEUTIC HEALTH BENEFITS OF EXERCISE.</u> Your allopathic doctor knows "<u>SQUAT</u>" about Squat. -☺

<u>YOUR DOCTOR IS UTTERLY IGNORANT ABOUT A BOAT-LOAD OF (non-drug) ESSENTIAL HEALTH CARE STRATEGIES!</u>

(That's another big reason that I wrote this book).

<u>YOU DESERVE TO KNOW HOW TO TAKE CARE OF YOURSELF AND YOUR HEALTH.</u>

<u>YOU DESERVE TO KNOW ABOUT DR. EXERCISE, DR. SUNSHINE, DR. SLEEP AND OTHER IMPORTANT DOCTORS.</u> -☺

<u>YOU DESERVE TO KNOW ABOUT THE MOST IMPORTANT DOCTOR OF ALL —</u>

<u>DR. KETOGENIC DIET!</u> Aka Dr. Ketosis

<u>MY NUMBER ONE REASON TO FIRE YOUR DOCTOR IS:</u>

<u>YOUR DOCTOR DOES NOT KNOW HIS ARSE FROM HIS ELBOW.</u>

<u>YOUR DOCTOR DOES NOT HAVE THE EXPERTISE AND KNOWLEDGE NECESSARY TO HELP YOU GET HEALTHY.</u>

<u>YOUR DOCTOR'S IGNORANCE MEANS THAT YOU MUST EDUCATE YOURSELF.</u>

<u>YOUR PRIMARY CARE PHYSICIAN'S IGNORANCE OF NUTRITION, BIOCHEMISTRY OF NUTRITION, HUMAN PHYSIOLOGY, HUMAN METABOLISM AND EXERCISE PHYSIOLOGY MEANS:</u>

<u>YOUR DOCTOR—</u>

DOES NOT KNOW HIS ARSE FROM HIS ELBOW—LITERALLY.

YOUR DOCTOR CANNOT HELP YOU GET HEALTHY—PERIOD.

REASON NUMBER TWO-

YOUR DOCTOR IS DOING MORE HARM THAN GOOD.

YOUR DOCTOR IS THE BIGGEST THREAT TO YOUR HEALTH!

YOUR DOCTOR IS A VERY DANGEROUS PERSON!

YOUR DOCTOR IS LIKELY KILLING YOU WITH HIS MEDICAL IGNORANCE AND WITH BIG PHARMA'S TOXIC DRUGS!

Are you willing to take that HUGE risk? You have a choice!Think about it. Every time you visit your doctor—he makes money. Every drug your doctor prescribes for you— improves HIS/HER finances— and puts money in the hands of Big Pharma. Together these DRUG BARONS are laughing all the way to the bank! Every pill, every shot, every injection you receive from your doctor puts cash in his bank account. It also makes the pharmacist and Big Pharma richer too.

The only way that these drug barons make money is by keeping sick—AND DEPENDENT ON THEIR POISONOUS "MEDICINE". If you get healthy- you would vanish as a customer!

PATIENTS OF ALLOPATHIC DOCTORS ARE PATIENTS UNTIL THEY DIE!

This is one of the reasons why there is a shortage of doctors. The number of patients increases daily while the number of allopathic clones or medical doctors decreases.

ALLOPATHIC DOCTORS KILL MORE THAN ONE MILLION PEOPLE EACH YEAR! (Death by Medicine- You can tell your doctor THAT you are firing him as your doctor... BECAUSE you have learned that your doctor KILLING PEOPLE and you do not wish to be his next casualty.

CHEMOTHERAPY USED BY DOCTORS KILLS ANOTHER MILLION PLUS PEOPLE EACH YEAR.

YOU SHOULD FIRE YOUR DOCTOR BECAUSE HE IS DOING MORE HARM THAN GOOD.

YOU SHOULD TELL YOUR DOCTOR THAT HE/SHE IS MORE DANGEROUS THAN CANCER AND HEART DISEASE COMBINED!

Are you prepared to risk your life by taking the poisonous pills that he prescribes to you? You must stop believing the medical propaganda and MEDICAL NONSENSE emanating from Big Pharma and conventional doctors. Here's an example.Doctors prescribe blood thinning drugs such as "Warfarin" literally 'RAT POISON and CHEMO DRUGS made from poisonous NERVE GAS which was used in the WW1 AS A CHEMICAL WEAPON TO KILL SOLDIERS!

HOW CAN DOCTORS BE LEGALLY ALLOWED TO USE A CHEMICAL WEAPON BANNED BY THE RULES OF WAR?

VACCINE DRUGS – ARE— THE WORST—THE MOST EVIL— THE MOST VILE— POISONOUS DRUGS EVER CREATED BY MAN!

ALLOPATHIC VACCINATORS SHOULD BE PROSECUTED FOR MEDICAL CRIMES AGAINST HUMANITY!

VACCINES NEVER HAVE BEEN EFFECTIVE AND THEY NEVER WILL!

THE JURY IS IN!

VACCINES SHOULD BE BANNED!

DOCTORS WHO –IGNORANTLY—AND ROBOTICALLY PRESCRIBE VACCINE DRUGS SHOULD BE JAILED!

ALL DOCTORS HAVE A LEGAL AND A MORAL DUTY TO DO NO HARM.

ALL DOCTORS HAVE A LEGAL AND MORAL OBLIGATION TO DISCLOSE THE DANGERS OF ANY DRUG, TREATMENT OR SURGERY. IF YOUR DOCTOR IS A VACCINE "JABBER"—YOU SHOULD FIRE HIS BUTT!

YOU WILL BE STRIKING A BLOW FOR THE HEALTH OF MANY PEOPLE WHEN YOU FIRE YOUR DOCTOR.

WHEN YOU FIRE YOUR DOCTOR YOU WILL INFLUENCE OTHER PEOPLE TO DO THE SAME!

WHEN YOU FIRE YOUR DOCTOR YOU CAN POST ON FACEBOOK AND THE SOCIAL MEDIA.

YOU CAN START A NEW HEALTH TREND!

SOON EVERYONE WILL FIRE THEIR DOCTORS AND TAKE CONTROL OF THEIR OWN HEALTH!

YOU ARE VERY POWERFUL!

YOU CAN MAKE THE MESSAGE "FIRE YOUR DOCTOR-HIRE YOURSELF" GO VIRAL ACROSS THE INTERNET!

DR. INTERNET ROCKS!

DOCTORS' FLAWED EDUCATION IS LIMITED TO DRUGS AND SURGERY.

VACCINATION "SURGERY" IS THE MOST DANGEROUS KIND OF SURGERY EVER INVENTED IN HUMAN HISTORY!

A ONE-SIZE DRUG FITS ALL—PROTOCOL—AND A ONE-SIZE SURGERY FITS ALL—PROTOCOL— IS THE MOST INSANE MEDICAL TREATMENT EVER CREATED BY HUMANS!

BIG PHARMA HAS CONVINCED AN ILL-INFORMED PUBLIC THAT VACCINATION SURGERY IS REQUIRED BY EVERYONE—ESPECIALLY NEWBORN BABIES! Yuk.

AN IGNORANT MEDICAL ESTABLISHMENT AND AN EVIL BIG PHARMA HAS DUPED 350 MILLION NORTH AMERICAN PEOPLE!

YOUR DOCTOR HAS BEEN BRAINWASHED TOO!

YOUR DOCTOR BELIEVES ALL OF THE MEDICAL DRIVEL THAT BIG PHARMA AND THE MEDIA SPEWS OUT!

YOUR DOCTOR IS A DRUG PUPPET CONTROLLED BY BIG PHARMA.

DOCTORS HAVE A LEGAL AND MORAL OBLIGATION TO EDUCATE THEMSELVES AND THEIR PATIENTS ABOUT VACCINES—ESPECIALLY ABOUT THEIR SAFETY AND EFFECTIVENESS.

YOUR DOCTOR HAS BREACHED A LEGAL AND MORAL OBLIGATION TO USE DANGEROUS VACCINATION SURGERY WITHOUT VERIFYING ITS DANGERS AND WITHOUT ADVISING YOU OF THOSE DANGERS.

YOUR DOCTOR IS DOING MORE HARM THAN GOOD!

DOING VACCINATION SURGERY WITHOUT HAVING EXAMINED THE DANGERS OF VACCINES IS CRIMINAL NEGLIGENCE.

DOCTORS HAVE A LEGAL AND MORAL OBLIGATION TO OBTAIN A PATIENT'S INFORMED CONSENT—BEFORE SELLING/ PRESCRIBING DANGEROUS DRUGS—OR EVEN TOUCHING A PATIENT!

HOW MANY MORE PEOPLE HAVE TO DIE BEFORE DRUG KILLERS ARE STOPPED!

ALLOPATHIC DOCTORS WHO ROBOTICALLY PERFORM VACCINATION SURGERY; PRESCRIBE DANGEROUS DRUGS OR ANY OTHER TREATMENT TO THEIR PATIENTS WITHOUT OBTAINING A VALID INFORMED CONSENT— SHOULD BE JAILED!

A DOCTORS' LEGAL AND MORAL DUTY TO OBTAIN A VALID INFORMED CONSENT –IS THE MOST IMPORTANT LEGAL OBLIGATION EXISTING BETWEEN A DOCTOR AND PATIENT.

ALLOPATHIC DOCTORS WHO BREACH THIS FUNDAMENTAL LEGAL OBLIGATION SHOULD BE STRIPPED OF THEIR MEDICAL LICENCE AND JAILED FOR FRAUDULENT MALPRACTICE.

DOCTORS WHO MAKE ANY KIND OF FRAUDULENT MISREPRESENTATION AND/OR OR FAIL TO OBTAIN A PATIENT'S VALID INFORMED CONSENT SHOULD BE JAILED.

DOCTORS WHO ENGAGE IN ILLEGAL CRIMINAL BEHAVIOUR HAVE NO LEGITIMATE LEGAL DEFENSE.

IGNORANCE OF THE LAW IS NO EXCUSE.

DOCTORS CAN EASILY LEARN ABOUT NUTRITION BY A CLICK OF A MOUSE. DOCTORS CAN LEARN ABOUT NUTRITION WITH THE CLICK OF A BUTTON—OR AT THE TAP OF THE SCREEN ON THEIR IPHONE.

ONCOLOGISTS AND CARDIOLOGISTS ROUTINELY ADVISE CANCER /HEART PATIENTS TO EAT WHATEVER THEY WANT OR TO EAT A HIGH-CARB-LOW FAT DIET WITH LOTS OF WHOLE GRAINS.

THESE IGNORANT DOCTORS ARE GUILTY OF CRIMINAL NEGLIGENCE!

MEDICAL CRIMINALS SHOULD BE HELD ACCOUNTABLE BY THE PUBLIC AUTHORITIES.

A SPECIAL WAR CRIMES TRIBUNAL SHOULD BE CREATED TO STOP THE BARBARIC PRACTICE OF MEDICINE AND KILLING AND SLAUGHTERING MILLIONS OF PEOPLE WITH POISONOUS DRUGS AND NEEDLESS SURGERY.

CRIMINAL DOCTORS SHOULD NOT BE PERMITTED TO HIDE UNDER THE LEGAL SKIRTS OF MOTHER PHARMA.

When you go to your conventionally trained doctor, you're playing "MEDICAL Roulette" with your health!

Unlike RUSSIAN Roulette played with ONE BULLET IN THE CHAMBER OF A PISTOL—when you play MEDICAL Roulette" — FIVE OF THE SIX CHAMBERS IN YOUR PISTOL CONTAIN BULLETS!

DO NOT PLAY MEDICAL ROULETTE WITH YOUR DOCTOR.

Fire his butt before you become one of his victims!

YOUR DOCTOR'S WAITING ROOM IS ONE OF THE MOST DANGEROUS PLACES IN THE WORLD!

A 13 YEAR STUDY OF 84,595 FAMILIES reported in the March (2014) edition of "Infection Control and Epidemiology" found that annual well-child exams and vaccinations were associated with a GIGANTIC INCREASED RISK OF FLU-LIKE ILLNESSES for children and their families within 2 weeks following their visit.

THIS ADDITIONAL RISK TRANSLATES TO 778,974 EXCESS CASES OF ILLNESS PER YEAR IN THE USA WITH A COST OF 500 MILLION DOLLARS!

YOU MUST FIRE YOUR DOCTOR TO PROTECT YOUR HEALTH!

YOU MUST FIRE YOUR DOCTOR TO START A HEALTH TREND TOWARDS A DO-IT-YOURSELF (DIY) APPROACH TO HEALTH.

YOU SHOULD AVOID TAKING YOUR KIDS AND YOURSELF TO YOUR DOCTOR'S SICKNESS-FILLED WAITING ROOM!

Your health is better served by avoiding your doctors' waiting room and eating NUTRITOUS FOOD.

You can be healthier when you AVOID your doctor's waiting room.

Your doctor is making you and your children SICK without even seeing them!

REASON NO. 2 TO FIRE YOUR DOCTOR IS:

YOUR DOCTOR IS DOING MORE HARM THAN GOOD.

REASON NUMBER THREE—

YOUR DOCTOR LIKELY IS AN ACTIVE PARTICIPANT IN WHAT HAS BEEN TERMED "MEDICAL CHILD ABUSE".

Medical Child Abuse is a controversial "catch-all" term for a wide spectrum of cases in which DOCTORS- DEEM PARENTS ACTING AGAINST THE BEST INTEREST OF THEIR CHILD IN A MEDICAL SETTING.

Here's how this medical scam typically works.

A child, often a teenager treated and/or diagnosed with some type of metabolic/physiological issue has occasion to be hospitalized and then treated by a new doctor who comes up with a new theory that the child's medical problem is PSYCHIATRIC rather than a metabolic medical problem.

Typically, parents then become sceptical because their child has undergone a BOATLOAD OF MEDICAL TREATMENTS, SURGERIES AND DRUGS.

NEXT- THE PARENTS DECIDE TO CHALLENGE THE DOCTOR (S) FINDING OR OPINION. SOMETIMES SCEPTICAL PARENTS EVEN REQUEST A SECOND MEDICAL OPINION!

CAN YOU IMAGINE THE AUDACITY OF A PARENT TO QUESTION A DOCTOR ABOUT TREATMENTS/SURGERY AND OR MEDIAL DIAGNOSIS OF THEIR CHILD???

QUESTIONING A PILL-PUSHER ABOUT HIS DIAGNOSIS AND/OR TREATMENT IS THE EQUIVALENT OF WAVING A FLAG IN THE FACE OF A MAD BULL!!

APPALLED BY PARENTS WHO DARE QUESTION GODS WEARING WHITE COATS- Here's what usually happens next...

NEXT- THE DOCTOR OR HOSPITAL CONTACTS THE STATE CHILD PROTECTION AGENCY. THE PARENTS ARE THEN CHARGED WITH MEDICAL CHILD ABUSE—

AND —IN A GROWING NUMBER OF CASES ARE LOSING CUSTODY OF THEIR CHILDREN TO GOVERNMENT AGENCIES! OMG!

ALLOPATHIC DOCTORS ASK CHILD PROTECTION SERVICES (GOVERNMENT AGENCIES) TO DEPRIVE PARENTS OF THEIR PARENTAL RIGHTS.

GOVERNMENT AGENCIES- ARMED WITH A HALF-BAKED AFFIDAVIT FROM SOMEONE WEARING A WHITE-COAT- PROCEED TO 'LEGALLY' SNATCH THE CHILD FROM CARING PARENTS WHO HAVE THE BRAINS

AND COURAGE TO QUESTION SOME DRUG-PUSHER'S OPINION ABOUT WHAT MEDICAL TREATMENT IS BEST FOR THEIR CHILD.

THIS IS SHEER MADNESS!

SO- DEAR PARENTS—IF YOUR CHILD HAS A DOCTOR OR IS HOSPITALIZED- YOU WOULD BE WELL-ADVISED TO FIRE YOUR CHILD'S DOCTOR BEFORE YOUR PARENTAL AUTHORITY AND YOUR CHILD ARE SNATCHED FROM YOU!

ALLOPATHIC DOCTORS SHOULD BE PROSECUTED AND JAILED WHEN THEY COMMIT CHILD ABUSE…NOT THE PARENTS!

THE THIRD REASON TO FIRE YOUR DOCTOR IS THAT HE LIKELY HAS NO HEART AND HIS ONLY CONCERN IS HIS INFLATED EGO—NOT YOUR WELL BEING OR THE WELL-BEING OF YOUR CHILD.

HERE'S A 'BONUS' REASON TO FIRE YOUR DOCTOR-☺

WHEN YOU FIRE YOUR DOCTOR YOU COULD BE DOING HIM A FAVOUR!

Having one less patient could actually help your doctor. There is an acute SHORTAGE of doctors. Research shows that the average doctor is overworked. Your doctor is probably stressed out even MORE than you are! Your doctor has likely seen his salary reduced— while his business expenses have increased.

THE AVERAGE ALLOPATHIC DOCTOR IS DEAD AT AGE 56!

Research shows that not only is the average doctor dead at age 56- MOST OFTEN BY SUICIDE! OMG!

According to the American Foundation for Suicide Prevention, the suicide rate among doctors is so high in the west, that "physicians" earned the number TWO spot on the Business Insider's list of the 19 jobs in which you are most likely to KILL yourself.(source: www.businessinsider.com)

Furthermore, according to the survey provided by The Doctor's Company, 9 out of 10 doctors in America are actively DISCOURAGING others from entering the medical profession!

Do you really want to take health advice from a doctor who WILL DIE BEFORE YOU? DO YOU WANT TO TAKE ADVICE FROM SOMEONE MORE STRESSED OUT AND DEPRESSED THAN YOU ARE?

YOUR DOCTOR LIKELY MIXED UP YOUR CHOLESTEROL NUMBERS WITH HIS GOLF SCORE! -☺

Do you really want to take health advice from a doctor WHO IS MORE UNHEALTHY THAN YOU ARE? Most likely your doctor is sicker, fatter, and less healthy than you are! You may have noticed that your doctor offers you very LITTLE HOPE.

Your doctor's bedside manner likely SUCKS because he's struggling to deal with his OWN health issues!

Your doctor probably needs to address HIS OWN HEALTH OR HIS OWN HEALTH ISSUES.—BEFORE YOUR DOCTOR CAN ADDRESS YOUR HEALTH ISSUES.You should have COMPASSION for your doctor. Your allopathic doctor has been DUPED BY BIG PHARMA! When you quit as a patient— you will provide your doctor more time to do FUN things like play golf or read about nutrition.

YOU COULD BE DOING YOUR DOCTOR A BIG FAVOUR IF YOU QUIT AS ONE OF HIS PATIENTS.

YOU WILL SEND A POWERFUL MESSAGE TO YOUR DOCTOR!

YOU MAY WAKE HIM UP FROM HIS MEDICAL SLEEP-☺

YOU MAY EVEN INSPIRE YOUR DOCTOR TO EXPLORE FUNCTIONAL MEDICINE!

Your doctor likely is very bitter at having been deceived by Big Pharma. Your doctor may have realized the FOLLY of his medical ways.

Perhaps an unhappy patient has already fired your doctor. You may wake up your doctor to realize that his medical approach is not only dysfunctional –but just plain OF ALLOPATHIC DOCTOR. I also relate the story about how I FIRED MY MOM'S DOCTOR.

Your doctor may wish to change the orientation of his/her medical practice. Your doctor may be VERY AFRAID of the medical establish-ment. Your doctor may be literally shaking in his/her boots. Your doctor probably is afraid to stand up to the iron-fisted conventional medical authorities. Your doctor may be under a lot of financial pressures and stress—too. Do you really want to assume any moral responsibility regarding your doctor's decision to commit suicide?

Do you really want to consult a negative, frightened, depressed, sad, stressed out individual regarding your health concerns.

You can help your doctor and you can help yourself.

Simply QUIT as one of his patients.

Just tell your doctor that you have decided to take a <u>DO-IT-YOURSELF (DIY) APPROACH TO YOUR HEALTH.</u>

Hey, your doctor may even be happy that you have taken <u>HIS HAPPINESS INTO CONSIDERATION!</u>

<u>YOU CAN TELL YOUR DOCTOR THAT YOU ARE PART OF THE NEW REVOLUTION IN HEALTHCARE.</u>

<u>YOU CAN EXPLAIN TO YOUR DOCTOR THAT YOU ARE ONE OF THE 80 PERCENT OF THE POPULATION THAT HAS MADE THE INFORMED DECISION THIS YEAR TO TAKE CONTROL OF YOUR HEALTH.</u>

<u>IN SUM- A BONUS REASON TO FIRE YOUR DOCTOR IS:</u>

<u>YOU COULD BE DOING YOUR DOCTOR A FAVOUR WHEN YOU FIRE YOUR DOCTOR.</u>

<u>HOW</u> I fired my allopathic doctor—

I've always been extremely healthy. At age 10 I had minor eye surgery to cut eye muscles to straighten my right eye. At age 2 I suffered nerve damage to my right eye when hit in the back of my head by as stone. At age 5, I had decided that I wanted to be a lawyer. For several years I wore an eye-patch over my left eye and then glasses in an effort to correct my vision and help might right eye. I suffered headaches and expert allopathic doctors told me that I would never be a lawyer due to the amount reading required. I have been a licenced attorney for more than 40 years.

That was my first experience with the allopathic medical profession. I never really had occasion to visit a doctor until I was about 50 years old. About 15 years ago, I began to half back pain so I consulted my Mom's family doctor. At that time, I had played about 2,000 competitive rounds of golf so back problems were not unexpected-☺.

I consulted Dr. T. Although my X-rays showed no serious pathology; I was worried and pretty stressed out. Dr. T took my blood pressure- it was 136 over 92. I was studying to be a personal trainer so I knew that these were not good numbers. Dr. T. referred me to a physiotherapist for an 8 week exercise program. Dr. T immediately wanted to put me on <u>blood pressure medication!</u> I categorically refused.

An appointment was made for 3 months later—after my back was healed. This time Dr. T took my blood pressure. My pressure was 120 over 80!

Dr. T almost fainted in surprise. I said to her—"I told you I was stressed when you took my BP". Then I asked Dr .T- "What is the

OPTIMUM BLOOD PRESSURE FOR A 50 YR. OLD GUY? She confessed to me that she had no idea. They never taught THAT in medical school! I then realized that this medical doctor with her allopathic colleagues learned VERY LITTLE in medical school about how to help people GET OR STAY HEALTHY!

Fast forward to several years ago when I moved to Ottawa; a friend of a friend managed to refer my former wife and myself to a family doctor here in Ottawa. The doctor, Dr. X agreed to add us to his patient list because "Gary is healthy as a horse" and would not need to take much of the doctor's time. I met with Dr. X for a 10 minute "meet and greet". Dr. X. was a pleasant young man about 40 years old. He scheduled an annual check-up but he cautioned me that it would likely be about 1.5 to 2 years for my annual check-up. I said "no problem"; I'm probably healthier than you are Doc". Btw: I am not a "patient"; I am a "client"!

I poked him gently in the stomach and said: "Doc- you're getting in a little soft in your gut"- ; your eyes look like two *** holes in the snow because you are stressed out".-☺ "I am a personal trainer—I should be examining YOU!

About 2 years later a check-up was scheduled for me; at 9:00 a.m. I was the first patient of the day. The nurse put me on the scale. The phone rang. It was her boss- Dr. X. –HE was sick as a dog! All his appointments for the day were cancelled. His nurse apologized and told me my check-up would be re-scheduled. Six months later, I breezed into Dr. X's office. I told him not to waste his time taking my BP because it was likely better than his BP. Anyway, he gave me a scrap of paper to have the usual bloodwork and PSA test done. And he said- "If there is any problem with the results—we will call you. "Perfect" I said.

About 6 months later- I thought hey- I want to see the numbers for myself. I can read and understand bloodwork and cholesterol as well or maybe better than he can. So, I telephoned his medical office asking for a copy of the bloodwork results. The nurse said- Oh- you need an appointment with the doctor. I responded—"well make one!"

Three weeks later, I breezed into Dr. X's office. Dr. X was literally running between two examination rooms. I sat down for 2 minutes. He gave me a copy of my bloodwork tests and said "The results are very good. I said "no Doc- I want the bloodwork of a 30 year-old healthy guy! " I smiled and said seriously Doc-actually— I'm looking for an urologist or a prostate guy." "Do you know one?"

"Yes" he replied "that's me". So I looked him in the eye and said— "Doc- do you know that most men 70 years and older have <u>PROSTATE CANCER</u>? Do you know that? He answered "Yes."

I said to him "Doc- do you also know that men over 50 years old should closely check their testosterone levels and take supplements— if necessary?"

Dr. X answered: "Well...the <u>STUDIES</u>" show... I immediately interrupted... "<u>YOU WANT STUDIES- DOC...YOU CAME TO THE RIGHT PLACE!</u>" I whipped out a two-inch wad of studies that I had brought to show him. Dr. X started taking notes.

<u>FOR THE FIRST TIME—I REALIZED THAT MY DOCTOR WAS CLUELESS ABOUT NUTRITION AND SUPPLEMENTS!</u>

I immediately stood up and said: "<u>DOC- YOU'LL HAVE TO EXCUSE ME BUT I HAVE A VERY BUSY DAY!</u>" That was the last time I saw or spoke to my allopathic doctor.

<u>THAT WAS HOW I FIRED MY DOCTOR.</u>

<u>THIS EXPERIENCE PROVIDED ME WITH CONFIRMATION THAT ALLOPATHIC DOCTORS HAVE INSUFFICIENT KNOWLEDGE AND "MEDICAL" EXPERTISE TO HELP ME GET AND STAY HEALTHY.</u>

<u>THAT DAY—I QUIT AS MY DOCTOR'S PATIENT—NEVER TO RETURN.</u>

<u>ON THAT DAY—I REALIZED THAT HAD FIRED MY DOCTOR WHEN I HIRED MYSELF AS MY DOCTOR SEVERAL YEARS PRIOR TO THAT WHEN I CAME TO UNDERSTAND THAT NO ONE CAN DOCTOR YOU- BUT YOURSELF!</u>

<u>YOU MUST FIRE YOUR DOCTOR AND HIRE YOURSELF!</u>

<u>YOU WILL FEEL EMPOWERED AND HAPPY WHEN YOU DO!</u>

<u>Sidebar:</u>

<u>How I fired my mother's doctor—</u>

My mother is an 87 years old "breast-cancer" survivor. I fired her <u>ONCOLOGIST</u>—but let's save <u>that</u> story for another day. About 15 years ago, I accompanied my mother to consult her allopathic physician. Dr. T, her doctor, wanted to prescribe her a <u>CHOLESTEROL-LOWERING DRUG</u> (a Statin called Lipitor) to my mother to lower her cholesterol.

I looked Dr. T straight in the eye and I softly uttered these words:

"DR. T — YOU SHOULD NOT BE PRESCRIBING STATIN DRUGS TO ANYONE!!

"IF YOU ARE FOOLISH ENOUGH TO PRESCRIBE LIPITOR TO ANYONE—YOU ARE GUILTY OF MALPRACTICE—YOU ARE CIVILLY NEGLIGENT".

"AND DR. T.- IF YOU ARE FOOLISH ENOUGH TO PRESCRIBE STATIN DRUGS TO A PATIENT WITHOUT PRESCRIBING COQ10 ENZYME SUPPLEMENT AT THE SAME TIME—

BY DOING THAT — DR. T—

"YOU ARE CRIMINALLY NEGLIGENT!

My mother's doctor has never prescribed **STATIN** or any other kind of poisonous drugs to my mother. **MY MOTHER REMAINS A DRUG-FREE SURVIVOR OF THE CRIMINAL CANCER INDUSTRY.** That's how I fired my mother's allopathic doctor.

I am sure that you have a boatload of personal reasons to fire your doctor. Be that as it may- either way- **YOU MUST HIRE YOURSELF AS YOUR OWN PRIMARY DOCTOR!**

IF YOUR DIE-TICIAN LACKS APPROPRIATE NUTRITIONAL KNOWLEDGE- YOU SHOULD PROBABLY FIRE YOUR DIE-TICIAN AND CONVENTIONALLY TRAINED DENTIST…TOO.

HERE ARE MY REASONS WHY YOU SHOULD HIRE YOURSELF.

C. REASONS TO HIRE YOURSELF.

MY NUMBER 1 REASON IS:

PRIMARY CARE PHYSICIANS ARE BECOMING OBSOLETE!

MANY PEOPLE IN THE MEDICAL ESTABLISHMENT PERCEIVE TECHNOLOGY AND THE ELECTRONIC REVOLUTION AS A DIRECT THREAT TO THEIR LIVELIHOOD.

THE TRUTH IS: THEY DARNED WELL SHOULD!

THE DEMAND FOR PRIMARY CARE PHYSICIANS' SERVICES IS SHRINKING!

ON-LINE TECHNOLOGY AVAILABLE IS SIMPLY AMAZING!

LIVE ON-LINE MEDICAL DIAGNOSIS IS ALREADY BOOMING!

YOU CAN GET DOZENS OF MEDICAL APPS/MEDICAL DEVICES ON-LINE.

WHO NEEDS TO MAKE AN APPOINTMENT WITH A PRIMARY CARE PHYSICIAN?

YOU CAN BOOK AN APPOINTMENT ON-LINE 24/7!

YOU CAN GET AN APP LIKE—"YOUR. MD." WHICH IS SUPER-CONVENIENT!

THESE SYSTEMS OFFER A RAPID, INEXPENSIVE, AUTOMATED ALTERNATIVE TO VISITING A PHYSICIAN ON-LINE OR IN PERSON!

THIS IS A PRACTICAL-FUNCTIONAL (DIY) APPROACH WHEREBY YOU CAN TAKE CONTROL OF YOUR HEALTH.

NO PHYSICAL DOCTOR VISIT IS REQUIRED!

IMAGINE HOW MUCH TIME, MONEY, INCONVENIENCE—AND STRESS-THAT YOU WILL SAVE!

JUST GRAB THE "8 FUNCTIONAL MEDICINE DOCTORS" FROM THIS BOOK!

HALLELUJAH!

FORGET YOUR PRIMARY CARE PHYSICIAN. YOU CAN KISS YOUR DOCTOR GOOD-BYE…-(PERHAPS EVEN VIRTUALLY-☺!

YOU HAVE A BETTER SAFER, LESS EXPENSIVE ALTERNATIVE TO GOING TO SEE A DOCTOR OR GOING TO A HOSPITAL.

YOUR DOCTOR DOESN'T KNOW WHY YOU GOT SICK IN THE FIRST PLACE.

YOUR DOCTOR DOESN'T HOW TO PREVENT YOU FROM GETTING SICK.

EXISTING HEALTH CARE SYSTEMS ARE ONLY USEFUL FOR MEDICAL EMERGENCIES—TO REPAIR BULLET WOUNDS AND PUT CASTS ON BROKEN BONES- and the like-☺

HOSPITALS WERE BUILT AS MACABRE "PLACES TO DIE".

Example: "COUMADIN" IS THE NUMBER ONE DRUG THAT'LL KILL YOU IN THE EMERGENCY ROOM!

YOU MUST AVOID HOSPITALS AND IATROGENIC DOCTORS TO LIVE A LONG AND HEALTHY LIFE. HOSPITALS ARE A STEPPING STONE TO A PREMATURE DEATH.

WHEN YOU TAKE A DO-IT-YOURSELF (DIY) APPROACH TO YOUR HEALTH—YOU CAN AVOID HOSPITALS—AND A SLOW PAINFUL DEATH.

ANOTHER DIY APPROACH IS TO GIVE BIRTH AT HOME AND AVOID HAVING YOUR BABY DAMAGED DURING CHILDBIRTH OR THE CRUEL BARBARIC PRACTICE OF CIRCUMCISION.

YOU DO NOT NEED AN ALLOPATHIC DOCTOR TO BOTCH THE DELIVERY OF YOUR CHILD BY USING FORCEPS. THE MID-WIFE- (DIY) APPROACH HAS BEEN SAFELY AND EFFECTIVELY USED FOR CENTURIES IN MOST PARTS OF THE WORLD. THE ONLY PERSON WHO BENEFITS FROM HOSPITAL BIRTHS IS DOCTORS.

YOU CAN CONSULT DR. INTERNET TO LEARN A BOATLOAD OF OTHER KINDS OF NATURAL EMERGENCY CARE THAT YOU CAN SAFELY DO AT HOME.

DIY: EXAMPLES OF EMERGENCY HEALTH CARE:

- YOUR BEST HEART MEDICINE (DIY) APPROACH IS:

    - BUY AN AED (Automated External Defibrillator)—A SMALL TALKING BOX THAT CAN BE USED BY A 10 YEAR OLD CHILD TO SAFELY REVIVE A HEART ATTACK PATIENT.

    YOU CAN SAVE THE LIFE OF DYING FROM A SCA (Sudden Cardiac Arrest)!

    YOU CAN SAVE A LIFE FOR $1,000 BUCKS!

    RESEARCH SHOWS THAT OF EACH YEAR 350,000 PEOPLE SUFFER SCA's IN THE UNITED STATES.

    RESEARCH ALSO SHOWS THAT IF AN AED IS NOT USED WITHIN THE FIRST 5 MINUTES OF A HEART ATTACK—

    80 PERCENT OF HEART ATTACK VICTIMS WILL DIE!

    WHY WAIT FOR A PARAMEDIC TO ARRIVE TO USE HIS AED TO TRY TO REVIVE YOU OR A LOVED PERSON?

    WHY NOT SPEND A $ 1000 BUCKS ON A TALK-ING BOX THAT A CHILD CAN SAFELY USE?

    INVESTING IN AN AED COULD BE THE SMARTEST $ 1000 BUCKS THAT YOU WILL EVER SPEND TO TAKE CARE YOUR HEALTH.

    YOU COULD EVEN SHARE IT WITH YOUR NEIGHBOUR-

IS $500 BUCKS WORTH THE COST OF A HUMAN LIFE?

- **YOU CAN USE ORGANIC CAYENNE PEPPER TO STOP BLEEDING FROM A BULLET OR KNIFE WOUND—IN LESS TIME THAN THE AMBULANCE TAKES TO ARRIVE AT YOUR HOME!**

- **YOU CAN USE A BOATLOAD OF OTHER SAFE-NON-TOXIC EMERGENCY HOME-REMEDIES THAT ARE AVAILABLE FROM DR. INTERNET.**

    - **YOU CAN USE HERBS OR GINGER TEA TO HEAL STOMACH UPSET, NAUSEA, ETC.**

    - **YOU CAN—NAY- YOU SHOULD— USE FOOD AS YOUR MEDICINE.**

THROUGHOUT THIS BOOK YOU WILL FIND DOZENS OF HEALING FOODS THAT CAN BE USED TO HEAL AND REVERSE HEALTH PROBLEMS.

DIY: EXAMPLE OF MEDICAL DEVICES AND MEDIC AL PROSTHESES-

- **INSTEAD OF PAYING $ 50,000 DOLLARS FOR AN ARTIFICIAL LIMB (ARM)- IT APPEARS THAT YOU CAN PRINT A 3D PROSTHETIC ARM FOR A COUPLE HUNDRED DOLLARS!**

    MOREOVER –IT APPEARS THAT 3-D PROSTHESIS HAS A MUCH BETTER RANGE OF MOTION.

- **DO YOU NEED OTHER KINDS OF MEDICAL DEVICES?**

    JUST ASK DR. GOOGLE—YOU MAY BE ABLE TO PRINT'EM OUT-TO GET A BETTER LIMB AND SAVE YOURSELF TIME, STRESS AND A BUNDLE OF CASH!

A (DIY) APPROACH— DR. INTERNET AND HIS ASSOCIATES- (e.g. Dr. Google) PROVIDE A VAST ARRAY OF CHOICES OF ELECTRONIC MEDICAL AND HEALTH CARE DEVICES WHICH ARE VERY AFFORDABLE, FAR SAFER AND FAR MORE EFFECTIVE THAN THOSE SUPPLIED BY ALLOPATHIC aka DINOSAUR MEDICINE. -☺

JUST FIND THE DEVICES THAT ARE FUNCTIONAL FOR YOU…AND YOUR WALLET!

Who needs a doctor? JUST DO-IT-YOURSELF- (DIY).

EFFECTIVE PLATFORMS SUCH AS "YOUR MD" CAN BE USED TO BY-PASS THE NEED FOR HUMAN DIAGNOSIS.

THE FUTURE OF SURGERY AND SUPPLEMENTS BELONGS TO VIRTUAL AUTOMATED ROBOTS WHO WILL DISPENSE BOTH. IT APPEARS

THAT DRONES AND AUTOMATED ROBOTS WILL PERFORM SURGERY QUICKLY AND CHEAPER THAN SURGEONS.

ALLOPATHIC SURGEONS WILL SOON BE OBSOLETE! IMAGINE A ROBOTIC DRONE COMING TO YOUR HOME TO CUT AWAY A SMALL PIECE OF FLESH!

YOU NO LONGER ARE FORCED TO RELY ON BIG PHARMA AND YOUR ALLOPATHIC DOCTOR. YOU CAN DIY— RAPIDLY AND CHEAPLY OBTAIN (See chapter 3 below)

- ON-LINE LABORATORY TESTING

- ACCURATE ADVANCED DIAGNOSTIC TESTING

- ACCURATE ADVANCED MEDICAL INFORMATION

YOU CAN OBTAIN ESSENTIAL LABORATORY TESTS, TEST RESULTS, AND ACCURATE MEDICAL INFORMATION AT THE CLICK OF A MOUSE!

BIG PHARMA AND THE MEDICAL ESTABLISHMENT HAVE LOST THEIR OLIGOPOLISTIC CONTROL OF THE HEALTHCARE INDUSTRY.

YOU CAN CONSULT DR. INTERNET –YOUR PERSONAL ON-LINE VIRTUAL DOCTOR IS AVAILABLE 24/7

HALLELUJAH!

MANY FUNCTIONAL DOCTORS AND NATUROPATHS PROVIDE THE HEALTH INFORMATION THAT YOU NEED TO TAKE CONTROL OF YOUR OWN HEALTH.

RECOMMENDED WEBSITES/ ARE PROVIDED AT THE END OF THIS BOOK.

WELCOME TO THE AGE OF VIRTUAL- DO-IT-YOURSELF MEDICINE- WHERE YOU CAN OBTAIN HEALTH INFORMATION FROM A TO Z AT THE CLICK OF A BUTTON OR THE TOUCH OF YOUR IPAD OR IPHONE!

YOU CARRY YOUR OWN PERSONAL PHYSICIAN (DR. INTERNET) WITH YOU WHEREVER YOU GO ON THIS PLANET!

PRIMARY CARE "ALLOPATHIC DINOSAURIC" PHYSICIANS ARE OBSOLETE!

YOUR SUPERHEALTH BEGINS WITH YOUR DECISION GET OFF OF THE CONVENTIONAL HEALTH GRID AND TAKE A HANDS-ON (DIY) APPROACH TO YOUR HEALTH.

SUPERHEALTH BEGINS WITH SUPERFOOD.

SUPERHEALTH BEGINS IN YOUR KITCHEN CUPBOARD.

SUPERHEALTH BEGINS ON YOUR PLATE.

MORE REASONS TO HIRE YOURSELF AS YOUR OWN DOCTOR—

- **YOU MUST TAKE A (DIY) APPROACH TO YOUR HEALTH.**

- **YOU MUST ASSUME RESPONSIBILITY AND TAKE A PRO-ACTIVE APPROACH TO YOUR OWN HEALTH.**

- **YOU MUST DO YOUR OWN RESEARCH AND EDUATE YOURSELF.**

- **YOUR DOCTOR AND YOUR DIE-TICIAN CAN-NOT HELP YOU GET STRONG AND HEALTHY.**

- **YOUR DOCTOR AND YOUR DIE-TICIAN HAVE NOT RECEIVED NU-TRITIONAL TRAINING TO PROPERLY MANAGE YOUR HEALTH.**

- **YOUR DOCTOR AND YOUR DIE-TICIAN CAN-NOT TAKE CARE OF THEIR OWN HEALTH!!**

- **NO ONE WEARING A LAB-COAT CAN TAKE CON-TROL OF/ OR MANAGE YOUR HEALTH.**

- **NEITHER YOUR SPOUSE, NOR YOUR FAMILY MEM-BERS NOR YOUR FRIENDS CAN HELP YOU REACH SU-PERHEALTH AND PREVENT ILLNESS.**

- **NO ONE CAN DO IT FOR YOU.**

- **THE ONLY PERSON THAT CAN SAVE YOUR HEALTH IS YOU!**

- **YOU MUST BE YOUR OWN DOCTOR. YOU ARE YOUR OWN CLIENT!**

- **BY TAKING A DIY APPROACH TO YOUR HEALTH, YOU CAN AVOID BECOMING YOUR OWN PATIENT!-☺**

- **YOU MUST BE YOUR OWN NUTRITIONIST TOO! YOUR DOCTOR AND YOUR MEDICALLY TRAINED DIE-TICIAN HAVE NOT BEEN TRAINED IN NUTRITION OR THE BIOCHEMISTRY OF NUTRITION.**

- **YOU MUST LEARN HOW TO HEAL YOURSELF WITH HEALING FOODS.**

- **FOR THE FIRST TIME –EVER! WE LIVE IN A VIRTUAL WORLD WHERE WE CAN GET THE HEALTH INFORMATION WE NEED TO CONTROL OUR DESTINY AND TAKE CONTROL OF OUR HEALTH!**

- **YOU MUST LEARN TO BE SELF-RELIANT; YOU MUST LEARN HOW TO TAKE CARE OF YOUR OWN BODY. IT'S THE ONLY PLACE YOU HAVE TO LIVE!**

- **YOU MUST UNDERSTAND YOUR DIGES-TIVE SYSTEM AND HOW IT WORKS.**

- **YOU MUST APPRECIATE THE IMPORTANCE OF STARTING A COMPREHENSIVE WELLNESS PROGRAM AS SOON AS POSSIBLE!**

- **WITHOUT PRIORITIZING YOUR HEALTH, IT'S VERY EASY TO ALLOW THE HEALTH CHALLENGES YOU FACE TO BEAT YOU DOWN.**

- **YOU HAVE THE COURAGE, THE DESIRE, THE POWER AND THE MEANS TO DOCTOR YOURSELF AT YOUR FINGERTIPS!**

- **YOU AND YOUR FAMILY MUST DO WHAT IT TAKES TO IMPROVE YOUR HEALTH EVERYDAY –OTHERWISE—IT'S ONLY A MATTER OF TIME BEFORE A HEALTH CHALLENGE OCCURS.**

- **YOU SHOULD START A PERSONAL WELLNESS PROGRAM TODAY!**

- **WHEN YOU PRIORITIZE YOUR HEALTH YOU WILL HAVE MORE ENERGY AND RESPOND TO STRESS MORE EFFECTIVELY.**

- **WHEN YOU MAKE THE DECISION TO TAKE CONTROL OF YOUR HEALTH—YOU WILL FEEL A GREAT SENSE OF RELIEF. AAAH…**

- **YOU WILL FEEL THAT YOU ARE IN CONTROL OF YOUR HEALTH AND YOU ARE IN CONTROL OF YOUR OWN DESTINY.**

- **WHEN YOU BECOME THE CAPTAIN OF YOUR HEALTH TEAM YOU'LL BE ABLE TO HANDLE ANY HEALTH CHALLENGES THAT MAY ARISE.**

- **WHEN YOU ARE THE CAPTAIN OF YOUR HEALTH TEAM –YOUR FAMILY AND LOVED ONES WILL SEEK YOUR HEALTH GUIDANCE.**

- **YOU HAVE THE POWER TO BY-PASS AND ELIMINATE GREEDY BIG PHARMA AND ALLOPATHIC DOCTORS FROM YOUR HEALTH PROGRAM.**

- **YOU HAVE THE POWER, TOOLS AND MEANS TO ELIMINATE ANY AND ALL UNHEALTHY STRATEGIES FROM YOUR LIFE.**

The take-home message:

YOU SHOULD VIEW YOUR HEALTH—AS WEALTH!

> **"Real Wealth is Health—not pieces of gold and silver"**

> **(M. Gandhi)**

YOU MUST TAKE A HANDS- ON (DIY) APPROACH TO YOUR HEALTH.

To begin your personal journey to SUPERHEALTH- please read on…

CHAPTER THREE
YOUR SIMPLE (DIY) APPROACH TO SUPERHEALTH
"If you're not testing- you're only guessing"

A. INTRODUCTION

So-you've fired your doctor and hired yourself... Now what?

In this chapter I will analyze the <u>CONCRETE</u> steps that you need to take to become your own doctor. You will discover that what you need to do is <u>far simpler</u> and <u>far easier</u> than you might imagine. I employ the <u>MISS</u> (Make it simple- stupid) principle.☺

<u>BELOW- I EXAMINE THE ESSENTIAL HEALTH TESTS THAT YOU NEED TO KNOW</u>—and some tests that are nice to know.

Often I'll use several different explanations to describe the same biochemical processes. Everyone learns and understands differently. Sometimes certain words obfuscate new concepts while some "hot-button" words promote easier understanding and learning.

<u>THREE COLLOQUIAL TERMS THAT ARE USED THROUGHOUT THIS BOOK:</u>

- <u>"BUSTED CELLS"</u>

- <u>"BUSTED MITOCHONDRIA"</u> (Mitochondria are tiny power plants (think batteries) which manufacture energy from the food that we consume). And

- "BUSTED METABOLISM" (Metabolism is the process of making energy and cellular molecules from breaking down food.)

THESE 3 WORDS WILL HELP YOU UNDERSTAND SOME VERY COMPLEX HUMAN PHYSIOLOGY AND HUMAN BIOCHEMISTRY.

THESE 3 WORDS ARE USED TO DESCRIBE A VARIETY OF DIFFERENT KINDS OF CELLULAR DYSFUNCTION, MITOCHONDRIAL DYSFUNCTION AND/OR METABOLIC DYSFUNCTION/DYSREGULATION. (These concepts will be demystified later-so no need to worry-☺)

MOST CHRONIC DISEASES ORIGINATE FROM "BUSTED CELLS" WHICH SOMETIMES MORPH INTO METABOLIC DISORDERS AND/OR A "BUSTED METABOLISM".

INDEED—MOST CHRONIC DISEASES-such as Obesity, Diabetes, Cancer etc. ARE METABOLIC DISORDERS DUE TO DAMAGED MITOCHONDRIA AND/OR DISEASED CELLS/AND/OR A DAMAGED METABOLISM.

The present chapter consists of two sections. SECTION B- analyzes:

"MY PLATINUM KEY TO SUPERHEALTH: IS: drum roll please-☺

" YOU MUST MAINTAIN STABLE, LOW BLOOD SUGAR LEVELS, AND STABLE, LOW INSULIN LEVELS TO ELIMINATE INSULIN RESISTANCE"

SECTION C- examines the principles and tools YOU NEED FOR SELF-ASSESSMENT.

THESE ARE THE BLOOD AND LABORATORY TESTS YOU CAN EASILY AND QUICKLY OBTAIN TO EVALUATE YOUR OVERALL HEALTH.

PRIOR TO BEGINNING THE KETOGENIC NUTRITIONAL PROGRAM, THESE ARE THE BLOOD AND LABORATORY STUDIES THAT YOU SHOULD HAVE PERFORMED IF POSSIBLE.

THESE TEST RESULTS WILL PROVIDE YOU WITH AN EXCELLENT EVALUATION OF YOUR CURRENT STATE OF HEALTH.

IDEAL AND OTHER NUMBERS ARE PROVIDED WITH EXPLANATIONS SO THAT YOU CAN DECIDE FOR YOURSELF THE TESTS THAT YOU PERSONALLY NEED TO PRIORITIZE.

YOU WILL DISCOVER THAT COSTS FOR THESE LAB/BLOOD TESTS ARE REASONABLE.

MOREOVER, YOU CAN CHECK WITH YOUR HEALTH INSURANCE PEOPLE TO VERIFY WHETHER YOUR INSURER WILL DEFRAY THESE COSTS. (The chances are excellent that these blood tests will be covered under your existing policy.

B.   MY PLATINUM KEY TO SUPERHEALTH

TO REPEAT—MY PLATINUM KEY TO SUPERHEALTH IS:

" YOU MUST MAINTAIN STABLE, LOW BLOOD SUGAR LEVELS AND STABLE, LOW INSULIN LEVELS TO ELIMINATE INSULIN-RESISTANCE"

TO BE HEALTHY— WE ARE "SUPPOSED TO HAVE" ABOUT (1) ONE TEASPOON OF GLUCOSE (BLOOD SUGAR) CIRCULATING IN OUR BLOODSTREAM.

HERE IS MY "COLES NOTES VERSION" OF MY PLATINUM KEY TO SUPERHEALTH. Here are some sugary facts.

- **95 PERCENT OF THE POPULATION EAT TOO MANY CARBOHYDRATES.**

- **95 PERCENT OF THE POPULATION ARE AD-DICTED TO CARBOHYDRATES (SUGAR).**

- **95 PERCENT OF THE POPULATION ARE SUGAR (CARB) BURNERS.**

- **95 PERCENT OF SUGAR (CARB) BURNERS HAVE TOO MUCH (GLUCOSE) SUGAR IN THEIR BLOOD.**

- **95 PERCENT OF THE POPULATION UTILIZE GLUCOSE (SUGAR) AS THEIR PRIMARY FUEL AND AS THEIR PRIMARY ENERGY SOURCE.**

- **80 PERCENT OF AMERICAN ADULTS HAVE BLOOD GLUCOSE LEVELS THAT ARE OUT OF THE SAFE HEALTHY RANGE!**

- **AN ABERRANT CARB- BURNING STRATEGY KEEPS OUR HORMONES DEREGULATED, CAUSING SUGAR (CARB) CRAVINGS AND STRESS!**

- **CARB (SUGAR) BURNERS SLOWLY POISON THEIR PAN-CREAS AND DESTROY THEIR BRAIN CELLS!**

- **THE MORE GLUCOSE (SUGAR —IN THE FORM OF CARBOHY-DRATES) THAT YOU BURN—THE SOONER THAT YOU WILL DIE!**

- **THE MORE FAT THAT YOU BURN FOR EN-ERGY- THE LONGER YOU WILL LIVE!**

<u>These are the sugary facts of life.</u> You have a very simple choice. You can fuel your body with carbs and die- OR you can fuel your body with healthy fats and live a long healthy, joyful life. You must accept the fact that you <u>ARE ADDICTED TO SUGAR.</u>

You have a choice. You can continue with eating your typical bad North American diet OR <u>YOU CAN DECIDE TO GO COLD TURKEY AND KICK YOUR SUGAR ADDICTION.</u>

<u>BUT- YOU SHOULD HAVE NO FEAR!</u> I make a solemn promise.

<u>A KETOGENIC DIET WILL MAKE YOU STRONG, HEALTHY AND SMART!</u>-☺

<u>TO BE HEALTHY—WE REQUIRE A HEALTHY PANCREAS, LIVER, KIDNEYS AND BODIES THAT PROPERLY REGULATE OUR BLOOD SUGAR LEVELS.</u>

- <u>OUR PANCREAS, (OUR SECRET FAT-BURNING ORGAN), THROUGH ITS BETA CELLS- PRODUCES A HORMONE CALLED—"INSULIN".</u>

- <u>INSULIN IS THE "MAIN" HORMONE THAT REGULATES THE AMOUNT OF BLOOD SUGAR IN OUR BODY.</u>

- <u>INSULIN HELPS YOUR BODY USE SUG-AR FROM FOODS THAT YOU EAT.</u>

- <u>THE HORMONE INSULIN— EITHER:</u>

<u>PUSHES SUGAR INTO YOUR CELLS TO BE USED/BURNED AS ENERGY—</u>

—OR—

<u>INSULIN STORES SUGAR (GLUCOSE) AWAY—AS FAT!</u> Yuk!

- <u>INSULIN IS ONE OF OUR MOST IMPORTANT BIO-LOGICAL SUBSTANCES AND IS A CRITICAL REGU-LATOR OF CELLULAR METABOLISM.</u>

- <u>INSULIN'S MAIN JOB IS TO FERRY GLUCOSE FROM THE BLOOD-STREAM INTO MUSCLE, FAT, AND LIVER CELLS. ONCE IN-SIDE OF OUR CELLS GLUCOSE CAN BE USED AS ENERGY.</u>

- <u>NORMAL HEALTHY CELLS HAVE A HIGH "SENSITIVITY" TO INSULIN.</u>

- <u>BUT —WHEN HEALTHY CELLS ARE BOMBARDED WITH HIGH LEVELS OF INSULIN CAUSED BY AN EXTREME INTAKE OF GLUCOSE CAUSED BY EATING TOO MANY CARBS- OUR CELLS REACT AND PROTECT THEMSELVES BY REDUCING THE NUMBER OF RECEPTORS ON THEIR SURFACES THAT CAN RESPOND TO EXCESSIVE INSULIN.</u>

- IN OTHER WORDS—OUR CELLS "DESENSITIZE" THEMSELVES TO INSULIN— WHICH IS TERMED "INSULIN RESISTANCE".

- THUS "INSULIN SENSITIVITY" IS THE OPPOSITE OF INSULIN RESISTANCE.

- WHEN DESENSITIZED CELLS IGNORE INSULIN AND FAIL TO ABSORB GLUCOSE FROM THE BLOOD. OUR PANCREAS DUTIFULLY RESPONDS BY PUMPING OUT EVEN MORE INSULIN!

- HIGHER LEVELS OF INSULIN BECOME NEEDED FOR SUGAR TO ENTER THE CELLS. THESE DESENSITIZED CELLS PROGRESS TO BECOME "BUSTED CELLS"(This is a technical term-☺)

- OUR AMAZING BODY THEN USES A BACK-UP FAIL SAFE METHOD TO HELP RESIST INSULIN. OUR CELLS PROTECT THEMSELVES FROM INSULIN BY REDUCING THE NUMBER OF "RECEPTORS" ON THE CELLS.

- OUR BODY ALSO LIKELY REDUCES THE NUMBER OF CELLS THAT HAVE INSULIN RECEPTORS.

- THIS VICIOUS CYCLE OF BUSTED CELLS CULMINATES UNTIL IT CAUSES A "BUSTED METABOLISM". (another technical term -☺). OFTEN THIS ULTIMATELY MORPHS INTO FULL-BLOWN TYPE 2 DIABETES

- EATING TOO MANY CARBS CAUSES "BUSTED" CELLS"; CARBS DON'T BUILD OR REPAIR ANYTHING. CARBS CAUSE BUSTED CELLS AND INSULIN RESISTANCE—PERIOD. MOST CARBS ARE TOXIC TO YOUR PANCREAS- AND MOST CARBS ARE TOXIC TO YOUR BRAIN!

- WHEN THESE BUSTED CELLS CAN NO LONGER ABSORB BLOOD SUGAR—WE HAVE WHAT IS CALLED "INSULIN RESISTANCE".

IN OTHER WORDS—INSULIN RESISTANCE OCCURS WHEN YOUR BODY'S RESPONSE TO A REGULAR LEVEL OF THIS HORMONE IS REDUCED CREATING A NEED FOR—EVEN MORE INSULIN!

WHEN BLOOD SUGAR BUILDS UP IN OUR BLOODSTREAM, OUR BODY REALIZES THAT THERE IS TOO MUCH GLUCOSE (SUGAR)IN OUR BLOOD WHICH IS TOXIC...SOOOO—OUR BODY RESPONDS BY TURNING ON THE PANCREAS PUMP TO FLOOD OUR BLOODSTREAM WITH AN EVEN BIGGER FLOOD OF INSULIN.

OVERWEIGHT PEOPLE HAVE A "BUSTED" METABOLISM. OBESE PEOPLE ALSO HAVE A BUSTED METABOLISM. FAT PEOPLE PRODUCE TOO MUCH INSULIN. (Too much insulin is called "HYPERINSULINEMIA").

PUT ANOTHER WAY—

WHEN INSULIN RECEPTORS ON OUR CELLS REFUSE TO ACCEPT THE BLOOD SUGAR OFFERED – THESE CELLS BECOME NON-FUNCTIONING OR "BUSTED CELLS". THESE CELLS AND/OR TISSUE BECOME INSULIN RESISTANT. (Think of insulin as the orchestra playing music but the damaged cell receptors have put on their earmuffs because they no longer wish to hear the music-☺)

Here's a simple way to remember what causes "insulin resistance"...

Here's a pop quiz!

Question:

What causes "insulin resistance"?

Answer:

INSULIN!!

NOW YOU UNDERSTAND WHAT CAUSES INSULIN RESISTANCE!

IT'S THAT SIMPLE!

YOU NOW HAVE A FAR BETTER UNDERSTANDING OF INSULIN RESISTANCE THAN MOST ALLOPATHIC DOCTORS! OMG! Now you have the essential information YOU NEED TO DOCTOR YOURSELF!

(Most chowder-headed doctors think that insulin resistance is a blood- sugar problem.) Just think- AHA- THE 99 PERCENT RULE!

Throughout this book I will constantly refer to insulin resistance.

You will read more explanations and more definitions defining insulin resistance.

UNDERSTANDING THE CONCEPT OF INSULIN RESISTANCE AND HOW TO MAINTAIN A LOW STABLE BLOOD SUGAR- WITH NO INSULIN RESISTANCE IS YOUR PLATINUM KEY TO SUPERHEALTH.

Below in the Sugar Factory chapter, especially in the context of DIABETES- the concept of insulin resistance will be examined in more detail...so please stay tuned.-☺

FACT:

CARBS EQUALS= INSULIN EQUALS= DISEASE!

THIS FACT IS SO IMPORTANT- IT BEARS TO BE REPEATED-

CARBS EQUALS INSULIN EQUALS DISEASE!

NO ONE CAN EVEN DISPUTE THIS FACT!

ANOTHER SIMPLE TWO PART EQUATION DEMONSTRATES:

"THE DIABETIC PROCESS"

Part A of this EQUATION SAYS:

BAD FOOD (CARBS) =HYPERINSULINEMIA=OBESITY=INSULIN RESISTANCE.

Part B of this EQUATION SAYS:

INSULIN RESISTANCE=PANCREAS EXHAUSTION= TYPE 2 DIABETES.

THIS DIABETIC PROCESS IS ANALYZED IN GREATER DETAIL—BELOW.

ALMOST ALL CHRONIC DISEASES ARE CAUSED BY "BUSTED MITOCHONDRIA" (another technical term-☺. **MITOCHONDRIA ARE THE LITTLE POWER FACTORIES INSIDE OF MOST CELLS. THE SCIENTIFIC TERMS ARE DYSFUNCTIONAL MITOCHONDRIA OR IMPAIRED MITOCHONDRIA.**

BUSTED MITOCHONDRIA LEAD TO BUSTED CELLS. BUSTED CELLS CAN LEAD TO BUSTED METABOLISM AND A BOATLOAD OF METABOLIC DISORDERS AND CHRONIC DISEASES.

DIABETES (TYPE 2) BASICALLY IS A "BUSTED CARB METABOLISM" (aka "Impaired Glucose Metabolism".

CANCER IS ALSO A METABOLIC DISEASE COMPRISING BUSTED CELLS AND A BUSTED METABOLISM.

INSULIN RESISTANCE LAYS THE FOUNDATION FOR VIRTUALLY ALL CHRONIC DISEASES FROM A TO Z!

INSULIN CAN BE A VILLAINOUS HORMONE-OR A GOOD HORMONE-☺

YOU GET TO CHOOSE IF INSULIN IS GOOD GUY OR A BAD GUY.

ITS MAIN JOB IS TO FERRY GLUCOSE INTO OUR CELLS —BUT—INSULIN ALSO IS AN ANABOLIC HORMONE –i.e. IT STIMULATES GROWTH, PROMOTES FAT FORMATION AND STORAGE AND INFLAMMATION! (That's the bad guy part).

HIGH INSULIN LEVELS CAUSE OTHER HORMONES TO BE "OUT OF WHACK (another technical term for **OUT OF BALANCE-☺)**

INSULIN CAN BE A DOMINEERING BULLY! TOO MUCH INSULIN CAN EITHER CAUSE TOO MUCH OR TOO LITTLE OF OTHER IMPORTANT HORMONES.

HORMONAL IMBALANCES THEN PLUNGE THE BODY INTO HEALTH CHAOS.

INSULIN RESISTANCE PROMOTES "CHRONIC INFLAMMATION" WHICH THEN SPEEDS UP THE ENTIRE AGING PROCESS THAT TRIGGERS A BOATLOAD OF ASSOCIATED HEALTH PROBLEMS.

A recent study on **LONGEVITY** concluded that:

- **HAVING VERY LOW LEVELS OF INFLAMMATION IN YOUR BODY IS THE MOST POTENT PREDIC-TOR OF LIVING BEYOND 100 YEARS OLD!**

- **INFLAMMATION LEVELS CORRELATED WITH PEOPLE'S ABILITY TO LIVE INDEPENDENTLY AND MAINTAIN COGNITIVE FUNCTIONS.**

YOU MUST UNDERSTAND THAT HIGH INSULIN LEVELS WILL MAKE YOU OLD, FAT, SICK and maybe even ugly.-☺

Can you guess which nutritional approach will make you melt off excess weight and make you lean?

Can you guess which nutritional approach best reverses insulin resistance and diabetes?

You guessed it!

IT'S THE KETOGENIC DIET! HALLELUJAH!!

THE KETOGENIC DIET IS THE BEST ANTI—INFLAMMATORY DIET IN THE WORLD! DELICIOUS "FAT" FOODS ARE VERY POWERFUL, ANTI-INFLAMMATORY FOODS.

OPTIMUM HEALTH BEGINS AT THE CELLULAR LEVEL. SUPERHEALTH BEGINS WITH OPTIMIZING OUR MITOCHONDRIAL HEALTH.

WE MUST REDUCE CELLULAR/ TISSUE/ INFLAMMATION TO RESTORE OUR MITOCHRONDRIAL HEALTH AND PREVENT DISEASE.

EATING A FAT KETOGENIC DIET BUILDS CELL MEM "BRANES".

A KETOGENIC DIET BUILDS BRAIN CELLS TOO!

CARBOHYDRATES ARE TOXIC TO YOUR BODY. CARBS EAT YOUR BRAIN CELLS AND DESTROY YOUR PANCREAS CELLS TOO.

A KETOGENIC DIET PROVIDES OPTIMUM INSULIN AND LEPTIN "SENSITIVITY." (Leptin is a satiety hormone.)

A KETOGENIC DIET REGULATES GHRELIN (hunger hormone) AND REGULATES YOUR THYROID HORMONES TOO!

THIS MEANS THAT YOU WILL BE EASILY SATISFIED SIMPLY BY EATING RICH SUCCULENT MOUTH-WATERING FATTY KETOGENIC FOODS.

THERE ARE 3 BASIC MACRONUTRIENTS:

CARBS====Long-chains of SUGAR MOLECULES.

FAT=======Chains of FATTY ACIDS.

PROTEINS==Chains of AMINO ACIDS

THINK OF CARBS AS A SECOND-RATE FUEL (think cheap low octane fuel) WHICH IS BURNED BY OUR BODY.

CARBS (make glucose which is sugar) CAUSE INFLAMMATION IN OUR CELLS.

- CARBS ARE GLUCOSE— A SECOND RATE FUEL WHICH DO NOT BURN COMPLETELY AND THEY DAMAGE OUR CELLS- ESPECIALLY THE MITOCHONDRIA- aka BUSTED CELLS, BUSTED MITOCHONDRIA AND THEN BUSTED METABOLISM.

- FAT—THE MAIN COMPONENT OF OUR CELLS—IS OUR BODIES' PREFERRED FUEL TO PRODUCE ENERGY.

- FAT IS THE PREFERRED FUEL OF HUMAN METABOLISM!

- FAT IS ALSO THE SECRET LOVE OF YOUR BRAIN! (Your brain is 75 % FAT!)

- FAT— (UNLIKE CARBS) BURNS CLEAN AS A WHISTLE!-☺ FAT LEAVES NO DIRTY CARBON DEPOSITS IN OUR CELLS-☺

- CARBS BURN AND LEAVE "deposits" IN THE FORM OF FREE RADICALS.

- THINK OF HEALTHY FATS AS HIGH-OCTANE SUPER FUEL THAT BURN CLEANER, FASTER AND PRODUCE MUCH MORE ENERGY FOR THE SAME AMOUNT OF FOOD COMPARED TO CARBS.

BLOOD SUGAR REGULATION

There are many factors that affect your body's ability to properly regulate and control blood sugar. DIET AND PHYSICAL ACTIVITY are important and other important factors include:

RESTORATIVE SLEEP, STRESS MANAGEMENT, GUT HEALTH AND HORMONE BALANCE. These and other factors are analyzed in greater detail in subsequent chapters.

Are you one of the TENS OF MILLIONS of Americans who struggle to maintain HEALTHY BLOOD SUGAR METABOLISM OR BLOOD SUGAR REGULATION?

Most often- a blood sugar issue first manifests with symptoms, like fatigue, mood swings, food cravings and weight gain. If you fail to heed warning signs—this condition can lead to insulin resistance. This will cause your blood sugar to FLUCTUATE WILDLY—leading to your doctor prescribing a DRUG-or even worse-a COCKTAIL OF DRUGS!

The consequences of living with a serious BLOOD SUGAR IMBALANCE CAN BE TRAGIC!

THE TRUTH IS there's an EASY, inexpensive way to maintain healthy BLOOD SUGAR LEVELS—SAFELY AND PERMANENTLY!

THE CURRENT MAINSTREAM MEDICAL MENTALITY ON BLOOD SUGAR MANAGEMENT HAS CREATED BIG PHARMA'S MOST LUCRATIVE CLASS OF DRUGS.

THEY WILL STOP AT NOTHING TO KEEP THEM ON THE MARKET.

THEY HAVE LIED TO YOU ABOUT THE SAFETY OF THESE DRUGS!

THERE ARE NO REASONS FOR YOU TO JEOPARDIZE YOUR HEALTH TO MAKE THEIR PROFITS SOAR WHEN THERE ARE SAFER—MORE EFFECTIVE OPTIONS.

BIG PHARMA WANTS TO HIDE THE TRUTH FROM YOU.

THE GOOD NEWS IS THAT IN MOST CASES—

IT'S EASY TO CORRECT A BLOOD SUGAR IMBALANCE WITH NATURAL SUBSTANCES SUCH AS —CINNAMON, APPLE CIDER VINEGAR (ACV) AND BERBERINE (analyzed when discussing Type 2 Diabetes below.)

FURTHERMORE, THE BEST, SAFEST METHOD TO REGULATE BLOOD SUGAR IMBALANCE IS BY USING A KETOGENIC DIET.

BESIDES INSULIN— THE THYROID HORMONES (esp. T-3) CAN HAVE THE MOST PROFOUND IMPACT ON BLOOD SUGAR.

THYROID HORMONES SERIOUSLY IMPACT BLOOD SUGAR LEVELS.

A study in the Journal of Diabetes Complications demonstrated the association between LOW T-3— HYPERINSULINEMIA AND ELEVATED BLOOD SUGAR. The good news is that if you follow a Ketogenic Diet- your insulin and thyroid hormones will be balanced as they are intended to be.

INSULIN AND THYROID HORMONE WORK TOGETHER LIKE A "SEE-SAW".

AS THYROID HORMONE (T-3 LEVELS) GO DOWN—INSULIN LEVELS RISE.

LIKEWISE—AS INSULIN LEVELS INCREASE DUE TO INSULIN RESISTANCE—THYROID HORMONE IS SUPPRESSED.

SINCE THYROID IS THE MAIN FAT" BURNING" HORMONE—AND SINCE INSULIN IS THE MAIN FAT "STORAGE" HORMONE—THIS LEADS TO A METABOLIC DOUBLE-WHAMMY! OMG!

LOW THYROID AND HIGH INSULIN LEVELS GUARANTEE YOU WILL STORE FAT —NOT BURN FAT EFFECTIVELY. Yuk!

ANOTHER THING INSULIN DOES IS TO TELL THE KIDNEYS TO HOLD ONTO SODIUM.

* THE TAKE-HOME MESSAGE IS:

THE HEALING KETOGENIC DIET (KD) AND "NUTRITIONAL KETOSIS" PERFORMS THESE MAGICAL FEATS:

1. KD RESTORES NORMAL BLOOD SUGAR LEVELS AND INSULIN SENSITIVITY.

2. KD AND (LOW-CARB DIETS) KEEP YOUR INSULIN LEVELS DOWN.

3. KD REVERSES INSULIN RESISTANCE AND DIABETES.

4. KD LOWERS INFLAMMATORY MARKERS.

5. KD OPTIMIZES METABOLISM AND METABOLIC FUNCTIONS.

6. KD IMPROVES BLOOD SUGAR LEVELS- STARTING WITH YOUR FIRST MEAL

YOUR FIRST MEAL!

How cool is that?

MY PLATINUM KEY TO SUPERHEALTH IS:

YOU MUST MAINTAIN STABLE, LOW BLOOD SUGAR LEVELS—STABLE, LOW INSULIN LEVELS AND ELIMINATE INSULIN RESISTANCE. (Restore insulin sensitivity).

C. SELF-ASSESSMENT

YOU MUST EDUCATE YOURSELF. NO ONE CAN DO THAT FOR YOU— NO ONE—NOT your physician, no government agencies, no dietician, no coach, no spouse, (not even your mother-in- law-☺)

YOU CAN TAKE THE PRACTICAL STEPS DISCUSSED BELOW TO BECOME YOUR OWN DOCTOR- SO YOU CAN HEAL YOURSELF!

TO OBTAIN THE ESSENTIAL HEALTH TESTS YOU NEED—YOU CAN ORDER THEM YOURSELF! YOU ARE MASTER OF YOUR OWN HEALTH DESTINY!

You can't rely on your doctor to properly **EVALUATE YOUR HEALTH NEEDS.**

To rely on your doctor to evaluate your health needs is illogical and foolish.

Your doctor does not even know how to evaluate his **OWN** health needs.

HOW IN THE WORLD CAN YOUR DOCTOR ASSESS YOUR HEALTH NEEDS?

YOUR DOCTOR'S FLAWED NUTRITIONAL EDUCATION MEANS YOUR DOCTOR IS TOTALLY IGNORANT ABOUT THE HEALTH TESTS THAT YOU REQUIRE.

SADLY- MOST ANNUAL MEDICAL CHECK-UPS AND TESTS THAT MOST PHYSICIANS ORDER AND USE ARE SIMPLY OLD-SCHOOL BLOOD TESTS.

THESE ANTIQUATED/ QUASI-USELESS TESTS DO NOT EVEN TEST FOR THE MOST IMPORTANT "MARKERS" OF DISEASE! Markers is a scientific word which means indicators of disease.

THE CHOLESTEROL TESTS (AND HEART TESTS TOO) USED BY CONVENTIONAL DOCTORS ARE THE WRONG ONES!

(The 99 percent rule again-☺) OMG!

How can allopathic doctors get a medical licence? Your grandmother is a medical genius compared to most doctors. Most medical doctors are clueless as to what they should do for you so they just dope you up...and leave you alone to suffer in misery.

In chapter one, you learned that cholesterol testing is the greatest health scam of this century. Cholesterol has been demonized by doctors and Big Pharma to make <u>MONEY</u>. <u>PERIOD!</u>

<u>THE TOTAL CHOLESTEROL TEST WILL TELL YOU VIRTUALLY NOTHING ABOUT YOUR DISEASE RISK</u>...unless over 350). Research shows that the higher your cholesterol levels- the longer you will live!

And conversely, the lower your cholesterol- the sooner you will die!

<u>SO—CHOLESTEROL TESTING IS NOT A GOOD BIOMARKER OF POSSIBLE DISEASE. THERE ARE MUCH BETTER LAB/BLOOD TESTS THAT YOU CAN OBTAIN.</u>

<u>YOU HAVE REASON TO REJOICE!</u>

<u>THANKS TO DR. INTERNET-</u>

<u>YOU CAN NOW COMPLETELY BY-PASS THE MEDICAL ESTABLISHMENT AND PHARMACEUTICAL COMPANIES BY PUTTING THE POWER OF KNOWLEDGE INTO YOUR HANDS!!</u>

<u>YOU HAVE A GREAT HEALTH SOLUTION AT THE CLICK OF A MOUSE— ANYWHERE—ANYTIME 24/7!</u>

<u>YOU MUST TEST-TEST-AND TEST!</u>

Unless you know what blood looks like under a microscope, you have no way to identify with <u>100 PERCENT CERTAINTY AND WHAT STEPS YOU SHOULD TAKE TO EAT THE RIGHT DIET/ OR WHAT SUPPLEMENTS YOU SHOULD TAKE.</u>

<u>FEW PEOPLE REALIZE THAT YOU CAN BY-PASS YOUR PHYSICIAN AND MANAGE THE ENTIRE PROCESS OF GETTING YOUR BLOOD WORK DONE YOURSELF!</u>

<u>AND YOU DON'T HAVE TO PAY THOUSANDS OF DOLLARS AT A LONGEVITY INSTITUTION OR HEALTH CLINIC OR CONSULT SOME SELF-PROCLAIMED HEALTH GURU!</u>

<u>YOU NOW CAN OBTAIN COMPLETE BLOOD TESTING ON LINE FROM REPUTABLE LABORATORIES—FAST!</u>

<u>YOU CAN EASILY GET YOUR OWN LABS ON LINE AT SITES SUCH AS:</u> DirectLabs.com and Wellness Fx.

<u>YOU CAN USUALLY GET YOUR LAB RESULTS IN ONE (1) DAY!</u>

YOU CAN TAKE CHARGE OF YOUR OWN HEALTH AND MONITOR YOUR TEST RESULTS YOURSELF.

QUICK –SIMPLE- EASY-AND INEXPENSIVE- AND BEST OF ALL-

WITH NO DOCTOR REQUIRED!!

YOU CAN GET YOUR LAB TEST RESULTS IN YOUR HAND IN LESS TIME THAN IT TAKES TO GET AN APPOINTMENT SEE YOUR DOCTOR!

YOU CAN PURCHASE THE MOST COMPLETE BLOOD-TESTING PACKAGES THAT MONEY CAN BUY. ALSO- MOST INSURANCE COMPANIES WILL PAY FOR THESE TESTS SO YOU CAN ORDER ANY TESTS THAT YOU REQUIRE.

BLOOD TESTING IS THE MOST IMPORTANT PRACTICAL STEP YOU CAN TAKE TO IDENTIFY AND PREVENT LIFE-THREATENING DISEASES— BEFORE THEY HAPPEN TO YOU.

TO REALLY KNOW WHAT CHEMICALS ARE IN YOUR BODY—YOU MUST LOOK AT YOUR BLOOD UNDER A MICROSCOPE.

ONCE YOU OBTAIN YOUR BLOOD TEST RESULTS- YOU CAN CATCH AND PREVENT CRITICAL HEALTH ISSUES IN YOUR BODY BEFORE THEY MANIFEST AS DIABETES, CANCER, HEART DISEASE-ETC.

INTIMATE- PERSONALIZED KNOWLEDGE OF WHAT'S GOING ON INSIDE "YOUR CHEMISTRY SET" EMPOWERS YOU—SO THAT YOUR CAN INITIATE AND MANAGE YOUR OWN HEALTH PROGRAM.

THIS PREVENTATIVE HEALTH PROGRAM CAN LITERALLY ADD DECADES OF QUALITY, HEALTHY YEARS TO YOUR LIFE.

You will be able to add LIFE to your YEARS and YEARS to your LIFE.

YOU CAN OBTAIN A COMPLETE (CUSTOMIZED) BLOOD AND/OR LIPID PANEL THAT EVALUATES OVERALL METABOLIC FUNCTIONING FOR OPTIMAL LONG-TERM HEALTH AND LONGEVITY.

YOU CAN BY-PASS THE MEDICAL SYSTEM AND BIG PHARMA!

YOU CAN TAKE THIS DIY APPROACH TO ATTAIN SUPERHEALTH!

BLOOD PANELS INCLUDE inter alia:

- Thyroid function, stress response, blood-glucose regulation, sex-hormone balance, heavy metals, inflammation, organs of detoxification (liver, kidneys, gallbladder and lungs); proteins, electrolytes, blood-oxygen and nutrient delivery, immune system status, Vitamin D-3 status, as well as

- **Apolipoprotein A-1 and B;**

- **Blood lead**

- **Blood mercury**

- **Cardio Q Lipoprotein fractionation**

- **Ion mobility**

- **A complete blood count with complete metabolic panel,**

- **Copper**

- **Cortisol**

- **Dehydroepiandrosterone**

- **Sulphate**

- **Ferritin,**

- **folate**

- **free fatty acids**

- **Hemoglobin Alc**

- **Homocysteine**

- **C-reactive protein**

- **IGf-1 (growth hormone surrogate)**

- **INSULIN**

- **Iron**

- **Lipid PANEL Lipoprotein (a), Luteiniz- ing Hormone, Omega-3 fatty acids;**

- **RBC Magnesium**

- **Selenium**

- **SHBG (sex hormone binding globulin)**

- **Thyroid hormones, Reverse T-3, T-4 (Thyroxine) T-3 free, T-4 free, & T-3 total, T-3 uptake; thyroid peroxidate AB & TSH;**

- **Testosterone & free testosteronew**

- thiamine

- Thyoglobulin antibodies

- Uric acid

- Zinc

- Vitamin A, B-12;

- Estradiol

IF your goal is not just to stop DISEASE- but also to perform at your PEAK PHYSICAL AND COGNITIVE CAPACITY—

BLOOD TESTING IS ABSOLUTELY CRITICAL TO ADDRESS YOUR DIETARY DEFICIENCIES.

BLOOD TESTING IS A GREAT DIAGNOSTIC TOOL THAT CAN BE USED TO PROTECT YOUR HEALTH; ENHANCE YOUR WELL-BEING AND PERMIT YOU TO PERFORM AT YOUR PEAK CAPACITY TO ENJOY A LONG HIGH-QUALITY LIFE.

THE FOLLOWING TESTS ARE PARAMOUNT:

Fasting Blood Glucose

* This common diagnostic tool is used to check for pre-diabetes and diabetes.

This test measures the amount of sugar (glucose) in your blood after you have not

eaten for at least 8 hours. The normal "range" is between 70 and 100 milligrams   per deciliter (mg/dl)

* 6 millimoles per liter(6 mmol/L) (108 milligrams per deciliter are considered normal.

- 6 mmol/L and below 7 mmol/L (108 to 128 mg/dl) are considered elevated or pre-diabetic;

- 7 mmol/L or greater are diagnosed as full-blown Diabetes 2;

- Above 100 mg/dl) shows signs of INSULIN RESIS-TANCE AND DIABETES/BRAIN DAMAGE;

- Recent study published in New England Journal of Medicine proved that a mild elevation of blood sugar levels (105-110 mg/dl) was associated with an elevated risk of developing DEMENTIA;

- Studies show that a Fasting Blood Glucose (FBS) of 100 to 125 mg/d had a WHOPPING 300 PERCENT higher risk of cardiovascular disease vs. people with a FBS level BELOW 79 mg/dl!

- 95 mg/dl/ means URGENT to address your blood sugar level!

- Less than 85 mg/dl is a good blood sugar level;

- OPTIMUM OR IDEAL fasting blood sugar level is 65 to 75 mg/dl ((2.5 – 3 mmol/L) i.e. HALF of what conventional doctors say)

- Keto-adapted level should be below 70 mg/dl)

Hemoglobin A1C

This test reveals an "average of blood sugar over a 90 day period:

It is a far better indication of overall blood sugar CONTROL.

Hemoglobin A1C IS THE BEST LAB REPORT TO REFER TO IN DETERMINING YOUR OVERALL HEALTH STATUS- NOT CHOLESTEROL!

- Hemoglobin A1C is the protein found in the red blood cell that carries oxygen and binds to blood sugar, and this binding is increased when blood sugar is elevated.

- It is well documented that 'GLYCATED HEMOGLOBIN' is a powerful risk factor for diabetes, stroke, cardiovascular diseases, brain health problems and DEATH from other illnesses. (Glycation is he biochemical term for the binding of sugar molecules-to proteins, fats, and amino acids;(aka Maillard reaction).

- N.B. A HIGH-CARB DIET SPEEDS UP THE GLYCATION PROCESS!

- Above 6.0 Percent is very dangerous for all of the above.

- IDEAL LEVEL IS 4.8 TO 5.3 percent.

Fasting Insulin TEST

THIS TEST IS "THE KEY TEST" YOU MUST GET TO ATTAIN SUPERHEALTH AND TO ASSESS YOUR BODY'S INSULIN LEVELS AND BLOOD SUGAR REGULATION.

YOUR PLATINUM KEY TO SUPERHEALTH IS TO ELIMINATE INSULIN RESISTANCE AND MAINTAIN STABLE LOW BLOOD SUGAR LEVELS.

TO ELIMINATE INSULIN RESISTANCE (aka IMPAIRED INSULIN SENSITIVITY)—

YOU MUST SHUT DOWN EXCESS INSULIN PRODUCTION IN YOUR PANCREAS.

THE BEST WAY TO FIND OUT HOW MUCH INSULIN YOUR PANCREAS IS PRODUCING IS TO TEST IT!

THE BLOOD TEST USED IS CALLED "THE FASTING INSULIN" TEST.

This blood test is done first thing in the morning before eating a meal; (in a FASTED state). An elevated level of insulin in your blood at this time is a HUGE RED FLAG—a sign YOU MAY HAVE SERIOUS METABOLIC PROBLEMS!

Here's the thing. You may have your fasting blood sugar level tested and find that your test numbers fall within the normal range. BUT—if you could take a peek inside of your pancreas, you might be appalled at what's going on. You might be shocked to learn that your pancreas is working overtime and struggling to pump out insulin to keep your blood sugar level balanced. Having normal blood sugar levels may mean that your pancreas is working overtime to keep your blood sugar normal. You have to find out what is really happening inside of your pancreas-☺

THIS IS HOW INSULIN LEVELS CAN RISE AND A PERSON BECOMES DIABETIC EVEN THOUGH BLOOD SUGAR NUMBERS APPEAR NORMAL.

THIS IS WHY IT IS ABSOLUTELY CRITICAL TO CHECK YOUR FASTING INSULIN LEVELS—AS WELL AS YOUR FASTING BLOOD-SUGAR LEVELS.

Elevated insulin levels prove two things. One- your pancreas is trying hard to normalize blood sugar. Two- this is clear proof that YOU ARE EATING TOO MANY CARBOHYDRATES.

IF YOUR BLOOD SUGAR HAPPENS TO BE "NORMAL"- THE ONLY WAY YOU WILL KNOW IF YOU ARE INSULIN RESISTANT IS TO HAVE YOUR FASTING BLOOD INSULIN LEVEL CHECKED. PERIOD.

YOU CAN BE LEAN AND INSULIN-RESISTANT!

"IF YOU'RE NOT TESTING- YOU'RE ONLY GUESSING!

THE FASTING INSULIN BLOOD TEST IS THE MOST IMPORTANT TEST THAT YOU MUST HAVE DONE –TO ENSURE THAT YOU ARE NOT INSULIN RESISTANT!

**NOTE BENE-

THE HIGHER YOUR FASTING INSULIN LEVEL—THE GREATER YOUR INSULIN RESISTANCE! IT'S THAT SIMPLE!

MOREOVER— IF YOUR BODY PRODUCES TOO MUCH INSULIN—

YOU WILL NOT BE ABLE TO PRODUCE KETONES (fat bodies).

And-

YOU WILL NOT BE ABLE TO BECOME A FAT-BURNING BEAST!-☺

TO ENSURE THAT YOU ARE HEALTHY AND TO STAY HEALTHY YOU MUST ELIMINATE INSULIN RESISTANCE.

INSULIN RESISTANCE IS THE PRECURSOR AND THE HALLMARK OF DIABETES AND A BOATLOAD OF OTHER CHRONIC DISEASES.

THAT'S WHY INSULIN RESISTANCE IS AN ESSENTIAL PART OF YOUR PLATINUM KEY TO SUPERHEALTH.

Most conventional doctors do **NOT** test for fasting insulin levels. Why is that?

There are at least three reasons.

1. If they tested your insulin levels and dis-covered elevated insulin levels—

    HOW IN THE WORLD WOULD THEY BE ABLE TO SELL YOU ANY POISONOUS SYNTHETIC INSULIN MAKING DRUGS?? OMG!

2. If they diagnosed you with elevated insulin levels—**THEY WOULD HAVE TO TELL YOU THE TRUTH AND- THAT IS TO EAT LOW CARB. ALL OF THE FOODS BEING PROMOTED ON THE "UNHEALTHY" FOOD PYRAMID WOULD BE BANNED FROM YOUR DIET!**

3. **DOCTORS WANT TO KEEP YOU INSULIN-RESISTANT!**

Doctors make money from your so they **WANT YOU TO REMAIN SICK.** Doctors profit by disease management. Wellness and good health do not generate profits for doctors. Would you kill the goose that laid the golden egg?

HONESTLY—HAVE YOU EVER HEARD OF EVEN ONE PERSON CURED OF ANYTHING BY A CONVENTIONAL DOCTOR?

YOU NEED TO KNOW THAT—

* THE IDEAL FASTING INSULIN LEVEL IS BETWEEN 2 AND 3 AND PREFERABLY BELOW 2.

Cholesterol TESTS

As discussed in chapter one, the main reason conventional doctors use cholesterol tests is so that they can sell you STATIN drugs under the fraudulent guise that statins can prevent heart disease. Statin drugs <u>CAUSE</u> heart disease- they don't prevent heart disease. (A classic example of the 99 percent Rule.)

Generally speaking— cholesterol tests used by conventional doctor are not good biomarkers or indicators of heart/health problems. However- research shows that:

<u>HIGH HDL LEVELS ARE BENEFICIAL AND CONSTITUTE A POWERFUL HEART DISEASE RISK FACTOR. You should know the following about cholesterol tests.</u>

<u>TWO RATIOS ARE VERY GOOD INDICATORS OF HEART DISEASE.</u>

1. Your HDL/Total cholesterol ratio.

   Just divide your HDL level by your total cholesterol. <u>IDE-ALLY</u>—this percentage should be <u>ABOVE 24 PERCENT</u>. (Below 10% is a significant risk factor for heart disease.

2. Your triglyceride /HDL ratio.

   To calculate your ratio- just divide your tri-glyceride level by your HDL.

   This ratio should be BELOW 2.

So while you strive to keep your HDLs high- you still want to <u>DECREASE YOUR TRIGLYCERIDES</u>.

One study found that people with the <u>HIGHEST</u> ration of triglycerides to HDL had A 16 <u>TIMES GREATER RISK OF HEART ATTACK</u> than those with the lowest ratio!

Another useful (functional) test is <u>THE NUCLEAR MAGNETIC RESONANCE TEST</u>. This lab test gives you <u>PARTICLE SIZE</u>. In cholesterol (and most things in life) <u>SIZE MATTERS</u>! Small LDL particles are more prone to <u>OXIDATIVE STRESS</u>…very small LDL particles hang around longer in your blood. These "little suckers" penetrate the linings of your arteries and your heart tissues—so they are dangerous!

<u>NMR LIPOPROFILE TEST</u> is an excellent test that tests your LDL PARTICLE <u>NUMBER</u>. Research shows that LDL particle number is an accurate predictor of heart disease risk. This test is easy to get and all major labs offer it. (e.g. Labcorp, Quest)

You can order TESTS directly for directlabs.com or on line from Healthtestingcenters.com etc. <u>YOU CAN ORDER YOUR TESTS ON LINE AND GET YOUR BLOOD DRAWN LOCALLY-WHERE YOU LIVE.</u>

<u>STEP NUMBER ONE:</u>

<u>YOU CAN OBTAIN ONE OF THE MOST POWERFUL DIAGNOSTIC TOOLS AVAILABLE!</u>

<u>BUY A GLUCOMETER TO TEST YOUR BLOOD SUGAR LEVELS.</u>

<u>YOU CAN PURCHASE ONE FROM YOUR LOCAL DRUGSTORE OR FROM</u> Abbot Laboratories for about $ 30.00.

<u>Here's how it works.</u>

A glucometer is a device that measures blood sugar (used by diabetics), You prick your finger with a sterilized lancet. Then you apply the drop of blood to a "test strip" that has been inserted into the glucometer—and it measures your blood sugar. The blood strips for testing are expensive in most places BUT- if you shop on-line or even at some department stores you can by 50 strips for about $ 10.00 or 20 cents each.

<u>MEASURING YOUR BLOOD SUGAR WITH A GLUCOMETER.</u>

<u>FOR STEP NO. 2-</u> Please see how to measure KETONES chapter 7 (infra.)

<u>Fructosamine test</u>

Similar to the Hemoglobin AIC test, a fructosamine test is used to measure an average blood sugar level but over a shorter time period—the past 2 to 3 weeks.

<u>Homocysteine Test</u>

Homocysteine is an amino-acid-like chemical that is known to be toxic to the brain.

<u>IDEAL LEVEL</u> OF Homocysteine is 8 micromoles per litre (8umol/L) or <u>LESS.</u>

<u>HAVING A LEVEL OF JUST 14 HAS BEEN FOUND IN THE JOURNAL OF THE NEW ENGLAND JOURNAL OF MEDICINE TO DOUBLE THE RISK OF ALZHEIMER'S DISEASE!</u>

Anything above a level of 10 is considered <u>ELEVATED</u>. Many drugs raise your levels of homocysteine - <u>BUT-</u>

YOU CAN ACTIVELY CORRECT YOUR LEVEL JUST BY SUPPLEMENTING WITH SOME B-VITAMINS AND FOLIC ACID.

TYPICALLY- YOU CAN TAKE A DOSE OF 50 Milligrams of Vitamin B-6, 800 micrograms of folic acid and 500 micrograms of Vitamin B-12. Typically, it's a good idea to re-test after three months.

High levels of homocysteine are associated with atherosclerosis, narrowing and hardening of the arteries, heart disease, stroke and dementia.

HOMOCYSTEINE LEVELS CAN BE RESTORED IN ABOUT 3 MONTHS TO HEALTHY LEVELS.

C-Reactive Protein Test

CRP is a marker of inflammation in the body.

AN IDEAL LEVEL IS LESS THAN 1.0 mg/L. You will likely see changes after a few weeks of being on a Ketogenic diet- but it may take several months on a KD.

Vitamin D- Test

THE IDEAL LEVEL OF VITAMIN D IS: 80ng/ml.

This test can be obtained from labs or from GrassRootsHealth. (see chapter Dr. Sunshine).

NOTE BENE! The Thyroid Tests THAT DOCTORS GIVE ARE WRONG ONES!

So- YOU MUST OBTAIN THE PROPER LAB TESTS FOR THYROID HORMONES!

THERE YOU HAVE THE INFORMATION THAT YOU NEED TO PERFORM A SELF-ASSESSMENT BY GETTING THE PROPER LABORATORY TESTS.

NOW YOU CAN BE YOUR OWN DOCTOR!

CHAPTER FOUR

EVIL NEUROTOXINS

A. INTRODUCTION

In this chapter we analyze <u>THE EVIL NEUROTOXINS</u> you need to eliminate from your air, your water, your food, and from <u>YOUR WHOLE ENVIRONMENT</u>.

<u>What is a "neuro-toxin?</u>

Neuro means brain; and toxin means poison.

In short— a neurotoxin is a <u>BRAIN POISON</u>.

Many of these neuro-toxins are causing you to be <u>FAT, SICK OR DIABETIC!</u>

<u>THE REAL REASON YOU ARE OVERWEIGHT IS DUE TO NEUROTOXIN (S)!</u>

<u>BEING OVERWEIGHT MAY NOT BE YOUR FAULT!</u>

<u>BIG GOVERNMENT, BIG PHARMA, BIG AGRICULTURE, BIG FOOD, BIG SUGAR AND MAINSTREAM MEDICINE SAYS THE REASON THAT YOU ARE OVERWEIGHT IS BECAUSE:</u>

"<u>YOU EAT TOO MANY CALORIES AND EXERCISE TOO LITTLE</u>".

<u>THIS IS A FRAUDULENT LIE!</u>

<u>THESE PEOPLE AND "THEIR TOXIC ADVICE" ARE ALSO NEUROTOXINS THAT YOU MUST ELIMINATE FROM YOUR LIFE.</u>

These toxic people have only <u>ONE GOAL</u>. That goal is:

<u>THEY WISH TO SEPARATE YOU FROM YOUR HARD-EARNED CASH!</u>

When these people look at you, they see you as: -$$$$$$$$$$$$$$$$$$$$$!

They do not give a darn about <u>YOUR HEALTH!</u>

<u>TO THEM –YOU ARE NO MORE THAN A CASH COW.</u>

When you eat processed <u>POISONS</u> aka <u>UNFOODS</u>—you're making yourself fatter and sicker. You get fatter and sicker and these people profit from your sickness and misery.

Their plan is simple. A typical scenario goes like this.

"Eat our tasty, good healthy food…-☺ Big Food says `Our food is low- fat, low-calorie, healthy protein. Your body needs healthy lean protein."

Eating their poisonous food makes you sick. Then you need to visit your doctor.

Maybe, you ate some commercial "<u>LEAN CHICKEN BREAST</u>" – (probably rotten) for supper. You cleverly checked the "best before date" on the package. But you did not think to consider what happened to that poor chicken before it went from the cage to your plate.

<u>RESEARCH SHOWS THAT 50 PERCENT OF STORE-BOUGHT CHICKEN CONTAINS BAD BACTERIA—USUALLY E-COLI!</u> Yuk!

You've heard of E-coli. It`s the bad bacteria which you get from your food when a restaurant employee fails to wash his hands… or is created by antibiotics fed to poultry or factory –raised animals. It may even have originated from the packaging or any one of a dozen other contaminated sources. Perhaps something fell from the hair of one of the store's employees…Who knows?

After your stomach felt sick and upset, you went to consult your local conventionally trained doctor.

He likely said: poor you; you have an upset tummy because you have been eating too many calories; your stomach has <u>too</u> much hydrochloric acid.

Then he typically says: Wow! You're in luck! – "I just got this latest new drug called "Super-duper Tummy Easer in a new liquid form so it is absorbed more easily by your body". You leave his office feeling that the new pill he has prescribed will make you feel better. You shell out $ 40.00 for a prescription at the pharmacy next door.

Two days later, you're rushed to the hospital by ambulance because you're violently ill. After profuse vomiting and having your stomach pumped, you felt horrific but lucky to be alive.

The next day, you throw the faulty medication in the garbage. You figure that there was something in that medication drug that did not agree with your stomach.

It never crosses your mind that your chowder-headed doctor used you as a guinea pig for a new drug. Gee- you thought—doctors go to medical school for 7 or 8 years...they should know what their doing... WRONG!

In all likelihood, there were **TWO** or more neurotoxins that poisoned you; and/or you got "leaky-gut syndrome" aka -**HOLE IN YOUR GUT LINING!**

E-COLI poisoning may **ONLY** have been "the straw that broke the pro-verbial camel's back,"

IF YOU HAVE BEEN EATING A TYPICAL WESTERN DIET OF PROCESSED JUNK FOOD—IT IS MORE THAN LIKELY THAT-

EITHER—

1. **YOU HAVE LEAKY GUT SYNDROME AND OR—**

2. **YOUR IMMUNE SYSTEM HAS BEEN SEVERELY DAM-AGED BY HARMFUL NEUROTOXIN (S).**

3. **YOU ARE EATING DRUG-LACED FOOD WHICH COM-BINES WITH OTHER POISONOUS DRUGS PRESCRIBED BY YOUR DOCTOR—AND YOUR BODY CONTAINS A BEVY OF DRUGS- KNOWN AS A DRUG- COCKTAIL.**

Either way—your health solution will not be to take a pill.

YOU MUST FIX YOUR GUT TO FIX YOUR HEALTH!

YOU NEED TO ELIMINATE ALL NEUROTOXINS FROM YOUR BODY AND FROM YOUR LIFE.

YOUR DOCTOR AND YOUR LOCAL GROCER ARE BOTH POISONING YOU WITH NEUROTOXINS AND DRUGS IN THE FOOD THAT YOU EAT!

WHEN YOU EAT PROCESSED FOOD—YOU ARE EATING POISONS THAT ARE DRESSED UP TO LOOK AND TASTE LIKE REAL FOOD.

95 <u>PERCENT OF THE WESTERN POPULATION ARE DRUG JUNKIES.</u>

<u>NEUROTOXINS ARE CONTAINED IN THE PILLS THAT YOUR DOCTOR SELLS YOU.</u>

<u>NEUROTOXINS ARE CONTAINED IN YOUR WATER AND BEVERAGES.</u>

<u>NEUROTOXINS ARE UBIQUITOUS IN YOUR ENVIRONMENT!</u>

<u>NEUROTOXINS DESTROY YOUR BRAIN- NERVOUS TISSUE AND PERIPHERAL NERVES.</u>

<u>MANY NEUROTOXINS ARE ENDOCRINE DISRUPTORS!</u>

These (neuro) toxins can kill your immune system is a variety of insidious ways. The neurotoxin BPA (Bis-phol A) is bad plastic.

<u>ALL PLASTIC IS BAD- BOTH FOR YOUR BODY AND FOR OUR ENVIRONMENT</u>

That fillet of mercury-loaded farmed salmon may have tasted good.

BUT- instead of making you lean and healthy—it will likely be stored in adipose (fat) tissue or in your reproductive glands. Mercury is not fussy. It can accumulate anywhere in your body it finds space. If your mouth is already mercury full —with your dental fillings, it finds another convenient place to accumulate...

By the way- your dentist is lying to you about silver fillings...silver fillings are 50 <u>PERCENT MERCURY!</u>

When the body ingests heavy toxic metals like mercury, your body has <u>GREAT</u> difficulty dealing with these `<u>FOREIGN INVADERS!</u> One of the sneaky things about these chemical neurotoxins is their <u>SMALL SIZE!</u>

Their small size is what makes them so powerful and evil; and allows them destroy <u>YOUR BRAIN AND YOUR IMMUNE SYSTEM.</u>

<u>YOUR BODY DOES NOT WANT TO STORE TOXIC HEAVY METALS LIKE MERCURY, ALUMINUM, ARSENIC, AND FLUORIDE.</u>

Your body is capable of excreting some of these metals through sweat, urine and feces. Unfortunately- <u>MOST OF THESE TOXIC METALS</u> (such as Mercury) are <u>LITERALLY VERY STICKY!</u>

They stick to your bodies' insides like <u>GLUE!</u>

<u>THE GOOD NEWS</u> is that when you eat the <u>PROPER FOODS</u> –

YOU CAN ELIMINATE MANY OF THESE TOXIC NEUROTOXINS.

You can eliminate them by eating certain `chelating`` foods.

MOTHER NATURE IS SO CLEVER!

YOUR BODY IS A CHEMISTRY SET!

YOUR FIRST JOB IS TO EAT HEALTHY NATURAL ORGANIC FOODS TO CLEAN OUT THE TUBES OF YOUR CHEMISTRY SET☺

For example if you eat food that contains MERCURY—Mike Adams-(aka Health Ranger) tells us that you can eat PEANUT BUTTER and STRAWBERRIES TO ELIMINATE MERCURY.

YOUR DOCTOR IS CLUELESS ABOUT NEUROTOXINS.

Your doctor is clueless that his tie and stethoscope ARE CRAWLING WITH BAD BACTERIA!

THE DOCTOR OF THE FUTURE WILL BE AN ENVIRONMENTAL DOCTOR who will be an expert in the ELIMINATION OF NEUROTOXINS.

As already mentioned; these neurotoxins are ubiquitous in our environment.

Any ONE of these neurotoxins can overwhelm your IMMUNE SYSTEM. Some neurotoxins work faster than others. Other neurotoxins may take years before they succeed in making us sick.

To further injure us, when these poisons work TOGETHER—THEIR EFFECTS ARE SYNERGISTIC!

Always remember your immune system works 24/7 to protect you from sickness. You need to protect your immune system from these neurotoxins before they wreak havoc on your body.

BEFORE putting in the good stuff (NUTRIENTS) into your body—

YOU MUST ELIMINATE NEUROTOXINS DESTROYING YOUR BODY.

Our Creator provided all humans with a HUGE SHIELD (OUR IMMUNE SYSTEM) to protect us. These neurotoxins shoot bullet-holes into our shield.

ONLY YOU HAVE THE POWER AND THE MEANS TO STOP THIS ATTACK ON YOU. YOUR FIRST STEP IS TO ELIMINATE THE FOREIGN INVADERS-THE NEUROTOXINS.

Wearing a Kevlar suit might protect you from a bullet—but it will not protect you from the toxins in your environment. Even Superman was powerless against Kryptonite-☺

YOU CAN LEARN TO BULLET- PROOF YOUR IMMUNE SYSTEM BY EATING SUPERFOODS. Your first step is to eliminate those poisonous things called neurotoxins.

You will preserve your brain and prevent illness.

Many neurotoxins cause your HORMONES to get "out of whack"(another technical term meaning "out of balance"-☺

Eliminating harmful toxins will help your body PRODUCE GOOD QUALITY HORMONES.

Eliminating toxic chemicals will help your body PRODUCE THE APPROPRIATE HORMONES RATHER THAN THE WRONG HORMONES.

The main hormones for women are estrogen, progesterone, and testosterone. For men, the main hormones are testosterone and estrogen. A big problem is that as we get older, women become more like men. Their bodies produce more testosterone!

Men become more like women. Their bodies produce too much estrogen and too little testosterone!

Ladies Do you really want that extra body hair!

Men- Do you honestly want to grow bigger breasts!

ONE BIG SOLUTION— ELIMINATE NEUROTOXINS THAT CAUSE HORMONAL DEFICIENCIES AND HORMONAL IMBALANCES.

IT'S A SCIENTIFIC FACT—

MANY NEURO-TOXINS ARE THE PRINCIPAL CAUSES OF CANCER; HEART DISEASE, ALZHEIMER'S AND MANY OTHER CHRONIC DISEASES!

Why is this so?

Again, the answer is simple.

ALL OF THESE NEUROTOXINS DESTROY OUR IMMUNE SYSTEM.

90 (EIGHTY) PERCENT OF OUR IMMUNE SYSTEM IS IN OUR GUT (or gastrointestinal tract).

Two more neuro-toxin examples:

   a) In 1931 Dr. Otto Warburg won a Nobel Prize in Medicine

when he discovered that

SUGAR feeds cancer cells. When you starve cancer cells by eliminating their fuel source- you literally STARVE them to death!

That's ONE reason SUGAR is labelled "QUEEN OF NEUROTOX-INS"; (infra).

SUGAR IS ONE OF THE BIGGEST NEUROTOXINS AND DE-STROYERS OF OUR IMMUNE SYSTEM- AND OUR BRAIN!

b) A MAJOR CAUSE OF CANCER IS MERCURY POISONING!

DENTAL AMALGAMS OFTEN CAUSE CANCER BY MERCURY POISONING. Often when they are ELIMINATED (REMOVED) BY A BIOLOGICAL DENTIST—CANCER IS REVERSED.

NEUROTOXINS ARE CHEMICAL POISONS in our air, water, soil or environment.

WE CAN TAKE THE NECESSARY MEASURES TO PHYSICALLY ELIMINATE THESE TOXINS TO PROTECT OUR IMMUNE SYSTEM AND OUR BODIES.

ELIMINATE NEUROTOXINS IN THE FORM OF NEGATIVE PEOPLE AND NEGATIVE THOUGHTS. Increasingly in the holistic community, these "neurotoxins" are recognized as EXTREMELY IMPORTANT FOR US TO HAVE SUPERHEALTH.

YOU MUST ELIMINATE ALL NEGATIVE NEUROTOXINS IN YOUR LIFE- INCLUDING ALL NEGATIVE THOUGHTS!

" A negative thought can kill you faster than a bad germ."

YOU NEED TO BECOME A CREATURE OF POSITIVITY!

Sidebar-

Another consequence of having an allopathic doctor is that he may (unknowingly) be PREVENTING you from reaching your goal of optimum health.

Any poisonous drugs that he prescribes for you (or encourages you to eat) "NEED" to be FLUSHED OUT AND/OR ELIMINATED from your body.

For example— in 2013 simple aspirin apparently killed about 12, 000 people— probably blinded thousands more!

If you are taking "UNDERLINE: MEDICATION(S)"— you "MAY" need to seek professional help IF YOU CANNOT WEAN YOURSELF OFF OF THESE DRUGS.

Whether you are an alcoholic, a heroin addict or taking any other kinds of poisonous drugs—you need to eliminate these "neuro-toxins" from your life—ASAP!

But- please be careful not to seek "chemical advice" from the same chowder headed doctor who encouraged you to put these toxic chemicals in your body in the first place!

Your allopathic doctor is very likely a creature of GLOOM AND DOOM.

Hope is usually not in his vocabulary. Instead of telling you not to worry and that you can overcome health problems—instead he usually frowns at you –as he tells you that you will have to take his pills for the rest of your life! YUK! Your doctor wants you to a patient for life so that you can finance his new car.

This is another major reason to fire your doctor. Your doctor destroys your immune system with his negative attitude. An honourable doctor instills optimism in his patient. A good doctor encourages and supports his patient. A good doctor has empathy and shows warmth and understanding to his patient/client. Your doctor may have had these qualities when he graduated medical school. But- your doctor has not learned proper bedside manner. Your doctor knows nothing about how to help people get strong and healthy. Your doctor became one of Big Pharma`s stooges.

A CARING- SUPPORTIVE DOCTOR WHO SHOWS A POSITIVE ATTITUDE AND OPTIMISM WILL INSTILL THIS OPTIMISM IN HIS PATIENT.

IT`S A PITY—ALLOPATHIC DOCTORS ARE NOT TAUGHT THE POWER OF THE `PLACEBO –EFFECT.

THE TRUTH IS ANY "BENEFIT" PRODUCED BY POISONOUS DRUGS ACTUALLY WORKS BY THE "PLACEBO- OR SUGAR PILL EFFECT".

IS IT REALLY IS POSSIBLE TO HEAL PEOPLE WITH A FEW KIND WORDS OR A GENTLE TOUCH ON THE SHOULDERS—ABSOLUTELY!

YOU MUST ELIMINATE ALL NEUROTOXINS –OF EVERY KIND AND SHAPE FROM YOUR LIFE! Your doctor could very well be a negative-neurotoxin that you need to eliminate from your life- oops another reason to fire your doctor-☺

YOU MUST ELIMINATE ALL NEGATIVE THOUGHTS, NEGATIVE EMOTIONS AND NEGATIVE ENERGY FROM YOUR BODY AND FROM YOUR LIFE!

YOUR FIRST PRIORITY IS TO ELIMINATE ALL NEUROTOXINS— which damage or destroy your **BRAIN!** That's why there called "neurotoxins"- they **KILL YOUR BRAIN!**

Some common **ADDICTIONS** (aka neurotoxins) everybody knows. You know some of the obvious ones such as nicotine (smoking), cocaine, heroin, morphine, alcohol and other poisonous drugs. Many other neurotoxins are less well known.

Each neuro-toxin is highly "neurotoxic" in its own right. BUT- when **COMBINED** with one or more of the other toxins—their synergistic effect together can be downright **HORRIFIC!**

JUST THINK OF ALL NEUROTOXINS AS BRAIN POISONS.

Once we have examined the neurotoxins (the bad stuff) that need to be eliminated; following chapters will examine the "good stuff". We can examine the **GREAT HEALTH BENEFITS** provided by our favourite doctors—Dr. Sunshine, Dr. Ketosis, Dr. Exercise, Dr. Sleep and so forth.

MAINTAINING AND BUILDING A STRONG IMMUNE SYSTEM IS THE FOUNDATION OF GOOD HEALTH.

Either we are building up our immune system OR we are destroying it by permitting powerful neurotoxins to destroy our health.

OUR BODIES' IMMUNE SYSTEM IS EXTREMELY POWERFUL!

YOU HAVE THE POWER TO SEIZE CONTROL OF OUR IMMUNE SYSTEM.

WE CAN TAKE CONTROL OF OUR LIVES. WE ARE NOT VICTIMS OF OUR GENETIC MAKE-UP—OUR DNA.

FOOD IS INFORMATION.

WHEN WE ELIMINATE THE BAD INFORMATION –NEUROTOXINS— FROM OUR BODIES AND OUR LIVES—

WE TAKE A VERY POWERFUL FIRST STEP!

YOU ARE THE ONLY PERSON WHO CAN DECIDE TO ELIMINATE TOXIC NEUROTOXINS AND OTHER TOXIC CHEMICALS FROM YOUR BODY.

YOU NEED TO DO WHATEVER IT TAKES TO ELMINATE ALL OF THESE NEUROTOXINS.

NO ONE CAN DO THIS FOR YOU!

IF YOU WISH TO BE HEALTHY AND FREE FROM ALL DISEASE—FIRST —YOU NEED TO PROTECT YOUR BODY.

YOU MUST INSULATE YOUR BODY FROM EVIL CHEMICALS CALLED DRUGS AND EVIL CHEMICALS CONTAINED IN YOUR FOOD, YOUR WATER,

YOUR AIR AND IN THE REST OF YOUR ENVIRONMENT.

NEUROTOXINS ARE PUBLIC ENEMY NUMBER ONE!

Every second of every minute of every day **OUR IMMUNE SYSTEM** is hard at work **FIGHTING OFF AND ELIMINATING FOREIGN PREDATORS** such as bad bacteria, viruses, toxic chemicals; and Heaven knows what else-☺

Our body's immune system silently works away doing its job—as it was designed and

Our immune system works 24/7 **NON-STOP PROTECTING US** from harmful things in ways that we may never fully understand.

Every living organism on Planet Earth (plants, animals & whatever) has a built-in immune system. Each organism—good or bad— has an immune system or some way(s) to protect itself from other predatory bacteria or viruses.

HUMANS HAVE THE MOST ADVANCED IMMUNE SYSTEM AMONG ALL OF THE LIVING CREATURES ON OUR AMAZING PLANET!

ALL DISEASE AND DISEASE PREVENTION STARTS IN OUR GUT!

TECHNICALLY —DISEASE AND DISEASE PREVENTION STARTS IN OUR COLON-☺

NINETY (90) PERCENT OF YOUR IMMUNE SYSTEM IS IN OUR GUT!

TECHNICALLY OUR GASTROINTESTINAL SYSTEM IS HOME TO QUADRILLIONS OF BACTERIA (BUGS-☺)(infra ch. 11)

OUR IMMUNE SOLDIERS ARE ACTUALLY THESE 'GOOD BUGS".

THESE GOOD BUGS CONTROL THE BAD BUGS- aka "The Bad Guys"(another technical term for bad bacteria/ bad fungi/bad viruses- etc.-☺

Dr. Hippocrates did not need microscopes and scientific instruments. He practiced real medicine. Not only did he advocate using food as our medicine- he recognized HOW AND WHERE DISEASE STARTED.

His words are as true today as when he uttered them almost 2,500 years ago. This brilliant man said:

"ALL DISEASE BEGINS IN THE GUT"

You will master your health when you follow his sage advice. He recognized that everyone has doctor in him or her. He said that we just have to help it in its work.

This means that we must eliminate all of the neurotoxins in our lives which are destroying our immune system and poisoning our bodies.

Dr. Hippocrates also said:

"The natural healing force within each one of us is the greatest force in getting well."

YOU ARE EITHER BUILDING UP/SUPPORTING YOUR IMMUNE SYSTEM OR YOU ARE WRECKING YOUR IMMUNE SYSTEM.

YOU GET TO CHOOSE.

AS MENTIONED-THE FIRST STEP TO TAKE CONTROL OF YOUR HEALTH IS TO MAKE THE DECISION TO DO THAT.

NEXT YOU MUST HAVE THE INTESTINAL (TESTICULAR-) FORTITUDE TO-

—Fire your Doctor and hire yourself as your own chief physician.

THE NEXT STEP IS TO ELIMINATE THE NEUROTOXINS IN YOUR LIFE AND

STOP SUPPRESSING YOUR IMMUNE SYSTEM!

THIS IS ABSOLUTELY ESSENTIAL- NO MATTER WHAT!

NO ONE ELSE ON THIS PLANET CAN DECIDE TO ELIMINATE THESE NEUROTOXINS.

THE QUALITY OF YOUR HEALTH WILL BE BASED ON THE QUALITY AND STRENGTH OF YOUR IMMUNE SYSTEM.

THE ELIMINATION OF NEUROTOXINS IS THE QUICKEST WAY TO SEE RESULTS OF AN IMMPROVED IMMUNE SYSTEM!

BUT- YOU ARE FOREWARNED.

TAKING PROPER CARE OF YOUR IMMUNE SYSTEM WILL REQUIRE WORK AND EFFORT.

YOU MUST MAKE A CONCERTED DELIBERATE EFFORT.

Wait until you hear what the other Health Doctors have to say! Their healthy dietary and lifestyle advice is a lot more **FUN TOO!**

Wait until you meet Dr. Ketosis!- ☺

B.   PHARMECEUTICAL DRUGS AND VACCINES

You don't need a degree in advanced biochemistry to realize that the human body was **NOT DESIGNED NOR CONSTRUCTED TO EAT POISONS.**

Is there any other living creature on this planet that gets healthy by eating drugs? Animals look to Mother Nature to fix their health issues. Unfortunately almost all factory farm raised animals are fed antibiotics and growth hormones to fatten them up before they are butchered.

When you walk in the forest, you are surrounded by Mother Nature's **MEDICINE.**

After all—Mother Nature works with Dr. Earth, Dr. Sunshine and the other Good Doctors.

Have you hugged a tree lately? Try it. See how it makes you feel-☺

How do you feel when you eat a piece of dark chocolate? or a venison steak?

Do you think that is what Dr. Hippocrates really meant?

If Hippocrates were alive today- this is what he would say:

LET FAT BE THY MEDICINE AND MEDICINE BE THY FAT!

THIS IS THE NO. ONE TAKE-HOME MESSAGE OF THIS BOOK!

Have you ever watched a cat or dog eat grass? Their instincts tell them to do that. They often eat grass not for food, but because it allows them to vomit hair or other unhealthy substances from their bodies. That's why humans are programmed to vomit— to rid our bodies of substances that we are not designed to ingest and do not belong there—PERIOD.

Everyone knows that rotten food or alcohol is EXTREMELY TOXIC to our bodies. Vomiting serves to rid our bodies from poisons. Our bodies' cure for a hangover is to vomit out the poisonous alcoholic drinks which have been imbibed. Drinking a rum and coke means that your liver has TWO POISONOUS CHEMICALS TO PROCESS!

One of the gatekeepers of our immune system is our liver which has to filter out all of the poisonous things that we eat or drink. And our poor kidneys! It's a good thing that we have two!

Do you have any idea how much toxic overload that you are placing on your liver? When you have your cocktail—then you smoke a cigarette or two—it's a miracle that our body's immune system doesn't IMMEDIATELY breakdown!

On a personal note— I have never smoked. FORTUNATELY— I realized the evil nature of tobacco at a tender age— thanks to common sense and my parents. My dad always said that if man were designed to smoke, humans would have been born with a cigarette-sized hole next to our mouth. I've not been a "social drinker" for many years. Today, I have the occasional glass of organic wine to celebrate s special occasion with family and friends. My imported "champagne of choice" is now "San Pelligrino" mineral water.

I personally get "jacked up" from eating my Ketogenic foods, (esp. my Ketogenic Coffee, infra) and by from hanging out with my loved family members and friends.

I confess that I was never a saint when it came to drinking alcohol. As a young man in university, I definitely attended my share of parties— replete with hangovers during my seven years at university.

As it turns out, at that time, distilled liquor was expensive— fortunately for me-☺

Besides the odd glass of beer after a round of golf, on most weekends I would have a few cocktails at our family parties. I became the bartender. When you're so busy making drinks for other people, it's actually a good thing. You have little time to make drinks for yourself… -☺ Also, hours of watching the ill-effects of alcohol on friends and family definitely had a cathartic effect on me. Eventually, one too many hangovers make me realize that feeling sick for a day or two afterwards was just not worth it.

I came to realize that alcohol was only a crutch for a weak mind. I came to realize that I could have fun with friends and family without relying on a chemical buzz. During my lifetime, I have witnessed too many people whose lives <u>have been ruined</u> and/or <u>shortened by cigarettes and alcohol.</u>

<u>Bottom line:</u>

You should eliminate as much ALCHOL (neurotoxin) from your life- as possible.

Research shows that <u>A GLASS OR TWO OF WINE DAILY IS VERY BENEFICIAL TO YOUR HEALTH—BUT-</u>

<u>—TOO MUCH WINE WILL LIKELY WRECK YOUR LIVER AND YOUR BODY.</u> Too much beer and distilled liquor will not help to keep your liver and body stay healthy.

As Aristotle said: "Moderation is best in all things."

<u>EVERYONE KNOWS THAT YOU SHOULD ELIMINATE SMOKING-</u> too.

Your brain and your body will be glad that you did.

<u>RESEARCH SHOWS THAT JUST QUITTING SMOKING DECREASES YOUR CHANCE OF HAVING A HEART ATTACK BY FIFTY (yes a) WHOPPING 50 PERCENT!!</u>

<u>HEALING BEGINS WITH YOU!</u>

<u>IT BEGINS WITH YOUR LIFESTYLE CHOICES AND YOUR ATTITUDE!</u>

If you attend a social gathering and you do not want people to think that you are a party-pooper… just have a Spritzer with lemon- or an extra Virgin Mary—or even have a glass of mineral or sparkling water. When asked why you are drinking THAT—just reply: I have to watch out. I have a very sensitive stomach.

I promise—very few people will criticize you for protecting your gut! Besides, at most parties, most people will not know or even care what you are drinking anyway!

The next morning you will be glad that you did not drink alcohol. That's because you will feel clear-headed and <u>GREAT</u>! Your friends will feel like they were run over by a truck.

Why would ANYONE want to take a chemo drug that makes you vomit profusely and lose your hair? And spend thousands of dollars of your hard-earned cash to take a drug that oncologists won't themselves or even prescribe for their family or friends! It's easy to understand why people drink beer and alcohol to self- medicate— to feel better... even if it's only for a short time. But why take toxic chemo drugs?

Where is the logic and common sense in that? This seems like sheer MADNESS!

<u>HOW IN THE WORLD CAN ANYONE TAKE DRUGS THAT MAKE THEM SICKER THAN BEFORE THEY TOOK THE DRUGS?</u>

<u>PLEASE EDUCATE YOURSELF AND JUST SAY NO TO DRUGS!</u>

It's much smarter to close the barn door before the cow gets out of the barn. For that matter you are likely to get better health advice from your local pet doctor. Your local vet likely kills fewer cats and dogs than your doctor kills people.

Frankly, it would not surprise me if conventional medicine starts using "blood-letting" as a remedy. Conventional doctors used to advertise cigarettes as being healthy! Doctors might decide that bloodletting seems like a good way to detox your blood.

The paradox is that donating blood is actually good for you!

<u>DONATING BLOOD SAVES LIVES AND MAKES YOU HEALTHIER AT THE SAME TIME</u>! You can reduce iron (ferritin levels) and help someone stay alive—it's a <u>SUPERHEALTH DOUBLE-WHAMMY</u>!

<u>DON'T LET BIG PHARMA</u> and some guy wearing a white coat <u>SELL YOU POISON CHEMICALS</u>.

<u>DO YOUR DUE DILIGENCE. REMEMBER ALWAYS</u>—

<u>CHEMISTS DRESSED IN WHITE COATS WILL NEVER OUTSMART MOTHER NATURE WHEN IT COMES TO PROVIDING GOOD FOOD AND MEDICINE!</u>

Her medicine cabinet will always supply you with medicine to heal your body. She will not provide you with a poison that will SUPPRESS and DESTROY YOUR IMMUNE SYSTEM. That's what Big Agriculture, Big Food, Big Pharma and conventional medicine DO BEST.

<u>OUR BODIES ARE SUCH AMAZING SELF-HEALING AND SELF-REPAIRING MACHINES!</u>

Do you know of any other self-healing self-repairing machines? You just have to give your body a chance to be strong and healthy. Eliminate the neurotoxins.

<u>ELIMINATE THE NEUROTOXINS TO ELIMINATE IMMUNE SYSTEM SUPPRESSORS AND DESTROYERS OF YOUR IMMUNE SYSTEM.</u>

ELIMINATE THOSE "IMMUNO-SUPRESSORS"!

We have already reviewed <u>SOME MAJOR HEALTH SCAMS</u> involving pharmaceuticals and vaccines. You already know that drugs <u>CAUSE DIRECT HORRIFIC EFFECTS TO OUR BODIES</u>. You've seen some of the pornographic statistics showing deleterious health results, including the HUGE numbers of deaths caused by pharmaceutical drugs and their dispensers—the white-coated crowd.

THE STATIN DRUG SCAM WILL BE SUPERSEDED IN THE NEXT 3 YEARS BY BLOOD DRUG SCAMS CALLED WARAFIN AND PRADAXA SCAM!

These are drugs used to thin blood. The general idea is to thin your blood-to prevent blood clots so you don't have heart attacks. All well and good you say but—

Did you know THAT—

<u>YOUR BLOOD IS 93 PERCENT WATER?</u>

<u>CAN YOU THINK OF A SAFER, CHEAPER EASIER WAY TO THIN YOUR BLOOD?</u>

<u>IF YOU GUESSED WATER—YOU'RE ABSOLUTELY RIGHT!</u>

In chapter one, you learned that Dr. Earth thins your blood much easier and far safer than <u>POISONOUS BLOOD-THINNING DRUGS LIKE COUMADIN.</u>

<u>NOW YOU KNOW THAT DR. CLEAN WATER ALSO THINS YOUR BLOOD!</u>

<u>Sidebar:</u>

<u>DID YOU KNOW THAT DR. CLEAN WATER ALSO LOWERS YOUR "BAD" CHOLESTEROL?</u>

<u>YOU CAN SAVE A BUNDLE OF YOUR HARD-EARNED CASH ON CHOLESTEROL/STATIN DRUGS AND BLOOD THINNER DRUGS!</u>

Best of all—<u>NO DOCTOR REQUIRED!</u>

<u>YOU ARE THE DOCTOR AND YOU ARE THE PATIENT!</u>

<u>DRINKNG A GALLON OF FRESH, PURE WATER EVERYDAY WILL NOT ONLY SOLVE YOUR BLOOD/CHOLESTEROL HEALTH ISSUES—</u>

<u>IT WILL GO A LONG WAY TOWARDS HEALING YOU AND HELPING YOU ATTAIN SUPERHEALTH!</u>

OMG!

Am I suggesting that your conventionally trained doctor does not know that <u>WATER IS MORE EFFECTIVE –FAR SAFER- AND FAR LESS EXPENSIVE THAN BLOOD DRUGS</u>? Yes- I am!

OMG! ANOTHER reason to fire your doctor and hire yourself. -☺) In reality— it's the same reason. You doctor does not know his arse from his elbow.-☺

The unfortunate truth is that your conventionally trained, allopathic doctor was taught very little about how your body actually works. But I digress. You can read about the reasons to fire your doc in chapter two. Let's return to the blood-thinners saga.

<u>BY 2018 —IT'S PREDICTED THAT BLOOD THINNERS WILL BE THE BIGGEST CASH COWS- OR MONEY MAKER FOR THE PHARMACEUTICAL INDUSTRY!</u>

But wait—"Houston- we have a problem!"

<u>BLOOD THINNERS</u>-(e.g. Warfin, etc.)<u>ARE THE LEADING CAUSE OF DEATH IN EMERGENCY ROOMS!</u>

<u>OMG</u>! How many more people are going to be killed by allopathic doctors in emergency rooms!

<u>WE MUST ALL WORK TOGETHER TO STOP THIS LEGALIZED MEDICAL KILLING THAT IS PASSED OFF AS MEDICINE!</u>

The suggestion that drugs cause "indirect effects" is simply clever marketing and good propaganda. Some people have even suggested that the medical mafia and Big Pharma should be prosecuted for crimes against humanity!

<u>MAKE SURE THAT YOU ARE NOT SUCKERED INTO BUYING POISONS THAT MAKE YOU EVEN SICKER WHILE DRAINING YOUR BANK ACCOUNT.</u>

Big Pharma hides the truth about toxic poisons called drugs. Their humble servants, (conventionally trained allopathic doctors) dispense their toxins for money. Don't finance anyone's pension plan but your own.

Do you know that DRUGS HAVE <u>TWO</u>" <u>OTHER</u>" "<u>DIRECT</u>" (not side effects) <u>TERRIBLE EFFECTS ON YOUR BODY?</u>

<u>VIRTUALLY ALL DRUGS—BOTH PRESCRIPTION AND OTC (Over-the-counter) DRUGS HAVE THESE 2 IMPORTANT " DIRECT EFFECTS":</u>

1. <u>DRUGS DESTROY YOUR IMMUNE SYSTEM!</u> (The technical expla-

nation is that drugs make you immuno-suppressed.) and—

2. DRUGS ROB YOUR BODY OF ESSENTIAL NUTRIENTS -it
   needs to function properly. (These two effects are conveniently missing from medical textbooks).

Pharmaceutical drugs, which a vast majority of North Americans are taking every single day ARE THE BIGGEST SUPPRESSORS OF NATURAL IMMUNITY!

This is clearly something you do NOT want to do.

When your gatekeeper (your immune system) is destroyed and/or suppressed—

Who will protect you? Certainly not some guy wearing a white green or blue smock!

DRUGS MAKE YOU VULNERABLE TO A BOATLOAD OF INFECTIONS AND DISEASES!

THESE EVIL NEUROTOXINS ROB YOUR BODY OF THE VITAL NUTRIENTS THAT YOU NEED TO BE HEALTHY!

HERE'S HOW DRUGS DEPLETE YOUR BODY OF ESSENTIAL NUTRIENTS:

- Statin drugs deplete your body of CoQ10 enzyme, Vitamin D etc. etc.

- Some women take hormone pills (menopausal) drugs that
  contain estrogens. These estrogens deplete ZINC, MAGNE-
  SIUM, & B-VITAMINS which are essential to good health.

- Diabetes medications rob the body of CoQ10 and Vitamin B-12;

- Blood thinner medications likely rob the body of Vitamin C
  because patients are told not to eat citrus fruits with them.

  Have you ever heard of anyone who died from mixing blood thinner medications with grapefruit?

  Have you ever heard of anyone getting sick or
  dying from eating   GRAPEFRUIT?

A THIRD DEVASTING EFFECT WHEN TAKING DRUGS:

- MANY GOOD FOODS CONFLICT OR DO MIX WELL WITH DRUGS!

- MANY DRUGS ARE SO POISONOUS THAT THEY OF-
  TEN CONFLICT WITH GOOD FOOD-

- **THIS IS ANOTHER WAY THAT DRUGS ROB YOUR BODY OF ESSENTIAL MINERALS-**

- **WHEN DRUGS CONFLICT WITH FOOD/SUPPLEMENTS- THEY CAN MAKE YOU VERY SICK—OR EVEN KILL YOU!**

One important scientific study is illustrative.

- **One scientific study shows that if you take Krill Oil (Omega 3 fatty acids obtained from little shrimp— AND TAKE STATIN DRUGS (e.g. LIPITOR)**

  AT THE SAME TIME—

- **YOU WILL NULLIFY OF THE ONE OF THE WORLD'S BEST FOODS/SUPPLEMENTS!**

- **IF YOU INGEST PHARMACEUTICALS, you are STRONGLY RECOMMENDED to obtain a copy of the book "Drug-Muggers."**

In her book, "Drug-Muggers", pharmacist Suzy Cohen examines this WHOLE ISSUE in great detail. She specifies which **DRUGS ROB WHICH NUTRIENTS and WHICH SUPPLEMENTS/ NUTRIENTS YOU CAN TAKE TO PREVENT THIS FROM OCCURRING**. It is beyond the scope of my book to explore the complexities involved in mixing FOOD with poisonous DRUGS.

VERY FEW PEOPLE IN THIS WORLD HAVE AN EXPERTISE REGARDING THE EFFECTS OF MIXING GOOD FOOD WITH POISONS.

Even most compounding pharmacists are clueless when it comes to mixing chemicals from food and poisonous drugs. Big Pharma taught pharmacists nothing about the effects of mixing food/nutrition with drugs. As already mentioned, supra, medical school teaches doctors nothing about **NUTRITION**.

Mixing chemicals from drugs and chemicals from food is a **WHOLE NEW BALLGAME!**

NO ONE KNOWS WHAT HORRIFIC EFFECTS MAY BE UNLEASHED ON OUR HUMAN BIOCHEMISTRY!

Most doctors learn about the **"DIRECT EFFECTS"** (aka '**THE SIDE-EFFECTS OF DRUGS FROM THE LOCAL DRUG SALESMAN WHO DELIVERS DRUGS TO THE DOCTOR'S OFFICE.**

Bottom line:

FIND A WAY TO ELIMINATE ALL DRUGS (prescription and OTC drugs) AND THEIR EVIL COUSINS— VACCINES FROM YOUR LIFE!

IT'S NEVER TOO LATE!

YOU AND YOUR IMMUNE SYSTEM WILL BE GLAD THAT YOU DID!

C.   CHEMTRAILS & LEAD POISON

What are chemtrails?

Chemtrails are technically called "stratospheric aerosol geoengineering" or SAG for short. What is happening is that our skies are being sprayed and systematically being poisoned with TOXIC CHEMICALS.

Tons of very tiny nano-sized particles of aluminum oxide, barium and strontium are being sprayed into our atmosphere every day. Where do they go? To our lungs of course—where they cause a wide variety of health issues, such as nausea, diarrhea, headache, eczema, upper respiratory diseases and even cardiac deaths. If you consult your conventionally-trained doctor; you will be told it's an "allergy"...here is a drug that will fix the problem"

OVER 100 MILLION PEOPLE WORLDWIDE SUFFER FROM ASTHMA.

These chemicals and toxic elements lodge deep inside of our bodies. They wreak havoc on our endocrine system and our emotional health. We know for example that aluminum, a major component of these chemtrails, accumulates in our body and can causes serious BRAIN disorders such as dementia, Alzheimer's disease and other neurological problems.

These toxic chemicals (which are a form of neurotoxins) are perhaps the most insidious of all because very few people are even aware of them. These chemtrails are poisoning our skies, our environment and represent A SERIOUS THREAT TO HUMANITY!

For more information, you can check out these resources:

> Youtube video- "What in the World are they Spraying" and

> Youtube video- "Why in the World are they Spraying".

How about lead poisoning?

North America is being doused <u>every minute of every day with the toxic heavy metal lead</u> which is burned in "avgas" (i.e. aviation gas) the fuel that powers any aircraft with a propeller.

According to the U.S Environmental Protection Agency, a total of 571 tons of lead are dumped into the air over our heads <u>from aircraft alone</u>. According to a scientific paper entitled "Lead and Halogen Contamination from Aviation Fuel Additives at Brackett Airfield", tests showed avgas contains the following:

- Lead: 48 ppm

- Bromine: 42.6 ppm

- Chlorine: 605.2 ppm

The big problem is that lead is a highly toxic heavy metal that causes bone diseases, BRAIN damage and cancer. Chlorine and bromine are also highly reactive chemicals

According to http://generalaviationnews.com 681,000 gallons of avgas were burned each day in 2013.

According to Mike Adams, The Heatlh Ranger, www.naturalnews.com , from ALL SOURCES—964 TONS OF LEAD were released into the air! (Does anyone remember that the EPA removed lead from automobile fuel?)

<u>Where does all of this lead end up?</u>

All chemicals sprayed and/or pumped into our skies ends up EVERYWHERE in our environment. From the air the chemicals go to our waterways, and to our soil. All of these poisonous chemicals, especially lead, ends up in our FOOD SUPPLY. That's because of course, plants absorb lead from soils, and grazing animals eat these plants.

<u>THAT IS WHY NUMEROUS TOXIC HEAVY METALS</u> (including lead) end up in our food supply. This is also why heavy metals are often HIGHER in milk or meat than in raw grass.

Mike Adams, the Health Ranger, supra, is <u>THE FIRST SCIENTIST IN THE WORLD TO TEST FOR AND IDENTIFY THE PRESENCE OF ALL KINDS OF HEAVY METALS IN ALL KINDS OF FOOD!</u>

He uses atomic spectroscopy in his ICP-MS laboratory. He has even identified (FOR THE FIRST TIME EVER) the presence of heavy metals even in some "organic "health foods!

<u>FINALLY—THE HARMFUL EFFECTS OF LEAD</u> are well- described by the National Institute of Health (NIH) as follows:

" Lead is a well-documented neuro-toxicant that is particularly harmful to children, who are typically exposed
when they ingest or inhale lead-containing dust in the
home. In recent years, serious harm to cognitive and
behavioral functions including intelligence, attention,
and motor skills has been demonstrated in children with
much less lead in their blood than previously thought
to cause harm, and now it is now understood there is no
safe level of lead exposure." (author's underline)

N. B. The word "neuro-toxicant" is another word for "neurotoxin."

WE MUST STOP POISONING OUR SKIES AND OUR ENVIROMENT WITH
THESE POISONS CALLED NEUROTOXINS OR NEUROTOXICANTS.

D. GLYPHOSATE- THE KING OF NEUROTOXINS!

A study published on April 1st, 2014 in the Journal Environmental
Toxicology has described glyphosate as:

"A NEW ENVIRONMENTAL NEUROTOXIN!"

Glyphosate (N-phosphonomethyl glycine) is registered as a herbicide
for many food and non-food crops as well as non-crop areas where
total vegetation control is desired.

The predominating uses of glyphosate, in descending order are
stubble management, pre-sowing application and pre-harvest application (dessication).

Glyphosate is also used to prevent weeds in fields with glyphosate
resistant genetically modified (GM) crops like soybean, rapeseed,
corn, etc.

Since 1996 the amount and the number of genetically engineered
crops dramatically increased worldwide. It is estimated that 90% of
the transgenic crops grown worldwide are glyphosate resistant.

The rapidly growing problem of glyphosate-resistant weeds is
reflected in steady increases in the use of glyphosate on crops.
Steams, leaves and beans of glyphosate resistant soy are contaminated with glyphosate. Moreover due to the intensive use of glyphosate it has frequently been detected in WATER, RAIN and AIR.

Researchers detected glyphosate concentrations in air and rain up to
2.5ug/L in agricultural areas in Mississippi and Iowa.

In Europe GM soybean for food and feed was admitted in 1996. All animals and humans eating this soy chronically incorporate unknown amounts of this herbicide. Residues of glyphosate in tissues and organs of food animals fed with GM feed (soybean, corn, etc.) are not considered or are neglected in legislation.

The influence of glyphosate residues on the quality of animal Products intended for human consumption is almost unknown.

In the above-referenced study, the authors provided technical explanations as to how GLYPHOSATE IS KILLING US:

They stated:

> " ...glyphosate has been reported to inhibit other enzymes, e.g. enzymes of the cytochrome P450 (Cyp) family. Other inhibition pathways are reported. Richard et al. reported that such as glyphosate inhibits Cyp450 aromatase inhibition, indicated crucial for sex steroid hormone synthesis.
>
> Glyphosate also interferes with cytochrome P450 enzymes which include numerous proteins able to metabolize xenobiotics. This may also act synergistically with disruption of the biosynthesis of aromatic amino acids by gut bacteria, as well as impairment in serum sulfate transport."

THIS PROCESS IS COMPLICATED—but—IN ESSENCE GLYPHOSATE DESTROYS OUR BACTERIAL AND GASTROINTESTINAL TRACT.

In my Dr. Sunshine chapter, infra, I discuss how glyphosate DESTROYS the body's production of Vitamin D.

The Jury is in once again.

Earlier studies have shown that GLYPHOSATE is strongly linked) CAUSES GASTROINTESTINAL DISORDERS, OBESITY, DIABETES, HEART DISEASE, DEPRESSION, AUTISM, INFERTILITY, CANCER, ALZHEIMER'S AND PARKIINSON'S DISEASES!

BLUNTLY PUT—

IF YOU ARE EATING PROCESSED FOODS—OR CONVENTIONALLY GROWN CROPS OR GMO CROPS—

YOU ARE EATING FOODS LACED 100 PERCENT WITH THE HERBICIDE CALLED GLYPHOSATE.

Cancer, diabetes, IBS (Irritable Bowel Syndrome) or maybe Leaky Gut Sydrome can be the consequence if you scarf down that pizza or hamburger!

Did you know that the pizza that you ate last week is likely still rotting somewhere in your intestinal tract?

Do you need more science?

There are several recent studies which are both compelling and conclusive.

In the May 2014 issue of EMBO Molecular Medicine, phosphate food additives have been linked with high blood pressure and heart disease.

Phosphates, called phosphorous additives are customarily added to processed meats, processed cheeses and various kinds of soda to increase shelf life and to intensify flavours. These additives also appear at high levels in fast food.

Researchers found that large quantities of added phosphates cause the body to produce a hormone called "fibroblast growth factor 23- or FGF23 for short. This hormone controls the excretion of phosphate through the kidneys. When phosphate levels are too high, FGF levels go up as well, as our kidneys struggle to excrete the excess phosphate.

When even more phosphates are ingested—the devastating effect on your body is like THOWING GASOLINE ON A FIRE!

The levels of both phosphate and FGF increase even more—a vicious cycle that leads to SERIOUS health problems, including damaging the cardiovascular system.

FGF23 levels are so important for KIDNEY patients, that researchers say they can serve as an INDICATION OF LIFE EXPECTANCY!

If this is not damaging enough, high phosphate levels also cause an increased uptake of calcium, which can lead to ventricular calcification.

Researchers warn that even young healthy men are at risk of coronary calcification if they ingest high phosphates. So while that pizza rots, it will also calcify your arteries and make you hard-hearted—if you are not now. –☺) Yuk!

In 2012, an alarming German study, published in Deutsches Arztebatt, researchers stated that excessive phosphate consumption causes higher mortality rates in patients with kidney disease; increases risk of heart disease in otherwise healthy people, damages blood vessels and induces the aging process. They urgently called for labelling to identify phosphate additives, as well as the need for alerting both physicians and the general public to the dangers of phosphates.

Have you suddenly lost your appetite for that grilled cheesy hot-dog with onion rings?

More scientific studies—

- In 2011, researchers in the UK linked a high phosphate diet with atherosclerosis. They noted that a high phosphate consumption causes increased cholesterol deposits and narrowing of arteries.

- In an animal study in 2010 published in The FASEB Journal (a very prestigious biology journal) phosphates were found to be toxic to mice, reduced their lifespans drastically and caused accelerated signs of aging and worsened age-related diseases.

(Source: for all of above-referenced studies" www.sciencedaily.com)

Note bene:

When adjuvants (other chemicals) are added to glyphosate-based pesticides-

THIS CREATES A POWERFUL SYNERGISTIC- TOXIC EFFECT OF GLYPHOSATE AND ITS DAMAGING EFFECTS ARE GREATLY AMPLIFIED!

Do you remember the old business adage?

"Two working together can accomplish more than twice as much as one!?...

In this instance, you really don't want TWO evil substances accomplishing more than twice the amount of evil which either poison can do by alone!

There are dozens of ground breaking scientific studies DETAILING THE HORRIFIC EFFECTS OF GLYPHOSATE.

World re-known researcher and scientist— Dr. Stephanie Seneff says:

"AROUND THE WORLD—

PEOPLE ARE USING GLYPHOSATE TO COMMIT SUICIDE."

GLYPHOSATE MAY BE THE MOST EVIL NEUROTOXIN EVER CREATED BY HUMAN CHEMISTS!

YOU MUST ELIMINATE GLYPHOSATE (& ROUNDUP) collectively 'THE KING OF NEUROTOXINS' FROM YOUR DIET FROM YOUR ENVIRONMENT AND FROM YOUR LIFE.

E.   NEUROTOXINS UNLIMITED

This section is short and ugly. No one knows how many of these chemicals are neurotoxins. In the USA there are <u>EIGHTY THOUSAND CHEMICALS USED.</u>

<u>ONLY</u> a few hundred of these chemicals have been tested for safety— <u>AND</u> –most research is conducted by the <u>CHEMICAL INDUSTRY.</u>

Do you trust the chemical industry to tell us the truth? You can assume that <u>ALMOST ALL OF THESE CHEMICALS ARE NEUROTOXINS IN THEIR OWN RIGHT.</u>

<u>WHEN CHEMICALS ARE COMBINED- IT IS HIGHLY LIKELY THAT NEUROTOXINS ARE CREATED THAT NO ONE KNOWS ABOUT- YET!</u>

<u>JUST ASSUME THAT ALL CHEMICALS ARE NEUROTOXIC UNTIL SCIENTIFICALLY PROVEN TO BE SAFE</u>

E.G- DDT banned 30 years ago is now appearing in Alzheimer's patients <u>BRAINS!</u>

<u>BLOOD SAMPLES FROM UMBILICAL CORDS OF NEWBORN INFANTS ARE LOADED WITH TOXIC CHEMICALS!</u>

<u>STUDIES SHOW THAT MOST PEOPLE HAVE DOZENS OF TOXIC CHEMICALS IN THEIR URINE AND IN THEIR BLOODSTREAM!</u>

<u>YOUR BODY'S CHEMISTRY TEST TUBES ARE FILLED WITH TOXIC POISONOUS CHEMICALS CALLED NEUROTOXINS.</u>

In 2013 the EWG (Environmental Working Group) identified the "Dirty Dozen List" of the 12 <u>WORST ENDOCRINE DISRUPTORS</u>. These are:

Bisphenol –A (BPA) Dioxin, Atrazine, Phthlates, Perchlorate, Fire retardants, lead, sglycol ethers.

<u>GET RID OF THE GLUTEN!</u>

You have likely heard about the evils of gluten. If you have a vowel in your first name, you are likely allergic to gluten-☺- even if you are not a Celiac patient.

GLUTEN is a toxic compound. Gluten is a toxic, sticky GLUEY PROTEIN found in grain. It's most commonly used in baked goods. It makes dough stretchy; bagels doughy, and it holds cookies together.

You can find gluten in pa..sta, beer, soy sauce, certain medications, toothpaste, and even lipstick. It can also hide in sausage and hamburger filler, ketchup. Ice-cream, mayonnaise and pre-packaged grated cheese

GLUTEN is an evil EXORPHIN. Basically – grains-and milk from "conventional "cows have something in them that acts like MORPHINE! They're called EXORPHINS.

Exorphins trick you by acting like natural ENDORPHINS—but there's NATURAL ABOUT THEM! Exorphins replace your endorphins by binding to your OPIATE RECEPTORS INSTEAD.

Exorphins are fooling you and telling you to eat more.

GRAINS, AND PROCESSED FOODS CONTAIN EXORPHINS WHICH MAKE YOU FEEL PLEASED AND REWARDED IN AN ARTIFICIAL WAY!

EXORPHINS TRICK YOU. EXORPHINS ATTACH TO YOUR OPIATE RECEPTORS IN THE PART OF THE BRAIN CALLED—"The nucleus accumbens".

EXORPHINS TELL YOUR BRAIN:

"Feel bad, but go eat and drink more anyway".

AVOID THESE FILLERS THAT HAVE GLUTEN EXORPHINS:

- Distilled grain vinegar
- Malt/maltodextrin
- Hydrolyzed protein
- Yeast extract
- Food starch
- Rennet and Samolina

YOU WILL BE PLEASED TO KNOW THAT ALL OF THE INGREDIENTS IN THE DELICIOUS KETOGENIC RECIPES PROVIDED IN THIS BOOK ARE HEAL-THY AND ARE SERIOUS THERAPEUTIC FOOD☺

THE OTHER NEUROTOXINS THAT YOU WANT TO AVOID ARE:

GMOS- WHICH MAY BE THE GREATEST THREAT TO OUR PLANETARY CROPS. –GMOS ARE PURE EVIL. THERE IS NO NEED TO SAY MORE THAN THAT!

EMF- ELECTROMAGNETIC FIELDS ARE ELECTRONIC POLLUTION THAT IS KILLING THOUSANDS OF PEOPLE AND CAUSING THOUSANDS OF PEOPLE TO DEVELOP CANCER!

ONE MINUTE ON A CELL PHONE INFLAMES YOUR BRAIN FOR 4 HOURS!

THAT SAYS IT ALL!

EMF FROM ELECTRONICS, CELL PHONES ,COMPUTERS, WI-FI, IPADS AND CELL TOWERS AND SMART METERS- actually should be called DUMB METERS BECAUSE THEY DESTROY YOUR BRAIN CELLS!

YOU MUST DO ANYTHING AND EVERYTHING YOU CAN TO SHIELD YOURSELF FROM THE ELECTRONIC NEUROTOXIN CALLED EMF!

YOU MUST DO EVERYTHING IN YOUR POWER TO SHIELD AND PROTECT YOURSELF FROM GMO CROPS, AND EMF RADIATION!

YOU MUST EDUCATE YOURSELF ABOUT THE DANGERS OF THE UNLIMITED NUMBER OF NEUROTOXINS THREATENING LIFE ON OUR PLANET!

CHAPTER FIVE
SUGAR—THE QUEEN OF NEUROTOXINS!

"Evolutionarily, sugar was available to our ancestors as fruit only for a few months a year (at harvest time) or as honey, which was guarded by bees. But in recent years, sugar has been added to nearly all processed foods, limiting consumer choice. Nature made sugar hard to get; man made it easy.

Dr. Robert Lustig

Did you know that ONE TEASPOON OF SUGAR SHUTS DOWN YOUR IMMUNE SYSTEM FOR 4 HOURS?

That means one can of soda shuts down little Johnny's immune system for 24 hours. Hmmm...What 4 or 5 times that amount of sugar will do?

According to Dr. Kenneth Bock, M.D.an expert in nutritional and environmental health, two cans of soda (which contains 24 teaspoons of sugar) reduces the efficiency of the white blood cells IN YOUR IMMUNE SYSTEM BY 92 PERCENT.

All of the sugar experts (except those who are paid by the Sugar Industry) tell us CLEARLY — THAT SUGAR DESTROYS YOUR IMMUNE SYSTEM.

Sugar affects the immune system in a variety of ways—NONE of them good. Sugar has been proven to destroy the germ-killing ability of white blood cells.

Sugar also reduces the production of antibodies that inactivate foreign invaders in the body. It also interferes with the transport of Vitamin C, one of the <u>MOST IMPORTANT NUTRIENTS FOR ALL FACETS OF IMMUNE FUNCTION</u>.

You already understand the importance of protecting your immune system.

<u>ONE OF THE SHARED EFFECTS OF ALL NEUROTOXINS IS THAT THEY DESTROY OUR IMMUNE SYSTEM IN MANY WAYS.</u>

WE HAVE SEEN THAT DRUGS, SUGAR AND OTHER NEUROTOXINS ALSO ROB OR BODY OF ESSENTIAL VITAL NUTRIENTS. This occurs sometimes by depletion; sometimes by blocking absorption of vital minerals, or by inhibiting neural pathways, etc.

NEUROTOXINS, LIKE SUGAR DO THEIR DIRTY WORK BY CAUSING <u>INFLAMMATION</u> IN OUR BODIES.

<u>INFLAMMATION IS THE CORNERSTONE OF ALL ILLNESS AND DISEASES IN OUR BODIES.</u>

For this IMPORTANT reasons I will be advocating A <u>KETOGENIC DIET</u>. (infra).

<u>A KETOGENIC DIET IS THE BEST ANTI-INFLAMMATORY DIET IN EXISTENCE!</u>

<u>IT IS NEURO— PROTECTIVE. IT PROTECTS OUR BRAINS AND OUR BODIES. IT PREVENTS INFLAMMATION.</u>

Inflammation is the root cause of MOST cardiovascular diseases. Allopathic doctors mask the symptoms of inflammation with drugs. Holistic doctors treat the root causes of sickness and disease.

<u>ALLOPATHIC DOCTORS DO NOT UNDERSTAND NOR DO THEY TREAT THE REAL CAUSES of INFLAMMATION.</u>

<u>SUGAR (especially FRUCTOSE) CAUSES EXTREME DAMAGE TO OUR IMMUNE SYSTEM.</u>

What else does this evil neurotoxin do to our bodies?

Dr. Robert Lustig, a specialist in pediatric hormone disorders and the leading expert in childhood obesity at the University of California, School of Medicine argues a bullet-proof scientific case that SUGAR IS A "<u>TOXIN</u>" OR A "<u>POISON</u>", in several published scientific articles. He is also supported by Gary Taubes in his book in 2011 called Good

Calories, Bad Calories. He has also written an excellent article the New York Times called Ìs Sugar Toxic`

Later in this chapter, we shall return to Dr. Lustig's ground-breaking research.

Why is sugar a "neurotoxin'?

I have labelled SUGAR a NEUROTOXIN, Dr. Lustig, and other experts call it a "toxin" a "poison" or "neuro-toxicant". I prefer the term "neurotoxin`. Sugar is the king of neurotoxins.

THE VISUAL SCIENTIFIC PROOF IS IMPRESSIVE—MRI PROOF SHOWS HOW YOUR BRAIN IS ON FIRE WHEN IT IS SUGAR DAMAGED!

Everyone knows that a PICTURE is worth a thousand words.

THESE PICTURES SHOW CLEARLY THAT HUMANS ARE BRAIN DAMAGED BY EXCESSIVE SUGAR and CARBOHYDATES.

You must remember—SUGAR which is a simple carbohydrate that is found in virtually EVERY FOOD ON OUR PLANET!

We have neurologists like Dr. Daniel G. Amen, who in his book, "Use your brain, to change your age, describes how sugar damages the brain. He shows pictures from brain scans from fat people. Fat people's brains often resemble "Swiss cheese" compared to healthy brains of people who are normal weight. The brains of people who are not overweight are smooth as a baby's bottom-☺

He shows us the BEFORE AND AFTER PICURES. The before (Swiss cheese) pictures where a patient is fat—and then the after pictures of patients who have lost a lot of weight. These after pictures show that the smoothness and healthiness of the brain CAN BE RESTORED!

Both neurologists tell us that:

> "AS OUR BELLY GETS BIGGER- -OUR BRAIN GETS SMALLER!" OR –

> "THE FATTER YOU GET—THE SMALLER YOUR BRAIN GETS"

There is a direct positive relationship between the SIZE OF YOUR GUT and the SIZE OF YOUR BRAIN!

Dr. David Perlmutter, world re-known neurologist in his new book, "Grain Brain" tells us some remarkable things about our brain and our body. He also advocates a KETOGENIC DIET for treating neurological disorders and all kinds of mental disorders. As previously mentioned in our introduction, a ketogenic diet basically is a high-fat, low-carb and moderate protein diet. This was the diet eaten during 99 % of our days on planet earth. This was our diet before the dawn of agriculture.

The ketogenic diet SHOULD BE YOUR DIET NOW!

The main reason that we are hard-wired to use FAT AS OUR PRIMARY SOURCE OF FUEL IS BECAUSE:

SUGAR—IN THE FORM OF GLUCOSE, FOR ALMOST OUR ENTIRE HUMAN EXISTENCE HAS BEEN SCARCE ON PLANET EARTH.

IN THE LAST 100 YEARS SUGAR HAS BECOME UBIQUITOUS WORLDWIDE.

SUGAR—THAT EVIL QUEEN OF NEUROTOXINS IS TRYING TO CONQUER OUR PLANET. WE HAVE TO STOP THIS EVIL QUEEN—NOW!

In the year 1700 when the explorers were exploring the new world, the average Englishman consumed about 4 pounds of sugar in a year. Sugar was considered as valuable as gold. That's when the sugarcane wars began in the Carribean.

About 100 years ago, the average sugar consumption by North Americans was perhaps still about 4 pounds per person per year. Refined sugar was in its infancy. Honey and maple syrup were still more prominent as natural sweeteners.

Fast forward to 2014—the USDA and others ESTIMATE THAT THE AVERAGE ADULT CONSUMES ABOUT 160 pounds per year.

However, when you consider that SUGAR IS PUT IN VIRTUALLY IN EVERYTHING WE PUT INTO OUR BELLIES—AND OVER 100 WAYS THAT SUGAR IS HIDDEN IN THE AVERAGE WESTERN DIET—

IT IS NO WONDER THAT THE AVERAGE NORTH AMERICAN ADULT CONSUMES ABOUT 200 POUNDS OF SUGAR PER YEAR!

ON TOP OF THAT—NORTH AMERICANS ARE "CARBOHOLICS".

90 PERCENT OF THE WESTERN POPULATION IS SUFFERING FROM A SERIOUS SUGAR ADDICTION THAT IS 8 TIMES WORSE THAN A HEROIN OR COCAINE ADDICTION!

CARBOHYDRATES ARE ONLY SLOW-BURNING SUGARS.

You will find it difficult to find a FOOD OR BEVERAGE in some form—apparent or disguised-THAT DOES NOT CONTAIN SUGAR.

That form could be fructose, sucrose or a HFCS (high fructose corn syrup) or any of the 100 forms of sugar (see infra.) Also, if you check labels closely you will see that sugar shows as a food ingredient BUT because the food substance contains less than 1 gram per table-spoon—it will never show up on the label!

THE SUGAR INDUSTRY IS A MASTER OF CLEVER DECEPTION AND FALSE ADVERTISING. Oscar Wilde said: "advertising is legalized lying".

These people pay marketing people to come up with deceptive mar-keting…just little "white" lies—not big ones! Hey, how much can one little half gram of sugar hurt you? Well that's 15 grams of sugar every month-from just their product.

At the end of this section, we shall provide you with sugars 100 names—to help you identify this NEUROTOXIN.

BTW: ARTIFICIAL SWEETENERS/POISONS such as aspartame, Splenda, Sweet & Low etc.) ARE EVEN WORSE POISONS!

Whether it's a candy-bar, a soda or a slice of whole wheat bread, we know that these are ALL SUGARS, albeit in slightly different FORMS.

YOU MUST UNDERSTAND THAT:

CARBOHYDRATES(Slow-burning   sugars)   ARE   NOT ESSENTIAL   NUTRIENTS.

Technically speaking—

> OUR BODY'S REQUIREMENT FOR CARBOHYDRATES IS VIRTUALLY ZERO!
>
> We have been told that there are 3 macronutrients. This is only a "two-thirds" truth. Fats and Protein are really Essential Nutrients. Carbs should not even be consid-ered nutrients. They are only slow-burning SUGAR THAT ARE CONVERTED TO GLUCOSE IN OUR BODIES.
>
> CARBOHYDRATES DO NOT REPAIR OR BUILD ANYTHING!

Who knew? How can this be true?

BECAUSE—IT HAS ONLY BEEN IN THE LAST 10,000 YEARS THAT HUMANS HAVE BEEN EATING CARBOHYDRATES AS THEIR PRIMARY FUEL (ENERGY) SOURCE!

PRIOR to that point in our evolution as a species, CARBOHYDRATES WERE SCARCE. Glucose (the sugar- fuel made from carbohydrates was therefore also rare.

This little known fact is HUGE!

It completely underpins our entire our understanding of what our PROPER DIET (Ketogenic) SHOULD BE.

The details a LOW-CARB- HIGH-FAT DIET will be analyzed in detail in my KETOGENIC DIET chapter.

DR. KETOSIS PROVIDES YOU WITH ALL OF THE DETAILS OF HIS KETOGENIC DIET.

At this point, you only need to remember that:

CARBOHYDATES ARE ONLY SUGARS- some burn faster than others.

ALL EVIL MAN MADE SUGARS ARE CHEMICAL POISONS OR NEURO-TOXINS. Anything that is processed or refined in any way shape of form is POISONOUS to the human body.

ONLY NATURAL SUGARS IN some naturally occurring fruits, berries, and honey have been put on our planet as a source of SAFE sugars in our diet.

Once humans began to plant and cultivate food—that's when our dietary problems STARTED! For example, the Greek and Romans did not eat much sugar in their diets for the simple reason that apart from wine and seasonal grapes, fruits were not that plentiful. The Mediterranean diet that is relatively healthy does not contain a lot of sugar and fruits.

LAB-MADE SUGARS or sugar alcohols are nothing more than refined CHEMICALS cooked up in a lab. If Mother Nature didn`t make it—you are not programmed to eat it.

MAN- MADE (SUGARS) POISONS are sold to humans to exploit a human ADDICTION FOR SUGAR. This addiction has been created and fuelled by the Sugar Industry for profit- for the last 100 years!

SUGAR- ESPECIALLY FRUCTOSE IS FAR MORE ADDICTIVE THAN COCAINE OR HEROIN.

IT IS EVIL AND HARMFUL TO OUR BODIES IN A BOATLOAD OF WAYS.

FRUCTOSE, HFCS, ASPARTAME, SPLENDA AND ALL SUGAR PRODUCTS ARE ALL EVIL QUEENS.

THESE EVIL QUEENS ARE ALL NEUROTOXINS THAT ARE KILLING PEOPLE AND CAUSING DISEASES BY THE MILLIONS!

With the introduction of HFCS, (High Fructose Corn Syrup) the rates of diabetes and obesity in the American people SKYROCKETED!

Could this just be a coincidence? ABSOLUTELY NOT!

Big Sugar has used Big Tobacco-style tactics to ensure that government agencies would dismiss troubling health claims against their products. For years, the sugar industry's priority has been to shed doubts on the scientific studies suggesting that its product makes people sick.

This decades- long effort to OBSCURE the truth is why, even today, the USDA's (United States Department of Agriculture) dietary guidelines only speak of sugar in vague generalities. They say, for example:

("Reduce the intake of calories from solid fats and added sugars.")

This also explains why the FDA insists that sugar is "generally recognized as safe" despite considerable evidence suggesting otherwise. It's why some scientists' urgent calls for the LEGAL regulation of sugary products have fallen on deaf ears.

With a boatload of scientific evidence available—

HOW CAN THE FDA SAY THAT SUGAR IS SAFE?

THE Food and Drug Administration (FDA) SHOULD DISSOLVED-NOW!

THE FDA NO LONGER SERVES THE PURPOSE FOR WHICH IT WAS CREATED.

THERE'S AN EVER-GROWING BODY of SCIENTIFIC RESEARCH THAT PROVES THAT SUGAR—

>ESPECIALLY FRUCTOSE AND HFCS DEFINITELY CAUSE DISEASES

>THAT KILL HUNDREDS OF THOUSANDS OF PEOPLE WORLD WIDE EVERY YEAR!

Let's examine the science of Sugar 101.

Here is a simplistic explanation of SUGAR DIABETES – the DIS-EASE known technically known as Diabetes Mellitus from the Latin.

Here it is in simply CHRONOLOGY OF HOW DIABETES IS CREATED—

- Our body manufactures energy from the food that
  we put into our mouths. Our body can take fat, protein or carbohydrates and make fuel.

- As mentioned, from an evolutionary perspective, the
  body had to be very clever. Our bodies developed a
  brilliant way to use food for energy—to fuel us.

- For MOST of our entire human existence of the human species
  on planet earth—GLUCOSE—the body's major source of energy
  has been scare. This scarcity forced us to develop ways to STORE
  glucose and to convert other things into glucose. The body adapted to manufacture glucose from fat and protein. This process of
  turning these macronutrients into glucose by the body is called
  "gluconeogenesis." (Using fat and protein requires more energy
  than the conversion of starches and sugars into glucose for fuel).

- The process whereby or body puts glucose into our cells
  and how our cells accept glucose is QUITE COMPLEX. Our
  cells don't just suck up glucose from our bloodstream.

- The vital sugar molecule is absorbed into our
  cells thanks to the hormone INSULIN.

  Insulin is manufactured by our pancreas. As you likely know,
  insulin is one of the MOST IMPORTANT BIOLOGICAL SUB-
  STANCES which governs human cellular metabolism.

- Insulin's job is to transport glucose from our bloodstream
  into muscle, fat and liver cells. Once it is inside of our cells, it
  can be "burned" or used as fuel to provide us with energy.

- The more SUGAR and refined junk foods that we eat, the
  more our blood sugar is "spiked" or jacked up with sugar. Our
  body, being very smart, responds to this sugar overload by
  reducing the number of insulin receptors on our cells.

- Normal, healthy cells have a high sensitivity to insulin. But when
  our cells are BOMBARDED, to protect themselves these cells desensitize themselves to insulin, causing INSULIN RESISTANCE.

- This insulin resistance allows the cells to IGNORE the insulin. They fail to retrieve glucose from our bloodstream.

- The pancreas then responds by PUMPING OUT more
  insulin. Then higher levels of insulin become needed for our cells to absorb sugar (glucose).

- This cascade creates a CYCLICAL PROBLEM! Most often refined evil sugar also <u>OVERWORKS</u> the pancreas and adrenal glands. The pancreas goes into overdrive, making insulin to normalize BLOOD SUGAR LEVELS. This rapid release of insulin of insulin causes a sudden drop in blood sugar. As a reaction to falling blood sugar, excess adrenal <u>CORTI-SOL</u> is stimulated to raise blood sugar back to normal.

- A constant intake of DIETARY SUGAR keeps this cyclical <u>ROLLER COASTER</u>

  <u>EFFECT</u> going—overworks/and/or burns out the whole pancreas/sugar fuel system…

  <u>AND BINGO! ONCE INSULIN RESISTANCE REACHES A HIGH ENOUGH POINT—</u>

  <u>THE RESULT IS FULL-BLOWN TYPE 2 DIABETES,</u> OR

  (hypo or hyperglycemia, chronic fatigue, heart disease <u>INFLAMMATION</u>- ETC.

In essence, people with diabetes, have high blood sugar because their bodies cannot get sugar into cells where it can be metabolized; and/or safely stored as energy. We can see that excess <u>blood sugar</u> leads to all of the health problems mentioned in the above paragraph.

<u>For the record, Diabetes Type 1 is a separate disease thought to be an autoimmune disease whereby the pancreas makes no insulin so daily injections of insulin are necessary. It appears that about 5 % of diabetics have Type 1 for which there is no cure.</u>

<u>Type 2 Diabetes—IS REVERSIBLE THROUGH DIET AND LIFESTYLE CHANGES!</u> Infra.

<u>90 % OF NORTH AMERICANS HAVE INSULIN AND LEPTIN RESISTANCE!</u>

Does that include you? If your mid-section is carrying a few extra-pounds it likely does. Often excess weight takes years to put on. Unfortunately, you can't melt off fat overnight. Surprisingly though, our bodies allow us to rid ourselves of adipose tissue FASTER than you think! Our "feast or famine" genes allow us to store fat quickly before winter. The problem is that most North Americans are in <u>FEAST MODE 24/7!</u>

<u>A BIG PROBLEM IS THAT BLOOD SUGAR LEVELS ARE NOT INDICATIVE OF DIABETES.</u> Even if your blood sugar level is normal, you could be insulin resistant. Your insulin pump—your pancreas could be struggling to produce insulin.

Why does Fructose deserve the title of the "Queen of Neurotoxins"?

We know that Fructose— Queen of Neurotoxins destroys our immune system, causes diabetes, and many other diseases. Everybody knows and can readily understand that OBESITY is most often a precursor to DIABETES.

This is well-known common knowledge.

WHAT IS CAUSING THE OBESITY EPIDEMIC IN THE WORLD TODAY?

FRUCTOSE IS "THE LEADING CAUSE" OF THE WORLDWIDE OBESITY EPIDEMIC!

FRUCTOSE REALLY DESERVES THE TITLE OF A QUEEN OF NEUROTOXINS.

THERE ARE DOZENS OF SCIENTIFIC STUDIES CONFIRMING THIS.

Here's a typical health scenario.

First— you are stressed out. Next, you start to put on a few extra pounds around your mid-section. Next- you discover that you have high blood pressure and/or hypertension! Darn.

Perhaps you have been "diagnosed with "Metabolic Sydrome" this is a description of symptoms like high blood pressure, hypertension, carrying around a few extra belly pounds; feeling burned out, fatigued, stressed, etc.

You may also be diagnosed as a "pre-diabetic". This is a precursor to DIABETES!

Basically, this is your body's way of telling you—YOU MUST FIX YOUR BUSTED METABOLISM!

YOUR BODY IS TELLING YOU THAT YOUR BLOOD IS FILLED WITH TOO MUCH TOXIC SUGAR.

YOUR BODY IS TELLING YOU THAT YOU ARE LIKELY INSULIN-RESISTANT.

UNLESS YOU MODIFY YOUR DIET AND YOUR LIFESTYLE— YOU ARE ON THE PATH TO DIABETES OR WORSE.

You know that bad health STARTS with being OVERWEIGHT OR OBESE.

So- what's the "REAL "CAUSE OF YOUR OBESITY ANYWAY?

Could it just be too much sugar in your blood? The Sugar industry, Big Pharma and all of the other experts wearing white coats will tell you:

The <u>MAIN</u> reason that you are OBESE or overweight is <u>BECAUSE</u>:

"<u>YOU EAT TOO MANY CALORIES AND YOU EXERCISE TOO LITTLE</u>"

<u>THIS IS A BIG 'FAT' LIE!</u>

<u>THIS IS A TOTAL FRAUD! THIS IS COMPLETELY WRONG!</u>

I am here to tell you that it is <u>NOT YOUR FAULT!</u>

<u>YOU ARE NOT OVERWEIGHT BECAUSE YOU OVEREAT OR BECAUSE YOU DO NOT EXERCISE ENOUGH!</u>

<u>ONE OF THE BIGGEST CAUSES OF OBESITY IS: STRESS!</u>

<u>THE "BIGGEST" CAUSE OF OBESITY IS SUGAR—(aka THE QUEEN OF NEUROTOXINS).</u>

<u>TO GET LEAN- and HEALTHY – YOU MUST ELIMINATE ALL SUGARS OF EVERY KIND OR DESCRIPTION FROM YOUR LIFE!</u>

<u>ALL SUGARS ARE TOXIC POISONS!</u>

<u>FRUCTOSE IS THE BIGGEST CAUSE OF OBESITY AND DISEASE ON OUR PLANET TODAY!</u>

What is the <u>process</u> of obesity? What causes obesity?

In order for you to gain a significant amount of weight, you must first become <u>LEPTIN RESISTANT</u>.

LEPTIN is a hormone which regulates your <u>appetite</u>. When your leptin levels rise, it signals your body that you are FULL. Then your brain tells you to stop eating. But when you start to become increasingly resistant to the effects of leptin, you end up eating MORE.

Many people who are overweight also have a problem because their bodies cannot oxidize fats which results in a low energy and lethargic state.

<u>The big question is:</u>

<u>Why do you become LEPTIN RESISTANT?</u>

Dr. Richard Johnson, head of Nephrology at the University of Colorado has researched <u>FRUCTOSE AND OBESITY –RELATED DISEASES</u> for more than 25 years.

This eminent scientist/researcher says plainly:

<u>OBESITY IS NOT CAUSED BY EATING TOO MANY CALORIES AND LACK OF EXERCISE.</u>

He says:

<u>OBESITY IS PRIMARILY DRIVEN BY EATING TOO MUCH REFINED SUGAR—ESPECIALLY FRUCTOSE.</u>

Dr. Johnson's research <u>CLEARLY SHOWS THAT REFINED SUGAR</u> (especially <u>FRUCTOSE) IS EXCEPTIONALLY</u> effective at causing leptin resistance in animals, as well as blocking fat burning. He says:

<u>"When you give fructose to animals, they lose their ability to control their appetite, they eat more and they exercise less. Fructose looks like it's playing a direct role in weight gain".</u> he says.

His research also reveals that FRUCTOSE also induces metabolic syndrome by blocking the burning of fat. But it also does MORE. Even when your control caloric intake; fructose can affect body composition (i.e. you get fatter.) This is because when you eat FRUCTOSE, you actually generate <u>more fat in your liver</u> for the same amount of <u>ENERGY INTAKE</u> –compared to <u>OTHER TYPES OF SUGAR.</u>

So, if you <u>CALORICALLY</u> restrict an animal—but give it a high-fructose diet or a high-sugar diet—it will still produce A <u>FATTY LIVER AND INSULIN RESISTANCE.</u>

Thus, according to Dr. Johnson, <u>FRUCTOSE</u> has two main effects:

1. It stimulates weight gain by affecting your appetite AND by blocking the burning of fat and

2. It changes your body composition (read: you get more body fat EVEN when you are on a calorie-restricted diet.

For more proof, let's return to Dr. Lustig's science.

In March 2013, in the Advanced Nutritional Journal (An International Review Journal), (source htttp://advances.nutrition.org)—

Dr. Lustig, world renowned scientist in the Endocrinology department of the University of California published a block-buster article entitled:

In this article, Dr. Lustig exposes FRUCTOSE AS A CHRONIC, DOSE –DEPENDENT LIVER TOXIN". (He had previously published other articles).

Previously, he described FRUCTOSE AS A "TOXIN" OR "POSION"

In his latest article he describes and explains in very scientific language—

THE FRUCTOSE CONNECTION- OR— HOW FRUCTOSE CAUSES-

   OBESITY AND SERIOUS LIVER DAMAGE.

As you know, fructose is the sugar found in EVERYTHING from HFCS and to fruits, fruit juices to agave syrup and honey.

The harm comes says Dr. Lustig WHEN TOO MUCH FRUCTOSE IS CONSUMED.

As with ALL POISONS—THE GREATER THE DOSE- THE GREATER THE POISONOUS EFFECTS!

This is what MOST North Americans do of course.

He explains:

FRUCTOSE ACTS THE SAME AS ALCOHOL IN YOUR BODY AND IN YOUR LIVER!

JUST LIKE ALCOHOL—FRUCTOSE IS METABOLIZED DIRECTLY INTO FAT!

(NOT CELLULAR ENERGY AS CLAIMED BY THE SUGAR INDUSTRY!)

Dr . Lustig analyzes THREE SIMILARITIES between FRUCTOSE and its fermented by-product—ETHANOL (more commonly known as ALCOHOL.

1. Your liver's metabolism of fructose is similar to alcohol as they both serve as substrates for converting dietary carbohydrate into fat which promotes insulin resistance, dyslipidemia (abnormal fat levels in the bloodstream) and fatty liver.

2. Fructose undergoes the Maillard reaction with proteins, leading to the formation of superoxide free radicals that can result in liver inflammation, similar to acetaldehyde, an intermediary metabolite of ethanol.

3. By stimulating the "hedonic pathway" of the brain, both directly and indirectly",

Dr. Lustig adds:

"FRUCTOSE CREATES HABITUATION AND POSSIBLY DEPEN-DANCE—ALSO PARALLELING ETHANOL". (author caps)

Like many leading experts, Dr. Lustig argues that SUGAR—

IN THE FORM OF FRUCTOSE— MAKES US FAT.

It acts like ALCOHOL. IT DESTROYS OUR LIVER.

To add insult to injury—SUGAR may be the most ADDICTIVE substance in the WORLD. That's another reason I have dubbed sugar- the Queen of Neurotoxins.

Now you know how SUGAR is killing us in SO MANY ways. Sugar deserves the title of Queen of Neurotoxins.

***NOTE BENE

SUGAR'S NATURAL (HEALTHY) FORMS are— berries, maple tree syrup and raw honey.

ALL OF THESE SUGAR SOURCES RAISE YOUR BLOOD SUGAR AND SHOULD BE EATEN SPARINGLY!

STEVIA IS A UNIQUE PLANT-BASED NATURAL SWEETENER LIKE NO OTHER SWEETENER IN THE WORLD!

STEVIA IS 100 TIMES SWEETER THAN ORDINARY TABLE SUGAR!

STEVIA IS THE ONLY "SAFE" NATURAL SUGAR IN THE WORLD!

STEVIA IS THE ONLY PLANT-BASED SWEETENER THAT DOES NOT RAISE YOUR BLOOD SUGAR! (Please see Stevia References in appendix A).

STEVIA HAS BEEN USED BY INDIANS IN SOUTH AMERICA TO TREAT DIABETES FOR THE LAST TWO HUNDRED YEARS!

DIABETICS AND PEOPLE SUFFERING FROM INSULIN RESISTANCE CAN NOW REJOICE!

PUBLIC AUTHORITIES HAVE KNOWN ABOUT HOW BENEFICIAL STEVIA IS FOR THE LAST 20 YEARS AT LEAST!

THE SUGAR INDUSTRY LOBBIED HARD TO PREVENT FROM BEING IMPORTED INTO NORTH AMERICA!

But- Guess What?

IT'S NOW HERE! THE NUMBER OF COMPANIES SELLING STEVIA PRODUCTS IS EXPLODING!

BUT- MOST OF WESTERN SOCIETY-INCLUDING NATUROPATHIC DOCTORS ARE NOT FAMILIAR WITH THE HEALING EFFECTS OF STEVIA!

STEVIA IS MOTHER NATURE'S MAGIC BULLET!

STEVIA WILL NOT RAISE BLOOD SUGAR!

STEVIA IS THE SWEETER THAT IS USED IN MY KETOGENIC RECIPES- INFRA

ON TOP OF ALL OF THAT- THERE ARE A FEW SCIENTIFIC STUDIES THAT SUGGEST THAT STEVIA HAS HEALING THERAPEUTIC POWERS!

HEALTHY "SWEETS "ARE PROVIDED COURTESY OF MOTHER NATURE'S PANTRY-AND OUR CREATOR!

If Mother Nature made it—it's good for us.

IF MAN MADE IT IN A LAB AND/OR- IF IT'S PROCESSED—IT IS A CHEMICAL POISON- AND USUALLY A NEUROTOXIN.

BIG AGRA AND BIG FOOD WILL SELL YOU ANYTHING TO MAKE MONEY!

Do you remember- supra- Do you like poopy burgers? Lol.

Humans will sell anything to make money- so will Big Pharma. Big Pharma tells us it will make us healthier—WRONG!

Big Food tells us that it tastes great and will make us healthy- WRONG AGAIN! Don't be fooled by these scam artists.

More recent science—

A research team from New Zealand`s University of Otago, published a study in the American Journal of Clinical Nutrition. After conducting a mega review and mega-analysis of dietary studies, lead author, Dr. Lisa Te Morenga has uncovered solid evidence that eating sugar has a direct effect on risk factors for heart disease.

The learned doctor stated:

> Òur analysis confirmed that sugars contribute to cardiovascular risk, independent of the effect of sugars on body weight." (source: http:ajcn.nutrition. org)

101 COMMON NAMES FOR SUGAR IN FOOD

- Aguave syrup > Amasake > apple sugar> Barbados sugar> Bark sugar > Barley malt > Barley malt syrup > Beet sugar > Brown rice syrup > Brown sugar > Cane juice > Cane sugar> Caramelized foods > Carbitol > Caramel colouring > caramel sugars > Concentrated fruit juice > Corn sweetener > Corn syrup > Date sugar > Dextrin > Dextrox> Diglycerides > Disaccharides > D-taglose> Evaporated cane juice > Florida crystals > Fructooligo-saccrides (FDS) > Fructose > Fruit juice concentrate > Galactose > Glucitol > Glucoamine > Gluconoactone > Glucose > Glucose polymers > Glucose syrup > Glycerides > Glycerine > Glyercol > Glycol > Hexitol > High-fructose corn syrup > Honey > Inversol > Invert Sugar> Isomalt> Karo Syrups >Lactose > Light sugar > " Lite Sugar > Lo Han > Malitol > Malt dextrin > Malted barley >Maltodextrins > Maltodextrose > Maltose > Mannose > Maple syrup > Micrcocrystalline cellulose> Molasses > Monoglycerides> Monosaccarides > Nectars >Pentose > Polydextrose > Polyglycer-ides > Powdered sugar > Raisin juice > Raisin syrup> Raw sugar > Ribose Rice Syrup > Rice malt > Rice sugar > Rice Sweeteners > Rice syrup solids > Sacccharides > Sorbitol > Sorghum > Suc-canat > Sucanet > Sucrose > Sugar cane > Trisaccharides > Tur-binado sugar > Unrefined sugar > White sugar > Xylitol Zylose

ASPARTAME IS THE EVIL HALF-SISTER OF FRUCTOSE.

I will tell you how terrible Aspartame really is. (The European Food Safety Authority and the FDA will not tell you.)

HERE IS THE TRUTH ABOUT ASPARTAME-:

"It's the most dangerous food additive ever approved for human consumption"

Mark Stengler, N.D. America's Natural Doctor.

Many years ago, I learned about the EVILS OF ASPARTAME from an article published in the Harvard Law Review titled: "The History of Aspartame".

Briefly, aspartame was discovered by accident. A scientist was working in a lab. He dabbed in his finger in a chemical solvent and discovered that it had a sweet taste! Eureka said he!

In subsequent lab experiments, rats were fed aspartame. Some died and most developed HUGE TUMORS. An application for approval was nevertheless made to the FDA. The first time it was rejected. Guess What?

A second application was submitted to the FDA (different people) AND GUESS WHAT?

You guessed it!

ASPARTAME WAS APPROVED BY THE FDA!

The rest as they say is history. The Food and Beverage Industry has been making BAZILLIONS OF DOLLARS WITH ASPARTAME and its related artificial sweeteners.

THE SCIENTIFIC RESEARCH CLEARLY PROVES THAT ASPARTAME AND OTHER SWEET CHEMICALS ARE VERY TOXIC AND POISONOUS NEUROTOXINS.

RESEARCH SHOWS THAT ASPARTAME AND ARTIFICIAL CHEMICAL SWEETENERS WILL MAKE YOU FAT AND SICK.

RESEARCH SHOWS THAT ASPARTAME AND ARTIFICIAL SWEETENERS ARE ASSOCIATED WITH TYPE- 2 DIABETES.

RESEARCH CLEARLY SHOWS THAT ASPARTAME AND THE OTHER ARTIFICIAL SWEETENERS MAKE YOU FAT; EAT A HOLE IN THE LINING OF YOUR GUT.

Are you surprised?

The take-home message:

Avoid Aspartame and all other lab chemicals sold as sweeteners unless you want to get very sick.

ALL SUGARS AND SWEETENERS ARE TOXINS—BUT FRUCTOSE IS THE QUEEN OF ALL NEUROTOXINS.

THE TAKE-HOME MESSAGE IS:

YOU ARE STRONGLY RECOMMENDED TO ELIMINATE FRUCTOSE, SUCROSE AND ANY AND ALL FORMS OF SUGAR FROM YOUR DIET AND FROM YOUR LIFE.

YOU SHOULD USE STEVIA AS YOUR ONLY SWEETENER—IF YOU ARE SERIOUS ABOUT RE-GAINING CONTROL OF YOUR HEALTH.

STEVIA IS THE ONLY NATURAL SUGAR THAT WILL NOT RAISE YOUR BLOOD SUGAR!

IN SHORT STEVIA IS A MAGICAL BULLET THAT WILL ASSIST YOU TO GET YOUR BRAIN AND BODY FREE OF TOXIC NEUROTOXINS!

CHAPTER SIX
THE SUGAR FACTORY

"If I were to summarize in a single sentence what practice would best promote HEALTH— it would be this:

Health and Lifespan are determined by the proportion of fat versus sugar people burn through their lifetime...the more FAT that one burns as fuel, the healthier a person will be, and the more likely he or she will live a long time and the more SUGAR a person burns, the more disease-ridden and the shorter the life-span a person is likely to have "

Dr. Ron Rosedale M.D.

A. INTRODUCTION

The opening chapter examined the history of allopathic medicine, its flawed paradigm of "cut burn, poison", the Cholesterol Medical Scam, and other FRAUDULENT TOPICS RELATED TO THE DISEASE MANAGEMENT MEDICAL INDUSTRY.

BUT CHAPTER ONE CONCLUDED WITH AN EXCITING POSITIVE SECTION—THE MOST IMPORTANT HEALTH DISCOVERY- EVER!

Chapter 2 catalogued reasons TO FIRE YOUR DOCTOR AND HIRE YOURSELF.

Chapter 3 analyzed THE PLATINUM KEY TO SUPERHEALTH:

STABLE LOW-BLOOD SUGAR LEVELS AND THE ELIMINATION OF

INSULIN RESISTANCE.

Chapter 3 ITEMIZED THE LAB TESTS YOU NEED TO OBTAIN TO BEGIN YOUR HEALING JOURNEY TO SUPERHEALTH.

Chapter 3 PROVIDED YOU WITH THE HEALTH TOOLS AND INFORMATION TO BYPASS THE MEDICAL ESTABLISHMENT AND ESCAPE THE EVIL CLUTCHES OF BIG PHARMA=☺

YOU—AND ONLY YOU— ARE THE MASTER OF YOUR OWN HEALTH DESTINY.

YOU MUST TAKE A DO-IT-YOURSELF (DIY) APPROACH TO YOUR HEALTH.

NO ONE KNOWS YOUR BODY BETTER THAN YOU DO.

YOU ARE THE ONLY PERSON IN THE WORLD WHO CAN TAKE CHARGE OF YOUR HEALTH. NO ONE ELSE CAN DO IT FOR YOU!

In chapter 4 NEUROTOXINS WERE EXAMINED. You were advised to ELIMINATE ALL neurotoxins; ALL processed foods, ALL "Frankenfoods" (e.g. GMOs) grains, conventional dairy and meat, etc.

A good rule of thumb is— if it comes in a box, bag or can, DON'T EAT IT! (There are very few exceptions!) If Mother Nature didn't make it— YOU don't need it.

Chapter 5 examined SUGAR—THE QUEEN OF NEUROTOXINS.

It turns out the Queen of Neurotoxins (SUGAR) has devious evil half-sister called—CARBOHYDRATES!-☺

CARBS ARE NOT NUTRIENTS!

CARBOHYDRATES DO NOT BUILD OR REPAIR ANYTHING.

Our bodies use carbs to metabolize or manufacture GLUCOSE. Our body takes protein and its amino acids also to manufacture glucose. Glucose is SUGAR that our bodies CAN USE AS FUEL FOR ENERGY.

But- "Houston- we have a problem! -☺

When we consume CARBOHYDRATES AS OUR PRIMARY FUEL (ENERGY SOURCE) our bodies make too much SUGAR/GLUCOSE!

What happens then?

OUR INTERNAL SUGAR FACTORY BREAKS DOWN!

OUR INTERNAL SUGAR FACTORY BECOMES "BUSTED".

Our internal sugar factory consists of the metabolic pathways, cells, organs, tissues etc. that produce biochemical reactions that our body uses to metabolize <u>FOOD</u> to produce glucose for cellular energy.

OUR INTERNAL SUGAR FACTORY IS THE BIG SUGAR FACTORY.

Our "external" sugar factory is "managed" by Big Agriculture (Big Agra) and Big Food.

Big Pharma, Big MED and BIG GOVERNMENT have partnered up with SUGAR the Queen of Neurotoxins-☺ and with her slutty half-sister CARBOHYDRATES-☺

<u>**IT IS DIFFICULT TO FIND FOODS IN YOUR SUPERMARKET THAT DO NOT CONTAIN ANY SUGAR.**</u>

<u>**FINDING LOW-CARB FOODS MEANS THAT YOU NEED TO PUT ON YOUR CARB EYEGLASSES-**</u>☺

Most ill informed doctors (and oncologists) advise their patients to eat a <u>HIGH-CARB</u> <u>DIET</u>. These people are clueless about nutrition because they receive no training in <u>NUTRITION</u>. Prescribing a high carbohydrate diet is a prescription for disaster!

CARBS FIRE UP YOUR "INTERNAL" SUGAR FACTORY!

<u>**CARBS PRODUCE GLUCOSE THAT CAUSES YOUR PANCREAS TO PUMP OUT INSULIN— TO MOP UP THE EXCESS GLUCOSE THAT'S PRODUCED.**</u>

For example—SUGAR IS THE PREFERRED FUEL FOR <u>CANCER CELLS—GLUTINOUS CANCER CELLS FEAST ON SUGAR!</u>

It's the same thing for <u>DIABETES</u> patients.

Most conventionally trained doctors advise their patients to eat <u>A HIGH CARB DIET.</u>

<u>**A HIGH CARB DIET IS A PRESCRIPTION FOR DISASTER!**</u>

This ill-advised strategy turns on our <u>PANCREAS'</u> insulin pump. Blood sugar levels then start to <u>SKYROCKET!</u> Your internal sugar factory becomes totally overwhelmed. Excess sugar floats around in your blood and your BODY; (thanks to <u>INSULIN</u>) and this stores excess sugar as <u>BELLY FAT!</u>

Obesity is step one. Step 2 is usually MB (metabolic syndrome), Sydrome X, or pre-Diabetes. Step 3 could be <u>DIABETES</u> Type 2 or <u>CANCER</u> or anyone of a dozen <u>METABOLIC DISEASES</u>.

<u>**HIGH-CARB DIETS MAKE YOU FAT AND SICK.**</u>

YOU MUST SCRUTINIZE LABELS FOR SUGAR AND CARBOHYDRATES!

Sugar and carbs are evil twin sisters.-☺ The more sugar you burn in your life- the quicker you will die- (quote above.) You must <u>ELIMINATE THE QUEEN OF NEUROTOXINS FROM YOUR DIET</u>.

<u>YOU MUST "VIRTUALLY ELIMINATE"</u> her evil half-sister—<u>CARBOHYDRATES</u>.-☺

EVEN MANY ORGANIC FOODS CONTAIN ADDED SUGAR!

ONE GRAM OF SUGAR IS ONE GRAM TOO MUCH!

The average amount of sugar floating around in the bloodstream of a healthy person should be about <u>ONE TEASPOON WORTH</u>! More than that is <u>TOXIC</u> to your body.

SUGAR OUTSIDE AND INSIDE YOUR BODY IS PUBLIC ENEMY NUMBER ONE!

STARCHY CARBOHYDRATES THAT BECOME SUGAR/GLUCOSE IN YOUR BODY ARE PUBLIC ENEMY NUMBER TWO.

When you rid your body from endogenous/exogenous sugar –you will go a long way towards strengthening your immune system. Your self-healing machine will be given a good chance to repair "<u>ANY BUSTED CELLS</u>".

Ladies—the old adage about "a moment on your lips- a lifetime on your hips"—as regards bad carbs could be true. That bagel will eventually make you fat and cause wrinkles- ☺ The human body was <u>NOT</u> designed or programmed to eat bagels or any other processed food –<u>WHATSOEVER</u>! Even your chemically-laced lipstick will end up in your blood, your brain, liver and anywhere else your body is able to stash it.

<u>YOU NEED TO GET YOUR BRAIN OFF SUGAR—FROM EXTERNAL</u> (exogenous) <u>AND INTERNAL</u> (endogenous sources). <u>THIS MEANS ELIMINATING ALL SUGAR FROM EXOGENOUS SOURCES (FOOD) and SHUTTING DOWN ENDOGENOUS PRODUCTION OF SUGAR FROM YOUR INTERNAL SUGAR FACTORY</u>!

Glucose (sugar) manufactured <u>FROM CARBOHYDRATES BY YOUR INTERNAL SUGAR FACTORY MUST BE SEVERELY RESTRICTED</u>. Shutting down the manufacture of glucose by your internal sugar factory will both <u>ALLOW</u> and <u>TEACH</u> your body to <u>USE/ BURN FAT AS ITS PRIMARY FUEL SOURCE</u>.

OUR BRAIN'S HIGH-OCTANE SUPERFUEL IS FAT!

Your heart and major organs also work 25 (Twenty-five) <u>PERCENT MORE EFFECIENTLY ON FAT</u>! Who knew?

Now we shall delve into the physiology and the intricate workings of our <u>INTERNAL SUGAR FACTORY</u>. You will learn how our body metabolizes sugar and fat.

You will gain a deep understanding of the complex process called" <u>HUMAN METABOLISM</u>".

Our bodies <u>METABOLIZE</u> (i.e. breakdown) <u>FOOD SO THAT IT CAN MAKE ESSENTIAL FUEL REQUIRED BY OUR BODIES.</u>

<u>THIS FUEL THEN CREATES ENERGY THAT POWERS OUR BODIES.</u>

<u>OUR BODIES HAVE THE ABILITY TO</u>— BURN SUGAR OR— TO BURN FAT AS FUEL. <u>THE CHOICE IS ENTIRELY YOURS.</u>

You can choose to become a <u>FAT-BURNER</u> or to remain as a <u>CARB (SUGAR) BURNER</u>.

<u>YOU CAN CHOOSE</u> to eat carbohydrates; make sugar (glucose) from carbs to burn as <u>SECOND-RATE FUEL—OR-</u>

<u>YOU CAN CHOOSE FAT- THE PREFERRED FUEL OF HUMAN METABOLISM.</u>

<u>CARBS</u> (just another source of SUGAR) <u>ARE ACTUALLY TOXIC TO OUR BODIES</u>! Eating carbs damages <u>OUR METABOLISM AND CAUSES A "BUSTED SUGAR METABOLISM".</u>

At the cellular level eating carbs also damages our cells (aka" <u>BUSTED CELLS</u>").

<u>"BUSTED METABOLISM" AND "BUSTED CELLS" SOMETIMES KNOWN AS METABOLIC DISORDER AND BUSTED MITOCHONDRIA ARE TECHNICALLY CALLED:</u>

<u>"MITOCHONDRIAL DYSFUNCTION"</u>

<u>What really is "Mitochondrial dysfunction?</u>

Essentially it means that the "mitochondria" are "busted." Mitochondria are the "powerful little batteries" inside of most cells in our bodies. When these little power plants become damaged- or busted—<u>THEY STOP PRODUCING ENERGY</u>. The mitochondria become sick or diseased. And this messes up our <u>METABOLISM</u>.

Our bodies can no longer proper digest food and nutrients properly.

POOR METABOLIC HEALTH IS THE ROOT CAUSE OF MOST DISEASES AND CHRONIC ADVERSE HEALTH ISSUES.

"Mitochondrial dysfunction" simply means: **BUSTED CELLS AND BUSTED METABOLISM.**

THE END RESULT IS INFLAMMATION THAT CAUSES DISEASES AND SICKNESS.

Mr. Raymond Francis puts this **CONCEPT** eloquently:

> **"THERE IS ONLY ONE DISEASE: MALFUNCTIONING CELLS"(aka "BUSTED CELLS" (my words)**

> **AND- ONLY 2 CAUSES OF DISEASE:**

>   1. **NUTRITIONAL DEFICIENCY and**

>   2. **CELLULAR TOXICITY.**

>   **ALL DISEASES FROM DIABETES TO CANCER TO AR-THRITIS ARE INFLAMMATORY DISEASES"**

> **MY SUPERHEALTH SOLUTION IS:**

>   a) **ELIMINATE NEUROTOXINS FROM YOUR DIET AND LIFE.**

>   b) **EMPLOY THE NUTRITIONAL SOLUTION CALLED THE "KE-TOGENIC DIET"...**

>   c) **A WELL- CONSTRUCTED KETOGENIC DIET FIXES BUSTED MITOCHONDRIA, BUSTED CELLS AND BUSTED METABO-LISMS!**

HAVING HEALTHY, PROPERLY FUNCTIONING MITOCHONDRIA IS THE CORNERSTONE OF GOOD HEALTH. (Here's a secret that few people know... Your DNA cellular mitochondria you get from YOUR MOTHER! You can impress your colleagues, and friends with that one!-☺

TO ENJOY AND ATTAIN SUPERHEALTH-

YOU MUST HAVE SUPER CELLULAR HEALTH. TO HAVE GREAT CELLULAR HEALTH YOU MUST HAVE VERY HEALTHY MITOCHONDRIA.

YOU MUST BUILD HEALTHY MITOCHONDRIA BY EATING NUTRIENT-DENSE WHOLE, REAL FOOD.

TO REPAIR YOUR MITOCHONDRIA AND FIX BUSTED CELLS YOU MUST EAT THE RIGHT FOODS. YOU MUST FIX YOUR HEALTH BY FIXING A BUSTED SUGAR-BURNING METABOLISM.

I AM CONFIDENT THAT YOU WILL CHOOSE TO EAT FATS TO BURN AS YOUR PRIMARY NEW HIGH-OCTANE SUPERFUEL.

WHEN YOU EAT A KETOGENIC DIET YOU WILL ELIMINATE INSULIN RESISTANCE AND MAINTAIN LOW STABLE BLOOD SUGAR.

After all—that's the platinum key to SUPERHEALTH!

HEALING HEALTHY FAT IS YOUR FRIEND! (It's also your brain's secret love-☺)

NINETY-FIVE PERCENT OF NORTH AMERICANS ARE SUGAR BURNERS & NINETY PERCENT OF PEOPLE ARE INSULIN-RESISTANT!

How shocking is that!

Even your doctor may be insulin-resistant! OMG! The poor devil likely doesn't know. Most doctors erroneously believe that DIABETES is a disease of caused by elevated blood sugar. Your doctor likely is clueless about biochemistry and human metabolism.

WORSE YET- your conventionally trained doctor is likely hurting his patients because your doctor does not understand the physiological mechanisms underlying BUSTED CELLS AND BUSTED METABOLISM!

EVEN WORSE—MOST CONVENTIONALLY TRAINED DOCS ARE POURING GASOLINE ON THEIR PATIENTS' DIABETIC FIRES! (See below).

IGNORANT DOCTORS ARE KILLING PEOPLE WITH DIABETES TREATMENT DRUGS LIKE METFORMIN (See below).

SYNTHETIC INSULIN— IS AN HORRIFIC TREATMENT FOR TYPE 1 DIABETICS!

DRUGS LIKE METAFORMIN KILL THOUSANDS OF TYPE 2 DIABETIC PATIENTS AND/OR CAUSE CANCER OR CARDIOVASCULAR DISEASE!

This is sad news—BUT-

THE HAPPY NEWS IS THIS:

THE KNOWLEDGE GLEANED FROM THIS BOOK WILL ALLOW YOU TO ESCAPE BIG PHARMA'S EVIL DRUGS!

IF YOU ARE TAKING 'MEDS' TO CONTROL BLOOD-SUGAR AND/OR DIABETES- YOU WILL BE PROVIDED WITH THE INFORMATION AND EXPERTISE THAT YOU NEED TO WEAN YOUR SELF OFF OF THESE HORRIBLE POISONS.

YOU WILL LEARN HOW TO KISS THESE DRUGS GOOD-BYE-☺ or toss them in the recycle bin.

YOU CAN APPLY THIS KNOWLEDGE AND BE EMPOWERED!

YOU CAN ADOPT YOUR NEW DIY APPROACH TO HEALTH, WELL-BEING AND HAPPINESS. WITH THE HELP OF THIS BOOK, YOU WILL GAIN THE KNOWLEDGE TO KINDLE YOUR DESIRE, PASSION AND THE COURAGE TO TAKE CARE OF YOUR OWN HEALTH.

IT'S YOUR PERSONALIZED- TAILOR-CUSTOMIZED HEALTH CARE PROGRAM!

Most lean people (outwardly looking healthy people) are SUGAR-BURNERS. Most are one bagel away from becoming PRE-DIABETIC;- ☺

THE EXPERTISE IN THIS BOOK WILL TEACH YOU HOW TO BECOME A FAT BURNER! -

BECOMING A FAT BURNER WILL MAKE YOU LEAN, HEALTHY ; AND WILL REVERSE VIRTUALLY ANY AND ALL ADVERSE HEALTH CONDITIONS THAT YOU MAY HAVE!

FOLKS —THE JURY IS IN! AND THE VERDICT IS SUPER!

THE KETOGENIC DIET (high-fat- low carb- moderate protein) IS OUR ANCESTRAL MAGIC HEALING DIET. (It's been buried by modern civilization- that's why it's new to most of us).

It's only existed FOR ALMOST 3 MILLION YEARS!; — ☺... which just happens to be long as humans have roamed Planet Earth.

THE KETOGENIC HEALING DIET WILL HELP YOU REACH SUPERHEALTH STATUS WITHIN A VERY SHORT TIME.

A WELL-CONSTRUCTED KETOGENIC DIET WILL MAKE YOUR IMMUNE SYSTEM BULLETPROOF.

NOTE BENE!

When you adopt a healing Ketogenic Diet and a Ketogenic Lifestyle—

1. YOU WILL NOT BE ABLE TO LEAP BUILDINGS WITH ONE LEAP!

2. YOU WILL NOT BE ABLE TO STOP SPEEDING BULLETS!-☺

THESE FEATS ARE RESERVED FOR SUPERMAN-☺

THE BIGGEST DANGERS WHEN YOU FOLLOW A KETOGENIC DIET AND ENTER NUTRITIONAL KETOSIS IS THAT YOU COULD FEEL SOOO ENERGETIC AND SOO POWERFUL—

THAT—YOU MIGHT START TO "IMAGINE" OR YOU MIGHT START TO "BELIEVE" THAT YOU "CAN" STOP A SPEEDING BULLET OR EVEN THAT YOU CA N LEAP TALL BUILDINGS!-☺

SO—PLEASE BE CAREFUL!-☺

THE KETOGENIC DIET IS EXTREMELY POWERFUL! IT'S LIKE MENTAL DYNAMITE! A KETOGENIC DIET WILL PROVIDE YOU WITH EXCEPTIONAL NEURAL STRENGTH, FOCUS AND EXCEPTIONAL MENTAL CLARITY!

A FINAL WARNING: IF YOU'RE IN KETOSIS WHEN YOU ENTER YOUR DOCTOR'S OFFICE- IT'S O.K. FOR YOU TERMINATE HIS SERVICES WHILE LAUGHING.

BUT PLEASE BE CAREFUL! YOUR BIG CONFIDENT KETOGENIC GRIN MAY CAUSE HIM TO HAVE A HEART ATTACK! He might even ask you to tell him your Ketogenic secrets. -☺) **Tip:** Tell his nurse to have an **AED** (automated external defibrillator) handy— just in case.-☺)

Here on Earth, "Kryptonite" is Superman's ultimate danger. Kryptonite can kill or hurt Superman. You can learn from Superman.

THINK OF SUGAR AS—"KRYPTONITE" FOR HUMANS.

SUGAR/FAT METABOLISM QUESTION IS INEXTRICABLY LINKED to the "lipid hypothesis"—junk science propagated by Ancel Key's disciples.

Since that flawed study- there have been absolutely **NO** credible, solid scientific evidence or clinical studies of **ANY KIND WHATSOEVER** that support the **DEMONIZATION FAT**— (aka **FAT FOBIA**).

Au contraire—

Dozens of solid scientific studies prove that **HEALTHY SATURATED FAT IS ESSENTIAL FOR GOOD HEALTH AND SATURATED FAT IS THE BEST FOOD THAT YOU CAN PUT IN YOUR BELLY. PERIOD.**

e.g. Coconut oil has been dubbed "The Cure for all Diseases"! Coconut Oil is **92 PERCENT SATURATED FAT.** Ihe closest **FAT** in the world to coconut oil is **MOTHER'S BREAST MILK.**

Does anyone really believe that mother's breast milk is **UNHEALTHY?**

CONVENTIONALLY TRAINED DOCTORS AND CONVENTIONALLY TRAINED DIE-TICIANS HAVE NO KNOWLEDGE OF ESSENTIAL NUTRIENTS!

These "health-care"/dis-ease care providers" BELIEVE THAT CARBOHDRATES ARE NUTRIENTS. Sheesh!

THESE SAME 'HEALTH CARE' PROVIDERS KNOW LITTLE ABOUT HUMAN METABOLISM!

Should you take advice from these people? ABSOLUTELY NOT!

Has their dietary advice been useful or helpful in the last HALF CENTURY? NOPE.

FOLLOWING CONVENTIONAL DIETARY ADVICE HAS MADE PEOPLE FATTER AND SICKER WITH EACH PASSING YEAR.

Since its creation, 100 years ago, the ALLOPATHIC PROFESSION IS A TERRIBLE EXPERIMENT GONE WRONG. 99 PERCENT OF WHAT ALLOPATHIC DOCTORS DO— IS SIMPLY WRONG.

THERE IS A BOATLOAD OF SCIENTIFIC AND CLINICAL STUDIES THAT PROVE THE TRUTH OF THIS STATEMENT. An esteemed colleague/ friend of mine is fond of saying: "Liars figure- but figures don't lie" (Dead doctors don't lie either).-☺

YOU MUST QUESTION EVERYTHING! My later father used to tell me- "Son- don't believe anything you hear and half of what you see".

It turns out that when we are in s fasted state—our brain actually eats our stored body fat as fuel. It makes ketone bodies (fat bodies) which actually builds brain cells and makes us smarter!

How cool is that? The word "ketogenic" comes from the word "ketones".

ONE MAGNIFICENT BENEFIT of a Ketogenic Diet is the MENTAL CLARITY AND CALMNESS it creates in your body.

YOU WILL BE AMAZED HOW GOOD YOU FEEL ON THE KETOGENIC DIET!

When you become keto-(or fat) adapted, you will have more com-passion for ill-informed health care workers who mistakenly believe they are helping patients— but fail to realize that they are actually hurting patients.

The latest 2015! Dietary Guidelines (still badly flawed) continue to wage a 60 year old WAR ON SATURATED FAT AND CHOLESTEROL. A diet high in carbohydrates is still being touted as HEALTHY.

MAINSTREAM HEALTH CARE PROVIDERS STILL DEMONIZE HEALTHY FATS AS FOOD THAT CAUSES CARDIOVASCULAR DISEASE etc.

THE TRUTH OF THE MATTER IS: that slice of wholewheat toast or ham sandwich ACTUALLY CAUSES HEART DISEASE; CANCER; (Leaky Gut Syndrome and Heaven knows what else)!

The happy news is- you're reading this book! Soon you will be able to extricate yourself from the clutches of incompetent allopathic doctors, ill-informed die-iticians.

HELP as many people as possible to get HEALTHY AND HAPPY. We can make the world a better, happier place— one person at a time.

Be warned. Most allopathic doctors and die-ticians refuse to even EXAMINE the benefits/merits of a KETOGENIC (LCHF) DIET. Doctors have been taught—

"KETONES ARE BAD AND DANGEROUS!

DOCTORS ARE COMPLETELY WRONG ABOUT KETONES AND THE KETOGENIC DIET! Conventional doctors confuse the concept of "ketosis" with the concept of ketoacidosis. Please see chapter.

THIS IS ANOTHER CLASSIC CASE OF THE 99 PERCENT RULE.

YOUR DOCTOR IS WRONG 99 PERCENT OF THE TIME.

THAT'S THE REASON THAT YOU SHOULD FIRE YOUR DOCTOR.

Most allopathic doctors still take their marching orders from Big Pharma. They have what you might call "fragile egos". Most have tunnel vision when it comes to examining/and/or considering the merits of another opinion and/or approach.

ONCE YOU ARE KETO-ADAPTED—YOU WILL THINK VERY DIFFERENTLY ABOUT YOUR HEALTH.

YOU WILL THEN REALIZE THAT MOST CONVENTIONAL DOCTORS AND DIETICIANS HAVE BOARDED THE WRONG HEALTH TRAIN. They sense it but they are afraid to acknowledge it.

Guess what?

ONLY TWO MONTHS AGO— SOME DIE-TICIAN "EXPERTS" CONFESSED THAT THEY WERE PARTIALLY WRONG ABOUT CHOLESTEROL. WOW! THEY'VE ONLY BEEN WRONG FOR THE LAST HALF-CENTURY!

JUST IMAGINE HOW BIG PHARMA AND BIG FOOD MUST BE PANICKING!

As this book goes to press- it's likely grocery stores are being inundated by consumers looking for THOSE TASTY HIGH CHOLESTEROL FOODS LIKE EGGS, BUTTER, SAUSAGES, BACON; etc.

SAVVY EDUCATED CONSUMERS ARE WAKING UP!

PEOPLE NOW KNOW THAT THEY HAVE BEEN MISGUIDED AND MIS-INFORMED ABOUT CHOLESTEROL.

People are starting to question spending $ 1,500 dollars per month on useless statin drugs to lower their cholesterol. People will soon begin ditching these poisons.

THOUSANDS OF PEOPLE HAVE BEGUN TO FLOOD MOTHER NATURE'S FARMACY FOR THOSE RICH SUCCULENT FATTY—HEALTHY FOODS.

MOTHER NATURE'S WHOLE FOOD PRODUCTS ARE A LOT CHEAPER –FAR SAFER AND FAR MORE EFFECTIVE FOR GOOD HEALTH.

AS AN ADDED SURPRISE—

OUR NEW KNOWLEDGE OF EPIGENETICS SHOWS THAT WHEN YOU EAT DELICIOUS NUTRIENT DENSE WHOLE FOODS- YOU IMPROVE YOUR OWN HEALTH AND-

YOU ARE IMPROVING THE HEALTH OF YOUR CHILDREN AND YOUR GRAND-CHILDREN FOR MANY YEARS TO COME!

YOU ARE LITERALLY CONTRIBUTING TO THE HEALTH OF HUMANITY AND HUMANS ON THE ENTIRE PLANET!!

How cool is THAT??

How can Big Pharma's toxic pills compare with THAT?

YOU CAN FEED YOUR ENTIRE FAMILY FOR THE COST OF A PRESCRIPTION FOR STATIN DRUGS! Wouldn't you rather spend money on delicious fatty foods?

In the '50's doctors were proud to extoll the Health Benefits of SMOKING CIGARETTES. You will not see many doctors advertising smoking cigarettes these days. It seems most of them died from lung cancer so- they decided that it wasn't such a healthy thing to do.

Paradoxically, in recent years the USE OF MEDICAL GRADE CANNIBIS (aka Marijauna) HAS SKYROCKETED AS A TREATMENT FOR MANY CHRONIC DISEASES. Is it really true that plants can help make you healthy?

Gee- Who knew? Actually, most people outside of North America have known FOR CENTURIES ABOUT THE HEALTH BENEFITS OF PLANTS, HERBS, & SPICES. It's called Ayuredic and Chinese Medicine.

Virtually, ALL of the health-care providers in North America—including doctors, cardiologists, nurses, die-ticians, and nutritionists still desperately cling to Ancel Key's frayed apron strings.

MOTHER NATURE AND HER FARMACY IS STILL UNDER ATTACK.

When you eat her medicine- you are promoting your own health .You are helping Mother Nature fight Big Pharma's, Big Chem's, Big Agra's, Big Food's POISONING AND DESTRUCTION OF OUR GLOBAL ENVIRONMENT.

Men, women, and even some dogs-☺ are waking up to realize that "Ancel Key's/ medical dietary approach" HAS BEEN AN UTTER DISMAL FAILURE.

Who can tell how many people HAVE DIED or WHO HAVE SUFFERED SERIOUS CHRONIC DISEASES BECAUSE OF THIS FLAWED APPROACH!

Just look around at the local shopping centre. THE EVIDENCE IS SHOCKING AND SELF –EVIDENT. North Americans have witnessed a sky-rocketing increase in obesity, diabetes, heart disease and many other chronic diseases.

Three decades ago, in 1986, Everett C. Koop the Surgeon-General of the United States authored a lengthy 300 page report specifically indicating that 85 percent of all diseases were related to dietary and nutritional problems.

ALMOST ALL HEALTH CARE PROVIDERS IGNORED THIS REORT. That ground-breaking NUTRITIONAL report issued by the head honcho- U.S. Surgeon-General really was relegated to the trash heap.

ALL DISEASES ARE REALLY CAUSED BY NUTRITIONAL DEFICIENCIES. The Surgeon-General gave an ACADEMY PERFORMANCE AND NO ONE ATTENDED-☺

Almost NO ONE in the healthcare community paid any attention to this report. However, one plausible explanation is likely because this report did not come from the BIG "BOSSMAN"- Big Pharma. Why believe the Top Surgeon whose report was supported by dozens of top scientists and several leading nutritional gurus? Gee- do you think it's because there's no money to be made from selling healthy nutritious foods? Yes ...I think you may be onto something.-☺

YES- IT'S TRUE. The big bucks are not made in promoting good health. The big money is made from dis-ease management. When people have a monopoly in any industry- they never want any competition!

In the days of Wild Wild West, and the American frontier, bounty hunters adopted the legal mantra of "Wanted Dead or Alive." Sometimes, where life had no value- sometimes death had some.

Are Big Pharma and the medical establishment just modern- day bounty hunters? Well...not really.

Western frontiersmen bounty hunters did not care how criminals were brought to justice- DEAD OR ALIVE. They received the same dollar reward. Big Pharma does not want to kill the goose that lays the golden egg! You are the golden goose-☺ Big Pharma and your conventionally-trained doctors don't want you to die! If you die too soon—they will lose money. They want your money. It's in their interest to KEEP YOU ALIVE! All they see is your wallet and big $$$! The longer you live- the more DRUGS THEY CAN SELL TO YOU!

If you are "unlucky"   and die from your toxic medications- the death certificate will likely say "Mr. X- died from pulmonary heart failure". The family is told- gee- the poor guy must have died from walking too fast on the treadmill.

No death-certificate EVER MENTIONS that the poor deceased was taking FIFTEEN POISONOUS DRUGS at the time of his" untimely" death. A typical explanation by the medical people to the grieving survivors might be something like:

> "Gee- poor Harry:-I cautioned him about going on a treadmill. His medications were supposed to work to thin his blood and lower his cholesterol, but I guess his heart was just too weak. Hey- If I remember correctly, George mentioned that there was a history of cardio-vascular problems which ran in his family. In any event, his death could not have been caused by his medications. Have a nice day,"

Allopathic doctors KILL MORE THAN ONE MILLION PEOPLE PER YEAR. Given that death certificates rarely mention DRUG- INDUCED heart attacks, cancer etc. -you can judge for yourself. Gee- maybe the iatrogenic death count is probably much too low!

<u>IT'S PROBABLE THAT ANOTHER 50 THOUSAND MORE HEART DEATHS DUE TO DRUGS GO UNREPORTED.</u>

Gee... Good Luck proving in Court that George died from a drug cocktail. Everyone knows that George had no business even walking to the gym. ...yeah sure... poor George never did follow his doctor's orders.-yada, yada, yada.

<u>IT'S ALMOST IMPOSSIBLE TO PROVE THAT DRUG COMBOS CAUSE HEART ATTACKS - DESPITE WHAT SCIENCE AND COMMON SENSE MIGHT SUGGEST.</u>

<u>MEDICAL MALPRACTICE IS ONE OF THE TOUGHEST THINGS TO PROVE IN A COURT OF LAW.</u> The medical business is rotten to the core and they protect their own. Large corporations employ hundreds of lawyers. Monsanto- for example has more than 300 lawyers.

<u>THERE WILL NEVER BE ANY CLINICAL STUDIES DONE ON THE SYNERGISTIC EFFECTS OF DRUG COMBOS.</u> Do you think that Big Pharma will pay for that study?

But- I digress.

<u>MOST CONVENTIONAL DOCTORS STILL PUBLICLY STATE THAT VITAMINS AND SUPPLEMENTS ARE A WASTE OF MONEY.</u> Well, sayeth the immortal Bob Dylan "the times they are a changin". It appears that consumers are starting to throw their medications down the toilet in favour of supplements.

<u>RESEARCH SHOWS THAT 50 PERCENT OF AMERICANS ARE TAKING SUPPLEMENTS.</u>

<u>SUPPLEMENTS ARE SAFE.</u>

<u>RESEARCH SHOWS THAT SINCE 1940's SUPPLEMENTS HAVE NOT CAUSED ONE DEATH. NIL. NADA!</u>

Last year the global Supplement Industry had sales of 300 billion dollars! Today— given the <u>WELL</u>- documented scientific research about the Therapeutic/Nutritional <u>POWER OF VEGETABLES and NUTS</u> such as coconuts, turmeric and chocolate, one can only speculate about the panic in the backrooms of Big Pharma.

<u>Do you see why Big Pharma is starting to panic?</u> People like you are reading books like this. The truth is getting out. <u>THE TRUTH WILL SET YOU FREE</u>—from the evil grasp of the pharmaceutical corporate giants and the medical mafia.

Do you believe Mother Nature is winning the hearts and minds of consumers?

Have you checked the numbers that show that fast-food and soft-drink sales are plummeting? Consumers are catching on—FAST! Many consumers are fed up (pun intended) with the food tyranny of Big Agriculture, Big Food, Big Chemical and Bi g Pharma.

WELCOME TO THE FOOD REVOLUTION!

(Please visit www.foodrising.org where you can learn how to GROW YOUR OWN NUTRITIOUS FOOD PENNIES ON THE DOLLAR!

HERE YOU HAVE THE BEST DO-IT-YOURSELF- (DIY) FOOD PARADIGM EVER!

THIS CONCEPT WILL REVOLUTIONIZE THE GROWING OF FOOD ON OUR PLANET! YOU CAN GROW YOUR OWN FOOD FOLKS- FOR PENNIES ON THE DOLLAR. YOU CAN PLUCK THE HEALING MEDICINE FROM MOTHER NATURE'S FARMACY!

A BIG THANK YOU TO ITS CREATOR- MR. MIKE ADAMS (aka THE HEALTH RANGER)!

Did you know that recently the FDA sent a warning letter to a walnut company? It seems that according to the FDA the walnut people cannot extoll the proven nutritional value of walnuts. They look like our brain- but are they really good food for your brain?

TRUTH IS: WALNUTS ARE ONE OF MOTHER NATURE'S FINEST SUPERFOODS!

Can you see why the FDA wants to control walnuts and OTHER INFORMATION ABOUT NUTRITOUS FOODS?

DO YOU KNOW NOT ONE PERSON HAS DIED AS A RESULT OF TAKING SUPPLEMENTS? NO ONE! NADA! In 2008, 27 people died when struck by lightning. NOT ONE SINGLE DEATH FROM SUPPLEMENTS. Compare that with the number of deaths by drugs! (A few reported "mysterious" deaths have been allegedly associated with a toxic combo of POISONOUS DRUGS TAKEN WITH SUPPLEMENTS.

What likely happened is that blood thinners like Coumadin (aka rat poison) were taken with grapefruits or other citrus fruits.

Gee- Have you ever heard of someone DYING FROM EATING A GRAPEFRUIT?

Let's return to the latest 2015- Dietary "Unhealthy" Guidelines.

The last Dietary Guidelines were issued in 2010. These guidelines are issued every 5 years. The 2015 Dietary Guidelines are due in the next few weeks. You'll never guess what! A few days ago, the Committee responsible for the 2015 Guidelines—

DROPPED A HUGE NUTRITIONAL BOMBSHELL!!

They stated in their draft report these <u>EARTH- SHATTERING</u> words:

"<u>CHOLESTEROL IS NOT CONSIDERED A NUTRIENT OF CONCERN FOR OVERCONSUMPTION!!</u> OMG!

THIS ADMISSION OF BEING WRONG HAS SHOCKED THE MEDICAL WORLD AND MOST REGISTERED DIETICIANS! (Gee…it's enough to make poor Mr. Keys roll over in his grave!-☺) The white-coated crowd must be in full-fledged panic mode!

ON TOP OF THAT- BIG FOOD-BIG AGRA- AND ESPECIALLY BIG MEAT ARE LIKELY BUZZING AROUND LIKE ANGRY HORNETS!

BIG FOOD IS TRYING TO DISCREDIT THESE DIETARY GUIDELINES – AND CALLS THEM NONSENSICAL.

CAN YOU IMAGINE HOW MUCH MONEY IS AT STAKE FOR BIG FOOD AND BIG AGRA? KA- CHING—KA-CHING!

Cardiologist, <u>Dr. Steve Nissen, Chairman of Cardiovascular Medicine</u> told USA Today:

<u>"It's the right decision. We've got the Dietary Guidelines wrong. They've been wrong for decades."</u>

(author's underlines)

Medical Journalist, Larry Husten stated:

<u>" The proposed change reflects a major shift in the scientific view of cholesterol that has taken place in recent years.</u>

<u>Although serum cholesterol is still considered an important risk factor, cholesterol consumed as food is now thought to play a relatively insignificant rile in determining blood levels of cholesterol."</u>

The Washington Post on February 10th, 2015 also ran an article covering the report. The Post suggested that the new stance on cholesterol would remain in the final Report.

This same message was repeated in <u>TIME MAGAZINE</u>, which reported that:

> "In the latest review of studies that investigated the link between dietary fat and causes of death, researchers say the guidelines got it all wrong. In fact, recommendations to reduce the amount of fat we eat everyday should never have been made."

(author's underline)

As mentioned, low-fat diets saw a real upswing in 1977. Do you remember the Declaration of the War on Fat?

The fat-phobic white-coated crowd recently received <u>ANOTHER NAIL IN THEIR "PHAT PHOBIC"- COFFIN</u>.

According to research published in the (2015) Open Heart Journal, conducted by Zoe Harcombe PhD.—

> "THERE WAS NO SCIENTIFIC BASIS FOR THE RECOMMENDATIONS TO CUT FAT FROM OUR DIET IN THE FIRST PLACE."

(Author's underlines)

<u>BELOW- THE MAGICAL HEALING PROPERTIES OF HIGH-FAT- LOW-CARB DIET (aka THE KETOGENIC DIET) ARE EXTOLLED.</u>

<u>A BOATLOAD</u> of scientific studies and literature support the view that <u>VIRTUALLY EVERYONE ON PLANET EARTH</u> should be eating a <u>Ketogenic Diet</u>.

We need to return to our ancestral KETOGENIC diet and lifestyle.

<u>YOU SHOULD STOP BURNING SUGAR AND START BURNING FAT IN YOUR FAT BURNING MACHINE!</u>

<u>IT'S TIME TO GET RID OF YOUR SUGAR ADDICTION AND DITCH THE CARBS!</u>

B. GLOBAL OBSESITY

Global obesity is now worse than smoking. 2.1 billion people— <u>30 PERCENT</u> of the global population are overweight or obese. That's more than <u>DOUBLE</u> the number of adults and children who are undernourished.

<u>70 PERCENT OF NORTH AMERICAN ADULTS ARE OVERWEIGHT OR OBESE</u>. It's an <u>EPIDEMIC</u> and it's having a major effect of on the North American economy.

According to a report by The McKinsey Global Institute, the global cost of obesity is now <u>TWO TRILLION</u> dollars annually. This is almost as much as the global cost of smoking— (2.1 trillion dollars.)

Obesity now causes <u>HALF A MILLION CANCERS</u> every year. Two-thirds of these cancers – colon, rectum, ovary, womb, post-menopausal breast cancer occur in North America.

The latest <u>obesity study</u> done on 5 <u>MILLION</u> adults in the UK and published in the Journal The Lancet on August 26th, 2014 found that there is a direct link between obesity and cancer. Being overweight or obese resulted in <u>INCREASED</u> risk of cancers as follows:

Cancer of uterus – 62 % increase; cancer of gallbladder- 31% increase; cancer of kidney 25 %; cancer of liver- 19 %; cancer of cervix- 10%; cancer of thyroid 9 %; leukemia- 9% increase; cancer of colon- 10% increase; ovarian cancer 9 % and breast cancer a 5 % increased risk.

Estimates say:

<u>50 PERCENT OF THE WORLD'S POPULATION WILL BE OVERWEIGHT OR OBESE BY 2030.</u>

<u>86 PERCENT OF AMERICANS WILL BE OVERWEIGHT OR OBESE BY 2030.</u>

8 out of 10 <u>PEOPLE</u> (45% women and 30% of men) <u>ARE ATTEMPTING TO LOSE WEIGHT.</u>

Obese children as young as 8 often display signs of heart disease. MRI scans and studies show that the hearts of obese kids had 27 percent more muscle mass in the left ventricle of their heart and 12 percent thicker heart muscles- both of which are signs of heart disease. These kids are at high risk because the thickening of their heart wall is associated with a reduced ability to pump blood.

According to a study published in 2013, ONE IN FIVE AMERICAN DEATHS IS NOW ASSOCIATED WITH OBESITY. OBESITY IS A MARKER FOR ALMOST ALL CHRONIC AND DEADLY DISEASES.

OBESITY IS MORE DANGEROUS THAN LACK OF FITNESS! A Swedish study of 1,317,713 men for 29 years published on December 21, 2015 in the International Journal of sbut fit" was debunked. The study concluded that the protective effects of high aerobic fitness are greatly reduced in obese people. Men in top 20% percent of aerobic fitness had a 48 % lower risk of all cause mortality vs. those in bottom 20 %. You can't exercise your way out of a bad diet. There is a strong relationship linking obesity with increased chances of premature death- which is not mitigated much if you are very fit.

Research shows that fat tissue secretes an inflammatory factor called CXCL5 which is linked to INSULIN RESISTANCE AND PARTICIPATES IN THE DEVELOPMENT OF DIABETES.

OBESITY PLACES FAR GREATER STRESS ON YOUR CELLS WHICH MAKES INSULIN RESISTANCE MORE LIKELY. (BUT- you can be lean and still be insulin-resistant!) People who are obese are metabolically damaged. These people have a busted carbohydrate metabolism.

The average human body contains about 30 billion fat cells;(about 30 lbs). For adults, the number may not increase. The cells expand like a balloon. There are two different types of fat cells- white and brown. In white cells, the excess energy unused by the body becomes stored in a semi-liquid state. Brown fat cells (often called "Baby Fat") is used by the body to generate heat. After weight loss, the same number of cells remain- waiting to be re-filled.-☺ Once filled and emptied, it is much more challenging to maintain a steady healthy weight (unless of course you are on a Ketogenic Diet!). It appears that about 10 % of adult storage cells are renewed...

The estimated annual MEDICAL COST OF OBESITY IN THE USA WAS $147 BILLION IN 2008- AND THE "SICK-CARE MODEL" OF MEDICINE HAS NO WAY OF REDUCING THESE COSTS.

THERE IS EXCITING NEW RESEARCH THAT SHOWS THAT GUT BACTERIA IS AN IMPORTANT CAUSE OF OBESITY. In the penultimate chapter, the entire subject of gut bacteria and digestive health is examined extensively. Scientific evidence proves that intestinal "bugs" inherited can be a cause of obesity.

Multiple studies have shown obese people have large numbers of bacteria called babies have lower risk of obesity because good bacteria called "bifidobacteria" flourish in the guts of breast-fed babies. Obese people have increased levels of Staph bacteria on their skin and this bad bacteria in turn exposes them to the toxins this (staph) bacteria produces.

RESEARCH SHOWS FAT PEOPLE'S BODY ARE COLONIZED BY STAPH BACTERIA IN LARGE NUMBERS! Large numbers of these bacteria are living on the surface of their skin. These obese people are chronically exposed to the SUPERANTIGENS that the Staph bacteria are producing.

Conventionally trained doctors are CLUELESS ABOUT BACTERIA AND DIGESTIVE HEALTH. Please read my chapter "The diseases your doctor cannot diagnose." You cannot disregard or underscore the importance of a healthy diet because THE FOOD YOU EAT IS INFORMATION. THE FOOD THAT YOU EAT CAN TURN 'ON' AND TURN 'OFF' THE GENETIC EXPRESSION OF OUR GENES.

Bacteria have been linked to certain diseases. Other microbes are involved in preventing certain diseases. For example, by eliminating/eradicating 4 species of bacteria—lactobacillus, allobacculum, rikenelleceae, candidatus arthromitus, researchers were able to trigger metabolic changes in lab animals that led to obesity.

OBESITY IS HUGELY INFLUENCED BY GUT BACTERIA.

Certain foods can pack on the pounds- but-certain bacteria play a major role in facilitating that process.

THE FOODS KNOWN TO PRODUCE METABOLIC DYSFUNCTION AND INSULIN RESISTANCE- (SUCH AS PROCESSED FOODS, FRUCTOSE/ SUGAR AND ARTIFICIAL SWEETENERS ALSO DECIMATE BENEFICIAL GUT BACTERIA.

THIS APPEARS TO BE A KEY MECHANISM BY WHICH THESE FOODS PROMOTE OBESITY. CHEMICALS also contribute to your weight gain by way of you gut microbiome (gut flora).

e.g. A study published in the July 2015 issue of Environmental Perspectives found that Persistent Organic Pollutants (POP's) found in food altered the gut microbiome (in mice) thereby contributing to the DEVELOPMENT OF OBESITY, DIABETES AND METABOLIC DYSFUNCTION.

Another study found that one microbe- "Akerrmansia Muciniphilia" helps ward off OBESITY, DIABETES, AND HEART DISEASE BY LOWERING BLOOD SUGAR, IMPROVING INSULIN RESISTANCE AND PROMOTING A HEALTHIER DISTRIBUTION OF FAT.

HEALTH AND WEIGHT LOSS IS NOT AS COMPLICATED AS YOU HAVE BEEN LED TO BELIEVE. IT COMES DOWN TO UNDERSTANDING AND APPLYING SOME VERY BASIC PRINCIPLES—BECAUSE—

YOUR BODY WAS ACTUALLY DESIGNED AND PROGRAMMED TO STAY HEALTHY!

YOUR BODY WANTS TO BE HEALTHY! YOUR BODY DOES NOT WANT TO BE DISEASED OR TO RELY ON DRUGS.

ONCE YOU GIVE YOUR BODY WHAT IT CRAVES (NEEDS!)—YOUR BODY WILL GO INTO SELF-REPAIR MODE AND HEAL VERY EFFICIENTLY!

THE UNDERLYING PROBLEM THAT LINKS OBESITY TO SO MANY OTHER CHRONIC DISEASES AND ADVERSE HEALTHY PROBLEMS IS:

"METABOLIC DYSFUNCTION" AKA
" BUSTED METABOLISM"

Metabolic dysfunction is a fancy term that means that the mitochondria of your cells are messed up. "Messed-up" is a technical term that means that cells are disturbed/impaired OR "BUSTED"-☺ Throughout this book, the words, busted cells, busted mitochondria and busted metabolism are used almost interchangeably.

THE TAKE-HOME MESSAGE IS:

YOU ARE ONLY AS HEALTHY AS THE HEALTH OF THE MITOCHONDRIA OF YOUR CELLS.

The Boston Medical Center says that 45 MILLION AMERICANS DIET ANNUALLY and that of those who lost weight—78 PERCENT DEVELOPED FEELINGS OF DEPRESSION.

These dieters became UNHAPPY because they were eating the WRONG FOODS!

The Psychology of Eating

Mot people have lost their connection to body intelligence. There's a brilliant wisdom that's activated once we start to clean up our diet and eat healthier food. Most people also eat TOO FAST. This cuts you off from your body's innate intelligence. So- slowing down the pace at which you eat is a very important part of restoring this natural connection. If you're a fast eater-you're not paying attention to the food you're eating and you're missing what scientists call 'THE CEPHALIC PHASE DIGESTIVE RESPONSE' (CPDR).

The Cephalic Phase Digestive Response is a fancy term for <u>TASTE, PLEASURE, AROMA AND SATISFACTION,</u> including the <u>VISUAL STIMULUS</u> of your meal.

Researchers estimate that about 40 to 60 <u>PERCENT OF YOUR DIGESTIVE AND ASSIMILATIVE POWER OF ANY MEAL COMES FROM THIS ' HEAD-PHASE' OF DIGESTION!</u> i.e. you look at food and your mouth starts to water. You think of food and your stomach starts to churn.

<u>THAT'S DIGESTION BEGINNING IN YOUR MIND.</u>

When we are not paying attention to our meal, our <u>NATURAL APPETITE IS DEREGULATED</u> (messed up). On top of that, eating very fast puts your body in a <u>STRESS STATE.</u>

<u>STRESS STOPS WEIGHT LOSS!</u>

<u>STRESS IS THE BIGGEST CULPRIT IN OUR LIVES! STRESS IS A TRIGGER FOR A BOATLOAD OF HEALTH PROBLEMS.</u>

<u>STRESS MAKES US FAT, SICK, DEPRESSED, FEARFUL, SAD AND UNHAPPY...GRUMPY TOO.</u>-☺

<u>ELIMINATE ALL THE BAD STRESS AND BAD STRESSORS FROM YOUR LIFE. AS THE OLD ADAGE SAYS—YOU SHOULD BE COOL, CALM AND COLLECTED.</u>

<u>EVEN TOO MUCH GOOD STRESS IS NOT HEALTHY EITHER!</u>-☺ So, while you may enjoy working hard doing whatever floats your boat...you must be careful not to overdo... even fun things... can be <u>TOO MUCH STRESS!</u> Stress and emotional health is discussed further in the final chapter, "Listen with your Ketogenic Heart".

<u>WHEN YOU PUT YOUR BODY IN A STRESSED) STATE, YOU HAVE SYMPATHETIC NERVOUS SYSTEM DOMINANCE, INCLUDING INCREASED INSULIN, INCREASED CORTISOL AND INCREASED STRESS HORMONES!</u>

<u>THE LAST THING IN THE WORLD THAT YOU WANT TO DO IS TO TURN ON YOUR INSULIN PUMP!</u>

<u>ALL TO SAY—WHEN WE EAT, WE MUST SLOW DOWN, BE CALM AND APPLY THE PRINCIPLE OF CPDR. WHEN YOU ARE STRESSED OUT- YOU WILL DEREGULATE YOUR APPETITE...</u>

<u>WHEN YOUR BRAIN IS NOT FOCUSED AND WHEN YOUR BRAIN DOES NOT HAVE ENOUGH TIME TO SENSE THE TASTE, AROMA AND</u>

PLEASURE FROM YOUR FOOD; YOUR BRAIN THEN KEEPS SIGNALLING THAT HUNGER HAS NOT BEEN SATISFIED.

Everyone has experienced this at some point. You <u>QUICKLY GORGE</u> yourself on a <u>HUGE MEAL</u>. But then when you are finished, your belly becomes DISTENDED AND YOU STILL FEEL THE URGE TO EAT MORE! OMG!-☺ Your stomach is telling your brain that your throat has been cut-☺

DEAR READERS—THIS PROBLEM IS CAUSED BY EATING TOO QUICKLY…WHICH CAUSES STRESS, STRESS AND MORE STRESS!

<u>The importance of chewing your food</u>

The chewing process is known as "<u>MASTICATION</u>". Chewing is the second step in the digestive process. Digestion actually begins when your "mouth waters" and your body produces saliva and digestive enzymes which are produced in your mouth. Chewing is done to break up food from larger particles into more easily digested smaller particles. Humans are carnivores. This seems to explain why we have large molars for ripping up and chewing meat. Our small teeth are better suited to eat rabbit food (plants)-☺

Chewing up food into smaller pieces makes it easier for our intestines to absorb nutrients from the food particles as they pass through the digestive tract. (Is there any more alarming sensation than to swallow a piece of food improperly chewed which becomes lodged in our esophagus…YUK!)

<u>PARTICLE SIZE IS EXTREMELY IMPORTANT</u>. Size matters… chewing size particles too…-☺

PARTICLE SIZE AFFECTS THE BIO ACCESSIBILITY OF THE ENERGY OF THE FOOD THAT IS BEING CONSUMED. THE MORE YOU CHEW—THE LESS IS LOST AND THE MORE NUTRIENTS ARE RETAINED IN THE BODY.

FOR MORE ENERGY CHEW YOUR FOOD MORE!

The longer your food remains in your mouth, the more time that the digestive enzymes in your mouth have to start breaking down (digesting) your food. Saliva also helps to lubricate your food so that it is easier on our esaphagus. (One enzyme called "lingual lipase" is really important for Ketomaniacs… because it helps break down FATS!)

<u>YOUR GOAL SHOULD BE TO CHEW YOUR FOOD UNTIL IT IS A GOOEY LIQUID MASS.</u>

<u>CHEWING LONGER HELPS YOU EAT MORE SLOWLY TOO!</u>

Weight lost tip—note bene!

COUNT YOUR BITES! This is a SUPER weight loss tip. Count your bites can help you lose weight. A "bite" is defined as "each time that your hand goes to your mouth".

In a recent 4 week study, reducing BITES BY 20 TO 30 PERCENT CAUSED AN AVERAGE WEIGHT LOSS OF 3.5 lbs among study participants.

THE REDUCTION OF BITES BY 20 PERCENT IS THE MOST EFFICACIOUS WAY TO LOSE WEIGHT! PERIOD!

You should follow a healthy ketogenic Diet out of INSPIRATION—NOT OUT OF FEAR!

Eat in a relaxed non-distracted environment-not on the run- not while you're watching the idiot box (aka T.V.)-☺ Watching T.V. or playing on your computer is not conducive to proper chewing and proper digestion.

TASTE your food...better yet SAVOUR YOUR FOOD. Turn eating into active meditation. SLOW DOWN; BECOME AWARE OF YOUR FOOD. YOU SHOULD FOCUS ON HOW YOUR BODY AND YOUR BRAIN RESPONDS TO THE FOOD YOU CONSUME.

A CALORIES IN—CALORIES OUT MENTALITY CREATES FEAR AND ANXIETY.

Constantly being worried about your intake of calories creates A CONSTANT STATE OF STRESS AND WORRY ABOUT OVEREATING AND GAINING A FEW POUNDS. When you're like most people and are following a program to lose weight by UNDER-EATING FOR YEARS...

Guess what happens?

YO-YO DIETING, DIETING AND CONSTANTLY UNDER-EATING FOR YEARS TRYING TO SHED THOSE FEW EXTRA POUNDS CREATES GREAT STRESS AND UPSET TO YOUR BODY AND TO YOUR BRAIN.

Have you ever notice how grumpy dieters are? Our ancestors never had to go on diets to lose belly fat. Constant dieting and counting calories causes low-level CHRONICALLY ELEVATED INSULIN LEVELS. When we are constantly in "fight-or-flight" mode, we cannot maintain low, stable blood sugar levels. Chronically elevated insulin and elevated cortisol levels has serious long-term impacts on your body; your sympathetic nervous system—ADVERSE EFFECTS ON YOUR BRAIN!

Eat slower to lose weight; you will eat less; it takes your brain about 15 to 20 minutes to signal your stomach that you are full. Research shows eating your food more slowly and chewing your food more completely leads to decreased intake, better absorption of nutrients, better appetite regulation and improved SATIETY.

SKIPPING MEALS SHOULD IMPROVE YOUR ABILITY TO LOSE WEIGHT—

BUT—

FEAR AND STRESS OVERRIDES THE PROCESS BY UP-REGULATING YOUR SYMPATHETIC NERVOUS SYSTEM. PLUS- THERE IS THE FACTOR OF CIRCADIAN NUTRITION.

What is "Bio-circadian nutrition"?

I confess that this is my personal terminology. We know that our bodies are built to work according to circadian rhythms (see Dr. Sleep, infra). For example, our bodies are designed to wake up when the sun rises and when darkness descends, we are programmed to get sleepy and to go to bed. There is a lot of truth to the old adage- "early to bed, early to rise makes a man, healthy, wealthy and wise".

The TIMING OF OUR MEALS is extremely important. Some people find it easier to lose weight in the 1st half of the day- rather than in the latter half of the day. We know that our body temperature is highest right around solar noon—and THAT'S when your body is metabolically operating at peak efficiency. It is likely burning many of its calories at that time.

Are you on a Sumo diet?

Sumo wrestlers get big by eating a LOT of food in the middle of the night. So- if you're eating the bulk of your calories late at night— you're on the SUMO diet. You will likely pack on the pounds with this eating approach. I absolutely love doing Sumo Deadlifts- but I loathe an unhealthy Sumo eating approach-☺

You have probably heard the advice to make your mid-day meal the biggest of the day and to have a lighter meal at dinner (supper). Allegedly this takes some stress off your body and allows time to wind down for bedtime- rather than digesting a heavy meal.

BUT THIS IS WRONG!

Some experts (including this author) believe that eating your main meal at night is more in tune with your innate biological clock- (biological circadian rhythms). Routinely eating at the wrong time may not only damage your biological clock and interfere with your sleep—it will <u>DEVASTATE</u> vital body functions and contribute to disease.

Your body is programmed for nocturnal feeding. All of your activities, including your eating are controlled by your autonomous nervous system that operates around the circadian clock. During the day, your sympathetic nervous system (SNS) puts your body in energy spending mode; whereas during the night your parasympathetic nervous system (PSNS) puts your body in an energy replenishing, relaxed and sleepy mode. At night, your different parts of your brain do other tasks. The glymphatic waste system in our brain literally takes out the trash- for example. During daytime, and wakefulness, other parts of our brain are active and perform different functions.

These two parts of your autonomic nervous system complement each other; like yin and yang. Your (SNS) which is stimulated when you eat supper at night, makes you relaxed and sleepy, with a much better capacity to digest food and nutrients before the early a.m. This is how your autonomic nervous system functions under normal circumstances.

<u>BUT</u>—that system is highly vulnerable to disruption, if you eat at the wrong time-such as having a large meal during the day—you will <u>MESS</u> with your autonomic nervous system- and you will inhibit your (SNS); and instead- turn on and fire up your (PSNS), which will make you sleepy and fatigued, rather than alert and active during the waking hours of the day.

<u>AND INSTEAD OF SPENDING ENERGY AND BURNING FAT, YOU WILL STORE ENERGY AND GAIN FAT!</u>

<u>YOU SHOULD NOT ADOPT A SUMO DIET. LATE-NIGHT EATING TENDS TO GENERATE EXCESS FREE RADICALS, WHICH PROMOTES DNA DAMAGE THAT CONTRIBUTES TO CHRONIC DEGENERATIVE DISEASES AND PROMOTES ACCELERATED AGING.</u>

<u>IN SHORT—YOU SHOULD STOP EATING AT LEAST 3 HOURS BEFORE BEDTIME.H</u>

The Academy of Nutrition and Dietetics, (AND), formerly the American Dietetic Association) receives <u>MILLIONS</u> of dollars from multinational Junk Food Corporations each year for "corporate-sponsored" education"(aka brainwashing) to teach registered dieticians about the value of everything from sugary beverages to chewing gum.

As noted by Dr. Greger (AND) "their official position is that there is no "good" or "bad" foods,—<u>THIS FLIES IN THE FACE OF NUTRITIONAL SCIENCE!</u>

What is considered these days as a "normal" diet is:

AN ABERRATION/PERVERSION BASED ON THE CORRUPTION OF SCIENCE THAT BENEFITS BIG AGRA, BIG FOOD, BIG PHARMA AND BIG MEDICAL.

IF WE COULD GO BACK IN TIME —TO THE DAYS BEFORE THE MODERN DIET WAS DESTROYED BY CORPORATE AND AGRICULTURAL INTERESTS;—WE WOULD FIND THAT "KETOSIS" WAS THE NORMAL METABOLIC STATE.

TODAY'S HUMAN METABOLIC STATE IS ABERRANT!

IT'S TIME TO CHANGE THAT!

5 Top Factors that affect your weight and contribute to obesity and poor health:

- **Processed Food**

- **Chemicals in food, environment and everyday household products**

- **Antibiotics**

- **Inactivity**

- **Lack of sleep**

Obesity, diabetes, high cholesterol, hypertension, and heart attacks are all diseases associated with a PROCESSED FOOD DIET- (aka junk food with NO NUTRITION).

Many chemicals promote obesity. A number of chemicals promote obesity by DISRUPTING YOUR HORMONES. This includes but is not limited to: BISPHENOL- A (BPA), PCB's, PHTHALATES, TRICLOSAN, AGRICULTURAL PESTICIDES AND FIRE (FLAME) RETARDANTS.

GLYPHOSATE (ROUND-UP AND OTHER PESTICIDES MAKE YOU FAT BY OBLITERATING GUT BACTERIA. THESE SUBSTANCES ALSO EAT A HOLE IN YOUR GUT LINING AND HELP CAUSE AUTOIMMUNE DISEASES.

ENDOCRINE- DISRUPTING CHEMICALS MAKE YOU FAT.

POLYCHLORINATED BIPHENOLS, ORGANOPHOSPHATES, PHTHALATES AND BIPHENOL- A. MAKE YOU FAT.

LACK OF SLEEP MAKES YOU FAT. Research shows people who sleep less than 7 hours a night tend to have a higher BMI. The biological mechanisms linking sleep deprivation and weight gain are numerous. Lack of sleep alters your metabolism.

When you are sleep deprived- LEPTIN—THE HORMONE THAT SIGNALS SATIETY FALLS; WHILE—GHRELIN- THE HORMONE THAT SIGNALS HUNGER RISES.

This combination leads to an increase in appetite. Also, sleep deprivation results in food cravings, especially sweet and starchy foods. Due to an increase in the stress hormone CORTISOL-sleeping 6 hours per night also radically decreases the sensitivity of your insulin receptors, WHICH RAISES YOUR INSULIN LEVELS.

This too is a sure fire way to gain weight (get fat) because ELEVATED INSULIN LEVELS WILL SERIOUSLY IMPAIR YOUR BODY'S ABILITY TO BURN AND DIGEST FAT. This also increases your risk of diabetes.

IN SUM—sleep deprivation puts your body in a PRE-DIABETIC STATE.

Writing in The British Journal of Sports Medicine, researchers stated:

"POOR DIET NOW GENERATES MORE DISEASE THAN PHYSICAL INACTIVITY, ALCOHOL AND SMOKING COMBINED. "

The false perception that exercise matters more than healthy eating is due to how the Food Industry markets food— (-as does the tobacco industry). Up to 40 PERCENT of those with normal body mass index will harbour METABOLIC ABNORMALITIES- typically associated with obesity, which include hypertension, dyslipidemia, non-alcoholic fatty liver disease (NAFLD) and cardiovascular disease (CVD).

RESEARCH has revealed that for every EXCESS 150 CALORIES OF SUGAR- there was an 11 FOLD INCREASE IN TYPE 2 DIABETES- in comparison to 150 calories obtained from healthy food sources.

MAINSTREAM MEDIA STILL PROMOTES JUNK FOOD AND DRUGS. That's how lamestream media makes money. Advertising is legalized lying said Oscar Wilde.

A MENTIONED SUPRA- OBESITY IS A DYSFUNCTIONAL METABOLISM; (aka Busted Metabolism). Obesity is a metabolic disease. Obesity is an inflammatory disease; like brain disease. MRI brain scans show that if you are fat or obese, your brain looks like Swiss cheese; BUT if you are lean, your brain is smooth as a baby's bottom-☺

Sugar (carbohydrates) eats holes in your BRAIN. Carbohydrates also destroy your BRAIN AND YOUR PANCREAS; CAUSE INSULIN RESISTANCE AND A BUNCH OF CHRONIC DISEASES.

YOU ARE PROBABLY OVERWEIGHT NOT BECAUSE YOU OVEREAT OR BECAUSE YOU EXERCISE TOO LITTLE...

YOU ARE OVERWEIGHT BECAUSE YOU ARE EATING THE WRONG FOODS!

FOOD EITHER SUPPORTS HEALTH OR IT DOESN'T.

A (2015) study proved that eating JUST ONE JUNK FOOD TREAT PER DAY IS ENOUGH TO TRIGGER METABOLIC SYNDROME IN HEALTHY PEOPLE! That "treat" consisted in an assortment of candy bars and pastries.

CALORIES ARE NOT THE ENEMY. CARBOHYDRATES ARE THE ENEMY. Research shows that women who ate at least one serving of full-FAT dairy a day gained 30 PERCENT LESS WEIGHT OVER A 9 YEAR PERIOD—(vs. women who ate only low-fat dairy or no dairy products.

YOU MUST EAT FAT TO GET LEAN...AND SMART TOO!!

As mentioned supra, one of the key mechanisms by which sugar promotes cancer and other chronic diseases is through mitochondrial dysfunction (aka busted cells). Since sugar is not our ideal fuel- it burns DIRTY and it creates far more reactive oxygen species (ROS) than fat does. This generates far more free radicals that in turn cause mitochondrial and nuclear DNA damage together with cell membrane and protein impairment (other kinds of busted cell damage).

Research has shown that chronic overeating in general has a very similar effect. Most people who tend to overeat also tend to overeat a lot of sugar-laden foods- a DOUBLE CANCER WHAMMY!!

Chronic overeating places AWFUL stress on the cellular part called the endoplasmic reticulum (ER), which is the membrane network found inside of the mitochondria of your cells. When the ER receives more nutrients (fuel) than it can process- it signals the cell to dampen the sensitivity of the insulin receptors on the surface of the cell.

SO- WHEN YOU CONTINUOUSLY EAT TOO MUCH (ESPECIALLY CARBS)— YOU DESTROY THE BETA CELLS IN YOUR PANCREAS WITH TOXIC CARBS.

BUSTED CELLS (AKA INSULIN RESISTANCE) AND BUSTED METABOLISM ARE THE RESULT.

INSULIN RESISTANCE IS AT THE CORE OF MOST CHRONIC DISEASES SUCH AS DIABETES AND CANCER. That is why it is the platinum key to SUPERHEALTH.

Obesity caused by a combination of eating too much refined fructose/sugar and (rarely –if ever fasting)- can also promote cancer via other mechanisms, including chronic inflammation and excess

FIRE YOUR DOCTOR—HIRE YOURSELF!

production of certain hormones such as estrogen—which is linked to breast cancer.

90 PERCENT OF PEOPLE HAVE INSULIN RESISTANCE- AND/OR LEPTIN RESISTANCE. YOUR BEST OPTION IS TO EAT REAL FOODS.

BY REDUCING PEOPLE'S WEIGHT EVEN SLIGHTLY, AN ESTIMATED 274,000 TO 309,000 CASES OF TYPE 2 DIABETES COULD BE PREVENTED IN THE NEXT 20 YEARS!

People who follow a Ketogenic Diet shed **TONS OF BELLY FAT**. One of the biggest "side effects" of being leaner is that you will feel better and **YOU WILL BE HAPPIER!**

You can do it. There's no more reason to struggle with dieting and counting calories. **CALORIES IN AND CALORIES OUT IS MEDICAL/ NUTRITIONAL NONSENSE.**

A properly- constructed Ketogenic Diet will solve your overweight or obesity issues. When you adopt a Ketogenic diet, the pounds will melt off effortlessly. It's your ticket to **SUPERHEALTH- AND FEELING GREAT!**

MOTHER NATURE CREATED HER FARMACY- A LONG TIME AGO!

Mother Nature's Superfoods will provide you and your bodies with the **HEALING DIET AND THE HEALING SUPERFOODS THAT YOU NEED TO EAT.**

Hurrah for Mother Nature! Boo to Big Pharma!

THE KETOGENIC DIET was eaten by our ancestors for 99 percent of the time that humans have roamed Planet earth.

IT'S NOT A PALEO DIET. IT'S NOT A VEGETARIAN DIET. THE KETOGENIC DIET IS A HIGH-FAT LOW-CARB, MODERATE PROTEIN DIET.

A PALEO DIET-

Research indicates that a "Paleo Diet" as generally understood by most proponents is unhealthy for 2 reasons. Firstly, Paleo recommends **TOO MUCH PROTEIN.** Too much protein damages our mTOR (mammalian pathway). The Paleo Diet also advocates eating **TOO MANY CARBS.** Most carbs are toxic un- nutrients. Most Paleo diets are **TOO LOW IN FATS.** Paleo Diets will not permit you to enter Ketosis —see below. Ultimately following a Paleo Diet will make you fat, sick and unhealthy. Research shows that a high carb diet leads to Alzheimer's Disease, Obesity, Diabetes, etc.

A MEDITERRANEAN DIET-

This diet is QUITE healthy as most people think. Obviously, olives and olive oil are healthy and good for you. <u>BUT</u>- remember— the Greeks are no. 5 on the <u>OBESITY</u> top 10 list. This diet is laden with <u>A LOT OF STARCHY CARBS</u>. Too much pasta/breads will often make you fat and sometimes sick. This diet lacks also often lacks enough good <u>FATS</u>. The Mediterranean Diet is <u>BETTER</u> than the Standard American Diet (SAD)-but <u>NOT</u> necessarily as healthy as most people think.

<u>VEGETARIAN DIETS</u>-

I cannot recommend vegetarian OR vegan diets either. Our ancestors did not thrive on these diets. With all due deference to vegetarians, no human society has every thrived as a meatless society.

<u>AT THE CELLULAR LEVEL-WE ARE MADE OF FAT. WE ARE DESIGNED TO BURN FAT. MOST VEGETARIANS SOONER OR LATER COME TO REALIZE THAT ELIMINATING MEAT/FISH FROM A DIET HAS HEALTH CONSEQUENCES.</u>

Why? The biggest challenge for most vegetarians is to get enough B vitamins, esp. B-12. Also, <u>our brain is 70 percent FAT. ANIMAL FATS ARE THE BEST SOURCE OF OMEGA-3 FATTY ACIDS.</u> Omega 3 fats <u>ARE</u> converted from flaxseed, hemp and plant sources to DHA and EPA. <u>BUT</u>-plant-sourced fatty acids NOT easily or well –converted to DHA and EPA (two essential fatty acids- elaborated hereinafter).

One recent Clinical study clearly found that a <u>VEGETARIAN DIET</u> — (both varieties) <u>ARE DANGEROUS AND NOT HEALTHY</u>.

I realize that many vegetarians may <u>NEVER CHANGE FROM THEIR DIETS</u>. I've heard "I love my juicing line" hundreds of times. There really is no one diet for <u>EVERYONE</u>... so if you are happy with a veg-etarian diet- best of luck. You will be given nutritional, physiological and metabolic information in this book. This information might per-suade you to consider the Ketogenic Diet. For all of the vegetarian readers, here are a few questions to think about:

> <u>Why do we have large teeth in our mouth anyway?</u>

> <u>Are you sure that plant sources of Omega 3 are suf-ficient? Are you sure that you are getting enough daily animal-based (wild caught salmon, or grass=fed beef) Omega 3 FATS in your diet?</u>

> <u>What dietary approach has permitted the human brain to grow so large and so fast since humans have roamed Planet Earth?</u>

Did you know that the human brain's secret love is FAT? Our brain is 75 % FAT and 50 % cholesterol.

Do you really believe that your brain runs best on veggies?

Are you aware of the benefits of a Ketogenic Diet?

Are you aware that your ENERGY LEVELS on a Ketogenic Diet are GREATER? Are you willing to compare?

Did you know that animal fats are necessary to build the membranes of all of our cells?

Do you honestly believe that a plant-based diet is best for the sustainability of our Planet?

THE MIND DIET

A recent study examined the effects of eating a "mind diet". This diet, (SOMEWHAT similar to a Ketogenic Diet) revolves around eating 10 BRAIN-HEALTHY FOOD GROUPS.

In the mind diet study, these 10 foods included: Nuts, berries (especially blueberries and strawberries), green leafy veggies, olive oil, poultry. fish, wine, beans and whole grains.

Here is what this study about the "Mind Diet" found:

- THE MIND DIET MAKES YOUR BRAIN 7.5 YEARS YOUNGER and

- THE MIND DIET REDUCED THE RISK OF ALZHEIMER'S DISEASE BY A WHOPPING 53 PERCENT!

Note bene:

THE MIND DIET IS HEALTHIER THAN THE "SAD" DIET…

BUT -THE KETOGENIC DIET IS THE HEALTHIEST DIET IN THE WORLD.

THE CLINICAL, SCIENTIFIC STUDIES AND EVIDENCE PROVIDED IN THIS BOOK PROVIDES SCIENTIFIC PROOF OF THE HEALING PROWESS OF THE KETOGENIC DIET.

HUMAN BEINGS DO NOT HAVE THE DIGESTIVE SYSTEM/METABOLIC MACHINERY TO DIGEST AND METABOLIZE 'WHOLE GRAINS' … That's why WHOLE GRAINS DO NOT FORM PART OF A KETOGENIC DIET.

OTHER MAJOR PROBLEMS WITH THE MIND DIET IS THAT THE STUDY DID NOT SPECIFY THAT THE VEGGIES SHOULD BE ORGANIC

AND THAT THE FISH SHOULD BE THE HEALTHY VARIETY- (NOT THE MERCURY POISONED KIND) THE STUDY DID NOT SPECIFY WHAT TYPE OF POULTRY (e.g. poisoned drug-laced chicken) or PASTURED HEALTHY CHICKENS etc.

THE MIND DIET STUDY SIMPLY LISTS 10 BRAIN FOODS USED IN THIS STUDY.

PERIOD. CLEARLY- THE SCIENCE SAYS THAT GRAINS AND BEANS ARE NOT BRAIN FOODS. GRAINS AND BEANS ARE SUGAR WHICH EATS HOLES IN YOUR BRAIN!

A WELL-CONSTRUCTED KETOGENIC DIET AND THE RECIPES PROVIDED IN THIS BOOK WILL GROW YOUR BRAIN; MAKE YOU LEAN, STRONG AND SMART.

SUPERHEALTH STARTS AND ENDS WITH BRAIN HEALTH! YOU ARE EITHER BUILDING BRAIN CELLS OR YOU ARE KILLING THEM-☺

WITHOUT BRAIN HEALTH—THERE IS NO HEALTH.

RICH –FAT- DELICIOUS RECEIPES - KETOGENIC RECEIPES- WILL SUPERCHARGE YOUR BRAIN AND SATISFY YOUR PALATE.

MY FAVOURITE RECIPES ARE PROVIDED- DOZENS MORE ARE AVAILABLE ON LINE FROM DR. INTERNET.

NO OTHER DIET CAN MAKE KETONES. Other diets do not properly nourish your BRAIN. Your brain simply does not run so well on veggies…

WHEN YOU BECOME KETO-ADAPTED—YOU WILL ASSUREDLY DECIDE TO DITCH YOUR 'OTHER' DIET— FOREVER— IN FAVOUR OF A HEALING KETOGENIC DIET!

The Take-home message:

NO DOCTOR CAN MAKE HUNGER BEARABLE.

NO DOCTOR CAN HELP YOU LOSE WEIGHT- (Your doctor lacks the knowledge and expertise required- -your doctor doesn't know his arse from his elbow-☺)

YOU MUST BE YOUR OWN DOCTOR.

TO BECOME LEAN AND HEALTHY YOU MUST STOP EATING SUGAR IN THE FORM OF FRUCTOSE, GLUCOSE AND STARCHY CARBOHYDRATES.

A study in the Journal "Cell Metabolism" concludes:

" Too much fat-storing insulin is the necessary cause of common diet-induced obesity".

INSULIN IS THE CAUSE OF COMMON OBESITY. IT'S THAT SIMPLE.

IN HUMANS- THE MAIN CAUSE OF ELEVATED INSULIN IS EATING TOO MANY CARBS.

IT'S THAT SIMPLE.

C. CARBOHYDRATE ADDICTION

"Carbohydrate is the bad guy, you have to see that".

Dr. Robert C. Atkins

A carbohydrate craving can be described as a compelling hunger, craving or desire for "CARBOHYDRATE— RICH FOODS". This is an escalating, recurring need or drive for starches, snack foods, junk foods or sweets.

The term "carbohydrate craving" is used in a theory about the relationship between CAROBOHYDRATE, INSULIN AND APPETITE.

EATING CARBS RAISES INSULIN WHICH RAISES BLOOD SUGAR.

This causes a desire (or craving) for more food, and for most people, carbs in particular. Sugary starchy CARBS INCREASES THE SUGAR ADDICTION.

These junk foods jack up BLOOD SUGAR AND HIGH INSULIN LEVELS. This leads to EVEN MORE CRAVINGS! They also produce higher levels of the brain chemical neurotransmitter called SERATONIN (aka feel good hormone).

SIDEBAR: SERATONIN—

When our serotonin levels drop; so do our feelings of SELF-ESTEEM. Dieters become depressed; dieting is the worst way to raise self-esteem; it makes us self-critical.

"SERATONIN" IS MOTHER NATURE'S "PROZAC"! 95 Percent of our serotonin is made in our gut. Some people who have low serotonin levels become obsessive-compulsive. They need to wash their hands 50 TIMES PER DAY!

Seratonin is made from the amino acid L-tryptophan. When serotonin levels drop with 7 hours of tryptophan depletion, depression and compulsive bulimia or anorexia can occur. When using amino acids to end emotional eating, we should look at 4 important BRAIN CHEMICALS OR "NEUROTRANSMITTERS".

These include:

- DOPAMINE/NORINEPHRINE, which is a natural ener-gizing chemical which helps with mental focus;

- GABA (gamma aminobutryric acid), our natural sedative;

- ENDORPHINS, our natural pain-killers;

- SERATONIN, our natural mood stabilizer and sleep promoter;

WHEN WE HAVE ENOUGH OF ALL FOUR OF THESE—OUR EMOTIONS ARE STABLE. When they are depleted or out of balance, we get "pseudo-emotions." These false moods can be very disturbing and stressful. They can drive us to relentless overeating and can exacerbate our "carb addiction".

THESE 4 KEY NEUROTRANSMITTERS ARE MADE OF AMINO ACIDS. 22 AMINO ACIDS ARE CONTAINED IN HIGH-PROTEIN FATTY FOODS- e.g. fish, eggs, chicken and beef. These complete foods contain all 22 amino acids, including the "9 ESSENTIAL AMINO ACIDS.

In sensitive people, particularly those who have low serotonin level to begin with, a "carbohydrate binge" is the equivalent of SELF-MEDICATION.

You may remember Dr. Robert Lustig describe how sugar actually makes ethanol or alcohol in our liver. "A CARBOHYDRATE BINGE" IS ACTUALLY JUST GETTING A"SUGAR-HIGH". SUGAR IS 8 TIMES MORE ADDICTIVE THAN HEROIN!

CARBS ACT LIKE ALCOHOL TO YOUR BRAIN! Remember the old adage- "Candy is dandy but liquor is quicker"-☺

The science behind the "Alternative Hypothesis" can be called Endocrinology 101. This requires an understanding of how carbs affect insulin and blood sugar levels and in turn fat metabolism and appetite. This is basic endocrinology; which is the study of hormones. The low-fat hypothesis (Ancel Keys) is the study of the effect of fat on cholesterol and heart disease.

Grain products and concentrated sugars were absent from human nutrition until the invention of agriculture about 10,000 years ago. In late 1984 Americans were told to curb their intake of fat; the National Institute of Health (NIH) recommended that Americans EAT LESS FAT

<u>TO ABATE AN EPIDEMIC OF KILLER DISEASES</u>. Americans were told "<u>DITCH THE BACON AND EGGS!</u>

<u>THE NIH SPENT</u> (wasted) <u>SEVERAL HUNDRED MILLION DOLLARS trying to prove Ancel Keys' false theory</u> in an attempt to demonstrate a link to prove <u>EATING FAT CAUSES HEART DISEASE</u>.

<u>METABOLIC SYNDROME</u>—

Metabolic Syndrome characterized by insulin resistance has become a <u>MAJOR HEALTH THREAT IN THE LAST 20 YEARS</u>. Metabolic syndrome and associated diseases are one of the major burdens in health care systems in most industrialized nations.

In 1923, the concept "metabolic syndrome" was invented by Kylin. The concept described a cluster of medical conditions, such as hypertension, hyperglycemia and gout. The concept did not attract much attention until Dr. Gerald Reaven, an endrocinologist introduced the Syndrome X in 1988; which is similar to metabolic syndrome.

The following are the accepted experts' opinion of the elements of MetS, namely: central obesity, hyperglycemia, insulin resistance, hypertension, elevated triglycerides, decreased HDL, fatigue, etc.

A study in the Journal of Internal Medicine in 2000 stated:

"The metabolic syndrome is synonymous to an iceberg with glucose intolerance   above the surface but a group of other key cardiovascular disease risk factors   lurking below."

The <u>BIGGER</u> part of the iceberg is <u>OBESITY</u>. There are other "conditions" associated with metabolic syndrome and Type 2 Diabetes. (abbreviated as T2D):

- NAFLD (non-alcoholic fatty liver disease
- sdLDL (small dense LDL cholesterol)
- Oxidative stress
- Inflammation
- Hyper-coagulability
- Polycistic Ovary Syndrome (POS)
- Gastroesophageal reflux disease (GERD)
- Sleep Apnea

- Asthma

- Depression

- Osteoporosis

- Alzheimer's Disease (AD)

- Cancers

EATING CARBOHYDRATES CAUSES METABOLIC SYNDROME (&/OR ABOVE CONDITIONS LEADS TO INCREASED PRODUCTION OF INSULIN AND HYPERINSULINEMIA (too much insulin).

THE CURRENT ALLOPATHIC APPROACH IS THE SHOTGUN OF MEDICATION-or "THE POLYPILL".

There are about 25 classes of DRUGS used to treat METABOLIC CONDITIONS SUCH AS:

*Blood sugar control

sulfonylureas, meglitinides, biguanides, T2D's, alpha-glucosidanen inhibitotrs, Selt 2, DPP-4 inhibitors, insulin;

* Blood pressure control

Ace inhibitors, diruretics, beta-blockers, vasodilators, calcium channel blockers,;

- Cholesterol control

Statins, niacin, bile-acid resins, fibric acid derivatives, cholesterol inhibitors;

Aspirin

* Inflammation control

statins

- Weight control

SNRI, pancreatic lipase inhibitors, appetite suppressants;

What advice does your hard-core calorie-counting doctor give?

Your doctor tells you "eat less; count your calories; make sure you eat low-fat foods, be sure to drink sodas sweetened with Aspartame, Splenda and other artificial sweeteners; AND EXERCISE MORE! "(For a good belly laugh- ask him how often he goes to the gym.) Have a look at his belly under his white coat…it may be bigger than yours! -☺

YOUR DOCTOR DOES NOT KNOW HIS ARSE FROM HIS ELBOW WHEN IT COMES TO OBESITY, HEALTHY FOODS …OR HEALTH FOR THAT MATTER-☺

Chowder-headed allopathic doctors ARE IGNORANT OF THESE BASIC NUTRITION FACTS:

1. CARBS EQUALS INSULIN EQUALS DISEASE. NO-BODY CAN DISPUTE THIS FACT.

2. EATING CARBS-NOT FAT— IS CAUSING IN-SULIN RESISTANCE AND DIABETES.

3. CARBS AND PROTEIN IS METABOLIZED IN OUR BODY TO SUG-AR. FAT IS METABOLIZED TO FAT BODIES CALLED KETONES.

4. FAT IS THE PREFERRED FUEL OF HUMAN METABOLISM.

5. AN IMBALANCE OF HORMONES IS AT THE ROOT OF THE ABOVE-MENTIONED CONDITIONS/PROBLEMS.

6. THERE ARE DOZENS OF RESEARCH STUDIES THAT PROVE THAT EATING LOW-CARB DIETS MAKE YOU LEAN.

7. SUGAR IS TOXIC OUT OF THE "NORMAL RANGE" IN THE BLOOD.

Our body works amazingly hard to (goes to extraordinary lengths) to keep SUGAR NORMALIZED AND STABLE. This is referred to as GLUCOSE HOMEOSTASIS.

EVERY PERSON HAS HIS OWN METABOLIC HOMEOSTATIC STATE.

This is a state where blood sugar (glucose) levels have reached a steady state (lower level in the blood) and ketones (fat bodies) have reached a correspondingly steady state in the blood also. You want (need) to know when your body has achieved a new metabolic state. Basically, we use ketones and glucose as the simplest measures of this new state.

Glucose numbers should about 55 to 65mg/dl (about 2.5 mmol or 3) and ketones should be about 3 or 4mmol.

LOW-CARB DIETS have been extensively studied since 2002. There have been over 20 randomized controlled well-documented studies detailing the efficacy of low-carb diets.

CUTTING DOWN ON CARBS WAS ALSO FOUND TO BE THE SINGLE MOST EFFECTIVE INTERVENTION FOR REDUCING ALL OF THE FEATURES OF THE METABOLIC SYNDROME.

RESTRICTION OF CARB INTAKE AS A MECHANISM FOR REVERSAL OF METABOLIC SYNDROME AND REVERSAL OF INSULIN RESISTANCE AND REVERSAL OF DIABETES SHOULD BE YOUR NUMBER ONE FIRST APPROACH!

PERIOD.

CARBOHYDRATE METABOLISM FOR ALL PRACTICAL PURPOSES IS THE METABOLISM OF GLUCOSE (SUGAR).

RESEARCH PROVES HANDS-DOWN THAT LOW-CARB DIETS CAUSE THE MOST WEIGHT LOSS-AND—IMPROVE ALL MAJOR RISK FACTORS FOR DISEASE- INCLUDING BLOOD SUGAR LEVELS, TRIGLYCERIDES, HDL AND MANY OTHER BIO-MARKERS.

RESEARCH STUDIES SHOW THAT DIABETES MANAGEMENT BENEFITS OCCUR EVEN WITHOUT WEIGHT LOSS!

The executive who can't resist the bagels eventually falls prey to his sugar addiction. He opens up the doors of his internal sugar factory when he has his breakfast sandwich. Bread is "carbs"—albeit more slow-digesting carbs than candy; but—it's just another form of sugar. ½ of a bagel has 10 grams of carbs. Adults should have 5 grams of sugar (1tsp) in their entire bloodstream. An adult has 5 litres of blood.

FOOD IS INTIMATELY CONNECTED TO OUR EMOTIONS. FOOD IS THE CAUSE OF THE VAST MAJORITY OF OUR HEALTH PROBLEMS…AND FOOD IS ALSO THE SOLUTION.

Biology is not the only reason that we eat. For many people, the mere thought of a favourite food evokes strong associations that blend image, senses, emotion and memory into a mixture that is nearly impossible to separate into different parts. Some of us eat when we are tense, but tension hurts our weight loss efforts in several ways. Tension not only triggers carb cravings; it also makes it difficult for us to lose additional weight.

CORTISOL (our "fight or flight –STRESS HORMONE) ALSO STIMULATES INSULIN that leads to blood sugar dips and fat storage.

SUGAR INCREASES STRESS AND STRESS INCREASES CARB CRAVINGS!

It's a vicious cycle that "feeds on itself" over and over. The more we try to ignore a feeling –the stronger it grows.

Let's take an example. You have an important business meeting scheduled. You leave home; grab a take-out coffee and a breakfast sandwich at the local coffee shop. You scarf that down and rush off to your big meeting. On the road a careless driver cuts you off and you jam on your brakes to narrowly avoid a bad car accident. You arrive at five minutes after 10 at your meeting. You are still breathing heavily and you stressed out to your mind.

You quickly sit down at the boardroom table. A beautiful young secretary brings in a huge plate of bagels, croissants, and other assorted pastries. She also brings a dozen large take-our coffees (commercial brands) from the local coffee shop. You grab some more pesticide-laced coffee with the usual poisonous sugary additives.

Then, your brain says, "I know I shouldn't eat the sugary stuff". Then you look at the bagels— and your brain says "no- I don't need one; I've had breakfast and I'm not hungry". Then you hear your wife/girl-friend's voice- "Dear- you've got to cut back on the sugary, unhealthy foods and lose a few pounds". Then your reptilian brain says "go on... just have <u>half</u> a bagel; it won't hurt". Your "smart brain" says "no"— again. This process is repeated every 10 seconds for the next 30 minutes. Finally- your reptilian brain wins out. You give in and eat only <u>half</u> of a bagel- slathered with some cream cheese. During the entire 30 minutes, instead of concentrating on your important business meeting—you spent most of the time debating with yourself. Your brain was more focused on eating a half of a bagel than thinking about business. Most likely, you had brain-fog and low-energy during the entire meeting.

Why did you really eat that half-bagel? Was it because you just weak-willed and you're a glutton by nature? <u>ABSOLUTELY NOT! YOU HAVE A SERIOUS CARB ADDICTION!</u>

You've programmed your body, your brain and your nervous system to fire up production of your internal sugar factory. Just at the sight of the bagels- your digestive system starts to mobilize. Enzymes are produced in your mouth and your internal sugar factory doors starts to open. When you ingested that second cup of sugar coffee-you were pouring gas on your internal sugar fires. Then you ate that <u>half</u>- bagel.

At 10:30 A.M. your internal sugar factory is now <u>IN FULL BLOWN SUGAR PRODUCTION</u>. Your internal sugar factory had fired up when you ate your breakfast sandwich. Your sugary coffee also helped to jack up your brain.

If you would have eaten, say, eggs and sausages (healthy kind) for breakfast (no nbread); there's an excellent chance your reptilian

245

brain might have been silenced by your smart brain. You ate that half-bagel because your brain/body was not satisfied. Your brain and your body crave healthy <u>FAT</u>. Instead you fed your brain <u>SUGAR</u> (unhealthy carbs) for breakfast. Your entire breakfast fuelled your <u>CARB/SUGAR ADDICTION</u>. On top of that you arrived in full fight and flight mode. You needed something sweet to comfort your nerves. When you have trained your body to burn sugar as its primary fuel you are a sugar addict.

The more we ignore a <u>feeling</u>- the <u>stronger</u> it grows. It's so much easier to deal with an issue while the emotion is still in a "fixable stage." But our denial system is extremely effective I shielding us from honestly facing ourselves.

Denial stems from a fear of admitting "Yes- this bothers me". The consequences of this admission are even more frightening. Now, the brain says "Now, I must take responsibility for making changes to correct the situation." But- honestly admitting to ourselves "Yes- this is the emotion underneath my food craving" is a tremendous relief.

If you realize that <u>EMOTIONS</u> are often the reason you eat- not hunger- then <u>THAT</u> emotional relief will help reduce or even eliminate the urge to eat. If the food you <u>CRAVE</u> is associated more with pleasure and immediate gratification than it is with pain—it's going to be hard to stop eating it.

This question needs to be asked:

> <u>"Is the short-term pleasure worth the long-term pain</u>
> <u>and guilt of eating food that keeps you FATTER than</u>
> <u>you'd like to be?"</u>

What is really causing this "<u>carbohydrate craving/addiction</u>" anyway?

The short answer is your body is <u>STARVING FOR REAL FOOD</u>! The more carbs (sugar-glucose) that you eat—the more carbs your brain and body demands. When you ditch the carbs in favour of <u>RICH WHOLE SATISFYING FAT FOOD</u>—you will reach <u>SATIETY</u>.

Do you feel incomplete in the morning without eating some bread or cereal? Do you often think of food…and eating… you're not alone!

<u>95 PERCENT OF THE WESTERN WORLD IS ADDICTED TO CARBOHYDRATES!</u>

<u>BINGE EATING CAN WREAK HAVOC ON YOUR INSULIN AND BLOOD SUGAR LEVELS!</u>—especially-if your meal includes a lot of <u>CARBS</u>. After eating a large, carb-heavy meal, your body's glucose level shoots up quickly and that causes <u>AND INSULIN SURGE</u>. This insulin

surge makes your blood sugar drop rather quickly as well. It can lead to a relative <u>HYPOGLYCEMIA.</u> You experience that low hypoglycaemia as hunger. This probably explains why you feel you can't eat another bite after a big meal—but then you become <u>RAVENOUSLY HUNGRY</u> again by your next meal.

<u>THEN – LATER WHEN YOU LOAD YOUR BODY WITH CARBOHYDRATES, THE WHOLE CYCLE FIRES UP AGAIN.</u>

<u>NINETY-FIVE (95) PERCENT OF PEOPLE IN THE WESTERN WORLD ARE ADDICTED TO THE SHORT-TERM ENERGY-BOOSTS THAT CARBS PROVIDE.</u>

Since refined foods are heavily processed and supply our bodies with little more than excess sugar; we often end up <u>CRAVING THEM FOREVER</u>- with serious long-term consequences for our health.

<u>HERE ARE THREE NUTRIENTS (SUPPLEMENTS) PROVEN TO MINIMIZE OR EVEN ELIMINATE UNWANTED CARB CRAVINGS.</u>

1. <u>GLUTAMINE</u>. Glutamine is an amino acid that plays an important role in protein metabolism. However, it is also a neurotransmitter. It fuels our brain along with <u>FAT</u> and <u>GLUCOSE</u>. When lacking in glutamine, our brain resorts to glucose for its fuel; triggering that all-too-familiar craving for carbs and sugary foods. Glutamine reaches our brain within minutes; it quickly satisfies the carb/sugar cravings. Glutamine powder can be purchased on line or in health-food stores. It is a good supplement to take temporarily when dealing with "emergency" cravings. One or two grams of glutamine powder taken with water will usually stop carb cravings. <u>GLUTAMINE</u> is also widely used to <u>HEAL GUT ISSUES</u>.

2. <u>MAGNESIUM</u>. Magnesium is the 4th most abundant mineral in our bodies. It is a co-factor in more than 300 biochemical reactions ranging from protein synthesis to nerve function. <u>RECENT STUDIES PROVE THAT IT PLAYS AN ENORMOUS ROLE IN REGULATING INSULIN SENSITIVITY.</u>

   One study by the American Diabetic Association in 2013 showed that higher magnesium intake could lower the risk of impaired insulin and glucose metabolism.

   Another 2013 study published in Nutrients found that dietary magnesium intake could improve insulin resistance among <u>NON-DIABETIC</u> subjects. Poor insulin health is directly related to acute and repeated carb cravings. Sufficient magnesium supplementation can help end them.

The most bioavailable types of <u>MAGNESIUM ON THE MARKET TODAY ARE</u>: Magnesium glycinate; Magnesium malate; also good are: Magnesium citrate, thurate, chloride and carbonate.

3. <u>CHROMIUM</u>. Chromium is an essential trace mineral which plays a beneficial role in regulating insulin activity; improving glycemic control; and assisting glucose metabolism.

   A study published in 2008 Diabetes Metabolism Research and Reviews showed that overweight and diabetic subjects who supplemented their diets with 600 micrograms daily of <u>CHROMIUM PICOLINATE</u> (along with B Vitamin Biotin) demonstrated improved glycemic control compared to non-users. <u>CHROMIUM PICOLINATE</u> is one of the best supplements to take for fixing carb cravings.

<u>REMEMBER—INDIVIDUAL RESPONSES TO CARBS VARY CONSIDERABLY.</u>

<u>YOU NEED TO DETERMINE YOUR PERSONAL LEVEL OF CARB-TOLERANCE.</u>

Carbs consumed fire up your internal sugar factory. When you eat fewer carbs you will be shutting down production of sugar in your internal sugar factory.

<u>YOU HAVE THE POWER TO BECOME A FAT BURNER INSTEAD OF A CARB BURNER.</u>

<u>CARB RESTRICTION</u> is your key to successful implantation of the <u>LOW-CARB-HIGH-FAT KETOGENIC DIET</u>. An important health principle says to eliminate <u>all</u> neurotoxins. The Queen of Neurotoxins is a sly devil. She not only tries to do her evil work with refined sugar and <u>HFCS</u>; she also has an <u>EVIL</u> half-sister (aka Carb Queen)-☺

The Carb Queen has secretly seduced your <u>BRAIN</u>. She has convinced your brain to eat and be addicted to <u>CARBS</u>. Your brain asks for its preferred fat fuel.

<u>BUT THERE'S A BIG PROBLEM</u>. Your brain and body have become addicted to <u>CARBS/SUGAR</u>. Your brain needs to be re-educated. Your brain needs to become "addicted" to eating good fats.

<u>YOU MUST KICK YOUR SUGAR (CARBOHYDRATE) ADDICTION.</u>

<u>YOU MUST GET YOUR BRAIN OFF SUGAR!</u>

<u>IT'S NOT YOUR FAULT.</u>

LIKE MILLIONS OF OTHER PEOPLE- YOU ARE CARB ADDICTS. IT'S THE FAULT OF MAINSTREAM EXPERTS- AND THE "SO-CALLED" HEALTH-CARE SYSTEM.

CARBS ARE NOT NUTRIENTS— CARBS DON'T REPAIR OR BUILD ANYTHING!

YOU MUST CUT YOUR CARBOHYDRATES "TO THE BONE"-☺ CARB ELIMINATION/RESTRICTION IS YOUR FIRST STEP TO BECOME "FAT-ADAPTED."

Guess what happens when you become fat-adapted on a Ketogenic Diet?

YOUR FOOD CRAVINGS FOR CARBOHYDRATES & SUGAR MAGICALLY DISAPPEAR! YOU CAN CURE YOUR CARBOHYDRATE ADDICTION!

ONCE YOU BECOME FAT / KETO-ADAPTED- YOUR APPETITE WILL PLUMMIT. YOU WILL FEEL FULLY SATISFIED AND COMPLETELY SATED.

FOOD CRAVINGS / CONTINUAL THOUGHTS ABOUT FOOD AND EATING WILL MAGICALLY DISAPPEAR!

WHEN YOU ARE KETO-ADAPTED YOU MAY EVEN FORGET TO EAT. OMG!

D. SHUTTING DOWN SUGAR PRODUCTION

"There is no sincerer love than the love of food."

-George Bernard Shaw,

To shut down sugar production, you must shut down your CARB-burning metabolism. You must switch metabolic "horses". You must switch from a "carb-burning horse" approach and switch to a "FAT-burning horse"-☺

YOU MUST START BUILDING YOUR FAT-BURNING MACHINERY.

YOU MUST MAKE THE DECISION TO CREATE NEW METABOLIC MACHINERY AND NEW NEURAL PATHWAYS.

TO ATTAIN SUPERHEALTH- YOU MUST SWITCH FROM A CARB-BURNING (SUGAR FACTORY) METABOLISM TO A FAT-BURNING METABOLISM.

What are the "REAL" CAUSES OF OBESITY?

CONTRARY TO POPULAR BELIEF—

1. THE WORLD'S OBESITY EPIDEMIC IS NOT CAUSED BY GLUTTONY OR DOING TOO LITTLE EXERCISE.

2. RATHER— OBESITY, DIABETES AND MOST RELATED AILMENTS ARE CAUSED BY HIGH-CARB DIETS. (These diets raise blood sugar levels and send insulin spikes through the roof).

3. THE OBESITY EPIDEMIC IS LARGELY CAUSED BY EATING THE WRONG KINDS OF FOODS! (The RIGHT foods are rich- nutrient dense, fat-rich whole foods eaten as RAW as possible.

4. OVEREATING (gluttony) SHOULD BE SEEN AS A "MANIFESTATION" OF OBESITY—NOT A ROOT CAUSE OF OBESITY.

So what should we eat?

YOU HAVE BEEN BRAINWASHED TO BELIEVE THAT THERE ARE

3 MACRONUTRIENTS— carbohydrates, protein, and fat. But—

CARBOHYDRATES ARE NOT NUTRIENTS!

FOR 60 YEARS YOU'VE BEEN TOLD THAT CARBOHYDRATES ARE GOOD FOR YOU. THIS IS A BIG LIE!

YOU'VE BEEN LIED TO BY DOCTORS AND DIE-TICIANS- BIG AGRA, BIG GOVERNMENT AND BIG PHARMA!

THIS 'CARB-LIE" KILLS MILLIONS OF PEOPLE EVERYDAY!

You have a CHOICE. You can burn SUGAR, suffer disease, & die prematurely— OR

YOU CAN BECOME A FAT BURNING MACHINE—ATTAIN SUPERHEALTH, AND LIVE A LONG, HEALTHY AND PROSPEROUS LIFE.

Are you still munching on that gluten, glyphosate GMO breakfast sandwich? Are you enjoying that antibiotic-laced burger and GMO fries? Perhaps you prefer e-coli chicken? How 'bout an all-dressed pesticide-laden GMO pizza?-☺

You might want to re-consider frequenting Macdonald's golden arches- otherwise you may visit the "real" golden arches sooner than you wish to…-☺ Human beings were not put on planet Earth to eat PROCESSED FOODS.

MOTHER NATURE'S REAL FOODS ARE ALL THAT YOU NEED TO BE HEALTHY AND SATISFIED.

PLEASE UNDERSTAND- YOU DO NOT HAVE TO GIVE UP ALL OF YOUR RICH DELICIOUS MOUTH-WATERING FOODS! EXACTLY THE OPPOSITE!

Humans were not placed on Planet Earth to eat on bland, unappetizing food. We are not designed to eat bird food. Nor are we programmed to eat wild grass and plants. We are designed to eat a wide variety of natural foods—not those coming from a factory farm, a fast-food restaurant or a cereal box.

DOZENS OF PHENOMENAL KETOGENIC RECEIPES AND KETOGENIC FOODS ARE AVAILABLE FROM DR. INTERNET!

AFTER YOU UNDERSTAND THE KETOGENIC NUTRITIONAL APPROACH IN THIS BOOK YOU WILL BE LIGHT YEARS AHEAD OF MAINSTREAM CONVENTIONAL MEDICINE AND CONVENTIONAL DIE-TICIANS.

MOREOVER— YOU WILL HAVE A SUPERIOR COMPREHENSION OF OUR BODY'S METABOLISM AND PHYSIOLOGY. You do not need to take a course in molecular chemistry; physiology. You will learn more about molecular biochemistry, human metabolism and physiology than conventional doctors learn from 200 hours of biochemistry they receive in medical school.

VIRTUALLY ALL DISEASES ARE THE RESULT OF DYSFUNCTIONAL MITOCHONDRIA. DYSFUNCTIONAL MITOCHONDRIA MEAN DYSFUNCTIONAL CELLS (aka busted cells). DYSFUNCTIONAL CELLS OFTEN ARE A PART OF A DYSFUNCTIONAL METABOLISM;(aka busted metabolism).

YOU WILL LEARN THE NUTRITIONAL AND METABOLIC KNOWLEDGE TO HEAL YOURSELF BY MEANS OF THE HEALING KETOGENIC DIET.

YOU CAN ESCAPE THE DISEASE MANAGEMENT SYSTEM- YOU CAN BY-PASS THE MEDICAL ESTABLISHMENT AND SAVE THOUSANDS OF DOLLARS!

WHY NOT SPEND YOUR HARD-EARNED CASH ON SOME DELICIOUS FOOD THAT WILL HELP YOU ATTAIN SUPERHEALTH?

YOU DON'T HAVE TO BE A ROCKET SCIENTIST TO KNOW HOW TO EAT. IT'S ACTUALLY QUITE SIMPLE.

If you own a Ferrari—would you put cheap fuel in your car and expect high-performance? Well, your body is the same. If you put in second quality fuel—i.e. toxic carbohydrates your car will likely stall or even worse. You could cause your engine to burn out, throw a ring or even a piston. That would be the end of a very expensive high-performance vehicle. You can always add a new engine to your Ferrari- or buy a new one.

Your body is only car you'll ever have. Many people scrupulously take care of their cars. Here in Canadian wintertime, many people line up for a drive thru for a 20-30 minute to get the chemicals and salt washed off of their cars.

Do they take 15 minutes each day to take care of themselves? Nope. Can they find 15 minutes to take care of THEIR bodies? Do they have 15 minutes a day to do a bit of exercise or go for a walk? Nope. But they have 2 hours to sit to in front of the idiot box (aka TV) and eat some poisonous fast food. Now you likely have an Internet/e-mail addiction that sucks up even more of your valuable time.

Sadly, most people (doctors included) still believe that a pill can fix any health problem. They just start receiving more and more pills as their health deteriorates. People are brain-washed to believe that your aging body is like a car- it breaks down and wears out with age.

Then— after several years of eating junk food and never getting off of their hind-sides, suddenly, most people wake up to the sad reality about THEIR OWN BODIES RUN-DOWN CONDITION. They find them-selves with shiny new clean car—but a rusted body.

Most people let their body ROT AND RUST from the inside.

IN SIMPLE TERMS- OUR BODY RUSTS FROM THE INSIDE.

Most people take better care of their car; (aka bucket of bolts). Most people cannot find 15 minutes a day to do something valuable to nourish or heal their bodies.

> "Most people spend a lifetime trying to get wealthy-
> then they spend that money trying to get healthy."

Are you going to remain a victim of a failed experiment BY THE PHARMACEUTICAL INDUSTRY AND THE MEDICAL PROFESSION?

YOUR LIFE EXPECTANCY IS MORE THAN 90 PERCENT DEPENDENT ON WHAT YOU EAT-AND- HOW WELL YOU TAKE CARE OF YOURSELF.

SUPERHEALTH STARTS WITH PROPER NUTRITION. Bad health is not due to an absence of pills. Bad health is caused by a lack of proper nutrients from a bad diet.

FIX YOUR FOOD — YOU WILL FIX YOUR BODY—YOU WILL FIX YOUR HEALTH.

If you don't take care of yourself— who will? Certainly not some pill-pusher dressed in a white coat.-☺

Here is my modernized Dr. Hipprocate's <u>HEALTH MANTRA</u>:

"<u>LET YOUR FAT BE YOUR MEDICINE- LET YOUR MEDICINE BE YOUR FAT</u>"
— Dr. Gabriela Segura, MD.

<u>YOUR BODY IS THE BEST HIGH- PERFORMANCE SELF- HEALING VEHICLE ON THE PLANET!</u> If plants, animals and pets do not have good nutrition- they get sick and die.

Unlike other living creatures—<u>HUMANS ARE THEIR OWN WORST ENEMIES!</u> Humans are at the top of the food chain. When it comes to taking care of their health- most humans are at the bottom of the health ladder. They blame their poor health on poor genes, family history or bad luck. Most adverse health issues are caused by <u>STRESS; A CRAPPY DIET & POOR LIFESTYLE CHOICES</u>.

<u>THE BEST PERSON IN THE WORLD TO HELP YOU GET HEALTHY IS YOU!</u>

<u>CAN YOUR MERCEDES REPAIR ITSELF?</u> Nope. Any repairs must be done by a skilled mechanic. High-performance vehicles require highly- trained mechanics who have studied all mechanical, systemic and computerized skills and knowledge needed to fix your car.

<u>YOUR BODY IS AN AMAZING- SELF –HEALING MACHINE!</u> <u>YOUR BODY IS FAR SMARTER THAN ANY CAR</u>. How many cars have the ability to self-repair themselves for more than 100 years?

<u>DO YOU KNOW ANY OTHER " MACHINE" OR ANIMAL THAT CAN REPAIR ITSELF?</u> Our bodies do not come with instructions of how and what we should do to make sure that we are healthy and strong. Did our ancestors need to read an instruction manual?

Would you hire a mechanic who suggested that mud on your windshield should be resolved by replacing your windshield? Would you go to your mechanic to fix your car's engine problem with a petrochemical?

When you go visit your doctor with blood sugar problems- what does he do? He sells you some Big Pharma poiso is marketed as "medication". Your doctor tells you that a pill will lower your blood sugar. That is the equivalent to your car mechanic telling you that your engine is overheating because there's not enough oil in your crankcase. Your mechanic has the common sense to assume that he should at least lift the hood of your car! What if several days later, your car engine burns out? Would you be content with your car mechanic's diagnosis that your car was a missing a quart of oil?

YOUR DOCTOR'S APPROACH IS WORSE THAN A BLIND MECHANIC DIAGNOSING YOUR CAR'S ENGINE PROBLEM WITHOUT LIFTING THE HOOD!

YOU MUST DIAGNOSE YOURSELF. YOU MUST BE YOUR OWN BODY MECHANIC! YOU ARE ONLY WASTING YOUR TIME, MONEY AND YOUR HEALTH BY TRUSTING THAT YOUR DOCTOR HAS THE KNOWLEDGE, TOOLS AND/OR EXPERTISE TO FIX YOUR HEALTH.

YOUR DOCTOR IS CLUELESS ABOUT METABOLIC DYSFUNCTION AND CELLULAR DYSFUNCTION. YOUR DOCTOR DOESN'T WHAT TO DO SO HE JUST DOPES YOU UP—OR SUGGESTS THAT THE PROBLEMATIC BODY PART CAN BE KILLED WITH RADIATION OR CUT OUT WITH SURGERY.

THIS BOOK IS YOUR "HOW TO DO IT YOURSELF" (DIY) GUIDE TO SUPERHEALTH & FITNESS.

THIS BOOK TEACHES YOU HOW TO BE YOUR OWN HEALTH MECHANIC. YOU WILL LEARN HOW TO REPAIR AND FIX YOUR BODY WITH HEALING FOODS.

THE KETOGENIC NUTRITIONAL APPROACH supported by science speaks for itself. As a World-Class Strength coach, I'm thrilled to provide you with my EXERCISE expertise. I have had the good fortune to learn from the foremost coaches in the world.

You don't need to go to medical school; you don't need an advanced degree in Physiology or an advanced degree in Nutrition (the latter would not likely help you anyway.)

You do not need to consult a Registered Dietician- or any white-coated person to learn and understand WHICH FOODS AND NUTRIENTS ARE ESSENTIAL TO PUT INTO YOUR BODY.

DOCTORS AND DIETICIANS HAVE NOT BEEN TAUGHT ABOUT THE SCIENCE AND BIOCHEMISTRY OF LOW-CARB NUTRITION

YOU NEED TO BE YOUR OWN NUTRITIONIST. YOU NEED TO HIRE YOURSELF AS YOUR OWN DOCTOR! Your health destiny is in your hands!

PILLS WILL NOT FIX YOUR HEALTH PROBLEMS! They will only rob your body of nutrients; wreck your immune system and make you fat, sick and diseased. You must eat anyway so why not eat the MOST NUTRITIOUS FOOD THAT YOU CAN FIND?

YOU MUST GIVE YOUR BODY THE NUTRITION THAT IT SCREAMS FOR!

GIVE YOUR BODY THE HEALTHY FOOD THAT IT CRAVES AND IT WILL REPAIR ITSELF! NO DOCTORS AND/OR DIE-TICIANS REQUIRED! Let Big Pharma scam someone else.

YOU NEED TO BE YOUR OWN HEALTH COACH.

YOU ARE THE EXPERT ON YOUR BODY AND YOUR OWN PERSONALIZED HEALTH REQUIREMENTS!

YOU NEED TO DO YOUR OWN DUE DILIGENCE.

IN THE UNLIKELY EVENT THE INFORMATION IN THIS BOOK DOES NOT RESOLVE YOUR HEALTH ISSUES—YOU CAN RESEARCH THE AREAS OF YOUR OWN HEALTH CONCERNS. If you are the Lady of your Castle, it is likely that you can apply THE KETOGENIC DIET for yourself; your spouse, your kiddies and your loved ones. (You may even decide to put your dog/ cat on a Ketogenic diet)-☺)

SUPPLEMENTAL INFORMATION AND/OR HEALTH ADVICE REGARDING YOUR HEALTH ISSUES can be obtained on-line. You can consult some of the online resources- such as consulting www.GreenMedInfo.com ; PUBMED or even Dr. Google-☺) No white-coats needed. Spending money for good electronics to access the health resources of the Internet may be SMARTER AND CHEAPER than consulting some white-coated individual.

SHOULD YOU HAVE A SERIOUS HEALTH ISSUE WHICH SURPASSES YOUR NUTRITIONAL OR OTHER EXPERTISE—

BY ALL MEANS —CONSULT ONE OR MORE NATURAL MEDICINE DOCTORS- e.g. NATUROPATHS.

Just Google up: "NATUROPATHS, OR FUNCTIONAL MEDICINE DOCTORS".

These functional doctors have expert knowledge and know how to help you overcome serious health issues—if you need to... Many of natural/functional doctors even post a lot of information on their websites too! These people are the good guys. Their passion to help people get better is not driven by profit/greed. These doctors are the people you should consult—NOT the allopathic crowd- who are only greedy pill-pushers.

THANK GOD FOR THE INTERNET! Now you don't have to suffer in misery- there's good competent alternative medical help out there. You just need to search it out. You will be glad that you did. Your body will be glad that you did.

BEST OF ALL- YOU CAN GET A VIRTUAL CONSULTATION AND ASK THE NATUROPATHIC PHYSICIAN ABOUT SOMETHING YOU READ ABOUT IN THIS BOOK!

IF YOU APPLY A WELL-STRUCTURED KETOGENIC DIET—THE CHANCES ARE EXCELLENT THAT THIS DIET WILL RESOLVE YOUR HEALTH ISSUES.

YOU SHOULD EAT THE ANCESTRAL KETOGENIC DIET THAT HAS BEEN ALREADY PROGRAMMED INTO OUR GENES!

Do you think that our ancestors ate dead bland tasting low-fat nutrient –deficient food? They didn't roast hot-dogs or a marshmallows over an open fire or make popcorn. They roasted some wild animal flesh or fish- or nuts, wild plants, herbs or anything else that tasted good and was plucked from Mother Nature's Farmacy.

FAT IS YOUR BRAIN'S SECRET LOVE! -☺)

FUEL YOUR BRAIN WITH ITS PREFERED FUEL—FAT AND KNOW THAT:

> **YOU WILL SUPERCHARGE YOUR BRAIN—**
>
> **YOU WILL SUPERCHARGE YOUR BODY AND YOUR ENTIRE LIFE!**
>
> **YOU WILL FEED YOUR SPIRITUAL SOUL!**
>
> **YOU WILL ADD LIFE TO YOUR YEARS AND YEARS TO YOUR LIFE!**

GIVE YOUR BODY THE NOURISHMENT IT REQUIRES AND YOU WILL BE DISEASE-FREE AND ACQUIRE SUPERHEALTH. (However—if you choose to eat crappy, poisoned, chemically-laced, dead-food- You'll likely leave planet earth pre-maturely.

DITCH THE (SAD) DIET (THE STANDARD AMERICAN DIET. ADOPT THE "HAPPY HEALING" DIET — THE KETOGENIC DIET!

Shutting down your sugar factory- more thoughts… If you drink that glass of **ORANGE JUICE—PLEASE BEWARE!**

That innocent glass of orange juice is **NOT INNOCENT! IT IS EXTREMELY UNHEALTHY!!**

ORANGE JUICE WILL DYNAMITE OPEN THE DOORS OF YOUR SUGAR FACTORY AND FIRE UP YOUR PANCREAS' INSULIN PUMP!

THIS WILL PUT YOU ON THE FAST TRACK TO DIABETES, HEART DISEASE, ALZHEIMERS DISEASE AND CANCER! OMG!

How does orange juice do that? That syrupy juice enters your body; fires up your pancreas' insulin pump. Some sugar syrup is burned as glucose to make energy.

MOST OF "THIS GLUCOSE" IS STORED AS FAT. THEN YOU GET OBESE.

THEN YOU ARE ON THE FAST TRACK TOWARDS TYPE 2 DIABETES. Often diabetes causes heart disease, cancer and Alzheimer's Disease.

SUGAR CAUSES INSULIN RESISTANCE. IT "GLYCATES" (sticks to proteins) and then FERMENTS...serious health problems then ACCELERATE! For example,

ONE ROOT CAUSE OF ALZHEIMER'S DISEASE IS:

> THE BRAIN'S INABILITY TO PROCESS SUGAR TO PRODUCE ENERGY and

> THIS DEFICIENCY ROBS YOUR BRAIN OF THE ENERGY THAT YOUR BRAIN NEEDS TO REPAIR BRAIN CELLS AND STIMULATE THE GROWTH OF NEW CELLS.

SIDE-BAR—

In my lifetime I have drank only one small glass of "REAL ORANGE JUICE".

It was fresh-squeezed orange juice from a small tree on a small Carribean Island. It had the colour of lemon juice and it tasted AMAZING! It tasted as Mother Nature intended. It tasted neither sour nor sweet. I just tasted good. THAT ORANGE CAME FROM A WILD ORANGE TREE planted by Mother Nature- not by a commercial USA orange grower. If Mother Nature doesn't make it –YOU don't need it!

Thirty-five years ago, I tasted field—ripened pineapple in the fields of Hawaii. It had an AMAZING TASTE! Organic pineapples sold in North America cannot compare (taste or nutrition-wise) with fresh field-ripened pineapples. BTW- The most nutritious part of a pine-apple is found in the core and the white part next to the skin. This is where a compound called "bromelain" is found. This fibrous com-pound is even used for THERAPEUTIC PURPOSES- TO HEAL THE BODY AND PREVENT DISEASES.

SUGAR FACTORY SHUTDOWN FACTS:

- CARBOHYDRATES are metabolized (bro-ken down) to GLUCOSE (sugar).

- FATS are used to make KETONE BODIES WHICH ARE FORMS

OF FAT FUEL- (except the glycerol backbone of triglyceride which is conjugated to the liver to make glucose. (Don't worry-the entire metabolism process is explained below-☺)

- CALORIES- most of them usually come down to GLUCOSE (sugar).

- IN SHORT— THERE ARE ONLY TWO FUEL SUBSTRATES WHICH OUR BODY USES-GLUCOSE AND FAT. (Our body actually uses several organs to manufacture these fuels).

Let's take another example: Eat a whole wheat muffin, or a bowl of oatmeal. Both of these turn into the EXACT SAME THING AS— a can of soda, or a handful of candy. That fructose (sugar) in fruits and those carbs in veggies end up the same way (in the same place too), as a piece of chocolate cake-☺

CARBS are substances that are converted to GLUCOSE (sugar) IN YOUR BODY.

To take another example—if you eat a teaspoon of coconut oil or butter- it will be quickly METABOLIZED by your liver to make KETONES; (fat bodies used as fuel.). These healing bodies will be sucked up by your brain very quickly!

YOU WILL ABSOLUTELY LOVE THOSE HAPPY HEALING KETONES!

Please take a moment to re-read Dr. Ron Rosedale's quote supra.

IN SIMPLE TERMS—EITHER YOU ARE BURNING SUGAR—OR— YOU ARE BURNING FAT AS YOUR PRIMARY SOURCE OF FUEL.

THE WHOLE FAT PHOBIA & THE LOW-FAT PARADIGM IS A BUNCH OF SCIENTIFIC NONSENSE! IT'S JUNK SCIENCE!

CALORIE COUNTING IS TOTALLY UNNECESSARY.

CALORIE COUNTING IS AN ARCHAIC WASTE OF TIME-BEST LEFT TO YOUR HARD-CORE CALORIE-COUNTING DOCTOR AND YOUR HARD-CORE CALORIE-COUNTING DIE-TICIAN.

BOTH OF THESE "HEALTHCARE PROFESSIONALS" ARE CLUELESS ABOUT LOW-CARB NUTRITION AND METABOLISM.-☺

YOU WOULD BE WELL-ADVISED TO LET THEM PLAY WITH THEIR CALORIE COUNTER TOYS. YOU CAN WATCH YOUR DOCTOR AND YOUR DIETICIAN AS THEY GET FAT.-☺

However—not all calories are ugly. All calories are not to be feared. Yes- SOME SPECIFIC FOODS COULD BE CONSIDERED EVIL. They don't call it Devil's cake for nothing!-☺ But calories themselves are not evil.

You need calories or you would die! Moreover, it is possible to live without eating food (only drinking nutrient-dense <u>WATER</u> for about 60 DAYS!) Mention that to your doctor...but please be careful...you don't want to give the poor devil a heart attack-☺

<u>WATER IS NUMBER ONE ON THE SUPERFOODS LIST!</u> Does water have any calories? It's "thermogenic". Drinking water actually burns about 93 calories per day!

When you reduce calories, your <u>SERATONIN</u> (happy hormone) levels drop. Low-calorie gurus then become depressed and obsessed with <u>UNDEREATING</u>. Moreover, you will almost always find that people on restricted calorie diets become irritable, grumpy and depressed. That's because those little critters (bacteria) in your gut that make serotonin become <u>VERY</u> disenchanted. When these little critters can't feast on say nice piece of raw cheese or dark chocolate, they go on strike-☺...well not exactly but...-☺

These critters become downright <u>ANNOYED</u>! They refuse to make serotonin and you become depressed. Have you ever noticed how you feel when you have a nice small square of dark chocolate?

A recent study that found that 50 percent of women preferred choco-late to <u>SEX</u>! Are you one of those ladies? Guys- smarten up and take care of your ladies or you'll have to compete with chocolate for your lady's affection. -☺)

<u>FORGET LOW-FAT/HIGH CARB NUTRITION.</u>

<u>YOUR DOCTOR'S ADVICE IS A SCAM!</u> Aka <u>THE 99 PERCENT RULE!</u>

<u>FAT IS NOT JUST YOUR FRIEND.</u> <u>FAT IS YOUR BEST FRIEND!</u>

On a positive note —a few real doctors are actually doing produc-tive research.

Dr. David Ludwig, Director of Obesity Prevention Center at Boston Children's Hospital, has joined an increasing number of functional nutritionists <u>DISPELLING</u> the notion that good health comes from limiting fat and counting calories overall. Most dieticians and nutri-tionists are still telling people to count calories. But, there are a <u>few</u> bright nutritional lights out there.

<u>WHEN YOU ADOPT A KETOGENIC DIET—YOUR CALORIE-COUNTING DAYS ARE OVER!</u>

This statement makes most people uncomfortable.

<u>THE TRUTH OFTEN DOES</u>.

In life, you can never go wrong when you take the <u>HIGH</u> road and tell the <u>TRUTH.</u> Being a good person is mostly about doing the right thing. You don't need to be a religious zealot to be a person of high moral character.

The healthcare community and the general public have been <u>BRAIN-WASHED FOR THE LAST HALF-CENTURY ABOUT ALMOST EVERYTHING IN THE HEALTHCARE DOMAINE.</u>

Big Pharma constantly bombards the public with advertisements extolling the wondrous qualities of medications. Most consumers believe the advertisement that they see or hear on TV- from talking head.

Mainstream media, doctors and most people go around extolling the safety of <u>VACCINES.</u> <u>MOST</u> have never even read the Vaccine Insert. Only one copy is provided for each of 10 vials...ask the pro-vaccine zealots to explain that one. Most people would be appalled about the dangers of vaccines listed on the insert!

<u>CAVEAT EMPTOR! —A MOST IMPORTANT RULE IN LAW- AND IN LIFE-LET THE BUYER BEWARE!</u>

I strongly believe that most people are inherently good. Sometimes people lose their way and unwittingly do bad things. We need to have compassion for these people.

Doctors are doing- perhaps blindly— what they have been taught to do—by an <u>EVIL CORRUPT BIG PHARMA AND CORRUPT MEDICAL ESTABLISHMENT.</u> Doctors do not need to be denigrated. They need your compassion. At some point in their lives most conventional doctors will have an AHA moment and realize that the allopathic "medical profession" is a big failure.

The low-calorie craze and processed food packages have been marked "diet" "fat-free", "low-fat" "lean cuisine", "for weight –watchers"- ad nauseam. These foods will <u>NOT</u> make you thin or lean. These kinds of foods are <u>VERY UNHEALTHY.</u> They are far more likely to make you <u>FAT AND SICK.</u> They are nutrient-deficient and laced with chemical additives.

The truth is: <u>YOU NEED SOME CALORIES! SOLID SCIENCE DOESN'T LIE.</u>

<u>WHEN YOU BECOME KETO-ADAPTED YOU WILL NEVER HAVE TO COUNT CALORIES FOR THE REST OF YOUR LIFE!</u> Caloric restriction will happen automatically because your <u>FOOD/VOLUME/INTAKE</u> will decrease.

How cool is that?

What is a calorie?

A calorie is a unit of heat energy. It's a term plucked from physics. Do you think that our ancestors counted calories? Do you think that they were concerned about losing weight or losing a few extra pounds -Of course not.

The WORLD'S HEALTH PROBLEMS began about 10 thousand years ago. The dawn of agriculture started the snowball of obesity and related health problems that have now skyrocketed to epic numbers. Eating bread may have been okay for the slaves building the pyramids. Firstly it contained a lot less additives and poisons like gluten. Secondly, slaves died young from exhaustion not type 2 Diabetes. Sugar was only a small factor in the pre-diabetic centuries.

It has been preached for 60 to 70 years by the supposed experts- "weight-loss gurus" that a calorie is a calorie. Just do the math they say. More calories burned than taken in equals weight loss.

NOT SO FAST!

A CALORIE IS NOT CALORIE. All calories are NOT created equal. The old adage "Garbage in-garbage out" also applies.

THE AVERAGE NORTH AMERICAN IS OVERFED AND UNDERNOURISHED.

MOST PEOPLE EAT DEAD – POISONED- GMO- FOODS, (ACTUALLY NON-FOODS) WHICH ARE LOADED WITH NEUROTOXINS- AND DEVOID OF NUTRIENTS.

Some of us call these foods "FRANKENFOODS" Imagine Frankenstein in a white lab-coat fiendishly concocting tasting new foods to sell to uninformed, unsuspecting, naive consumers? I know what you're thinking.

How can malnourishment be the problem when the problem is excess weight and eating too much?

The problem begins with the soil. It has been depleted of nutrients. It no longer contains the trace minerals that used to be absorbed into our produce (fruits, and veggies- even grains). The majority of what people eat is GMO foods. This means that they are really no longer food. They are "UNFOODS".

Today, there's probably more nutrition in the cardboard of your cereal box—than in the contents!

The reason that crops have been altered is to maximize food production. More crops produced faster CREATES MORE MONEY—and…and

261

more resistance to bugs. Growing faster actually means less actual maturation and <u>LESS NUTRITION!</u>

Oh yes- one other small point- some plants produce their own cellular pesticide internally which we consume as well. Eating non-organic, poisonous, non-nutritious produce will make you sick and kill you in ways <u>THAT HAVE NOT YET EVEN BEEN DISCOVERED!</u> For example, broccoli now contains only <u>50 PERCENT</u> of the nutrition that it contained a half-century ago.

If your meat that is laced with growth- hormones and antibiotics from Confined Animal Feeding Operations (CAFO's) you are eating diseased unhealthy meat. These animals are treated <u>VERY CRUELLY</u> before slaughter. This animal flesh is <u>STRESSED</u> to put it mildly. Often animals stumble and break legs on the way to the slaughterhouse...

It turns out that <u>HUMANS AND ANIMALS HAVE TRAPPED EMOTIONS IN OUR BODIES?</u> Enough said; I think you get the picture. Conventional poisonous animal flesh contains little nutrition but is pumped full of bright red dyes to look yummy! Or I should say <u>YUKKY?</u>

So when you're eating unhealthy meat and unhealthy produce- you're not only <u>POISONING</u> yourself with chemicals. Worse yet -you are eating <u>DEAD FOOD</u>. When you eat nutritionally deficient food— guess what happens?

<u>YOU EAT TOO MANY CARBS AND TOO MANY EMPTY CALORIES.</u>

<u>THIS IS BECAUSE YOUR BODY IS SCREAMING AT YOU FOR HELP!</u>

Your body knows intuitively; your body is <u>HUNGRY</u> despite eating mountains of food!

<u>YOUR BODY AND YOUR BRAIN ARE BEGGING FOR REAL WHOLE FOOD!</u>

<u>"PLEASE GIVE ME SOME REAL FOOD- SOME NATURAL NUTRIENT-DENSE WHOLE FOOD!"</u> Your body is saying...

<u>"PLEASE GIVE ME SOME DELICIOUS, MOUTH-WATERING RICH SATISFYING FATS!</u>

Which sounds more <u>APPETIZING?</u>

<u>TWO DELICIOUS PASTURED SAUSAGES, TWO PASTURED EGGS – LIGHTLY FRIED —SLATHERED IN BUTTER, WITH A FEW SHITAKE CANCER-FIGHTING MUSHROOMS, AND A PIECE OF RAW CHEDDAR CHEESE</u>

<u>OR –</u>

A BIG BOWL OF GMO SPAGHETTI PASTA TOPPED WITH 5 or 6 ANTIBIOTIC MEATBALLS COVERED SOME WITH PESTICIDE-LACED GMO PASTA SAUCE; ...HOW 'BOUT A SIDEORDER OF GLUTEN GMO FRENCH BREAD TO DIP IN YOUR PESTICIDE-LACED CANOLA OIL- Yummy...=☺

Pop Quiz- Which meal will satisfy your hunger longer? Which meal is healthier? Which meal will make you healthy and lean? Which meal will make you fat and sick? Not sure? Please read on.

LADIES AND GENTLEMEN—YOU ARE NOT "WHAT YOU EAT".

YOU ARE "WHAT YOU SAY YOU EAT!

NUTRITIONALLY SPEAKING— AMERICANS ARE A NATION OF DEAD PEOPLE!

WHEN YOU EAT ORGANIC non-GMO FOODS—YOU ARE NOT JUST GETTING CALORIES.

You are getting micronutrients, vitamins, minerals, phytonutrients, polyphenols, amino acids, etc. YOU ARE GETTING SUSTENANCE. Your body constantly strives to obtain what it is really wants. Your body is relentless in its search for delicious-tasting nutrient-dense foods.

Feeling SATIATED by food means that your CRAVINGS for food- especially JUNK FOODS and processed foods i.e. EVIL CARBOHYDRATES WILL GRADUALLY DIMINISH. After a few days/ or weeks- THESE EVIL CARB CRAVINGS WILL DISAPPEAR!

YOU WILL FIND THAT YOU HAVE NO NEED TO COUNT CALORIES.

Your body will naturally respond and work with you.

YOU WILL AUTOMATICALLY STOP EATING BECAUSE YOU WILL FEEL SATISFIED. YOUR BELLY WILL BE HAPPY AND FULL-☺

TO SHUT DOWN YOUR EXTERNAL SUGAR FACTORY...YOU'VE ELIMINATED THE QUEEN OF NEUROTOXINS (Fructose) (Sucrose) and artificial sweeteners from your DIET AND FROM YOUR LIFE.

CONGRATULATIONS!

YOU HAVE TAKEN A HUGE STEP TOWARDS ATTAINING SUPERHEALTH!

YOU WILL LIKELY STILL HAVE A FEW SUGAR (CARB CRAVINGS); BUT DON'T WORRY. THIS IS QUITE COMMON.

THIS IS PERFECTLY NORMAL. YOU ARE UP-REGULATING NEW GENES!

You are re-programming your body back to its factory setting. When you were born- you were actually in a STATE OF KETOSIS. NUTRITIONAL KETOSIS IS THE NORMAL STATE FOR HUMANS.

How cool is that?

YOUR BRAIN AND YOUR ENTIRE BODY NEEDS TIME TO ADJUST AND ADAPT. CHANGING YOUR PRIMARY FUEL SOURCE OF ENERGY FOR YOUR BODY IS A PHENOMENAL CHANGE FOR ANYONE.

YOU MUST HAVE PATIENCE TO MAKE THIS LIFE-SAVING CHANGE.

SHUTTING DOWN YOUR "EXTERNAL" SUGAR FACTORY IS NEXT IMPORTANT STEP TOWARDS SUPERHEALTH.

YOU NEED TO LEARN TO SHUT DOWN YOUR INTERNAL SUGAR FACTORY.

YOU SHUT DOWN THIS SUGAR FACTORY WHEN YOU ELIMINATE CARBS FROM YOUR DIET.

YOU NEED TO RE- PROGRAM YOUR FAT-BURNING MACHINE TO RUN ON HIGH-OCTANCE DIESEL FUEL i.e. FAT. YOU NEED TO REPROGRAM YOUR BRAIN AND SAVE YOUR PANCREAS-☺

YOU NEED TO STOP BURNING CARBS THAT ARE JUST A "DIRTY GASOLINE".

FOR YOUR ENTIRE LIFE—you've been a "sugar burner". As a result- your internal little recognized "SUGAR FACTORY" HAS BEEN BURNING OUT OF CONTROL CAUSING INFLAMMATION THROUGHOUT YOUR BODY!

YOUR INTERNAL SUGAR FACTORY AND CARB-BURNING METABOLIC MACHINERY HAS LIKELY WREAKED METABOLIC HAVOC IN YOUR BODY.

EATING TOO MANY CARBS HAS CAUSED "METABOLIC DISTURBANCE WITH CELLULAR INJURY" (Dr. Alex Vasquez)- aka busted mitochondria and busted cells.

- NO MATTER HOW MUCH TIME YOU SPEND DIETING—

- NO MATTER HOW MUCH TIME YOUR SPEND EXERCIS- ING YOUR HEART OUT- despite pounding that treadmill for years— Have you lost any weight in the last few years? All that you've received is tired joints for your efforts. You may even find that going to the gym starts to be stressful and you stop going. This is what happens to most people. They start an exercising regime the first week of January. Most times by the 2nd week of February they get stressed out/fed up and abandon their weight-loss program until the next time…

- <u>UNLESS YOU CHANGE YOUR FUEL SOURCE FROM CARBS TO FAT-YOU NEVER PERMANENTLY LOSE THAT STUBBORN BELLY FAT!</u>

<u>NO MATTER HOW MUCH YOU DIET OR HOW MANY CALORIES THAT YOU GIVE UP…</u>

That sneaky hidden internal Sugar Factory sabotages and defeats every effort that you make to shed those excess, unwanted pounds.

<u>Is there anything more frustrating?</u>

<u>AN ANTI-FLAMMATORY KETOGENIC DIET IS YOUR SOLUTION.</u>

Our ancestors ate food that killed inflammation automatically in their body. This is how we evolved as humans on Planet Earth. Our internal Sugar Factory can be <u>VERY DANGEROUS</u>. It is the white elephant inside all of us-☺

Our modern high-carb diets and sedentary lifestyle have spawned a kind of <u>"EVIL METABOLIC FRANKENSTEIN"</u> aka <u>'BUSTED METABOLISM"</u>, or 'BUSTED CELLS". Scientists describe this condition as <u>"METABOLIC DYSFUNCTION"</u>.

<u>AT THE CELLULAR LEVEL— THIS METABOLIC DYSFUNCTION IS TECHNICALLY CALLED 'MITOCHONDRIAL DYSFUNCTION"</u>. Those microscopic batteries in your cells or mitochondria <u>"GET BUSTED."</u> (a technical term-☺.

<u>OUR CELLS GET OXIDIZED, INJURED AND DAMAGED BY TOXIC CARBS</u> (esp. <u>NEUROTOXINS AND FREE RADICALS.</u>

<u>OUR CELLS ARE CONTINUOUS ASSAULTED BY THE HUNDREDS OF CHEMICALS (AND TOXIC AIR) IN OUR ENVIRONMENT.</u>

<u>Sidebar-</u>

This carb "rusting process" generates "free radical damage" called (ROS) or "reactive oxygen species". (ROS) is an important concept to remember because it occurs in so much of our bodies- at the cellular level. Think of (ROS) as: an internal kind of <u>OXIDATION OR INTERNAL RUSTING.</u>

Our bodies produce natural <u>"ANTIOXIDANTS"</u> to help combat (ROS) or free radical damage. You may have heard about the boatload of antioxidants or supplements that are available to slow down this "oxidation" or internal rusting.

Reactive Oxygen Species (ROS) is the new buzzword to describe this process. As we age our body often slows down its production of some kinds of antioxidants. If we can't make or get these from our diet- then we likely need to <u>SUPPLEMENT WITH ANTIOXIDANTS</u>.

("Astaxanthin" is an example of a very powerful antioxidant.) Sometimes you will hear <u>GLUTATHIONE OR ASTAXINTHIN CALLED THE MASTER ANTIOXIDANTS</u>. We need to ensure we are producing enough from our diet or we should supplement.

Your internal sugar factory has programmed <u>YOU</u> and <u>YOUR BODY TO STORE FAT AND TO BECOME SLOW AND TIRED</u>. <u>YUK!</u> No one has ever told you how evil carbs can be.

<u>TAKE HEART! THERE'S EXCITING NEWS!</u>

<u>YOU HAVE THE ABILITY TO REPROGRAM YOUR METABOLISM AND SHUTDOWN YOUR RUNAWAY "SUGAR FACTORY!!</u>

How can this done? I'll bet you can guess. You can adopt <u>THE KETOGENIC DIET</u>.

<u>OUR ANCESTORS WERE NEVER OVERWEIGHT</u>. Our Paleolithic-Neolithic ancestors evolved as a lean, strong, species of brilliant hunters, and fast sprinters. Hey you would learn to sprint <u>TOO</u> if you wanted to avoid being lunch for a lion -☺ Our ancestors were perfectly adapted to their environment. If our ancestors had belly flab- they would not have been able to run very fast- nor very far-☺

Your brain functioin determined whether you would eat lion for lunch OR whether he would eat you! Our ancestors had <u>SPORADIC</u> access to <u>DENSE NUTRIENT-RICH FOODS</u>. Their physical challenges were many and varied; they needed to be healthy, strong and fit. They <u>HAD</u> to move <u>WELL—OFTEN</u>; they had to move <u>FAST!</u> If you live in an urban area you can go weeks without seeing someone move fast- unless it's to jump in line at a local pizza parlour-☺

Researchers believe that the human brain became larger as a result of eating more diet-rich <u>ANIMAL FATS</u>. Indeed, when we are <u>FASTING</u>; we actually become <u>SMARTER!</u>

Say what? <u>YES</u>— <u>IT'S ABSOLUTELY TRUE!</u> Our mental focus, brain function and cognitive processes actually work better after 24 to 48 hours <u>WITHOUT FOOD!</u>

<u>How is this possible?</u>

The short answer is: DURING FASTING OUR BODY BURNS FAT!

FASTING- ESPECIALLY INTERMITTENT FASTING IS AN ESSENTIAL COMPONENT OF A PROPERLY STRUCTURED KETOGENIC DIET.

DURING FASTING— KETONE FAT BODIES PROVIDE US WITH HIGH-OCTANE-SUPERFUEL!

THE BRAIN'S PREFERRED FUEL IS FAT +FAT & MORE FAT!

Your brain is sub-consciously **BEGGING YOU TO EAT FAT!** You've have been taught to fuel your brain and your body with **CARBS**.

THE BIGGEST BRAIN MYTH – BELIEVED BY 99 PERCENT OF MAINSTREAM DOCTORS IS:

   "OUR BRAIN PREFERS GLUCOSE (SUGAR) FOR FUEL"

   THIS IS TOTAL PHYSIOLOGICAL NONSENSE! (Oops- another reason to fire your doctor and hire yourself-☺

FAT IS THE PREFERRED SUPERFUEL & SECRET LOVE-☺) OF OUR BRAIN!

FAT IS 25 PERCENT MORE EFFICIENT AND EFFECTIVE AS FUEL FOR OUR BRAINS AND OUR HEARTS! (I'll bet your doctor doesn't know that!)

OUR BODY BURNS SATURATED FATS LIKE GASOLINE BURNS ON AN OPEN FIRE! Our **FAT** greedy brain quickly grabs the lion's share of **FAT FOR FUEL.**

OUR BODY TURNS THESE FATS INTO KETONES— BUT THERE EXISTS A PARALLEL MECHANISM IN OUR BRAIN THAT ALSO MAKES KETONES!

Who knew?

WHY is FAT our preferred fuel- both in times of FEAST or FAMINE?

Well, imagine if after 2 days without finding any animals to kill for food our brains did not function properly. What if we couldn't remember where we killed that last wild caribou? What if we lacked the necessary strength and energy to track, find and kill our favorite wild animal? What if we lacked the necessary energy because of an empty stomach? What if we were so fatigued suffering mental brain fog" that we could not even remember where we left our spear? Seniors may believe that's its normal to forget where they put their keys-but imagine the consequences of not remembering where you left your spear! It's quite simple- the human body is programmed to have laser like senses and a strong nimble brain.

EATING A HIGH-CARB DIET IS A PRESCRIPTION FOR SICKNESS AND PRE-MATURE DEATH. Follow Ancel Key's low fat-dietary approach AT YOUR OWN RISK!

You will not starve if you do not eat for 24 hours!—provided you hydrate properly (& take appropriate electrolytes). And when you fast, your liver can do some (house-cleaning) detoxing; and your pancreas can take a well-deserved holiday (rest)-☺

OUR KEY ORGANS AND OUR BODIES- NEED SUFFICIENT REST AND THE OCCASIONAL VACATION TOO!

OUR BODY IS AN AMAZING SELF-HEALING MACHINE! WHAT WE NEED TO DO IS TO PROVIDE OUR BODY WITH THE NUTRIENTS REQUIRED SO THAT IT CAN REPAIR ITSELF. THEN WE NEED TO ALLOW OUR BODIES TO REST AND RECOVER.

OUR BODY IS CONSTRUCTED AT THE CELLULAR LEVEL TO BURN FAT! NOT CARBS THAT TURN INTO GLUCOSE (SUGAR).

OUR BODY REQUIRES FAT FOR 2 BIG REASONS:

1. FAT IS THE BODY'S PRIMARY SOURCE OF SUPERFUEL

   and-

2. FAT IS ESSENTIAL TO BUILD STRONG HEALTHY CELLULAR MEMBRANES.

THE ONLY SUGAR OUR ANCESTORS HAD ACCESS TO— CAME FROM NATURE. This natural sugar consisted of wild veggies, seasonal berries and the occasional BIT OF RAW HONEY. Our ancestors were not overweight or disease-ridden. Numerous archaeological studies of ancient populations, including Paleolithic populations PROVE THIS.

GENETICALLY- WE ARE 99.99 PERCENT DNA IDENTICAL TO OUR ANCESTORS. OUR HUMAN GENOME (our genes/DNA) has NOT changed. Our bodies and our brains are not designed to wear out like an old car. Our body can rebuild itself and regenerate new healthy cells. Our body can repair and rebuild our cellular mitochondria.

SUPERHEALTH BEGINS WITH HEALTHY CELLS AND HEALTHY MITOCHONDRIA. SUPERHEALTH MEANS HEALTHY MITOCHONDRIA. WE CAN FIX OUR HEALTH WHEN WE FIX OUR BUSTED CELLS. WE CAN REPAIR OUR BUSTED DYSFUNCTIONAL CARB METABOLISM.

TO FIX OUR BUSTED METABOLISM WE NEED TO ATTAIN "GLUCOSE HOMEOSTASIS"-aka low stable, steady blood sugar levels with great insulin sensitivity and cells that have healthy insulin receptors).

AS HUMANS WE STILL HAVE EXACTLY THE SAME NEEDS AS OUR ANCESTORS. BUT- According to Discovery Magazine, arguably

"WE MADE THE WORST MISTAKE IN THE HISTORY OF THE HUMAN RACE". THAT MISTAKE WAS:

> **THE TRANSITION FROM A HUNTER-GATHERER TO BECOMING A RACE OF FARMERS! Humans left the rural countryside and moved into towns and cities. The dawn of Agriculture meant the growing of GRAINS, RICE and POTATOES.**

When we moved away for our ancestral hunter-gatherer traditions, we started eating **STARCHY GRAINS**.

THIS FUNDAMENTAL TRANSITION HAD HORRENDOUS CONSEQUENCES FOR HUMANS:

- **We became shorter and weaker;**

- **We fell prey to infectious diseases caused by crowd-ed conditions and poor sanitary conditions;**

- **We lost bone strength and density;**

- **We developed dental diseases, cavities and gum diseases;**

- **We started to have shorter lifespans'**

- **WE GOT FAT FOR THE FIRST TIME- Fast-forward to the last 100 years OUR EXTERNAL AND OUR INTER-NAL SUGAR FACTORIES FIRED UP PRODUCTON.**

OUR DAILY REQUIREMENTS DO NOT INCLUDE GRAINS. Bread is not the "staff of life". Bread is a quick SUGAR FIX. PERIOD.

OUR BODIES DO NOT NEED BAD CARBS OR CARB-RICH DIETS.

THE HUMAN DIETARY REQUIREMENT FOR CARBS IS VIRTUALLY ZERO!

OUR BODIES DID NOT EVOLVE TO PROCESS THE ENORMOUS AMOUNTS OF SUGAR AND HIGH-FRUCTOSE CORN SYRUP (HFCS) THAT SATURATE ALMOST ALL OF OUR FOODS.

SUGAR FILLS OUR LIFE AND THE BLOOD IN OUR BODIES!

OUR BODIES HAVE BEEN TRANSFORMED INTO GIANT SUGAR FACTORIES!

TO BE HEALTHY—YOU MUST SET YOURSELF FREE FROM SUGAR—THAT INCLUDES THE QUEEN OF NEUROTOXINS AND HER EVIL HALF-SISTER- MADAM CARBS-☺

THESE 2 VILLAINS CAUSE OUR BODIES' "INTERNAL" SUGAR FACTORY TO BE OVERWORKED AND BREAKDOWN. OUR BODIES HAVE BECOME FLOODED WITH TOO MUCH BLOOD SUGAR.

OUR PANCREAS WORKS OVERTIME PUMPING OUT INSULIN IN AN ATTEMPT TO MOP UP THE EXCESS BLOOD SUGAR.

WE MUST SHUT DOWN OUR INTERNAL SUGAR FACTORIES—NOW!

YOU MUST SHUT DOWN YOUR INTERNAL SUGAR BY CUTTING OFF THE SUPPLY OF CARBS. YOU MUST STOP BEING A "CARBOHOLIC"!

OUR BODIES CAN EITHER BURN SUGAR OR FAT. You may "think" that your brain/body prefers a bowl of ice cream. You may be pleasantly surprised to learn that it actually prefers a piece of raw cheese or 2 pastured eggs- and some green beens slathered with grass-fed butter...yummy -☺

Paradoxically—**YOU CAN ACTUALLY EAT (in moderation) COCONUT ICE-CREAM WHICH IS 'REASONABLY' HEALTHY FOR YOU-☺**

FOR THE LAST 10 THOUSAND YEARS WE HAVE BEEN DEPRIVING OUR BODY OF ITS FAVOURITE FUEL—FATS- especially SATURATED FATS- THE MOST IMPORTANT FOOD TO MAKE US STRONG AND HEALTHY!

> **SUGAR (as in a small piece of fruit will likely not open up the doors of your internal sugar factory TOO wide—**
>
> **One apple a day might be okay—BUT—**

TWO APPLES A DAY WILL EVENTUALLY LEAD TO OBESITY AND DIABETES!

Too much sugar is too much sugar! No matter how you calculate it...

This is not an exaggeration folks! Are you in shock or disbelief? Read on.

Paradoxically—though **AVOCADOES ARE FRUITS-**

> **"AN AVOCADO A DAY—MAY KEEP THE DOCTOR AWAY" -☺**

Why is that? It's very simple.

AVOCADOES ARE LOADED WITH HEALTHY FATS! OUR BODIES AND BRAINS CRAVE HEALTHY FATS. OUR BODIES DO NOT NEED CARBS TO MAKE GLUCOSE.

THE WAY TO SHUT DOWN OUR INTERNAL SUGAR FACTORY IS QUITE SIMPLE.

JUST CUT CARBS TO THE BONE-☺

This strategy will help starve production of glucose in your internal sugar factory. You need to say to your brain- "Brain Baby…your sugar (CARB) eatin' days are gone"-☺

You need to verbalize: "I promise not to eat bad carbs which will literally eat away MY BRAIN, DESTROY MY THE MITOCHONDRIA OF MY CELLS, BUST MY METABOLISM CAUSE INSULIN RESISTANCE AND A SLEW OF METABOLIC DISEASES.

You should even write this down. Why? When you make verbal and/or written AFFIRMATIONS- YOU ARE SENDING A POWERFUL MESSAGE TO YOUR SUBCONCIOUS (95 %) and (5 %) to your CONSCIOUS MIND!

YOU ARE LITERALLY RE-PROGRAMMING AND RE-WIRING YOUR DNA! RUSSIAN RESEARCHERS HAVE PROVEN THAT WE CAN RE-PROGRAM OUR GENES IN 2 MINUTES!

I suggest writing this affirmation on your bathroom mirror. Each day you can read it.

THIS AFFIRMATION WILL HELP YOU ELIMINATE STARCHY CARBS FROM YOUR DIET. YOU CAN DITCH THAT SUGAR ADDICTION. IT JUST TAKES A BIT OF DISCIPLINE AND COURAGE.

WHEN YOU EAT FOOD- YOU'RE EITHER:

STRENGTHENING YOUR IMMUNE SYSTEM—OR YOU'RE DESTROYING YOUR IMMUNE SYSTEM. PERIOD.

WHEN YOU EAT CARBS YOU'RE "KILLING" BRAIN CELLS.

WHEN YOU EAT HEALTHY FATS—YOU ARE "BUILDING" BRAIN CELLS.

CARBS DO NOT REBUILD ANYTHING. WHEN YOU CONSUME STARCHY CARBS, YOU ARE SHORTENING YOUR LIFE. CARBS ARE NOT ESSENTIAL NUTRIENTS.

EAT FAT- GET LEAN AND HEALTHY— OR—EAT SUGAR/BAD CARBS YOU WILL FIRE UP YOUR INTERNAL SUGAR BURNING FACTORY;

and **DAMAGE YOUR CELLS**; (aka busted cells (**MITOCHONDRIAL DYSFUNCTION**) AND/OR "a busted metabolism". Busted metabolism means a metabolic disorder or metabolic disease such as diabetes, heart disease, cancer, Alzheimer's etc. etc.

How do we know this? Two ways:

FIRST: THE SCIENCE IS UNEQUIVOCAL AND CRYSTAL CLEAR.

SECOND: BRAIN MRI's/ BRAIN SCAN PHOTOS VISUALLY CONFIRM HOW BRAINS ARE DAMAGED BY SUGAR/CARBS.

A picture is worth a thousand words. If you are seriously overweight your brain likely looks like Swiss- Cheese. If you are lean and healthy, your brain is a smooth as a baby's bottom.-☺

THE BIG TAKE- HOME MESSAGE IS:

THE FATTER YOU GET- THE SMALLER THAT YOUR BRAIN GETS!

EATING TOO MANY CARBS (aka **CARB OVERLOAD/ADDICTION**)— **CAUSES OUR INTERNAL SUGAR FACTORY TO BREAKDOWN.**

THIS BREAKDOWN OR METABOLIC DISORDER OFTEN PROGRESSES TO METABOLIC SYNDROME, AND OTHER METABOLIC DISORDERS, ESPECIALLY:

"DIABETES MELLITUS- aka Type 2 Diabetes"

YOU WILL LEARN HOW TO — "RE-SET" — YOUR METABOLIC SWITCH "TO FAT BURNING MODE"!

ONCE YOUR METABOLIC DIAL IS RE-SET— IT CAN REMAIN PERMA-NENTLY ON "FAT-BURNING MODE". Our goal is to change you from a sugar/GLUCOSE BURNER into a FAT BURNER. Flipping this metabolic switch will change how your internal sugar factory processes food to make FUEL and ENERGY.

FLIPPING THIS METABOLIC SWITCH WILL ENSURE THAT YOUR BODY FUNCTIONS SAFELY AND EFFICIENTLY. I'll show you how to upregu-late your fat burning genes. You will effectively change your genetic profile— (food is information).

IT'S NOT YOUR FAULT that you're overweight; or you suffer symp-toms of metabolic syndrome, DIABETES or worse. You're not carrying around extra abdominal flab because you eat TOO MUCH. You're overweight because you have been MISINFORMED!

YOU HAVE BEEN LIED TO AND BRAINWASHED BY BIG FOOD. BIG GOVERNMENT, BIG PHARMA AND A CORRUPT MEDICAL ESTABLISHMENT.

YOU HAVE BEEN FUELING YOUR BODY WITH CARBS. YOU HAVE BEEN ERRONEOUSLY TOLD TO EAT SEVERAL SMALL MEALS PER DAY!

EATING SEVERAL CARB MEALS EACH DAY IS SHEER MADNESS! EATING FREQUENTLY CAUSES YOUR BLOOD SUGAR AND INSULIN LEVELS TO GO UP AND DOWN LIKE A YO-YO!

YOU MUST STOP TREATING YOUR METABOLISM LIKE A YO-YO!

Your digestive system and your sugar factory are working OVERTIME 24/7! Do you honestly believe that our ancestors scarfed down food several times a day? They didn't even have a constant assured supply of food. Before they could kill food; they had to track and find it. Wild game is tough to kill- even if you have a high-powered rifle. To get up close to kill an animal with a spear or knife is not an easy job. Our ancestors needed to be agile, quick and smart. Most Western urban dwellers have never killed anything bigger than a mosquito. They have no clue about the time and effort required to hunt wild game.

Getting off an addictive substance will not be easy for most people.

KICKING YOUR SUGAR ADDICTION AND SHUTTING DOWN YOUR SUGAR FACTORY WILL TAKE DISCIPLINE AND COURAGE.

DIETING CAN BE A LONELY BUSINESS—I PROMISE YOU WHEN YOU HAVE THE COURAGE AND DISCIPLINE TO EMBARK ON A KETOGENIC NUTRITIONAL APPROACH...YOU WILL FOREVER BE HAPPY THAT YOU DID!

You may have to endure the ridicule of friends and neighbours. Just wait until they see how effortlessly the pounds melt off...they will be envious...they will ask you what you are doing. Your friends and neighbours will to desperately know what your SECRET WEIGHT LOSS PROGRAM IS! You can reply you eat as much HEALTHY FAT AS YOU DESIRE. Scientists and researchers refer to this as eating FAT AD LIBITUM- aka freely and as much as you like.

If you're reading this book, I'm confident that you can get the job done. You have the necessary courage and discipline adopt the Ketogenic Diet and Lifestyle. Do you have the necessary intestinal fortitude TO MAKE A FUNDAMENTAL DIETARY CHANGE? Are you willing to change your genes?

ARE YOU READY TO TRANSFORM YOUR BODY & TRANSFORM EVERY PART OF YOUR LIFE? Imagine how great your life will be without headaches, upset stomachs, drugs, drugstores, hospital visits AND DOCTOR VISITS! Imagine how much time, IN

PROPER NUTRITION IS THE KEY TO SUPERHEALTH.

PROPER NUTRITION IS A LOW-CARB, HIGH-FAT MODERATE PROTEIN DIET.

THE WAY TO SHUT DOWN YOUR INTERNAL SUGAR FACTORY IS VERY SIMPLE-

"ELIMINATE AS MANY CARBS FROM YOUR DIET AS YOU CAN- AS SOON AS CAN.

YOU NEED TO MAKE YOUR MITOCHONDRIA HAPPY. YOU NEED TO FIX YOUR BUSTED MITOCHONDRIA. WHEN YOU DEPRIVE YOUR MITOCHONDRIA FROM TOO MUCH TOXIC BLOOD GLUCOSE YOU WILL FIX YOUR BUSTED BRAIN- YOU WILL ALSO GET YOUR BRAIN OFF SUGAR.

WHEN YOU CURE YOUR CARB ADDICTION- YOU WILL TAKE A GIANT STEP TOWARDS SUPERHEALTH.

E. DIABETES MELLITUS

Introduction

YOU CAN TAKE YOUR OWN HEALTH BACK INTO YOUR OWN HANDS. You can free yourself from the shackles of constant blood sugar readings, daily drug regimens and even prevent the horrible health complications that await diabetics down the road.

I have reviewed many scientific studies and powerful medical research—which has been used by smart healthcare professionals to help THOUSANDS OF DIABETICS AROUND THE WORLD.

I could not sit by idly, while diabetics SUFFER NEEDLESSLY THEIR WHOLE LIVES; waste their money on useless treatments, and then DIE A HORRIBLE DEATH FROM HORRIBLE COMPLICATIONS; while the greedy pharmaceutical companies line their pockets with your hard-earned cash.

YOU DESERVE TO KNOW THE TRUTH ABOUT OUR FRAUDULENT MEDICAL/DRUG SYSTEM AND THE QUASI-CRIMINAL BEHAVIOUR RAMPANT IN THE DIABETIC INDUSTRY!

THE TREATMENT OF DIABETICS BY ALLOPATHIC DOCTORS IS A MEDICAL CRIME AGAINST HUMANITY!

DIETARY INTERVENTIONS ARE FAR SAFER, FAR MORE EFFECTIVE AND MUCH LESS EXPENSIVE.

AM I A HEALTH ALARMIST? ABSOLUTELY!

THIS IS NOT A CONSPIRACY THEORY FOLKS. IT'S CALLED MEDICAL FRAUD.

IT'S TIME TO PUT AN END TO CRIMINAL NEGLIGENCE IN THE HEALTHCARE INDUSTRY/DIABETIC INDUSTRY.

THE ILL-TREATMENT OF DIABETICS HAS GOT TO STOP- NOW!

DIABETICS! THE TIME HAS COME TO RISE UP AND THROW YOUR POISONOUS DRUGS IN THE RECYCLE BIN! All diabetics who leave near Lake Michigan—kindly refrain with flushing YOUR METFORMIN diabetic drugs down your toilet. It appears that LAKE MICHIGAN has already over-dosed on metformin!-☺

YOU HAVE THE POWER TO WEAN YOURSELF OFF POISONOUS, TOXIC DRUGS AND REPLACE THEM WITH SUPERFOODS AND A KETOGENIC DIET.

RESEARCH SHOWS THAT TYPE 2- DIABETES CAN BE REVERSED IN A SINGLE DAY!

RESEARCH SHOW THAT TYPE 1-DIABETES CAN BE REVERSED IN 3 WEEKS (unless the cells have been damaged by strong antibiotics),

RESEARCH PROVES THAT A LOW-CARB, KETOGENIC DIET EASILY AND PAINLESSLY REVERSES DIABETES BY REVERSING INSULIN RESISTANCE!

Background

Diabetes Mellitus is often colloquially referred to as "sugar diabetes." The word "mellitus" in Latin means "of honey". The term diabetes mellitus appears to have been coined in 1745. In feudal times, sugar was very hard to obtain. It was treasured by the European nobility who obtained it from traders and explorers. Then in the 1600s sugar started to become more globally available with the start-up of tropical sugar plantations. Nevertheless, its scarcity and high price meant that it was not widely available to most people.

It appears that circa 1700, the average sugar consumption (among those having access to sugar) was about 3 <u>POUNDS PER YEAR</u>.

In 2015, THE <u>AVERAGE SUGAR CONSUMPTION</u> by North Americans was <u>A WHOPPING 185 POUNDS PER YEAR!</u>

<u>ADD A WHOPPING 150 POUNDS OF FLOUR CONSUMED also ALSO-AND YOU HAVE CREATED A PRESCRIPTION FOR DISASTER!</u>

In the 1880's in the United States diabetes began to increase very gradually.

Can you guess how diabetes (type 2) was treated by the "<u>PHYSICIANS</u>" <u>OF THAT ERA</u>?

<u>DIABETES WAS TREATED WITH A LOW CARB APPROACH!</u>

<u>Yes, it's true</u>— dear readers. Diabetes was treated in those days with "A LOW-CARB- HIGH FAT DIET. <u>OMG!</u>

What happened? Big Pharma came along with her drugs. If your business is selling drugs—do your really have any incentive to cure disease? The Flexner report changed the entire health care business er…sick-care business supra chapter one).

<u>THEN CAME THOSE "MARVELOUS" PHARMACEUTICALS TO THE RESCUE!</u> The only thing rescued has been the bank accounts of pill pushers.

Dr. Rath, a leading health researcher stated:

> "Throughout the 20<u>th</u> Century, the pharmaceutical industry has been constructed by investors, the goal being to replace effective but non-patentable natural remedies with mostly ineffective but patentable and highly profitable pharmaceutical drugs. The very nature of the pharmaceutical industry is to make money from ongoing diseases. Like other industries the pharmaceutical industry tries to expand their market—that is to maintain ongoing diseases and to find new diseases for their drugs."

Prevention and cures for diseases hurt the pharmaceutical business. The eradication of common diseases threatens its very existence. Therefore, the pharmaceutical industry fights the eradication of disease at all costs.

The Pharmaceutical Industry itself is the main obstacle. This is the real reason why most widespread diseases are further expanding— including heart attacks, strokes, cancer, high blood pressure, diabetes, osteoporosis, etc. etc. Pharmaceutical drugs are not intended to cure diseases. According to health insurers, over 24,000 pharmaceutical drugs are currently marketed and prescribed without any proven therapeutic value. (source: AK Magazine, 4/98)

100 years later after the creation of the new "allopathic medical profession" doctors and Big Pharma are making BAZILLIONS OF DOLLARS TREATING DIABETICS WITH DRUGS.

Here are some figures:

* THE DIABETIC/DRUG INDUSTRY EARNS 300 BILLION DOLLARS YEARLY!

According to a recent study: A PATIENT DIAGNOSED WITH DIABETES IS WORTH $ 750,000.00 FROM DIAGNOSIS UNTIL DEATH.

ARE BOATLOADS OF DIABETES DRUGS AND BLOOD-SUGAR PILLS HELPING? NO! NO!

POISONOUS DRUGS ARE KILLING THOUSANDS OF PEOPLE; CAUSING CANCER, CARDIOVASCULAR PROBLEMS ALZHEIMER'S AND A BOATLOAD OF OTHER DISEASES. Meanwhile, Big Pharma and its lackeys are getting rich from your misery.

What is Type 1 Diabetes?

Type 1 diabetes is a separate kind of disease from the other forms of diabetes. Type 1 appears to be an autoimmune disorder- which accounts for about 5 percent of all diabetes. People with Type 1 diabetes make no insulin (or very little) because their immune system attacks and destroys the beta-cells in their pancreas that make INSULIN. Type 1 Diabetics do not make insulin; the hormone required for processing carbohydrates and other nutrients. People with Type 1 Diabetes allegedly require insulin to deal with high blood sugar with an appropriate dose of synthetic insulin.

Most often allopathic doctors prescribe DAILY INSULIN INJECTIONS. Mainstream "medical" people theorize that these insulin (hormone) injections are required to balance blood sugar levels. Prescribing synthetic insulin aggravates TYPE 1 (and Type 2) Diabetes' health CAUSES EVEN MORE HEALTH PROBLEMS. Type 1 -diabetes is typically diagnosed in young children and in adolescents.

ESSENTIAL FACTS YOU NEED TO KNOW—

1. TYPE-1 DIABETES IS ANOTHER SYPHOSTICATED EXAMPLE OF "BUSTED BETA CELLS" aka- "MITOCHONDRIAL DYSFUNC-TION." DIABETES – LIKE OBESITY IS A METABOLIC DISEASE.

2. TYPE -1 DIABETES IS WIDELY PROMOTED AS "INCURABLE" BY THE CONVENTIONAL MEDICAL ESTABLISHMENT. Technically, this may not be true. TYPE- 1 DIABETES CAN BE REVERSED BY DIET AND LIFESTYLE CHANGES- e.g. THE KETOGENIC DIET.

3. TYPE -1 DIABETES HAS BEEN PEGGED AS– "AN AUTO-IMMUNE DISEASE".

4. RESEARCH SUGGESTS THAT THERE IS A STRONG POSSIBIL-ITY THAT IT IS CAUSED BY CHILDHOOD VACCINATIONS! There can be little doubt that there is a strong correla-tion between the development of Type 1 diabetes and IM-MUNIZATIONS IN INFANTS AND YOUNG CHILDREN.

   Science tell us how Type 1 is caused; human genetics play a very limited role. EPIGENETICS tells us that we can re-program most of our genes. Type 1 diabetes IS NOT THE DEATH SENTENCE AS MODERN MEDICINE CLAIMS.

5. TYPE -1 DIABETICS ARE EXTREMELY ILL-TREATED BY MOST AL-LOPATHIC DOCTORS! These ill-informed doctors are doing more harm than good with their poisonous pharmaceuticals.

6. YOU NEED TO KNOW THAT POPULAR NOTIONS ABOUT THE "LIFE-SAVING" VALUE OF SYNTHETIC INSULIN ARE MYTHS! ... Propagated by the Biotech Industry and Big Pharma.

7. PROTEINS BREAKDOWN INTO AMINO ACIDS AND THEIR SE-QUENCE CAN PROMOTE INFLAMMATION. Researchers are finding that although such triggers, as gluten cause an au-toimmune response in people with Celiac disease-or glu-ten sensitivity, it is the chain of amino acids that are con-tained in the gluten which damage the small intestine.

8. WHEAT, SOY, AND MILK HAVE ALL BEEN ASSOCIATED WITH TYPE-1 DIABETES DUE TO HOW THE BODY PERCEIVES THE PRO-TEIN CONTAINED IN THESE COMMON FOOD ALLERGENS.

9. COUNTRIES THAT CONSUME REFINED WHEAT FLOUR AS A MAJOR FOOD SOURCE FOUND THAT THERE IS A HIGHER INCIDENCE OF TYPE-1 DIABETES.

RECENT STUDIES SHOW THAT SYNTHETIC INSULIN IS KILLING PEOPLE; CAUSING CANCER AND MAJOR CARDIOVASCULAR "EVENTS.

"Events" is polite word used by Big Pharma to indicate **DEATH AND OTHER "BAD EVENTS"** which includes heart attacks, strokes; comas, and every kind a "horrific health problems"!

YOU NEED TO KNOW ABOUT THE HORRIFIC EFFECTS CAUSED BY DIABETIC DRUGS PRESCRIBED BY ALLOPATHIC DOCTORS.

In a recent study, 6,484 patients with type 2 diabetes who were prescribed "progressive" INSULIN MONOTHERAPY (only insulin) from 2000 for 3.3 years were tracked.

THE RESULTS not progressive; the results were HORRIFIC! The results were reported as follows: * DEATHS- 1,110, * MACE" (Major Cardiovascular Events: 342 and CANCER DIAGNOSES: 382;

The take-home message is:

Insulin monotherapy like ALL other drugs have HORRIFIC DIRECT EFFECTS! Drug effects are NOT SIDE EFFECTS!

HOW CAN DEATH BE CONSIDERED A SIDE EFFECT!!

In another 2013 study composed of 85,000 Type 2 Diabetic patients, it was found that INSULIN MONOTHERAPY DOUBLED THE RISK OF ALL CAUSE MORTALITY IN ADDITION TO SIGNIFICANTLY INCREASING THEIR RISK FO CANCER AND "OTHER DIABETES- RELATED " COMPLICATIONS.

In another Japanese study found that "Insulin administration may trigger TYPE 1 DIABETES in Japanese TYPE 2 DIABETES patients with Type 1 Diabetes High-risk HLA Class II and the insulin gene VNTR genotype."

Enough said about horrors of synthetic insulin and diabetes drugs. For more studies/information you can consult www. PubMed.com or sites such as www. GreenMedInfo.com

THERE ARE DOZENS OF CLINICAL STUDIES SHOWING THERAPEUTIC CLINICAL RESULTS OF HOW MANY PEOPLE ARE KILLED BY DIABETIC AND/OR BLOOD-SUGAR LOWERING DRUGS.

Type -1 diabetes (Juvenile-onset diabetes) primarily affects children and young adults. People with Type 1 diabetes are often of normal weight. In the months prior to being diagnosed they have lost weight inexplicably.

Type-1 diabetes is caused by death of most of the body's insulin-producing pancreatic beta cells (allegedly from an unknown cause). Severe deficiency of insulin causes high blood sugar and rapid weight loss. Standard treatment consists of self-administration of the insulin you lack using a syringe.

What is TYPE 2 DIABETES?

This most common form of diabetes is often abbreviated in the medical/ clinical literature as TD2—an acronym.

TD2 — A WORLDWIDE HEALTH ISSUE, IS A CLUSTER OF METABOLIC DISEASES CHARACTERIZED BY HYPERGLYCEMIA THAT RESULT FROM DEFECTS IN INSULIN SECRETION/ AND/OR ACTION.

TD 2 is another classic example of "BUSTED CELLS". People with TD2 are capable of producing insulin- but their bodies do not respond adequately. They are said to be "insulin-resistant". As a consequence, they have deteriorating function of the pancreas, the insulin producing organ that cannot keep up with the demands of an insulin-resistant body.

CONVENTIONAL MEDICINE HAS T2-D WRONGLY DIAGNOSED AS "A PROBLEM WITH ELEVATED BLOOD SUGAR". THIS IS A CLASSIC EXAMPLE OF A FLAWED UNDERSTANDING BY CONVENTIONAL DOCTORS.

It might be hard to believe but when you prick your finger with a meter and see a blood sugar reading of let's say 250- it's NOT NECESSARILY BECAUSE YOU HAVE DIABETES! Some people can walk around with blood sugar as high as 300- without having diabetes. Conversely, some skinny people are diabetics or pre-diabetics!

What causes Type 2 Diabetes? What is Type 2 Diabetes?

Diabetes today is diagnosed not by measuring the sugar in your urine. Today, diabetes is diagnosed by measuring glucose in the blood serum. The current diagnostic criteria uses blood glucose of 126 or greater to indicate diabetes. In addition, the haemoglobin A1C test, which measures the percentage of glycated (caramel sugar-coated) haemoglobin in the red cell is diagnostic of diabetes at 6.5% or greater in the blood); the condition is slightly more complex than that.

Diabetes is really <u>BLOOD-SUGAR DYSREGULATION</u> (aka busted carb metabolism). The body has lost its ability to regulate and control blood glucose levels. This can occur during a resting state, an active state, a fasting state or a post-prandial (after eating) state. It can be affected by numerous factors; sleep quality or disruption, physical activity level and fitness, STRESS, hormone balance, immune system health, organ function- such as liver, thyroid and kidneys, digestive system, AND THE STRUCTURAL INTEGRITY OF THE CELL MEMBRANE (aka busted cells and busted mitochondria).

At the end of the day, the cause of type 2- diabetes is loss in the ability of the body to regulate the complex blood sugar system. The reasons this happens vary from one person to the next. What appears to be universal are problems caused by insulin. Insulin's main job is to store sugar into cells and tissues. In particular insulin is released in the presence of glucose and amino acids in order to open the door to the cells and allow them to soak up and absorb glucose and important nutrients for energy production and storage.

In type 2- diabetes, the pancreas is typically producing <u>PLENTY OF INSULIN</u>. In fact, <u>MOST TYPE 2 DIABETICS ARE HYPERINSULINEMIC (i.e. TOO MUCH INSULIN IN THE BLOOD.)</u>

<u>WHAT CAUSES INSULIN-RESISTANCE?</u>

<u>TOO MUCH INSULIN!!</u>

<u>INSULIN AND LEPTIN RESISTANCE ARE THE REAL CULPRITS UNDERLYING DIABETES AND MANY OTHER METABOLIC DISORDERS.</u>

The cells- liver, muscle, kidneys, fat cells, etc. have become resistant to the effects of insulin. These cells have become desensitized to insulin. These cells have reduced the number of insulin receptors to protect themselves against insulin. After years of being bombarded by too many carbs, too much sugar, the wrong fats, and lack of physical activity the mitochondria of our cells become badly impaired.

<u>THE TOXIC BURDEN FROM OUR ENVIRONMENT, FOOD SUPPLY, OXIDATIVE STRESS, AND FREE RADICALS ALL CAUSE OUR CELL RECEPTORS FOR INSULIN TO STOP WORKING.</u>

A genius named Dr. Alex Vasquez, M.D. Ph.D says: "The Data is impressively clear"-

<u>"THOSE WITH TYPE 2 DIABETES, METABOLIC SYNDROME, AND HIGH BLOOD PRESSURE HAVE DYSFUNCTIONAL MITOCHONDRIA".</u>

He explains:

INFLAMMATION IS DIVIDED IN 3 DIFFERENT FORMS THAT EXIST ON A CONTINUUM AND OVERLAP EACH OTHER-namely:

1. 1. METABOLIC INFLAMMATION (conditions such as DIABETES and hypertension)

2. 2. ALLERGIC INFLAMMATION

3. 3. AUTOIMMUNE INFLAMMATION

CHRONIC, LOW-LEVEL INFLAMMATION which tends to underlie most chronic health conditions, Dr. Vasquez describes as:

"METABOLIC DISTURBANCE WITH CELLULAR INJURY."

MITOCHONDRIAL DYSFUNCTION (or "Busted Mitochondria-my technical term-☺ IS INVOLVED IN VIRTUALLY ALL DISEASES!!

This includes:

TYPE 2 DIABETES, OBESITY, METABOLIC SYNDROME, HYPERTENSION, CANCER, HEART DISEASE, AUTOIMMUNE DISEASES, ALZHHEIMER'S DISEASE, PARKINSON, DEPRESSION, CHRONIC FATIGUE SYNDROME, ASTHMA AND ALLERGIES, FIBROMYALGIA, ETC.

YOUR MITOCHONDRIA PERFORM MANY IMPORTANT FUNCTIONS IN YOUR BODY. These include, inter alia:

- MOST OF YOUR BODY'S ENERGY IN THE FORM OF ATP

- CELLULAR SIGNALLING

- AN IMPORTANT ROLE CONTROLLING INFLAMMATION

ALL OF THESE FUNCTIONS MAKE YOUR MITOCHONDRIA KEY PLAYERS IN ALL OF THE ABOVE-MENTIONED DISEASES-AND PERHAPS MORE.

Age-associated decline in mitochondrial function contributes to insulin resistance in elderly. Research shows that the elderly have a slightly higher plasma glucose concentrations and SIGNIFICANTLY HIGHER PLASMA INSULIN CONCENTRATIONS.

Oral glucose tolerance tests given to elderly patients show that the elderly are relatively insulin-resistant as compared to the younger controls. To determine what tissues were responsible for insulin resistance, hyperinsulinemic-euglycemic clamp studies were performed.

RESULTS SHOWED THAT MITOCHONDRIAL OXIDATIVE AND PHOSPHORYLATION ACTIVITY WERE BOTH REDUCED BY 40 PERCENT IN THE ELDERLY AS COMPARED TO THE YOUNG CONTROLS.

THIS MEANT THAT THERE WAS AGE-ASSOCIATED REDUCTION IN MITOCHONDRIAL NUMBER AND/OR FUNCTION.

BECAUSE MITOCHONDRIAL OXIDATIVE AND PHOSPHORYLATION ACTIVITY IS A MAJOR SOURCE OF ENERGY IN MOST ORGANS-INCLUDING THE BRAIN, ALL OF THE DATA SUPPORT THE HYPOTHESIS THAT A DECLINE IN MITOCHONDRIAL OXIDATIVE PHOSPHORYLATION ENERGY PRODUCTION PLAYS AN IMPORTANT ROLE IN AGING.

FURTHERMORE, BECAUSE MITOCHONDRIAL ENERGY METABOLISM PLAYS A CRITICAL ROLE IN GLUCOSE-INDUCED INSULIN SECRETION, SIMILAR AGE-ASSOCIATED REDUCTIONS IN PANCREATIC BETA-CELL MITOCHONDRIAL FUNCTION, IN THE SETTING OF PERIPHERAL INSULIN RESISTANCE HELPS EXPLAIN THE HIGH PREVALENCE OF DIABETES IN THE ELDERLY.

FOLKS —

THIS IS A FANCY WAY OF SAYING THAT ELDERLY PEOPLE HAVE BUSTED MITOCHONDRIA/BUSTED CELLS. Busted mitochondria cause insulin resistance that then causes—TYPE 2 DIABETES.

In February 2015, scientists and researchers at the University of California again proved that:

"TYPE 2 DIABETES IS CAUSED BY INFLAMMATION.

RESEARCHERS DISCOVERED THAT AN INFLAMMATORY MOLECULE CALLED LTB 4 CAUSES INSULIN RESISTANCE. AND— THEN INSULIN RESISTANCE LEADS TO HIGH BLOOD SUGAR AND DIABETES."

This is why treating your blood sugar with drugs and injecting insulin to combat insulin sensitivity will NEVER HEAL YOUR DIABETES!

DOCTORS ARE NOT TREATING THE ROOT CAUSE OF DIABETES—ONLY THE SYMPTOMS OF DIABETES.

HERE ARE COMMON SYMPTOMS OF DIABETES

- EXCESSIVE THIRST AND AN ABNORMALLY HIGH URINE PRODUCTION-This is because periodically your blood sugar is so high e.g. above 15 mmol/L or 270 mg/d/L – that it leaks out into urine- pulling fluid from the body

- A WORSENING VISION. Too high sugar makes the lens in the eye swell and you will become near-sighted

- FATIGUE

With Type 1 Diabetes you may inexplicably <u>LOSE WEIGHT AND YOUR BREATH MAY SMELL OF ACETONE</u> (nail polish remover). With milder forms of diabetes or pre-diabetes, you often don't notice <u>ANYTHING</u> but sugar may be damaging your body.

<u>DIABETICS USUALLY HAVE 10 TIMES MORE INSULIN IN THEIR BODIES THAN NORMAL HEALTHY PEOPLE.</u>

When you shut down your sugar factory, you will shut off your insulin pump. Maintaining a low stable blood sugar level and become insulin SENSITIVE is the paramount key to <u>SUPERHEALTH</u>.

Allopathic doctors treat diabetes the same way they treat a cold or the flu. How is a cold or flu treated? What are the symptoms of the flu? Fever and congestion- what is the cause of the flu itself?—a virus. If we treat the <u>SYMPTOMS</u> of the flu; bring down the fever; take some decongestants; will that <u>CURE THE FLU</u>? <u>NO</u>! <u>NO</u>!

It will make you feel a bit better but it will not in any way make the flu better; because you have not treated the <u>FLU ITSELF</u>. You have simply treated the <u>SYMPTOMS</u>. You are still sick with the FLU, but you now feel a bit better. Actually these decongestants slow down your body from its natural healing by producing a fever.

Let's take another example. Let's say you broke your leg. What are the <u>SYMPTOMS</u>? Bleeding and lots of pain- if you take pain killers and wrap your leg in a bandage to stop the bleeding- have you fixed your <u>BROKEN LEG</u>? <u>NO</u>! <u>NO</u>! You simply treated symptoms. You still have a problem; <u>A BROKEN LEG</u>!

SO- how does this compare to Diabetes? It's exactly the same.

<u>THE BIGGEST "SYMPTOM" OF DIABETES IS ELEVATED BLOOD SUGAR.</u>

What do chowder-headed doctors do? They prescribe pills to lower blood sugar and insulin to help with insulin resistance. Have you actually done anything to treat <u>DIABETES ITSELF</u>? <u>NO</u>! <u>NO</u>! <u>THIS MEDICAL TREATMENT IS LIKE POURING GASOLINE ON A FIRE!</u>

Doctors have simply treated the symptoms of diabetes; so again- you are still sick. You still sick. Any beneficial effect works because of the "placebo effect."(aka sugar pill/psychological effect). What your doctor says to you when he sells you a pill can actually greatly affect how well the sugar pill effect works. For example, your doctor likely knows that he can easily <u>SCAM</u> you by asking you whether you want diabetic drugs that cost 2 dollars each or whether you want to buy the new super-duper diabetic drugs that cost $ 20 dollars each.

Which pill do you think most naïve people will buy?

REMEMBER THE 99 PERCENT RULE?

YOUR DOCTOR IS A DRUG SELLING SCAM ARTIST. AT LEAST SNAKE-OIL SALESMEN SELL YOU SOMETHING THAT COULD POSSIBLY BE HEALTHY FOR YOU- SNAKE OIL!-☺

What if you have a problem during your sleep? Getting rushed to the hospital while the paramedics break all of your ribs giving you CPR WILL BE HELL ON EARTH!

Spending your last few moments with tubes, pumps and ventilators in unbearable agony—YOU WILL WISH THAT YOU DID SOMETHING SMARTER SOONER!

HERE ARE 3 BIG DIABETES LIES-

1. T2D is something that you're stuck with for life;

2. You must take Diabetes DRUGS, insulin injections and measure blood sugar until the day you die;

3. Prescription drugs are the best way to battle this disease; and as long as you take your prescribed medication, you are safe from an early death. NO! NO!

THESE ARE LIES- LIES-LIES!

THESE ARE LIES PERPETRATED BY BIG PHARMA TO KEEP YOU SICK AND HOOKED ON DRUGS! ; Just more Big Pharma medical "excreta"-☺

DIABETES CAN BE REVERSED IN A FEW DAYS! How?

BY EATING A LOW CARB KETOGENIC DIET- APPROPRIATE EXERCISE… and BY MAKING LIFE-STYLE CHANGES.

THERE ARE A BOATLOAD OF REPUTABLE SCIENTIFIC STUDIES THAT PROVE DIABETES CAN BE REVERSED-EASILY AND QUICKLY!

Diabetics have been kept in the dark about THESE POWERFUL LIFE-SAVING STRATEGIES, Can you hear that glorious sound KA-CHING! KA-CHING!

Big Pharma has netted themselves 370 million customers and trillions in profits.

BIG PHARMA HAS CONDEMNED HUNDREDS OF MILLIONS OF PEOPLE TO A CERTAIN EARLY DEATH- ALL IN THE NAME OF PROFITS.

DIABETES HAS MUSHROOMED INTO A 300 BILLION DOLLAR INDUSTRY!

HOT OFF THE PRESS – YOU HAVE THE DIABETES SOLUTION!

HERE IS THE LATEST DIABETES STUDY!-

PLEASE NOTE THE WORD "CURE"! OMG!

Dr. Gowen, a lead author explained:

> **"DIABETES IS A DISEASE OF CARBOHYDRATE INTOLERANCE"**
>
> **FOR MANY PEOPLE WITH TYPE 2 DIABETES—LOW-CARBOHYDRATE DIETS ARE A REAL CURE".**
>
> **They no longer need drugs. They no longer have symptoms. Their blood glucose is normal. And they generally lose weight"**

On July 24th, 2014, Dr. Barbara Gower PhD, Professor of Nutritional Sciences, joined a CONSORTIUM of 26 eminent Nutrition researchers and published this EARTH-SHATTERING STUDY!

The researchers also included some world- renowned KETOGENIC DOCTORS including, inter alia- Dr. Eric Westman, Dr. Mary C. Vernon and Dr. Jeff Volek.

These authors concluded:

LOW-CARBOHYDRATE DIETS SHOULD BE THE FIRST POINT OF ATTACK IN THE MANAGEMENT OF TYPE 1 AND TYPE 2 -DIABETES.

Dr. Gower continued:

> **"Reducing carbohydrates is the obvious treatment. It was the standard treatment before insulin was discovered. It is in fact practised with good results in many institutions".**

THESE AUTHORS say that their review of the medical literature shows that low-carb diets reliably reduce high blood sugar—the most salient feature of diabetes- and at the same time show general benefit for the risk of CARDIOVASCULAR DISEASE-(CVD).

12 POINTS OF EVIDENCE BACKED UP BY CLINICAL STUDIES ARE:

1. High blood sugar is the most salient feature of Diabetes. Dietary carbohydrate restriction has the great-

est effect on decreasing blood glucose levels.

2. During the epidemics of obesity and Type 2 Diabetes, caloric increases have been due almost entirely to increased carbohydrates.

3. Benefits of dietary carbohydrate restriction do not require weight loss.

4. Although weight loss is not required for benefit, no dietary intervention is better than carbohydrate restriction for weight loss.

5. Adherence to low-carb diets in people with Type 2 Diabetes is at least as good as adherence to other dietary intervention and frequently is significantly better.

6. Replacement of carbohydrates with proteins is generally beneficial.

7. Dietary total and saturated fats do not correlate with risk of cardiovascular disease.

8. Plasma-saturated fatty acids are controlled by dietary carbohydrates more than by dietary lipids.

9. The best production of microvascular and to a lesser extent, macrovascular complications in patients with Type 2 Diabetes is GLYCEMIC CONTROL (HbAlc).

10. Dietary carbohydrate restriction is the most effective method of reducing serum triglycerides and increasing high-density lipoprotein.

11. Patients with Type 2 Diabetes on carbohydrate restricted diets reduce and frequently eliminate medication. People with Type 1 Diabetes usually require less insulin.

12. Intensive glucose-lowering by dietary carbohydrate restriction has no side-effects comparable to the effects of intensive pharmacologic treatment.

Some people suggest that diabetics should seek help from a <u>physician</u> to help "tapering off drugs" to avoid dangerous low-blood sugar. If you were an alcoholic- would you ask for nutritional advice from your local bartender? If your doctor is a pill-pusher- he will not be pleased that you wish to replace his dope with good food. Didn't your physician tell you to eat a low-fat – high –carb diet?

<u>THAT HORRIBLE ADVICE TURNED YOU INTO A DIABETIC IN THE FIRST PLACE!</u> Then your brainwashed doctor prescribed a poisonous drug to you to counter the horrendous effects of the first/other drugs…

THAT POISONOUS DIABETES DRUG HAS MADE YOUR HEALTH WORSE!

DOES IT MAKE SENSE TO ASK FOR NUTRITIONAL ADVICE FROM A DOCTOR WHO PRESCRIBED A DIET THAT CAUSED YOU TO BECOME DIABETIC?

Does it make sense to ask a pyromaniac advice on how to extinguish a fire that <u>HE</u> has started?

My advice is—to use your common sense. Think for yourself. Taking advice from a doctor who prescribed poisonous food that made you sick; and then prescribed a drug that has made you even sicker... Asking the same doctor for medical advice is <u>SHEER LUNACY!</u>

Listen to your body. You know how you feel when you <u>EAT ANY KIND OF FOOD</u>. You also know how you feel when you <u>EAT DRUGS</u>.

Who determines if, when or how many drugs you have taken? Research shows that most people do not take their "meds" regularly. Sometimes, people get off drugs by accident. They forget to take their "medications" and then realize that they feel better without them.

Have you ever exercised and then felt good so that you took fewer drugs? Why is this?

<u>EXERCISE IS FAR BETTER MEDICINE THAN ANY CHEMICAL EVER INVENTED!</u>

IF YOU ARE TAKING ANY KIND OF DRUGS AND DO EXERCISE- YOU ARE AT RISK OF CAUSING SERIOUS HEALTH PROBLEMS!

<u>TAKING DRUGS WITH EXERCISE CAN KILL OR SERIOUSLY INJURY YOU!</u>

For example, if you take <u>STATIN DRUGS</u> – the research shows that <u>YOU ARE AT GREAT RISK FOR SUDDEN HEART ATTACKS, KIDNEY FAILURES,, etc. & ALL KINDS OF PROBLEMS! RHABDOMYLYSIS (a serious kidney disease IS OFTEN CAUSED BY MIXING STATINS AND EXERCISE!</u>

<u>ALSO</u>— good food and drugs do not mix well either. (e.g. Coumadin and blood pressure meds do not mix well with citrus fruit).

Did your physician warn you about the dangers of taking diabetes/ other drugs while doing strenuous exercise? Oops- another reason to fire your doctor.-☺ You should be very careful because exercise will lower your blood sugar (a good thing), but combined with the blood-sugar lowering of a toxic drug might overwhelm your body and cause a heart attack!

TAKING CARE OF YOUR HEALTH BEGINS WITH ELIMINATING POISONOUS DRUGS AND TOXIC FOOD FROM YOUR BODY.

ONCE THAT IS DONE- YOU NEED TO EAT DELICIOUS NUTRITIOUS FATTY FOODS TO HEAL YOURSELF.

YOU ARE THE PERSON WHO CAN BEST WEAN YOURSELF OFF OF POISONOUS DRUGS. Who knows your body best? Your doctor's best advice is to take a pill and call him in the morning.

YOU are your own doctor; YOU are your patient; YOU are your patient's advocate.

YOU ARE THE BOSS OF YOUR BODY AND YOU ARE THE BOSS OF YOUR OWN HEALTH! YOUR BODY IS A CHEMISTRY SET—AND YOU ARE THE CHEMIST.

MEDICAL DOCTORS SHOULD NOT LEGALLY BE PERMITTED TO GIVE NUTRITIONAL ADVICE! THEY HAVE NO TRAINING IN NUTRITION. They are hurting people with their bad nutritional advice! And the worst irony of all- the recommendation to speak to your doctor BEFORE YOU EXERCISE! What your doctor knows about exercise could fit on the end of a pencil.

The public is catching on fast to the nutritional incompetence of physicians. You can help spread the word. Tell your friends, neighbours and loved ones. Let's stop the madness of "a pill for every ill" approach to health. You have the POWER to help thousands of people who you will never even know. You CAN affect the lives of thousands of people.

MOST DOCTORS VIOLATE THE MOST SACRED RULE OF MEDICINE!

Dr. Hippocrates, the Father of Medicine said: "FIRST DO NO HARM."

An old adage says: "Fool me once, shame on you; fool me twice, shame on me."

Dr. Richard Feinman, (a Ketogenic proponent, lead author of this wonderful study above, concluded with these VERY POSITIVE WORDS:

> "We've tried to present clearly the most obvious and least controversial arguments for going with carbohydrate restriction. Here we take a positive approach and look to the future- while acknowledging this paper calls for change. The low-fat paradigm, which held things back is virtually dead as a major biological idea. Diabetes is too serious a disease for us to try to save face by holding onto ideas that fail."

From this study you can see that low-carb diets are <u>NOW</u> recognized as the key dietary approach to treat and reverse <u>DIABETES</u>.

<u>YOUR HEALTH SOLUTION TO REVERSE DIABETES IS A LOW-CARB DIET.</u>

<u>DIABETICS NEED TO GET DOWN TO LESS THAN 25 GRAMS/DAY OF CARBS. TYPE-2 DIABETES IS REVERSED 'CURED" BY INGESTING NO MORE THAN 25 GRAMS OF CARBS EACH DAY.</u>

<u>CLINICAL STUDIES AND SCIENTIFIC RESEARCH CLEARLY SHOWS THAT CONSUMING ABOUT 10 GRAMS OF CARBS PER DAY WILL REVERSE INSULIN RESISTANCE, REGULATE YOUR BLOOD SUGAR, FIX ANY METABOLIC DISEASES THAT YOU MIGHT HAVE.</u>

<u>WHEN IN DOUBT EAT FEWER CARBS. YOU WILL START TO ENJOY THE PLEASURES OF SUPERHEALTH BEFORE YOU CAN SAY HYPERINSULINEMIA-</u>☺

<u>THE KING OF LOW-CARB DIETS IS: THE HEALING KETOGENIC DIET! THE SCIENTIFIC STUDIES HAVE BEEN HIDING IN PLAIN SIGHT!</u>

<u>DEGENERATIVE DIABETES CAN BE COMPLETELY REVERSED AND IS PREVENTABLE THROUGH AN ANTI-INFLAMMATORY LIFESTYLE AND DIET. i.e. A~KETOGENIC DIET.</u>

<u>A RECENT STUDY (published on February 23, 2015) FOUND THAT LOW LEVELS OF VITAMIN D WERE A SIGNIFICANT CAUSE OF T2D, PRE-DIABETES, AND METABOLIC SYNDROME.</u>

<u>VITAMIN D DEFICIENCY CAUSED DIABETES REGARDLESS OF PATIENTS' WEIGHT!</u> You can be lean and have diabetes; or you can be overweight and <u>NOT</u> have diabetes.

<u>THE CONCEPT OF "INSULIN RESISTANCE" IS PARAMOUNT FOR ANYONE SEEKING TO ATTAIN SUPERHEALTH.</u>

Here's the concept of insulin-resistance explained again (you must be careful… there is sure to be a question about I.R. on your biology test-☺

Digestion starts with the production of enzymes in your mouth which breakdown food when you chew food. You then swallow this mush. This process fires up your internal sugar factory.

The <u>PANCREAS</u> is the main gland involved in diabetes. It is located behind the stomach. It secretes digestive enzymes and insulin; as well as helping with energy storage of glucagon, secreted by alpha cells in the liver.

The pancreas is one part of a whole system which includes the pituitary gland in your head, (Master Gland); the thyroid gland located in your throat, (helps with metabolism and calcium);the thymus, (sits behind the chest bone) acts with the immune and lymph systems); the adrenal gland, (located on top of each kidney) and help with regulating stress and the production of corticosteroids; the ovaries in women, and testes in men (producers of male/female hormones, estrogen, progesterone and testosterone).

The pancreas has several functions. It is directly connected with the pituitary gland through hormonal secretion. The vagus nerve from the brain (more on that below) directly connects to the pancreas too. The pancreas is most often thought of as the gland that secretes insulin and digestive enzymes. It works in conjunction with the liver by helping to regulate hormones and manufacture enzymes. It also works closely with the adrenal glands to regulate and modulate <u>STRESS</u>. Stress is the trigger for about 85 % of chronic health conditions/diseases.

<u>REVERSING/PREVENTING   DIABETES   IS   ALL   ABOUT   SAVING YOUR PANCREAS!</u>

Our body has developed a very sophisticated evolutionary mechanism to turn our food into fuel (energy) for our cells to burn. Our body can manufacture glucose from <u>FAT OR PROTEIN,</u> if necessary through a process called <u>"GLUCONEOGENISIS"</u>. This is pronounced <u>GLU</u>-<u>CO</u>-<u>GEN</u> –<u>ISIS</u>. This fundamental process you need to understand will be examined below. The concept of metabolism and how our body manufactures energy (ATP) from food will also be explained in greater detail below.

<u>INSULIN</u> as you now know, is one of most important hormones for cellular metabolism. Insulin is produced by the pancreas by beta-cells; assuming they're not busted of course☺

Insulin is a key player in the complicated metabolic dance shared by most human organisms. Insulin is a <u>REGULATOR AND A MODULATOR</u>. Its <u>primary job</u> is to ferry glucose from the bloodstream and get it into cellular tissues of muscle, fat and liver cells.

Dr. Mary Vernon succinctly describes insulin's job in our body:

> <u>"INSULIN'S ONLY JOB IS TO STORE FAT AND KEEP FAT FROM BEING BURNED".</u>

<u>"NORMAL"</u> cells have a <u>"HIGH SENSITIVITY"</u> to insulin. Insulin's job is to get glucose into our cells. Here's how busted cells (aka insulin resistance) is caused. When our cells are constantly "BOMBARDED"

with insulin— they get blunted or busted. Our tiny cell receptors get busted by insulin trying to allow glucose to enter our cells. Some receptors die off; some busted cells adapt by reducing the number of receptors on their surfaces to respond to insulin.

Either way- our cells become "desensitized". Our cells become non-responsive and just plain impervious to insulin- OR INSULIN-RESISTANT. Insulin-resistance is NOT A METFORMIN DEFICIENCY!

Next our cells continue to ignore insulin's "signals". Insulin can't do its job to transport glucose into our cells. Our pancreas then responds by TURNING ON ITS INSULIN PUMPS FULL BLAST! Your brain says— here's some more insulin-now go drive that glucose sugar into those unreceptive cells!

THIS CREATES A VICIOUS CIRCLE— FULL-BLOWN DIABETES TD2 IS THE END RESULT.

THE MAIN CULPRIT CAUSING (IR) IS OF COURSE DIETARY INTAKE OF SUGAR (sucrose, FRUCTOSE) AND STARCHY CARBS. You may have developed T2D by eating too many bagels/ pastas/ or other bad carbs.

FOLKS—NOW YOU UNDERSTAND WHY IT IS SO IMPERATIVE TO SHUT DOWN PRODUCTION OF GLUCOSE IN YOUR INTERNAL SUGAR FACTORY!

People with T2 D HAVE HIGH BLOOD SUGAR. THIS IS BECAUSE THEIR BODY CANNOT TRANSPORT GLUCOSE (SUGAR) INTO CELLS. The sugar cannot enter cells to be stored so blood- sugar levels continue to RISE. Elevated blood sugar levels produce a BOATLOAD of health problems. Elevated blood sugar is only a SYMPTOM. Allopathic doctors prescribe dangerous drugs under the FALSE belief that TYPE 2 Diabetes IS CAUSED BY ELEVATED BLOOD SUGAR LEVELS. THIS IS "STINKIN THINKIN".

THE ACTUAL CAUSE OF T2D IS: INSULIN RESISTANCE AND LEPTIN RESISTANCE. MANY CELLS ARE BUSTED. INSULIN RECEPTORS ARE BLUNTED, DAMAGED OR KILLED OFF. The pancreas is playing sugar music but many cells have turned a deaf ear to its music-☺

INSULIN- A PEPTIDE HORMONE HAS MANY JOBS INCLUDING:

- It alters the expression of numerous hormones;

- It stimulates your Sympathetic Nervous System (SNS);

- It promotes Vasoconstriction;

- It helps mobilize or signal a certain kind of protein

to mobilize glucose from outside of your cells;

- It's a satiety hormone that affects your hunger;

- It's also interconnected with another hunger-regulating hormone- leptin;

- It's part of the mTOR pathway that is part of the insulin pathway, (this mechanism builds protein in your muscles (called protein synthesis), which is part of the insulin pathway as well. To build protein in the muscle and to grow muscle you must choose to activate the mTOR mechanism which activates what's called the "eukaryotic initiation factor", that signals muscles to build protein.

Insulin is not only a transporter and a regulator hormone. Insulin does not only just escort glucose into our cells. Insulin is an ANABOLIC hormone. It can promote muscle growth- BUT it also promotes FAT FORMATION, RETENTION AND STORAGE.

If your insulin receptors are insensitive, like with Type 2 Diabetes-

MUSCLE WASTING IS INEVITABLE! INSULIN ALSO INCOURAGES INFLAMMATION! YOU MUST RESTORE YOUR INSULIN SENSITIVITY.

When insulin levels get too high; (aka "INSULINEMIA")—THIS CAN ADVERSELY AFFECT OTHER HORMONES TOO. These other hormones are thrown out of whack. Our bodies need to maintain a delicate balance among its various hormones.

THESE HORMONES ALL WORK TOGETHER—IN A SYNERGISTIC MANNER.

Too much or too little of insulin is not a good thing. Insulin is a major accelerant of the AGING PROCESS! SUGAR makes you OLD & WRINKLED TOO! -☺) Insulin affects MANY bodily processes all of which impact your longevity.

GLYCATION is a contributing cause of insulin resistance; (IR). It is very important to understand GLYCATION-

GLYCATION IS NOT WELL UNDERSTOOD BY THE MEDICAL ESTABLISHMENT. IT IS A PROCESS THAT AFFECTS MANY OF OUR CELLS AT THE CELLULAR LEVEL.

What is "glycation'?

A simple answer is this. Have you ever spilled fruit juice on your hands? Remember how sticky and glue-like that was? Well, this is what happens to your blood when you eat too much sugar (bad carbs) and develop elevated blood-sugar levels. Sometimes, naturopathic doctors will refer to glycation of cells as a sort of "caramelizing" of tissues. Think caramel popcorn—pretty to look at but not pretty inside your body-☺

The technical explanation of glycation is as follows. World-renown neurologist Dr. David Perlmutter describes it as follows:

> "Glycation is the biochemical term for the bonding of sugar molecules to proteins, fats and amino acids; the spontaneous reaction that causes the sugar molecule to attach itself to itself is sometimes referred to as the Maillard reaction....

Two good examples come to mind. In the case of LDL (aka as the "bad cholesterol); this molecule, a LIPO- PROTEIN if it becomes very dense (small) and /or if this protein becomes GLYCATED, it drastically increases its OXIDATION— (think 'rusting").

Another example is wrinkles caused by smoking. Smoking sucks out antioxidants in the skin. When advanced glycation occurs it produces end products called appropriately- (AGEs) more rusting...-☺ There is a very strong link between OXIDATIVE STRESS AND SUGAR. When proteins are glycated (think "caramelized")—the amount of FREE RADICALS (rusters/oxidants) is increased by MORE THAN 50 TIMES! OMG! That's a lot of rust makers!

The take-home message—

If you want to reduce oxidative stress and the production of FREE RADICALS, you must reduce the GLYCATION of proteins.

HOW? GET YOUR BRAIN OFF SUGAR! ASAP!

YOU MUST STOP MAKING STICKY CARAMEL-COATED BLOOD SUGAR!

YOU MUST SHUT PRODUCTION OF YOUR INTERNAL SUGAR FACTORY- TODAY!

SUGAR IS PUBLIC ENEMY NO 1 in the sugar bowl or as syrupy blood sugar in your bloodstream.

ARE THERE VARIOUS KINDS OF INSULIN RESISTANCE? YES=ABSOLUTELY!

As noted by Dr. Robert Lustig, many of our chronic diseases today are in fact INSULIN-RESISTANT METABOLIC DISEASES.

WHICHEVER ORGAN becomes insulin-resistant ends up manifesting ITS OWN METABOLIC SYNDROME/INSULIN RESISTANCE: THEREFORE—

- Insulin Resistance of Liver= Diabetes

- Insulin Resistance of Kidney= Chronic Renal Disease

- Insulin Resistance of Brain(aka ALZHEIM-ERS DISEASE (aka DIABETES 3)

TO BE HEALTHY AND DIABETES/DISEASE-FREE— YOU MUST KEEP YOUR INSULIN LEVELS AS LOW AS POSSIBLE—AND YOUR BLOOD SUGAR LEVELS STEADY AND LOW TOO.

MY PLATINUM KEY TO ATTAIN SUPERHEALTH IS LOW-STABLE BLOOD-SUGAR AND NO INSULIN RESISTANCE!

How do you do that? The secret is to:

1. ELIMINATE ALL SUGARS FROM YOUR LIFE AND RESTRICT YOUR CARB INTAKE;

2. GET ON A KETOGENIC DIET ASAP!

Here are some ALARMING NUMBERS:

- 29 million Americans have diabetes (source CDC) Predictions had been that that figure would only be reached in 2050!)

- by the year 2030 – 552 million people will have diabetes;

- By 2050 – 50 % of Americans will have DIABETES OR PRE-DIABE-TES. These people will develop PRE-DIABETIC HIGH BLOOD SUGAR.

THESE CONDITIONS ARE ALSO KNOWN AS IMPAIRED GLUCOSE METABOLISM

- Another 86 million people (18.8 %) have insulin-resistant PRE-DIABETES. (The vast majority of diabetes is Type 2 variety sometimes known as degenerative diabetes.)

DIABETES IS ENTIRELY PREVENTABLE THROUGH AN ANTI-INFLAMMATORY DIET (Ketogenic Diet) AND LIFESTYLE CHANGES.

Diabetes is common metabolic disorder that is associated with chronic complications such as neuropathy, angiopathy, and peripheral neuropathy. However, as early as 1922 it was recognized that diabetes also can lead to cognitive dysfunction. The observed cerebral manifestations of diabetes appear to develop insidiously; seemly independent of diabetes; associated with acute metabolic and vascular disturbances- such as severe hypo-and hyperglycemic episodes and stroke.

Nerve pain is called "Neuropathy". <u>DIABETIC NEUROPATHY IS VERY PAINFUL AND AWFUL</u>. Research shows that you can use <u>CAPSACIN the hot substance found in chilli peppers, ORGANIC CAYENNE PEPPER and liquid extract supplements to treat diabetic neuropathy</u>. Capsacin regulates <u>GLUCOSE HOMEOSTASIS by waking up RPV1 receptors</u>. These receptors pass the ball to signal GLP-1 secretion from your intestinal cells of your gastrointestinal tract; voila : <u>YOU CAN PUT THE FLAME ON THE PAIN!</u>

<u>HYPOGLYCEMIA</u> is a condition characterized toward abnormally low blood sugar; it's commonly associated with diabetes—<u>BUT</u> you can be hypoglycemic even if you're <u>not</u> a diabetic. Common symptoms of hypoglycemic crash include: headaches, weakness, tremors, irritability and hunger. As your blood glucose levels continue to plummet, more severe symptoms can set in. These include confusion, or abnormal behaviour, visual disturbances, seizures, and loss of consciousness.

<u>HYPOGLYCEMIA HAS BEEN CALLED –"THE CARB FLU".</u>

One key to preventing hypoglycemia is <u>ELIMINATION OF ALL GRAINS, FRUCTOSE AND BAD CARBS FROM YOUR DIET</u>. In reality, "carb flu" is the body's reaction when it is deprived of its favourite sugar supply. What happens when you take a lollipop from a small child? What happens to a heroin addict when you cut off his supply? What happens when you deprive an alcoholic from his liquor? What happens when an IV drip is pulled out of a patient in the hospital?

Folks—<u>WHEN YOU'RE CARB ADDICTED AND YOUR SUGAR IS TAKEN AWAY— YOUR BRAIN AND YOUR BODY GETS UPSET!</u> Your body begins to cry like a baby deprived of its lollipop…aww…-☺ no more sugar/ethanol for your brain… Hypoglycemic reactions and symptoms are like a hangover. Having a hangover is not fun…for anyone. The same thing happens when you start restricting carbohydrates. Everyone has a different carb tolerance level – so reactions vary.

<u>BUT— WHEN YOU SWAP OUT BAD CARBS FOR GOOD FATS—YOUR BODY ULTIMATELY FEELS MUCH BETTER!</u>

<u>WHEN WE EAT SUGAR, GRAINS OR CARBS, OUR DIGESTIVE SYSTEM CONVERTS THESE LARGE MOLECULES INTO GLUCOSE</u>. This glucose is then absorbed into our bloodstream and taken (in theory) to every cell of our body. Blood sugar fuels our cells to make them grow and be healthy.

FOR PROPER FUNCTIONAL HEALTH —IT IS IMPERATIVE TO MAINTAIN STABLE BLOOD SUGAR LEVELS. STABLE BLOOD SUGAR MEANS THAT THE BODY IS IN A STATE OF GLUCOSE HOMEOSTASIS.

Too low or too high blood sugar levels may cause depression or unhappiness. We need balance in balance in our body—and our lives.

Stabilizing blood sugar is mostly performed by the pancreas through the hormone INSULIN. When our body recognizes that blood sugar is elevating- the pancreas starts its insulin pump. Insulin provides the cellular key that fits into the cellular door of each cell. It permits blood sugar to enter our cells. When the cell receptors are busted; blunted or destroyed, this becomes insulin resistance which mushrooms into full blown diabetes.

Poor diet and a sedentary lifestyle are two big causes of diabetes. When we eat too many carbs our internal sugar factory gets overwhelmed. Increased elevated blood glucose levels and insulin produces MORE INFLAMMATORY PROSTAGLANDINS (cellular messengers). Advanced diabetes soon follows.

PREVENTION AND REVERSAL OF DEGENERATIVE DIABETES DEPENDS ON OUR ABILITY TO REDUCE INFLAMMATION; TO ENHANCE AND REPAIR OUR BUSTED CELLS/METABOLISM.

THE HEALING PROCESS BEGINS WITH A KETOGENIC DIET- RICH IN HEALTHY FATS, NUTRIENT DENSE VEGGIES AND CLEAN PROTEIN.

Typically, a doctor will check you out for possible diabetes. What does he do?

Most ill-informed doctors believe that blood glucose is the key to diagnosing diabetes. So- they order a fasting blood glucose test. That's a snapshot of sugar circulating in your blood.

- Fasting blood glucose: This test measures the amount of sugar (glucose) in your blood after you have not eaten for at least 8 hours. A level between 70 and 100 milligrams per deciliter (mg/dL) is considered "normal"; above this, your body is showing signs of insulin resistance and diabetes and an increased risk for brain disease.

- Studies have shown that people with a fasting blood sugar level of 100 to 125 mg/dL had a 300 PERCENT HIGHER RISK OF CVD COMPARED TO PEOPLE WITH A LEVEL BELOW 79mg/dL. A study suggests that the risk of stroke is 27 percent higher if your fasting glucose level is higher than 83 mg/dL.

- Above 126- usually means diabetes;

- Dr. Seyfried, (A proponent of the Ketogenic Diet) maintains that the IDEAL fasting blood sugar level is BETWEEN 55 to 65 mg/dL

THIS IS HALF OF WHAT CONVENTIONAL DOCTORS CONSIDER "GOOD" or "NORMAL"!!

A FASTING BLOOD GLUCOSE TEST—A fasting blood glucose will not DIAGNOSE your problem.

IT'S THE WRONG TEST!

What you really need is a FASTING INSULIN TEST! This is a simple blood test that you take first thing in the morning. A HIGH reading would be 10 to 15 micro international units per milliliter (pulU/mL). The "average" insulin level in the United States is about 8.8 for adult men and 8.4 for women.

PEOPLE HAVE DIFFERENT INSULIN LEVELS AND DIFFERENT METABOLISMS TO BEGIN WITH. A HIGH INSULIN LEVEL TELLS YOU THAT YOU'RE AT A HIGH RISK OF INSULIN RESISTANCE AND DIABETES— BUT—

EVEN IF YOUR TEST RESULTS ARE HIGH— YOU'RE NOT STUCK! YOU CAN STILL REVERSE INSULIN RESISTANCE NATURALLY!

YOU WON'T HEAR THAT FROM MOST DOCTORS! THEIR MOTTO IS: –"DRUGS R US"-☺

IF YOU ARE VERY CAREFUL ABOUT YOUR CARBOHYDRATE INTAKE-YOUR IDEAL INSULIN LEVEL ON YOUR LAB REPORT SHOULD BE LESS THAN 2.0!

When your insulin level is 2 or below, this is a sign that your pancreas is NOT being overworked; your blood sugars are under excellent control— AND THERE IS NO EVIDENCE OF INSULIN RESISTANCE AND —YOU HAVE A VERY LOW RISK FOR DIABETES AND OTHER RELATED BLOOD SUGAR PROBLEMS.

Have you ever why conventional doctors do not measure YOUR FASTING INSULIN LEVEL? It's quite simple.

How in heck could a doctor sell you synthetic insulin if your insulin test showed that you had FAR TOO MUCH INSULIN IN YOUR BLOOD!

A FASTING INSULIN LEVEL OF LESS THAN TWO MEANS THAT YOU ARE LIKELY ENJOYING SUPERHEALTH!

IF YOUR FASTING LEVEL IS ELEVATED—(ANYTHING OVER 5 should be considered elevated) AND YOU SHOULD BE CONCERNED.

Research shows that reducing people's weight EVEN SLIGHTLY COULD PREVENT AN ESTIMATED 274,000 TO 309,000 CASES OF TYPE 2 DIABETES IN THE NEXT 20 YEARS! PRESCRIPTION DRUGS AND SYNTHETIC INSULIN MAKE YOU FATTER AND SICKER SO THAT YOU REMAIN A SICK PATIENT AND DRUG USER FOR THE REST OF YOUR LIFE.

HAVE NO FEAR! YOU'RE IN LUCK! HERE ARE "SOME" FOODS/ NUTRIENTS THAT WILL HELP HEAL YOUR DIABETES.

- COCONUT OIL- aka "The King of Fat" (Coconut has been called the "Cure for all Diseases"!

  THERE ARE DOZENS OF STUDIES PROVING THE BENEFIT OF SUP-PLEMENTATION WITH COCONUT PRODUCTS. Coconut Oil in particular contains MCT'S or medium-chain-triglycerides. MCT'S are considered as ONE OF THE BEST SATURATED FATS IN THE WORLD!

  Research proves that Coconut Oil CAN REVERSE INSU-LIN RESISTANCE, LOWER BLOOD SUGAR AND LOWER MANY OTHER BLOOD BIOMARKERS. Below you will read about Dr. Mary Newport who reversed her husband's AL-ZHEIMER' S DISEASE WITH MCT'S FROM COCONUT OIL!

  THERE ARE DOZENS OF CLINICAL STUDIES PROV-ING THE EFFECTIVENESS OF COCONUT OIL. In Sri Lanka people eat about 144 coconuts per year and that country has a heart disease rate of one in 500 people!

  TO REVERSE DIABETES: The therapeutic dose is 4 to 6 TABLE-SPOONS PER DAY. You should ease your way into coconut oil. Start with 1 teaspoon per day to get used to it. You can cook with it. You can slather it on your body. You can add it to any food. You can even put it on your hair (as I do-☺).

  THE MAINTENANCE DOSE IS 1 TO 3 TABLESPOONS PER DAY! My personal favourite way to take coconut oil is in my Ketogenic Coffee and a PLETHORA OF MARVEL-LOUS KETOGENIC RECIPES IN BAKED GOODS, ETC. ETC. ETC. (Please see my Ketogenic Recipes- infra).

  THERE ARE HUNDREDS OF USES FOR COCONUT OIL!

  COCONUT OIL IS ANTIBACTERIAL, ANTIVIRAL, AND ANTIFUNGAL-

  No wonder it is called the CURE FOR ALL DISEASES!

- Krill Oil

(Shrimp based)- Omega 3 capsules containing <u>ES-SENTIAL FATTY ACIDS</u>; Krill Oil — DHA and EPA) – <u>AR-GUABLY THE BEST SUPPLEMENT ANYONE CAN TAKE FOR THEIR HEALTH</u>! (in my humble opinion).

- Tumeric

  Phenomenal for anyone- diabetics included. Check out the diabetes studies benefits on <u>www.GreenMedInfo.com</u>

- Apple Cider Vinegar

  There are several studies proving that <u>ACV DRAMATICALLY</u> reduces insulin and glucose spikes in the blood that occur after meals. One study showed that 2 TBSP of ACV before meals greatly benefited people with Diabetes AND pre-diabetics. In one study blood-glucose concentrations were cut by <u>50 PERCENT</u>! One study showed vinegar supplementation produced greater satiety; a <u>SIDE-EFFECT</u> was a LOSS OF 2 pounds in 4 weeks.

  In 2007, a study reported in The Diabetes Journal showed that ACV <u>supplementation caused a 4 to 6 PERCENT REDUCTION IN FASTING BLOOD GLUCOSE</u>. The study looked at Type 2 Diabetic patients with "waking hyperglycemia" – aka "dawn phenomenon."

  Another study involving only women found that there was a <u>55 PERCENT</u> <u>REDUCTION IN GLUCOSE RE-SPONSE</u> following morning meal containing ACV.

- Cinnamon

  There are many studies showing that cinnamon has a very <u>POWERFUL</u> effect by lowering blood glucose levels, and improved hemoglobin A1C levels in diabetics. It was also extremely effect at regulating blood sugar; fasting glucose levels and had a beneficial effect on glycemic control.

- Olive Oil

  Studies show that olive oil supplementation is <u>VERY EF-FECTIVE</u> to reduce insulin resistance and useful to regulate blood sugar for diabetics. It is effective to treat metabolic syndrome. It promotes weight loss too.

- Gamma-tocotrienol

  In a study in 2014 at the University of Florida, it was proven that gamma-tocotrienol (a substance found in from Red Palm Oil) greatly improved glucose tolerance and insulin sensitivity; it also reduced inflammation in adipose tissue and decreased macrophage MI activation.

- Biotin or B7 is Mother Nature's Insulin Helper. It improves insulin sensitivity. (2,000 to 4,000 mcg. daily for insulin-resistance/ Diabetes);

AND FINALLY- THERE ARE TWO SUPER-HELPERS FOR DIABETICS TO REVERSE AND PREVENT DIABETES!

THE FIRST SUPER SUPPLEMENT TO REVERSE DIABETES IS:

BERBERINE.

BERBERINE IS THE WORLD'S MOST POWERFUL SUPPLEMENT!

MORE THAN 2, 800 STUDIES ON BERBERINE ARE LISTED ON PUBMED AND PUBLISHED IN THE LAST 5 YEARS!

Berberine is a yellow-coloured compound alkaloid compound found in several different plants, including European berbery, goldenseal, golden thread, Oregon grape, phellodendron and tree turmeric.

Berberine has AMAZING ANTIBACTERIAL, ANTI-INFLAMMATORY AND IMMUNE-ENHANCING PROPERTIES.

Berberine IS EFFECTIVE AGAINST A WIDE VARIETY OF BACTERIA, PROTOZOA AND FUNGI! (Great for Travellers Diarrhea Too!)

RESEARCH IS THE LAST 5 YEARS CONFIRMS WHAT TRADITIONAL MEDICINE HAS KNOWN FOR CENTURIES—

BERBERINE IS THE MOST POWERFUL HEALING SUPPLEMENT IN THE WORLD!

BERBERINE REGULATES YOUR METABOLISM; BERBERINE INDUCES A CASCADE OF EVENTS THAT ARE ALL INVOLVED IN MAINTAINING ENERGY HOMEOSTASIS.

BERBERINE ACTIVATES AN ENZYME CALLED AMPK INSIDE YOUR BODY'S CELLS. AMPK STANDS FOR: "Adenosine Monophosphate Protein Kinase"

AMPK IS SOMETIMES CALLED "A METABOLIC SWITCH"

BERBERINE HAS BEEN CALLED BY RESEARCHERS- "A POTENT ORAL HYPOGLYCEMIC AGENT!"

DIABETIC STUDIES SHOW THAT IN PEOPLE WITH DIABETES AMPK ACTIVATION CAUSED BY BERBERINE

- Stimulates the uptake of glucose into cells;

- Reduces Glucose production in the liver AND-

MOST AMAZING OF ALL- BERBERINE IMPROVES INSULIN SENSITIVITY!

HALLELUJAH!

BERBERINE IS A DIABETIC'S DREAM COME TRUE!

BERBERINE REGULATES BLOOD SUGAR METABOLISM.

BERBERINE REVERSES (CURES) INSULIN RESISTANCE!

A review study published in the International Journal of Endocrinology stated these words verbatim:

" Modern Pharmacological effects of BERBERINE on glucose metabolism, ...include improving insulin resistance, promoting insulin secretion, inhibiting gluconeogenesis in liver, stimulating glycolysis in peripheral tissue cells, modulating gut microbiota, reducing intestinal absorption of glucose, and regulating lipid metabolism"

YIPPEE!

BERBERINE HAS BEEN SUCCESSFULLY USED TO REVERSE METABOLIC SYNDROME, DIABETES, HYPERGLYCEMIA, LIPID ANORMALITIES AND ENERGY IMBALANCES!

BERBERINE HAS BEEN SUCCESSFULLY USED TO TREAT DIABETICS!

BERBERINE HAS BEEN PROVEN TO CAUSE WEIGHT LOSS!

In one study, obese subjects who took 500 mg. of berberine 3x daily for 12 weeks lost an average of FIVE POUNDS. Blood levels of triglycrides and cholesterol were also reduced.

BECAUSE OF BERBERINE'S ABILITY TO INHIBIT FAT STORAGE AND IMPROVE THE FUNCTIONS OF HORMONES SUCH AS INSULIN, LEPTIN AND ADIPONECTIN IT IS PHENOMAL TO REDUCE OBESITY, VISCERAL FAT.!

BERBERINE'S ACTIVITY ALSO ENHANCES BROWN FAT- A HEAT GENERATING TYPE OF FAT THAT BURNS ENERGY INSTEAD OF STORING IT.

Sidebar: Brown fat is loaded with MITOCHONDRIA that convert the fat directly to energy to produce heat

BERBERINE ACTIVATES AMPK WHICH PRODUCES THE SAME BENEFITS AS EXERCISE, DIETING AND WEIGHT LOSS These lifestyle modifications are beneficial for a BOATLOAD of maladies.

BERBERINE PROTECTS YOUR HEART- STUDIES PROVE IT REDUCES APOLIPROTEIN B RISK FACTOR FOR CVD BY UP TO 15 PERCENT!

In clinical studies competing with the diabetic drug METFORMIN— BERBERINE KICKED METFORMIN's proverbial A** !

The take-home message:

In light of a boatload of scientific evidence-

DOCTORS WHO TREAT DIABETES WITH METFORMIN AND OTHER TOXIC DRUGS- SHOULD HAVE THEIR MEDICAL LICENCES STRIPPED AND BE PROSECUTED FOR MEDICAL FRAUD.

THE SECOND MAGICAL PLANT BULLET IS STEVIA-

STEVIA IS ONE OF MOTHER NATURE'S BEST-KEPT SECRETS.

STEVIA IS 100 TIMES SWEETER THAN REGULAR SUGAR!

BEST OF ALL—STEVIA IS SAFE FOR DIABETICS AND EVERYONE!

Can you guess what other magic quality that stevia has?

Research shows that stevia reduces blood sugar and blood pressure.

Research also suggests that STEVIA CAN REGENERATE BETA-CELLS IN THE PANCREAS! OMG!

You can read the referenced studies (Appendix A) to know more about stevia's healing properties for yourself.

STEVIA IS A MAGIC BULLET THAT WILL HELP YOU GET YOUR BRAIN OFF SUGAR AND REVERSE YOUR SUGAR ADDICTION! (You will see that stevia is the sweetener that I have used in many of the Ketogenic Recipes -infra.

Take-home message:

To reverse Diabetes/Metabolic DIS—EASES— YOU MUST FIRST ELIMINATE ALL TOXINS FROM YOUR DIET AND FROM YOUR LIFE.

T2D toxins include EXOGENOUS toxins; Examples are: research shows that gas station attendants are more prone to develop diabetes due to their environmental exposure to MANY ENVIRONMENTAL TOXINS; such as heavy metals. Are you living in and old house? Do you have

MOLD in the walls? Are you exposed to a lot of PLASTIC products? Are you drinking water from a BPA plastic bottle?

EVERY LITTLE TOXIC EXPOSURE INCREASES YOUR TOXIC LOAD THAT CAN TRIGGER DIABETES OR ANY OTHER HEALTH PROBLEM.

The doctor of the future will be an ENVIRONMENTAL DOCTOR. BUT FOR NOW—YOU MUST BE YOUR OWN EVIRONMENTAL DOCTOR!

No else in the world can figure out which toxins are making you sick with diabetes or some other dis-ease. You must hire yourself as your environmental detective/doctor. You can eliminate all neurotoxins. You need to give your body the support that it needs. Your body CAN THEN HEAL ITSELF—as it was designed to do.

You must also eliminate all ENDOGENOUS toxins. A good example is your GUT BACTERIA. Research shows that fixing these little critters will go a long way towards healing YOU AND YOUR GUT. Conversely, "bad critters" and bad bacteria (or absence of good bacteria) can lead to Diabetes; etc.

A recent study involving young children showed that the ONSET OF TYPE I DIABETES tends to be preceded by a change in gut bacteria. Microbes can prevent this disease. Gut Flora (gut microbiota) are often the cause for many diseases- including diabetes (all kinds) In short, you must eliminate all toxins; both exogenous and endogenous, from your diet and from your life. Other research discussed infra outlines the gut/brain connection and how gut microbial can be used to reverse diabetes.

In the Netherlands, a clever doctor (few and far between these days) HAS SUCCESSFULLY USED FMT (Fecal Microbial Transplants) TO REVERSE DIABETES!

Taking healthy fecal matter ("poop") from a healthy person to transplant it into the colon has now become A VERY EASY EFFECTIVE WAY TO REVERSE DIABETES AND MANY OTHER BACTERIAL PROBLEMS. FMT was used by the Yellow Emperor in the 4th Century B.C. Who knew?

DR. EARTH, DR. CLEAN WATER, DR. CLEAN AIR, DR. KETOGENIC DIET, DR. EXERCISE, DR. SLEEP, DR. SUNSHINE ARE THE DOCTORS WHO CAN REVERSE DIABETES; HEAL YOUR BODY AND HELP YOU ATTAIN SUPERHEALTH!

Examples: One recent study from the University of Chicago found that people in their 20's and 30's who slept fewer than 6.5 hours per night had THE SAME INSULIN SENSITIVITY AS SOMEONE OVER

<u>60</u>! The study also found that those people who slept <u>5 HOURS PER NIGHT WERE 73 PERCENT MORE LIKELY TO BECOME OBESE THAN THOSE WHO SLEPT 9 HOURS</u>!

Studies also show that diabetics typically have 30 percent blood serum levels of Vitamin D than non-diabetics.

Finally, when you start deliberately spending a <u>few minutes</u> each day to reduce the <u>STRESS/CORTISOL LEVELS</u> in your life—you may find that your health issues rapidly resolve themselves. You take 9 slow deep breaths in front of your mirror every morning. Beforehand, you can begin by writing these few words on your bathroom mirror; "I love and approve of myself; "<u>I AM GRATEFUL FOR THE LOVE AND EVERYTHING</u> that I have in my life. " I promise that I will let go of my ego—I promise that I will not take myself so g**damned seriously!"-☺ The famous comedian Red Skelton once said "Don't take life seriously- you will never get out of it alive.-☺

<u>ALL TYPES OF DIABETES CAN BE TREATED EFFECTIVELY WITH NATURAL HEALING.</u>

<u>DIABETES IS A METABOLIC DISORDER. THIS "BUSTED MITOCHONDRIA/ BUSTED METABOLISM" CAN BE FIXED! IT CAN BE HEALED.</u>

<u>IT'S NEVER TOO LATE!</u>

<u>The take-home message</u>:

To maintain low-stable blood sugar levels, become insulin-sensitive and attain SUPERHEALTH- you must shutdown production of sugar/ glucose in your internal sugar factory. This is your platinum key to attain SUPERHEALTH.

Prior to the advent of exogenous synthetic insulin for the "treatment" of diabetes Mellitus in the 1920's, the mainstay foundational approach was dietary modification. Diet recommendations in that era aimed at controlling glycemia, (actually glycosuria) were the <u>EXACT OPPOSITE OF CURRENT LOW-FAT HIGH-CARB RECOMMENDATIONS</u> s

<u>BIG PHARMA AND THE MEDICAL ESTABLISHMENT SUPPRESSED THE APPROPRIATE DIETARY PROTOCOL TO REVERSE AND ELIMINATE DIABETES</u>!

Dr. Elliot Joslin and Dr. Frederick Allen's <u>DIABETIC DIET IN 1923 con</u>sisted of:

<u>MEATS, POULTRY, GAME, FISH, CLEAR SOUPS, GELATIN, EGGS, BUTTER, OLIVE OIL, COFFEE/TEA</u>...

AND CONTAINED: <u>5 PERCENT ENERGY FROM CARBOHYDRATES:</u>

<u>20 PERCENT ENERGY FROM PROTEIN—and</u>

<u>75 PERCENT ENERGY FROM FAT! OMG! OMG!</u>

<u>THE KETOGENIC DIET WAS USED IN 1923 TO TREAT DIABETES!!</u> Who knew?

CHAPTER SEVEN
THE HEALING KETOGENIC DIET (Dr. KETOSIS)

A. INTRODUCTION

The Ketogenic Diet is not new. It is our ancestral diet which has been the human diet for almost 3 million years. However— it was pretty much abandoned when humans began planting crops; (see The Greatest Mistake in Human History, supra).

WE NEED TO RESPECT OUR GENOME;(aka our genetic make-up). Please see my penultimate chapter entitled: "Diseases that your doctor cannot diagnose."

FAT- NOT CARBOHYDRATE IS THE PREFERRED FUEL OF HUMAN METABOLISM. Our ancestral diet was changed about 10 thousand years ago when "hunter/gatherer" man became "farming man".

As a species, we are genetically and physiologically identical to our ancestors who lived before the dawn of agriculture. We are the product of an optimal design. We have been shaped by nature for thousands of generations. We don't consider ourselves hunters and gatherers anymore, but our bodies still function in accordance with our reptilian natures.

From a biological perspective, our reptilian nature leads us instinctively to 1. Seek safety- (or fight or flight response; 2. Next- feed our bellies; and 3.when we are in a safe environment, with full bellies, to seek sexual gratification. Today, modern humans do not need to seek safety. So then they eat. The big problem is that when carbs are the primary fuel—the brain is saying: "So where is my delicious mouth-watering greasy steak.

TO RESPECT OUR GENOME—WE NEED TO EAT TO BE SATISFIED. WE NEED TO FUEL OUR BRAINS AND OUR BODIES WITH DELICIOUS, NUTRITIOUS HEALTH FATS AS OUR ANCESTORS DID!

Eating healthy healing whole, natural animal/plant foods is what we were meant to do. Humans have been programmed to live a long and healthy life. We used to say that it's in our genes.

Today- WE UNDERSTAND THAT WE CAN CHANGE OUR GENES BY SWITCHING OFF THE UNDESIRABLE GENES AND TURNING ON THE GOOD DESIRABLE GENES-☺

TO BE HEALTHY, HAPPY AND DISEASE FREE- WE MUST RESPECT OUR GENOME. WE MUST EAT A KETOGENIC DIET- AS OUR ANCESTORS DID.

THERE ARE VERY FEW REMAINING CULTURES ON PLANET EARTH who practice this kind of ancestral diet.

One of the last populations on earth that had dietary habits closest to our ancestors—was extensively studied on the Island of KITAVA (in New Guinea). A famous study known as ("the Malinowski study), was published by anthropologist, Bromislaw Malinowski. He found that among the 23,000 people living on the island—THERE WAS NOT A SINGLE INSTANCE OF OBESITY, DIABETES, HIGH BLOOD PRESSURE, CVD OR ANY OTHER ADVERSE HEALTH PROBLEM! The Kitavans remained active and vital even in their late 80's and 90's!

What was their secret to SUPERHEALTH?

60 PERCENT OF THEIR DIET CONSISTED OF HEAL-THY TRANSFORMATIVE FATS! Despite an abundance of food, Kitavan islanders are lean and their blood pressure does not increase with age. Kitavans die of old age; or an occasional accident such as falling from a tree. A study by (Lindenburg- 1999) showed that THE INSULIN LEVELS of Kitavans are HALF of those Swedes living in Sweden. Kitavans eat a high-cholesterol diet- high in saturated coconut fat; fish, taro, some fruits and sweet yams. Kitavans exercise only at the level of a moderately active Westerner.

Another example is the TOKELAU ISLANDERS (among Cook Islands), in the South Pacific. The Tokelau islanders eat more than 40 PERCENT OF THEIR DIET AS SATURATED (COCONUT) FAT. Males 55 to 64 years old have cholesterol levels averaging 245! These peoples enjoy ROBUST CARDIOVASCULAR HEALTH- free from obesity and all of the other Western dis-eases.

East African nomadic peoples, and Innuit peoples are other good examples; (Cretans also).

The Innuit peoples, (once called "Eskimos" of the far north are the closest Western example. The Innuit culture has thrived on a **KETOGENIC DIET and LIFESTYLE**; possibly for thousands of years. As you know, on the frozen tundra, there are very few vegetables (plants) and even fewer fruits, except for some seasonal berries. So for these peoples—a plant-based diet was not an option.

THE TRADITIONAL INNUIT PEOPLES ATE THE MOST FAT OF ANY DIET EVER STUDIED.

The Innuit would basically follow their food supply during the year. They would eat fish seals, walruses and whales. They would carry their belongings on their backs and trek many miles each day If you've ever hiked 20 miles with 50 lbs on your back; you understand the necessity of eating the right foods for strength and endurance. The Innuit peoples are extremely clever people. They used to make skin bags to carry around pounds of animal fat. In the fall, they would kill caribou; when the caribou were nice and fat. They would make pemmican (strips of dry meat to carry). When they killed a caribou, they would preferentially eat the organ meats (liver, brains, heart, kidneys etc). The muscle meats they would usually be given to their dogs. (They also made butter, etc.) Essentially- their diet consisted of 80 percent good fats and about 20 percent protein. They knew that Mother Nature provided well- even in very cold parts of the world.

If the Innuit peoples had <u>been unable</u> to fuel their bodies properly; they would have <u>died out</u> a long time ago.

Another surviving "Ketogenic type" culture, existing today, is the **MASSAI** peoples of east Africa. The Massai warriors were known for their prowess in battle. Essentially, the Massai hunters (males) would go off in the woods for days at a time to kill wild animals. They also kept their own herds when possible. The Massai warriors would eat 3 to 5 pounds of meat, milk and blood every day. Massai peoples often lived to their 80's and 90's- being lean, healthy—and disease-free. They ate the right foods. Massai women (the gatherers) used to live mostly in small villages. Their job was to raise the children and gather nuts, berries or whatever limited plants that they could. Often other tribes would come to trade with the Massai women. Sometimes they would get bananas or perhaps sweet potatoes. It appears that occasionally Massai women sported a few extra pounds...perhaps from having a few too many sugar carbs-☺

IN SHORT- most of our ancestors had little access to carbohydrates. They certainly didn't have access to food 24/7. In practice, our

309

ancestors underwent alternating intervals of "FEAST OR FAMINE". Our human body has adapted to this type of eating pattern for hundreds of thousands of years. Our bodies and our GENOME are designed to eat in this feast or famine pattern. Humans understood that their bodies were hard-wired to be able to survive for 2 or 3 days at a time, without eating any food whatsoever. Most humans had little fear of starving to death. Many carb-burners today believe they can't survive without eating for 6 hours!

ABSTAINING FROM EATING (aka FASTING) ACTUALLY OPTIMIZES OUR BIOLOGICAL/BRAIN FUNCTION!

It turns out that humans can regenerate a new immune system by a 72 hour fast!

How cool is that?

INTERMITTENT FASTING IS A VERY IMPORTANT- INTEGRAL PART OF A KETOGENIC DIET; (infra).

Should we mimic the way our ancestors ate?

Should we eat a LOW-CARB- HIGH-FAT-MODERATE PROTEIN-KETOGENIC DIET? ABSOLUTELY!

Origin of the Ketogenic Diet

In 1921 Dr. Woodyatt in a review article about Diet Adjustments and Diabetes stated: "acetone, and beta-hydroxybutyric acid appear in a normal subject by starvation—or a diet containing too low a proportion of carbohydrate and too high a proportion of fat."

Descriptions of dietary restriction date back to the time of Dr. Hippocrates-and are mentioned in the New Testament. High fat diets were considered (and used) 140 years ago!

But- the first American use of the diet appears to have been in 1899- by a fitness guru named Bernard McFadden and an osteopath named Dr. Hugh Conklin. As metabolism as debunked—the concept evolved that a high-fat diet could mimic the "ketosis" during fasting.

In the early 1920's the Ketogenic Diet was used to successfully treat EPILEPSY in the has been used specifically for patients with deficiencies in the GLUT-1 glucose transporter, (where glucose cannot be transported into the cerebrospinal fluid for use by the brain) and pyruvate dehydrogenase (E1) deficiency, (where ketone bodies can by-pass the enzymatic defect.) It was noted early in history that FASTING could be used in the treatment of epilepsy.

What is known today as the Ketogenic Diet was the number one treatment for epilepsy until Big Pharma arrived with its dangerous cocktails of poisonous anti-epileptic drugs. The preferred anti-epileptic drug became " diphenylhydantoin". The efficacy of the ketogenic diet was suppressed for several decades- until 1994 when the public heard found out about the Charlie Foundation.

The father of a 20 month- old boy (Charlie) refused to accept the medical excreta propagated by his son's neurologists. The boy's father had to find out about the Ketogenic diet in a library. After only 4 days on the diet the boy's seizures stopped and never returned! (You can Google up the Charlie Foundation).

Working on the work of Dr. Woodyatt, Dr. Russell Wilder at the Mayo Clinic began using the ketogenic diet. Dr. Wilder confirmed that the benefits of fasting could be obtained if "ketonemia" was produced by other means. The ketone bodies...are formed from fat and protein. Whenever a disproportion exists between the amount of fatty acid and the amount of sugar actually burning in the tissues.

In any case, it has long been known, it is possible to provoke "ketogenesis" by feeding diets that are very rich in fat, and low in carbohydrate. As Dr. Wilder suspected, a "keto diet" should be as effective as fasting.

It was Dr. Wilder who coined the term 'KETOGENIC DIET."

Dr. Peterman and other paediatricians eagerly acted on Dr. Wilder's suggestions. Dr. Peterman first reported the calculation and effectiveness of the Ketogenic Diet. From the Mayo Clinic in 1924, Peterman's Ketogenic Diet composed of one gram of protein per kilogram of body weight in children, 10 to 15 grams of carbs per day— and the remainder of calories in fat.

THIS IS IDENTICAL TO THE KETOGENIC DIET USED TODAY AND ADVOCATED IN THIS BOOK.

Dr. Peterman documented the importance of teaching caregivers management of the diet before discharge; individualization of the diet, close follow-up and the potential for further adjustment at home. He observed that excess ketosis could lead to nausea and vomiting- symptoms that were quickly relieved by ORANGE JUICE!

This clinical caveat is still useful to know and is employed as needed during initiation of the Ketogenic Diet. Dr. Talbot also acknowledged the critical role of a "nutritionist" (dietician of the day). A clever nutritionist works (YOU!) and works out various little tricks to get enough fat into your body-☺ (4: 1- fats to carb ratio) is pretty much the common composition of today's ketogenic diet.

McQuarrie and Keith while studying the biochemistry of children on the Ketogenic diet in 1927 made the initial observation that the proportion of acetone bodies in the blood runs parallel to that in the urine.

62 YEARS LATER THIS WAS VALIDATED BY Schwartz et al. The Mayo Clinic investigators were the first to note variations during the day in the intensity of the ketosis- with a maximum in the late afternoon and the nadir in the early morning hours. Kids have a tendency to have seizures in the morning- when ketosis is minimal- and they suggested the addition of a midnight snack to maintain early ketosis.

As mentioned, when the anti-epileptic drugs came along in circa 1938—

DOCTORS ABANDONED THE KETOGENIC DIET. (The Ketogenic Diet was buried together with the thousands of dead people killed by allopathic doctors.)

In 1971, Huttenlocker et al. introduced an MCT Oil diet that was more Ketogenic per calorie- and supposedly to make the ketogenic diet "more palatable".

Some of the Ketogenic clinical studies that I have reviewed describe the ketogenic diet as "not palatable". Folks— this is another classic example of the 99 Percent Rule applying to allopathic doctors.

Allopathic doctors are "unpalatable". The Ketogenic diet is the most delicious tasty food that you will ever eat! (99 % of the advice allopathic doctors give is medical *#%$##%#%! We should always be professional and polite- even if the allopathic crowd are not… two wrongs never make a right.

YOU MUST TEST YOUR KETONE LEVELS.

1. Blood Ketone Meter

This measures BHB and is considered by many to be the most accurate way to measure ketone bodies. You have to prick your finger. You can get a Precision Xtra Blood Glucose and Ketone meter from Abbot Labs for about $ 30.00. Then you need to buy the ketone strips ($ 3 to $ 4 each but you can shop for a bargain on-line). Most people will enter light ketosis with a 0.5 to l mmol reading on the meter. It often takes from 3 days to 3 weeks to get into a stable an optimal ketosis level of 1.5 to 3.0 mmol/L

2. Breath Testing

This test is cheaper and non-invasive. This measurement technique has been shown in the literature to be an accurate way to test for NUTRITIONAL KETOSIS.

The Ketone Acetone Breathalyzer is an easy and inexpensive way to test your BREATH KETONE LEVELS.

Remember- breath ketones are not always a perfect reflection of blood ketones because they can be affected by several factors such as water intake, alcohol consumption, etc. When you blow into the Ketonix mouthpiece, the LED light goes on indicating a colour that corresponds to your LEVEL OF KETONES. You get an electronic program/ file and just plug the Ketonix into a USB port. The one time cost is about $ 200.00. You can consult Dr. Internet.

At the time of going to press for this book—the market for <u>KETONE DEVICES IS SKY-ROCKETING SO- YOU SHOULD DO YOUR RESEARCH AND SHOP AROUND!</u>

3. Urine Ketone Strips

You can test your urine (acetoacetate) with simple strips ($ 10 each?) These are cheaper strips but not as accurate and not considered a reliable analysis of blood ketone levels.

The take-home message is:

<u>YOU ARE IF SERIOUS ABOUT GETTING INTO NUTRITIONAL KETOSIS-</u>

<u>YOU MUST TEST- TEST- AND TEST SOME MORE!</u> (If you are diabetic- you may already have a GLUCOMETER from ABBOTT LABS or your local drugstore.

B.   THE SMART BRAIN—HEAL-THY DIET

> <u>"The chief function of the body is to carry the brain around"</u>
>
> <u>Thomas Edison</u>

If you want to stay <u>HEALTHY</u>—protecting and nourishing your brain should be one of the first things you should do. Every day with your diet and lifestyle habits, you are either <u>HELPING OR DAMAGING THE HEALTH OF YOUR BRAIN.</u>

<u>WITHOUT BRAIN HEALTH- YOU HAVE NO HEALTH!</u>

Your diet, habits and lifestyle determine how old your brain is; how long you will live and how <u>WELL</u> you will live. As your weight goes up- the size of your brain goes down.

THE FATTER YOU GET- THE SMALLER YOUR BRAIN GETS!

We have changed our diet so much in the past 100 years that the human brain is actually <u>SHRINKING!</u> <u>BUT</u>- That's the bad news. The good news: with every meal that we eat, the opportunity exists to make our brain <u>SIGNIFICANTLY HEALTHIER!</u> We may worry about obesity, heart disease and cancer. BUT—all of us have the <u>ABILITY AND THE POWER TO RE-PROGAM OUR GENES WITH FOOD!</u> The biggest benefit received from proper nutritional choices is a healthier brain. Food is Information. We need to provide our brains with the right information. When assessing a person's mental state, it's necessary to consider food—<u>FIRST</u>.

TWO BILLION PEOPLE ON PLANET EARTH ARE IRON DEFICIENT!

According to Dr. Drew Ramsey, (author of Fifty Shades of Kale), people would eat their <u>RDA</u> of <u>IRON</u>—

THE GLOBAL IQ WOULD INCREASE BY 13 POINTS! Zowie. We'd literally have smarter planet simply by eating the right food.

HEALTHY FOOD BUILDS BETTER BRAINS.

Dr. Ramsey continues: "When the brain is missing a single nutrient" he says, "it limps along; sputters...and it misfires."

We have evolved into a species that requires a <u>HIGH</u> portion of our dietary intake to be <u>FAT</u>. Fat is essential to our brain, body and to our <u>TOTAL HEALTH</u>. Very few people eat enough <u>FAT</u>. To make matters worse—most people eat massive amounts of <u>CARBS</u> that fuels their internal sugar factory-which ends up working 24/7.

If you worked 24/7...how long would you last before you would die?

HUGE AMOUNTS OF CARBS MAKE PEOPLE FAT, SICK AND INFLAMMED!

That next slice of "healthy "whole wheat toast will likely eat a hole in the lining of your gut. Humans do not have the metabolism to digest grains. Corn is a grain- not a vegetable. Neither humans, nor animals are able to properly digest grains—nor starchy vegetables!

TO HEAL YOUR BRAIN AND YOUR BODY—YOU MUST EAT A HEALING ANTI-INFLAMMATORY DIET— -THE KETOGENIC DIET.

Thomas Edison was 100 % right. Your brain health is where health starts; and ends; <u>LITERALLY</u>. Have you ever heard that fish is brain food? It's absolutely true.

<u>YOUR BRAIN IS THE FATTEST ORGAN IN YOUR BODY. YOUR BRAIN IS MADE UP OF MORE THAN 75 PERCENT FAT.</u>

<u>YOUR BRAIN IS COMPOSED OF 50 PERCENT CHOLESTEROL!</u>

When you understand that one fact alone—can you imagine that doctors prescribe statin drugs to <u>LOWER CHOLESTEROL! IS THAT CRIMINAL NEGLIGENCE OR WHAT?</u>

The brain has a consistency similar to Tofu. (Please do NOT eat Tofu! It's very unhealthy— <u>you might get Tofu "brain" and die!</u> -☺)

<u>OMEGA-3 FATTY ACIDS ARE THE BEST-DOCUMENTED FAT-DARLINGS OF OUR BRAIN.</u> I'm sure you've heard about the truly remarkable HEALING POWER of Omega-3's. The two big Omega-3's are Docosahexaenoic acid (DHA) and (EPA).

<u>NEW EVIDENCE SHOWS DHA IS SO POWERFUL</u> that it prevents your brain from <u>SHRINKING</u>- as you get older. Research shows t<u>he HIGHER YOUR DHA LEVELS IN YOUR BODY- THE LONGER THAT YOU WILL LIVE!</u>

- <u>DHA REPRESENTS MORE THAN 50 PERCENT</u> of the omega-3 fats in your brain. DHA is 1/3 of the dry weight of your brain.

- <u>50 PERCENT OF THE WEIGHT OF A NEURON'S PLASMA MEMBRANE IS COMPOSED OF DHA</u>; it is an important building block for the membranes surrounding brain cells, particularly at synapses which are the essence of efficient brain function;

- <u>DHA IS ALSO A KEY COMPONENT OF HEART TISSUE.</u>

- <u>DHA PUMPS UP THE VOLUME OF YOUR BRAIN'S GRAY MATTER— ESPECIALLY THE PART ASSOCIATED WITH HAPPINESS!</u>

- <u>DHA IMPROVES BLOOD SUGAR AND INSULIN!</u> In one study- 70 <u>PERCENT OF PEOPLE WITH BLOOD SUGAR CONCERNS TAKING DHA SAW A DRAMATIC IMPROVEMENT IN RESPONSE TO INSULIN!</u>

When you get a high-powered form of Omega-3 FAT DHA into your bloodstream, you grow, activate and nourish the part of your brain that makes you feel happy and at peace with the world. The trick is getting your blood levels high enough. Not only is DHA a reliable brain-booster—<u>IT ALSO IS AN "ESSENTIAL NUTRIENT".</u>

When I say "essential", I mean that your body needs it every day and your body cannot make enough of it on its own. You need to get enough of it in all the right places. DHA has the power to cushion your aching joints; it supports razor-sharp eyesight, and it can keep your oldest, most treasured memories safe for the rest of your life. Because DHA is a must have fuel source for every cell in your body; it has a broad, universal impact from head to toe, and everywhere else in between. You not only depend on it for survival, but you need it to repair, revive and <u>HEAL</u> your body.

Sidebar-

Mother's Breast Milk- is <u>THE MOST POTENT SOURCE OF DHA ON EARTH! IT CONTAINS 4 TIMES MORE DHA AS EPA</u>. Mother Nature will always outsmart anyone wearing a white coat! Shop at her natural Farmacy and you will never go wrong.

<u>DHA IS THE REAL HEALER AND CARE GIVER</u>. New research comparing DHA and EPA backs this up; it shows that DHA supports blood pressure.

<u>DHA</u> supports good circulation. It is the magic one that opens up your tiny blood vessels, called capillaries, that carry oxygen deep into your heart, brain and some hard to reach areas of your body.

<u>DHA</u> restores memory and ramps-up your brain power. A Tufts University study found that those with higher levels of DHA have a <u>47 PERCENT</u> lower risk of memory and brain difficulties.

<u>DHA</u> keeps your <u>HDL HIGH</u> and keeps your <u>TRIGLYCERIDES LOW</u>; in higher doses, it's DHA that catapults your HDL to super protective levels, while keeping bad blood fats low.

<u>DHA</u> supports keen eyesight and a spotless retina. Studies show DHA to be the real vision helper. Those with high levels were <u>40 to 50 PERCENT LESS LIKELY TO HAVE MACULAR VISION ISSUES</u>.

<u>DHA</u> lubricates joints. Studies show people taking highly –absorbable <u>DHA</u> saw their <u>PAIN SCORES DROP BY 22.9 PERCENT!</u>

<u>DHA IS A POWERFUL DETOXIFICATION WHICH ENHANCES GENETIC EXPRESSION! RESEARCH SHOWS THAT COMPOUNDS GENERATED FROM THE OXIDATION OF DHA AND EPA (in vivo) CAN REACH CONCENTRATIONS HIGH ENOUGH TO INDUCE NrF2 ANTIOXIDANT AND DETOXIFICATION DEFENSE SYSTEMS.</u>

<u>DHA</u> protects your brain from fuzzy memory and loss of focus. It keeps the messages in your brain moving fast and accurately. It signals your brain to maintain healthy function and quick thinking.

DHA is the main nutrient that helps your brain grow new branches, neural networks, and renew and rejuvenate itself.

In one study—known as the MIDAS (Memory Improvement with DHA study, 485 subjects averaging 70 years old with mild memory problems were supplemented with DHA for 6 months. Those subjects who consumed the most DHA had a 60 PERCENT REDUCTION IN RISK FOR DEVELOPING ALZHEIMER'S DISEASE.

In the Framingham 10 year study of 899 subjects the results showed that there was a 47 PERCENT REDUCTION OF ALZHEIMER'S DISEASE AMONG THE HIGHEST BLOOD LEVELS OF DHA.

MOREOVER- THE RESEARCHERS ALSO FOUND THAT CONSUMPTION OF MORE THAN 2 SERVNGS OF FISH PER WEEK WAS ASSOCIATED WITH A 59 PERCENT REDUCTION IN THE OCCURRENCE OF ALZEIMER'S DISEASE.

DHA IS MOTHER NATURE'S ANTI-INFLAMMATORY MAGIC BULLET.

DHA is an important regulator of inflammation. It naturally reduces the activity of the COX-2 ENZYME (which can turn on damaging brain chemicals. Low DHA is also a biomarker for brain aging. The famous (or infamous) Framingham study showed that people with LOW DHA levels have SMALLER BRAINS; and do worse on tests of visual memory, function and thinking.

DHA HELPS PREVENT METABOLIC DYSFUNCTION (aka busted metabolism) RESULTING FROM TOO MANY CARBS IN THE DIET.

Sidebar-

Because of its PHENOMENAL HEALTH BENEFITS; Krill Oil, (an animal-based Omega-3 fat) IS ONE OF THE FEW SUPPLEMENTS that I heartily recommend for virtually everyone to improve overall health. (Most days I take 400mg. of DHA / 1000mg of Krill oil). I-t is 47 times more anti-inflammatory than aspirin. But please be careful— research shows that statin drugs NULLIFY the health effects of Krill Oil.

MOST DRUGS BLOCK THE ABSORPTION OF ESSENTIAL NUTRIENTS!

BLOCKING ABSORPTION OF NUTRIENTS IS NOT A SIDE EFFECT- THE BLOCKING OF NUTRIENTS IS A DIRECT EFFECT OF MOST DRUGS!

One study published in the Journal Nutrition Research showed that people taking Krill oil for 4 weeks had their Omega-3 LEVELS SKYROCKET BY 178 PERCENT!

How cool is that?

Research indicates <u>MOST FISH OIL</u> is rancid. Fish oil is a triglyceride molecule that has to be broken down in your gut into DHA and EPA. About 80-85 percent is never absorbed and is eliminated in your intestine. (50 percent of people cannot tolerate fish oil which causes "fish burbs." Then, once the fatty acids are absorbed into your bloodstream, your liver has to attach "tophosphatidyl choline" (PC), for it to be used by the body.

The Beauty of krill oil is that it already is a <u>PHOSPOLIPID</u>. It's in the correct form in the capsule— so it is bioavailable; it crosses the blood-brain-barrier (BBB) readily and your body uses virtually all of it. Krill oil contains a powerful antioxidant called "Astaxanthin"; which is responsible for the pink colour of salmon and flamingos.

<u>OMEGA-3 DEFICIENCY IS THE 7th BIGGEST KILLERS OF AMERICANS-ESTIMATED AT ALMOST 100,000 PRE-MATURE DEATHS EACH YEAR!</u>

Squid oil also appears to a good source of DHA. Best food sources are wild-caught salmon, sardines, etc. Have you ever tried fresh calamari rings coated with shredded coconut and gently fried in coconut oil? Hmmm...Yummy! Your brain will love them too!

Recent research shows that animal-based Omega-3 fatty acids, (especially EPA) and Vitamin D improve cognitive function and behaviour associated with it- e.g. ADHD, bipolar disorder, and schizophrenia by regulating your brain's <u>SERATONIN LEVELS</u>. The Omega 3 fatty acid EPA reduces inflammation signalling molecules in your brain that inhibit serotonin release from pre-synaptic neurons, thereby <u>BOOSTING YOUR SERATONIN LEVELS</u>. DHA also has a beneficial effect on serotonin receptors by increasing their access to serotonin. According to researchers, optimizing your Vitamin D and animal-based fats EPA and DHA will help optimize your brain serotonin concentrations and function. This will/can prevent brain problems. Seratonin, a pre-cursor to the formation of <u>MELATONIN WHICH HAS MANY HEALTH BENEFITS</u>, such as reduced cancer risk, etc.

MCT OIL-

<u>MCT OIL- (Medium-chain-triglycerides) IS ABSOLUTELY AMAZING FOR YOUR BRAIN! RESEARCH SHOWS</u> that the administration of MCT oils caused a significant improvement in cognitive functioning in adults with memory disorders.

<u>THE BEST WAY TO ADD COCONUT/MCT OIL TO YOUR DIET</u> (without adverse gastrointestinal effects) <u>IS TO START WITH ONE TEASPOON EACH DAY AND WORK UP TO 1 to 3 TABLESPOONS PER DAY. 4 to 6 TABLESPOONS OF COCONUT OIL PER DAY IS THE THERAPEUTIC DOSAGE TO REVERSE DIABETES OR ALZHEIMER'S DISEASE.</u>

** Coffee drinkers may wish to try my <u>HIGH-OCTANE KETOGENIC COFFEE RECEIPE</u>- infra). This is my Ketogenic coffee inspired by Dave Asprey's "Bulletproof Coffee" name/recipe bears TM.

THE KETOGENIC DIET HAS AMAZING BRAIN-HEALTH BENEFITS!

SOME INCREDIBLE INFORMATION ABOUT YOUR BRAIN:

- The brain holds only 2 percent of the body's mass- but contains <u>25 percent</u> of the body's <u>CHOLESTEROL</u> which supports brain function and development;

- <u>TWENTY PERCENT OF YOUR BRAIN BY WEIGHT IS CHOLESTEROL!</u>

  (How much sense does it make to take a statin (cholesterol-lowering) drug which will make you dumber, poison your liver and slowly kill you?

  <u>BOTH FAT and CHOLESTEROL ARE SEVERELY DEFICIENT IN DISEASED BRAINS</u>; higher cholesterol levels in later life are associated with increased longevity; 75 percent of people admitted to hospitals have normal cholesterol levels;

- Remember for every <u>EXCESS POUND— PUT ON YOUR BODY</u>- your brain gets a little <u>SMALLER</u>! Remember- the FATTER you are- the smaller your brain! Eat fat to get lean. Who knew?

- Your brain can generate about 25 watts of power at any given time; you might be able to power a small light- but it might be difficult to wire it up. -☺

- The brain's immune system is composed of cells called <u>MICROGLIA</u>, which function similarly to the macrophages found in other parts of the body;

- You have as many microglia in your brains as <u>NEURONS</u>; They cover nearly all of your brain tissue; they are <u>MOBILE</u>; they move around to identify and destroy foreign particles; they can pose a threat to your neurons; Microglia play a key role in your brain's immune response by producing a number of inflammatory molecules. This inflammatory response is a double-edged sword; If inflammation doesn't resolve, it can damage cerebral tissue—<u>DAMAGE THAT CAN BE PERMANENT!</u> When microglia become confused; they sometimes become hyperactive and begin to attack everything. This can lead to cognitive deficiencies, demyelation, permanent brain damage or even <u>DEATH</u>.

- <u>YOU ACTUALLY USE</u> more than 10 percent of your brain- <u>YOU USE ALL OF YOUR BRAIN!</u>

- The human brain is estimated to contain about 100 billion neurons;

- Having a bigger brain though- does not mean necessarily mean that you are SMARTER; (Albert Einstein had a relatively small brain);

- Experts estimate that over the course of a lifetime, modern human brains will retain about a QUADRILLION pieces of information!

- There are more than 100,000 CHEMICAL REACTIONS happening in your brain every SECOND!

- Every day YOU have about 70, 000 thoughts; (I'm betting that most of them are not about your job...-☺) our brain will retain and hold up to 2.5 petabytes of information or the equivalent of 300 hours of television!

- Most of your brain is ACTIVE ALL OF THE TIME; your brain is MORE ACTIVE WHEN YOU ARE ASLEEP! During sleep your brain takes out the brain trash with its waste removal system called the GLYMPHATIC SYSTEM.

- You have MORE THAN 100,000 MILES of AXONS in your brain; - that's enough to wrap around the Earth 4 times!

- The brain has about 100 BILLION NEURONS;

- Information can travel in your brain at a speed of 260 MPH;

- Your brain does not have PAIN receptors—it can't feel anything- that's why your brain can't feel anything; (you have a headache because your "other brain says that you ate too much junk food or drank too much alcohol;

- You have as many MICROGLIA in your brain as NEURONS;

- Microglia cover nearly all of your brain tissue; THEY ARE MOBILE; they move about in order to identify and destroy foreign particles;

- Microglia play a key role in your brain's immune response; they pose a threat to your neurons because they produce a number of inflammatory molecules;

- This inflammatory response is a double-edged sword; if INFLAMMATION does not resolve, it can damage cerebral tissue- DAMAGE that can be PERMANENT; when microglia become confused- they sometimes become' hyperactive' and attack everything. This can lead to cognitive deficiencies; DEMETHYLATION, permanent brain death or even DEATH.

- ANY HIGH PERFORMANCE ENGINE NEEDS FUEL HIGH-OCTANE FUEL. OUR BRAIN IS OUR HIGH-PERFORMANCE ORGAN! IT HAS A VERY POWERFUL PATHWAY CALLED AN NrF2 PATHWAY-supra).

  The NrF2 pathway is activated by some foods- e.g. COFFEE; (coffee lovers will enjoy my Supercharged High Octane Coffee recipe infra). This pathway, the NrF2 pathway is also activated by CALORIC RESTRICTION AND EXERCISE; infra.

- EVERYDAY- WE HAVE ABOUT 70,000 THOUGHTS! FOOD and SEX likely account for a most of these. -☺)

- Our brain contains a memory boosting protein called BRAIN-DERIVED NEUROTROPIC FACTOR OR BDNF. BDNF IS THE MASTER MOLECULE IN YOUR BRAIN THAT HELPS BUILD THE COMPLEX INFRASTRUCTURE IN YOUR BRAIN

- THE MORE BDNF YOU HAVE, THE MORE BRAIN CELLS YOUR BRAIN MAKES AND THE STRONGER THE CONNECTION BETWEEN THEM. BDNF SHARPENS YOR MEMORY, FOCUS AND ALERTNESS. It improves skills like driving a car, boat or operating machinery.

- Studies show that your brain's BDNF LEVELS GET A BIG BOOST WHEN YOU DO VIGOROUS EXERCISE!

- Our brain has a MAGNIFICIENT WASTE DISPOSAL SYSTEM; called the "GLYMPHATIC SYSTEM." This system operates in a similar way to your body's LYMPHATIC SYSTEM; (Exercise chapter- infra), which is responsible for eliminating cellular waste products. The lymphatic system does not include your brain. The reason for this is that your brain is almost a closed system; protected by the blood-brain-barrier (BBB). The (BBB) controls what can go through to your brain and what cannot. The glymphatic system, controlled by "glia brain cells" ("G"), manages your brain's waste system.

  By pumping cerebral spinal fluid (CSF) continually through your brain's tissues, the glymphatic system flushes waste from your brain back into your body's circulatory system. (CSF) is your brain's "DRANO"-☺) The (CSF) flows from your arteries to brain to veins and from there the waste eventually reaches your liver where it's broken down and ultimately eliminated. The coolest part is this:

  YOUR GLYMPHATIC SYSTEM FIRES UP ITS ACTIVITY DURING SLEEP. This allows your brain to clear out TOXINS- including a VERY HARMFUL PROTEIN CALLED "AMYLOID-BETA". Research clearly shows that the build-up of this toxic substance causes the brain to be "clogged". This build-up of amyloid-beta is a main culprit which causes dementia, Alzheimer's and a host of brain-related diseases. During sleep, the glymphatic system is 10 <u>TIMES MORE ACTIVE</u> than during wakefulness. During sleep, simultaneously your <u>BRAIN CELLS SHRINK ABOUT 60 PERCENT</u>. This allows for greater efficiency of waste removal. During the day, the constant activity of your brain cells causes your <u>BRAIN CELLS TO SWELL IN SIZE</u>—until they take up 85 <u>PERCENT OF YOUR BRAIN'S VOLUME</u>. Ever been told that a swelled head is a good thing?-☺

- Recently researchers have discovered that the (BBB) naturally tends to become more permeable with age. This has a negative result. This increased permeability allows <u>TOXINS</u> to enter your brain more <u>EASILY</u>. But your body is <u>AMAZING</u>. Increased permeability of the BBB— <u>ALSO MEANS THAT THE GOOD STUFF</u>- e.g. neurotransmitters, good fatty acids <u>ETC. ARE ALSO ABLE TO GET THROUGH YOUR</u> (BBB) <u>EASIER TOO!</u> Who says that we become more hard-headed with age?-☺ In conjunction with reduced efficiency of the glymphatic system, damage in both your brain and your (BBB) can start to accumulate at an increased pace which can lead to brain problems like Alzheimer's disease.

In sum, if we do not eat the proper foods and nutrients; get at least 8 hours good sleep- the brain's "sewer system" will become clogged—and everyone knows that a clogged sewer is not a good thing. -☺)

<u>YOUR 75 PERCENT FAT BRAIN—NEEDS LOTS OF HEALTHY FAT! (CARBS NEED NOT APPLY-</u>☺

<u>SHOCKINGLY— DOCTORS AND DIE-TICIANS STILL RECOMMEND A LOW-FAT- HIGH -CARB DIET!</u>

When you adopt the brain-smart Ketogenic Diet; you will be <u>LIGHT YEARS AHEAD OF THESE POOR MISGUIDED SOULS! You can spread the word to your friends and loved ones.</u> You will have the knowledge and expertise to advise them of the benefits they will receive-from a Ketogenic- <u>BRAIN-SMART DIET</u>. This is diet for every person, young or old, who values good brain health—the fundamental key to <u>TOTAL SUPERHEALTH</u>.

<u>LET THY FAT BE THY MEDICINE. LET THY MEDICINE BE THY FAT.</u>

As you might have guessed- we are designed to be smart our entire lives. Conventional doctors believe our brain is supposed to deteriorate. You're reading this book so you likely believe that humans are programmed to be smart until our last breath.

Conventional doctors are taught that with age comes cognitive decline. They are taught and <u>BELIEVE</u> like most people, that the brain degenerates with age. These people erroneously believe that getting old; getting wrinkles, and getting sick is our human destiny.

THIS IS ANOTHER MONSTROUS BIG PHARMA LIE! IT'S A BIG WHOPPER!

THE TRUTH IS—YOU DO NOT NEED TO GET OLD, FEEBLE AND LOSE YOUR 'MARBLES"-☺ YOU HAVE THE POWER TO RE-GENERATE NEW MARBLES (aka BRAIN CELLS—YOU CAN GROW YOUR BRAIN!

YOU CAN RE-SET YOUR DNA BACK TO ITS FACTORY SETTING!

STUDIES PROVE OUR DNA CAN BE RE-PROGRAMMED IN TWO MINUTES!

This sounds incredible— but it's **TRUE!** You are not the victims of your genetic destiny. You have the **INCREDIBLE POWER** to change your **GENETIC DESTINY!** Our day-to-day lifestyle choices have profound effects on our **HEALTH AND OUR LONGEVITY.**

THE SCIENCE OF EPIGENETICS PROVES WE CAN CHANGE THE EXPRESSION OF MORE THAN 90 PERCENT OF OUR GENES!

THIS IS POSSIBLE IN TWO WAYS:

BY EATING THE RIGHT FOODS —AND BY EMPLOYING THE PROPER LIFESTYLE CHANGES.

We can enhance the expression ("turn on") of our **"HEALTHY GENES",** while "turning off" the genes that trigger bad things such as **INFLAMMATION AND PRODUCTION OF FREE RADICALS (ROS)** or **REACTIVE OXYGEN SPECIES.** The bad genes (bad guys) are **STRONGLY INFLUENCED BY OUR DIETARY APPROACH.**

FOOD IS INFORMATION. GOOD FAT IS THE BEST INFORMATION IN THE WORLD. YOUR BRAIN LOVES GOOD FAT. IT CRAVES GOOD FATS!

Conversely carbohydrates, (bad information) destroy our brain-by slowly eating it away—**LITERALLY.**

Our brain is a **DYNAMIC ORGAN.** It's constantly adapting, changing- **FOR BETTER** or **FOR WORSE.** A poor diet loaded with carbs will destroy your brain. A healthy fat rich diet will support your brain health. You must eat to maintain brain health. Healthy-brain rich nutrients will grow and maintain the physiology of your brain.

A KETOGENIC DIET HELPS YOUR BRAIN GROW NEW NEURONS.

All of us can grow new neurons throughout our entire lives. We can reinforce existing brain circuits and create entirely new connections and GROW NEW BRAIN CELLS!

THIS PROCESS WHEREBY YOU CAN GROW NEW NEURONS IS CALLED "NEUROGENESIS" (your doctor may not believe this-☺). THIS PROCESS IS ALSO CALLED –"NEUROPLASTICITY."

If you wish to stay healthy; protecting and nourishing your brain should be THE FIRST THING THAT YOU DO! The Ketogenic Diet is the brain-healthy diet.

EVERY DAY THROUGH YOUR BEHAVIOUR, YOUR FOOD AND WITH YOUR THOUGHTS-

YOU'RE EITHER HELPING YOUR BRAIN'S HEALTH —or— YOU'RE DAMAGING YOUR BRAINS' HEALTH.

YOU HAVE FAR MORE CONTROL OVER YOUR BRAIN, YOUR BODY AND YOUR MIND THAN YOU THINK!

ACTIVITY AND MOVEMENT STIMULATES PLASTICITY! Plasticity is what allows tissues to HEAL. YOUR BODY AND YOUR BRAIN ARE MALLEABLE- LIKE PUTTY!

TWO TYPES OF NEUROPLASTICITY EXIST:

- Functional Plasticity= your brain's ability to move functions from a damaged area to undamaged areas and-

- Structural Plasticity= your brain's ability to change its physical structure as a result of learning;

The take-home message:

YOU HAVE THE POWER TO CHANGE— YOUR BRAIN- YOUR BODY— AND EVERY ASPECT OF YOUR LIFE!

The foods you eat, exercise, emotional states, sleep patterns and your STRESS LEVELS all affect your BRAIN- CONTINUOUSLY EVERY WAKING MOMENT –even during your dreams too-☺ You should not eat at least 3 hours before going to sleep. Snacking before bed is not a good idea.

Your pancreas, liver and the rest of your digestive system NEED TO REST TOO! Three hours before bedtime you need to make sure that you've locked the doors to your internal sugar factory. You will learn how to train your body to FAST for 16-17 hours.

<u>WHEN YOU STOP RECEIVING HUNGER SIGNALS EVERY 5 or 6 hours-YOU ARE WELL ON YOUR WAY TO BECOMING KETO-ADAPTED.</u> You will be building new and better metabolic machinery. You will be <u>RE-BUILDING YOUR FAT- BURNING FURNACE</u>—(formerly called your Internal Sugar Factory.

All of us interact with our genome every moment of our lives.

<u>KEEPING YOUR BLOOD SUGAR LOW IS VERY POSITIVE!</u> Low blood sugar levels permit your genes to express <u>REDUCED INFLAMMATION WHICH INCREASES THE PRODUCTION OF NEUROTRANSMITTERS</u> (aka feel good chemical messengers) <u>AND ANTIOXIDANTS</u> (aka your body's natural rust-proofers).

<u>IN SUM –</u>

<u>YOU HAVE THE POWER TO RE-PROGRAM YOUR GENES &</u>

<u>YOU CAN GROW NEW BRAIN CELLS- AND A NEW BRAIN!</u>

<u>MY TOP 10—BRAIN SMART FOODS</u>

- **Coconut Oil**
- **Coffee (esp. High-Octane Buttered Coffee)**
- **Tumeric**
- **Wild Alaskan Salmon (or Sockeye)**
- **Broccoli & Cauliflower (cruciferous veggies)**
- **Blueberries**
- **Walnuts**
- **Celery**
- **Sprirulina**
- **Chorella**

<u>12 POWERFUL BRAIN NUTRIENTS</u>

- **Acetyl L- carnitine (ALC)-**

   This exceptional brain nutrient boosts your brain power! It promotes dendrite rejuvenation. It restores razor-sharp thinking. Studies show that if you're low on mental energy, your mitochondria could be deficient. Supplying your brain with ALC maintains and rebuilds brain cells; enhances your mind's power and energy; it gives you more stamina; maintains healthy moods; promotes short-term memory; promotes increase of dopamine from neurons and supports other beneficial brain factors; ALC stimulates your brain to grow more neurites (the branches that are extensions of your brain cells). These let brain cells communicate with each other. (ALC keeps the receptors of your growth factors, (NGF's) healthy and vital.

- Alpha-GPC- boosts your brain's memory fuel to limit "senior moments";

- Bacopa (also called Brahmi)

This is one of Mother Nature's most potent remedies for forgetfulness. It is a perennial plant with white or blue flowers and grows throughout southern Asia. It has been commonly cited as a nerve tonic in Ayurvedic Medicine. It has been traditionally used to enhance learning and memory through its neuroprotective and antioxidant properties. The active constituents for cognitive have been linked to saponin compounds called bacosides. They have been shown to improve neurotransmission among brain cells, repair damaged neurons and improve nerve synapse performance, as well as increase serotonin production.

Research trials suggest that bacopa can help provide relief for memory recall, comprehension, anxiety, depression, insomnia and ADD.

Bacopa is not addictive and has no reported side effects after CENTURIES OF USE IN AYURVEDIC MEDICINE. IT IS SAFE FOR EVERYONE.

- Baicalin

Baicalin is contained in an herb called Hoodwot. Baiclin travels to the hippocampus (power center of the limbic system responsible for forming, storing and processing memory.) Baiclin builds, rebuilds and maintains brain cells in the hippocampus. It supercharges cell production; it restores mental horsepower -☺; Studies also show Baiclin significantly alleviated memory-associated decreases in the hippocampus.

- Luteolin- to combat inflammation in the brain and restore working memory;

- Phosphatidylestrine (PS) – to support cell membranes;

- VINPOCETINE

Vinpocetine is phenomenal for your brain and your body's

health. Studies show that it can boost and speed up blood flow to your brain. It increases oxygen to your brain; it boosts memory; it supports CNS health generally; it reduces your risk of brain health problems; it produces lots of those "feel good" neurotransmitters like dopamine.

Vinpocetine helps direct your thinking and behaviour to stay motivated. It provides lightning recall; it floods your brain with FEROCIOUS THOUGHT-CREATING ENERGY! IT HARNESSES YOUR UNTAPPED INTELLECTUAL POTENTIAL FOR SUCCESS! How cool is that?

- Ginkgo biloba

The Ginkgo biloba tree is one of the oldest trees in the world and is native to China. They reach up to 40 metres in height and have greenish-yellow fan-shaped leaves. This herb helps improve memory and overall brain functions. The ginkgo leaves contain two chemicals- flavonoids and terpenoids, which are important antioxidants that inhibit free radical damage to the brain- and other areas of the body. Oxidative stress is a leading factor in the development of neurodegenerative brain diseases, like dementia, Parkiinson's and Alzheimer's disease.

The World Health Organization reports that gingko can help people suffering from cerebrovascular insufficiency, which can manifest as poor concentration, memory and headaches. ** N.B. Be careful when choosing a Ginkgo Supplement! Those from China could be laced with high levels of toxic heavy lead.

EVEN THE AIR COMING FROM CHINA IS CONTAMINATED!

- Acetycholine is an important neuro-transmitter (chemical messenger) which helps maintain memories and improve mental clarity. Two herbs which help to rejuvenate your brain are:

- Sage— try it; smell it; breathe it and eat it! It helps maintain normal healthy memory;

- TUMERIC- (Circumin)

This phenomenal orange (or white) coloured herb has Big Pharma quaking in its boots! -☺)

A recent Japanese Study (NishiKawa W. et al. from the Dept. of Neurology in Karniya Hospital in Tokyo discovered that 3 subjects experienced incredible

Brain health results after taking Tumeric Powder capsules for 12 weeks.

Tip: Look for a Circumin Supplement that contains Piper-
ine. This is a black pepper extract that greatly increases
the absorption of turmeric (and other nutrients). I recommend that you take ONE GRAM DAILY of turmeric, (major compound Curcumin) to get the most benefits.

- REISHI

  In Eastern Medicine, reishi is known as the "mushroom of im-
  mortality" and the "King of Herbs". It is a medicinal mushroom
  that grows in various regions of the world in damp and tem-
  perate conditions. Reishi is known to have multiple benefits
  to the immune system, cardiovascular, adrenal, nerve and
  mental functions. It is a great brain herb due to its strong anti-
  bacterial and fungal qualities. It helps the health of the vagus
  nerve/gut connection. (Our gut may be our first brain). This
  herb also has strong adaptogenic qualities which provide us
  with calmness and mental clarity in stressful situations.

N.B** This list is illustrative only; e.g. krill oil and brain (blue) berries
are not included.

What does it mean to have a KETOGENIC BRAIN?

(Glutamate and GABA)

GABA is the major inhibitory neurotransmitter in the mammalian
nervous system. GABA is made from glutamate. GLUTAMATE is the
major excitatory transmitter. You need both of these; BUT- trouble
arises if too much glutamate creates too much excitement in
the brain.

Too much excitement in the brain means NEUROTOXICITY- THE
EXTREME MANIFESTATION OF WHICH IS SEIZURES! Neurological
diseases (e.g. .depression, bi-polar disorder, migraines, ALS, and
dementia have been linked to NEUROTOXICITY.

GLUTAMATE can either BECOME GABA (Inhibitory);- OR- IT CAN
BECOME ASPARTATE. The latter is (Excitatory) and in EXCESS
IS NEUROTOXIC!

KETOGENIC DIETS SEEM TO FAVOR GLUTAMATE BECOMING GABA—
(as opposed to Aspartate). NO ONE KNOWS WHY THIS IS SO.

PART OF THE REASON HAS TO DO WITH HOW KETONES ARE
METABOLIZED –AND— HOW KETOSIS FAVOURS USING ACETATE FOR
FUEL. (Acetoacetate is a ketone body after all).

Acetate becomes glutamine, an essential precursor for GABA. It is less efficient to make ATP from glucose than it is to make ATP from ketone bodies. More garbage (aka cellular waste) is left over when glucose is burned. A more efficient energy supply makes it easier wwhe when trestore membranes (mem-brains) in the brain to their normal states. After a when a depolarizing electrical energy spike occurs; this means that energy is produced with fewer destructive free radicals left over. The brain needs a boatload of energy to keep all those membrane potentials maintained—to keep pushing sodium out of the cells and pulling potassium into the cells.

Our brain is only 2% of our body weight; but it uses 20 PERCENT OF OUR OXYGEN; AND 10% of glucose stores just to keep running. Some brain cells are actually too small (or have tendrils that are too small) to accommodate to accommodate the mitochondria. In those places, we must use glucose itself (via Glycolysis) to create ATP).

WHEN WE CHANGE THE MAIN FUEL OF OUR BRAIN FROM GLUCOSE TO KETONES, WE CHANGE AMINO ACID HANDLING AND THAT MEANS WE CHANGE THE RATIOS OF GLUTAMATE AND GABA.

The best responders to a Ketogenic Diet for EPILEPSY end up with the highest amount of GABA in the central nervous system. Our brain has to keep the reins on the amount of GLUTAMATE hanging out in the synapses. Too much GLUTAMATE in the synapse means BRAIN INJURY- OR SEIZURES; OR LOW-LEVEL EXCITOTOXICITY as you might see in depression. The brain is humming along(in ketosis-hopefully-☺ like a madman. Even a little bit more efficient use of energy makes it easier for the brain to pull the GLUTAMATE back into the cells. (That- dear readers is a good thing-☺)

In sum, we need to build a Ketogenic Brain; we need to build a brain then burns fat rather than glucose. A ketogenic brain produces BOATLOADS OF NEUROPROTECTIVE substances.

YOU SHOULD REPAIR BUSTED CELLS—YOU SHOULD GROW NEW BRAIN CELLS.

YOU SHOULD EAT A BRAIN-HEALTHY KETOGENIC DIET.

C.   FAT VS. CARB METABOLISM

What is metabolism?

Metabolism refers to the physical and chemical processes that syn-thesize energy. These chemical processes take place within the cells with help from enzymes and hormones. This process converts food and oxygen to the energy needed to run the body. Increasing or boosting your metabolism increases energy and enables weight loss. Everyone's metabolism is different. This is partly determined by your genetics. Your metabolism is also influenced by your age. Research shows that your metabolism slows down 5 percent each decade after age 40.

BUT—THERE ARE MANY LIFESTYLE/ DIETARY CHANGES THAT INCREASE METABOLISM FOR EVERYONE.

When you begin the process of digestion, your metabolism increases especially during the 1st hour after eating. Protein requires 25 % more energy. Higher protein/fats can help boost your metabolic rate. Each 100 calories of protein takes about 30 calories to digest.

What is energy production?

There are many man-made myths surrounding energy production on our body. There are also myths about which foods supply energy. Mitochondria or organelles are the little powerhouses or little "power engines" inside cells where they produce the cell's energy.

MAINSTREAM SCIENCE SAYS CARBS ARE USED AS FUEL FOR ENERGY PRODUCTION. This process is called "oxidative" metabolism because oxygen is consumed in the process. There's only one small problem.

MAINSTREAM SCIENCE DOES NOT UNDERSTAND THAT OUR MITOCHONDRIA ARE SPECIFICALLY DESIGNED AND PROGRAMMED TO USE "FAT" FOR ENERGY PRODUCTION!

If the power centers of our cells are made to burn fat—why does a FAT PHOBIA EXIST?

The energy produced by the mitochondria is stored in a chemical energy molecule called ADENOSINE TRIPHOSPHATE (ATP). Energy-packed ATP is then transported throughout the cell, and energy is released on demand with the help of specific enzymes. In addition the fuel that they produce, mitochondria also produce an oxygen by-product called "reactive oxygen species" (ROS) aka "FREE RADICALS".

THE TRUE FAT NATURE OF OUR METABOLIC MACHINERY HAS SUPPRESSED BY MAINSTREAM SCIENCE!

OUR MITOCHONDRIA, (little powerhouses of our cells) WERE SPECIFICALLY DESIGNED TO USE FAT FOR ENERGY- NOT CARBOHYDRATES!! OMG!

THIS IS SOOOO IMPORTANT!

THIS MEANS THAT OUR MITOCHONDRIA ARE PRIMARILY DESIGNED TO USE FAT AS ENERGY! DEAR READERS- THIS SCIENTIFIC TRUTH IS A GAME-CHANGER!

This is what Christian B. Allan, Phd and Wolfgang Lutz, MD said in their book titled "Life Without Bread":

> "Carbohydrates are not required to obtain energy. Fat supplies more energy than a comparable amount of carbohydrate, and low-carbohydrate diets tend to make your system of producing energy more efficient. Furthermore many organs prefer fat for energy.
>
> Mitochondria are the power plant of the cell. Because they produce most of the energy in the body, the amount of energy available is based on how well the mitochondria are working. Whenever you think of energy, think of all of those mitochondria churning out ATP to make the entire body function correctly. The amount of mitochondria in each cell varies, but up to 50 percent of the total cell volume can be mitochondria. When you get tired, don't just assume you need more carbohydrates; instead, think in terms of how you can maximize your mitochondrial energy production...
>
> If you could shrink to a small enough size to get inside the mitochondria, what would you discover? The first thing that you'd learn is that the mitochondria are primarily designed to use fat for energy!" (author's underline)

HEALTHY CELL MEMBRANES:

The cell membrane is the double outer layer of fatty acids. This structure is made of a blend of saturated, monounsaturated and highly unsaturated fatty acids (HUFAs). The cell membrane and particularly the HUFA's are very susceptible to free radical damage. This free radical damage causes something called "lipid peroxidation" which negatively affects hormone sensitivity.

Elevated lipid peroxidation leads to problems like INSULIN RESISTANCE AND POOR BLOOD SUGAR METABOLISM. Insulin resistance and poor blood sugar metabolism leads to FAT STORAGE and MUSCLE TISSUE BREAKDOWN. This is the exact opposite to healthy aging and a healthy body.

The TWO biggest dietary factors that REDUCE LIPID PEROXIDATION ARE:

A. <u>CARBOHYDRATE LEVEL OF THE DIET</u>

B. <u>THE ANTI-OXIDANT CONTENT OF THE DIET</u>

Abundant research proves that a low-carbohydrate, ketogenic diet reduces oxidative stress in our bodies. The reduction in oxidative stress on the cell membrane allows for the formation of <u>HEALTHY INSULIN RECEPTORS AND NORMALIZED BLOOD SUGAR REGULATION</u>. This, of course improves insulin sensitivity which further <u>REDUCES INFLAMMATION</u>. Better insulin sensitivity means that the body stores <u>LESS FAT</u>. Better insulin sensitivity means less <u>STRESS</u> on the rest of our body. This makes it easier TO <u>BURN FAT AND BUILD MUSCLE</u>.

Based on this information— how come you do not see <u>KETOGENIC DIETS RECOMMENDED UNIVERSALLY</u> by all our health care providers?

<u>THIS IS THE BIGGEST HEALTH/ NUTRITIONAL GAFFE IN THE LAST CENTURY!</u>

<u>THE WHITE-COATED CARB- PUSHING PEOPLE STILL ERRONEOUSLY RECOMMEND CARBS (aka SUGAR/GLUCOSE) AS THE MAIN STAPLE AND MAIN SOURCE OF OUR DIETARY INTAKE.</u>

<u>BUT NOW—YOU KNOW THE SECRET TO A SUPER-METABOLISM!</u>

<u>YOU WILL BE ABLE TO APPLY THIS FUNDAMENTAL PRINCIPLE OF HUMAN METABOLISM! THE KETOGENIC DIET WILL TRANSFORM YOUR ENTIRE BODY!</u>

<u>YOU WILL DISCOVER WHAT IT FEELS LIKE TO BURN HIGH-OCTANE FAT-FUEL!</u> Once you graduate from carb-school to fat -school—you will feel <u>BETTER THAN YOU EVER HAVE</u>!-☺

<u>YOU WILL BE AMONG THE FIRST HUMANS TO FUEL YOUR BODY AS OUR ANCESTORS DID.</u> A ketogenic diet respects our genome and our biochemistry. You will be powering your brain and heart with fuel that makes both work 25 to 28 percent more efficiently.

<u>FAT IS THE PREFERRED FUEL OF OUR BRAIN—THE PREFERRED FUEL OF OUR HEART—AND—THE PREFERRED FUEL OF HUMAN METABOLISM!</u> Who knew?

How does our body turn <u>FOOD</u> into <u>ENERGY</u> aka ATP.

<u>What are the 5 STEPS involved in making ATP within our mitochondria?</u>

The process is rather complicated but you only need to have a general idea. You do not need to focus on the terminology; you just need an idea of the five steps of ATP production. Then you will understand how energy is created within our mitochondria.

FATS ARE KEY TO OPTIMIZE MITOCHONDRIAL FUNCTION.

<u>First step</u>: Getting food fuel source into mitochondria (carbs or fats)-

Fuel must get into the mitochondria where the action happens. Fuel can come from <u>CARBS</u> or it can come from <u>FATS</u>. Fatty acids (chemical name for fat), medium and large-sized fatty acids are transported (think like a train) into the mitochondria with the help of a substrate called "L-carnitine". This word- L-carnitine is taken from the Greek word "carnis" which means meat of flesh. L-carnitine is chiefly found in <u>animal</u> foods/products.

Fuel coming from <u>CARBS</u> needs to get broken down; first, outside of the mitochondria and the product of this breakdown (<u>PYRUVATE</u>) is the substance that gets transported inside of the mitochondria- OR- it can be used in a very inefficient way <u>outside</u> of the mitochondria through <u>anaerobic</u> (without oxygen) <u>metabolism</u> which produces ATP .

Step 2- Fuel is converted into Acetyl-CoA

When <u>PYRUVATE</u> – the product broken down from CARBS enters the mitochondria- it must be first converted into acetyl-CoA by an enzymatic reaction. Fatty acids that are <u>ALREADY</u> inside the mitochondria are broken down into acetyl-CoA in what is known as BETA-OXIDATION. Acetyl-CoA is the starting point of the next step in the production of ATP inside of the mitochondria.

Step 3- Oxidation of Acetyl-CoA and the <u>KREBS CYCLE</u>.

The <u>KREBS CYCLE</u> (aka Tricarboxylic acid cycle or citric acid cycle) is the key step which oxidizes the Acetyl-CoA; thus removing electrons from Acetyl-CoA and producing carbon dioxide as a by-product in the presence of oxygen inside of the mitochondria.

Step 4 - Transport of Electrons through the Respiratory Cycle

The electrons obtained from Acetyl-CoA- which either come from <u>CARBS</u> or <u>FATS</u>- are shuttled through many molecules as part of the electron transport chain inside of the mitochondria. Some molecules are proteins; others are cofactors molecules. One of these cofactors is called CO- ENZYME Q-10. This enzyme is mainly found in animal foods. Without this key enzyme mitochondrial energy production would be minimal.

This essential enzyme CoQ10 is A CRUCIAL ONE THAT IS BLOCKED BY STATIN DRUGS! This cripples the health of people taking statin drugs. Does it sound surprising that people taking statin drugs have no ENERGY? In some cases, warnings are place on packages of drugs. To prescribe a statin drug to lower cholesterol is stupid. When a doctor does not realize that statin drugs BLOCK THE PRODUCTION OF THE BODY'S MOST IMPORTANT ENERGY ENZYME—THAT IS MALPRACTICE!

Sidebar

Many years ago, I was obliged to threaten my mother's doctor with criminal negligence. An allopathic MD, she had wanted to pre-scribe Lipitor to my mom and she never mentioned any side effects. Fortunately, my mother did not take statin drugs- even though I had my Mom take the natural supplement CoQ10 for a short time. This is a good natural supplement that can help with fatigue and lack of energy.

In this step 4- water is also produced when oxygen accepts the electrons.

Step 5- Oxidative phosphorylation

When electrons travel down the transport chain, they cause electrical fluctuations between the inner and outer membrane in the mitochon-dria. These electrical fluctuations or gradients are the active driving forces that produce ATP in what is called oxidative phosphorylation. Then the ATP is transported outside of the mitochondria for the cell to use as ENERGY for any one of a thousand biochemical reactions.

WHY is FAT superior to CARBS as fuel?

Mother Nature provides MITOCHONDRIA THAT SPECIFICALLY AND PREFERENTIALLY USE FAT FOR ENERGY!

THEY ARE DESIGNED AND PROGRAMMED TO BURN FAT AS FUEL.

Just think about that for a moment.

VERY FEW HUMANS ARE BURNING THE RIGHT FUEL!

PHYSIOLOGICALLY—OUR CELLS ARE DESIGNED TO USE FAT AS PRIMARY FUEL TO PROVIDE US WITH ENERGY!

Here's another MITOCHONDRIAL BOMBSHELL.

ALL OF YOUR MITOCHONDRIA (your cellular power engines) COME FROM YOUR MOTHER! Who knew?

There is what's known as the "process of endosymbiosis". In this process, mitochondria evolved from bacteria and became incorporated 1.5 billion years ago within anaerobic bacteria—allowing them to survive in an oxygen-rich environment. Mitochondria have become the key source of energy within our bodies. They are after all where oxidative phosphorylation takes place in the electron transparent chains, allowing us to make ATP molecules from glucose. Human mitochondrial DNA is a single-stranded configuration arranged in a ring just like bacteria.

All of your mitochondria come from your mother (even the most masculine of us...☺

THESE TINY ORGANELLES THAT ARE SO VITALLY IMPORTANT FOR OUR LIFE ENERGY!

Professor Enzo Nisoli believes that our MORE THAN 10 MILLION MITOCHONDRIA MAKE UP 10 PERCENT OF OUR BODY WEIGHT.

In some cells, like the heart, they account for up to 40 % of the cellular substance.

IT IS THOUGHT THAT WE HAVE A MILLION BILLION MITOCHONDRIA IN OUR BODIES! Wow!

MANY CHRONIC DISEASES—SUCH AS PARKINSON'S AND DEMENTIA, for example, ARE ACTUALLY THE RESULT OF MITOCHONDRIAL DAMAGE—AKA- BUSTED CELLS. Does this sound familiar?-☺

ALMOST ALL CHRONIC DISEASES IN OUR BODIES ARE LINKED TO BUSTED MITOCHONDRIA, BUSTED CELLS AND BUSTED METABOLISM...

Here's how you can nurture your mitochondria:

- Limit calorie intake; EXCESSIVE CALORIES lead to excessive free radicals (ROS) which can damage mitochondrial DNA. Caloric restriction has repeatedly been shown to reduce tumorigenesis; and to slow the aging process.

- Occasional FASTING, as well as regular exercise will promote the transcription of NRF2, which leads to enhanced production of endogenous antioxidants; (think GLUTATHIONE- Master Antioxidant), which helps protect mitochondria.

- Choose your FOODS in such a way as to enhance production of GLUTATHIONE, the most important and prevalent antioxidant within your cells. It is the primary free radical protector for mitochondria. Glutathione helps maintain he redox potential of the mitochondrial membrane. Glutathione is a tripeptide made of cysteine, glutamic acid, and glycine. M-Acetycysteine and alpha lipoic acid promote the formation of glutathione; so do <u>WHEY PROTEIN</u>, <u>MAGNESIUM</u>, <u>VITAMIN C</u>, <u>VITAMIN E</u> etc.

- Consume foods that contain the sulfur-containing building blocks for glutathione—<u>ONIONS, LEEKS, GARLIC, BROCCOLI, CABBAGE & ARUGULA.</u>

- Avoid destabilizing molecules such as neurotoxic pesticides, herbicides and volatile chemicals. The mitochondrial DNA is less protected tan nuclear DNA and is exquisitely sensitive to injury by these compounds. B vitamins, niacin – ubiquitous COQ10, (known as UBIQUINONE) is also a co-factor in the electron transport chain.

<u>MITOCHONDRIA</u> have interesting characteristics which differ from all other structural parts of our cells. Our mitochondria are made of <u>PHOSPHOLIPIDS</u>; the membrane that controls what comes in and what comes out. When you eat a diet high in sugar, fructose, gluten and casein, this causes your membrane to <u>OXIDIZE AND RUST</u>. Your mitochondrion cell membrane should be like a jelly-fish; nice and fluid. But when it becomes rusty; it causes free-radical damage causing mutation of your cell.

When you have a diet <u>LOW IN HEALTHY FATS</u> and low in choline, your mitochondria will go through oxidative stress. Oxidative stress is at the root of oxidized cholesterol, stiff arteries, brain damage, dementia and autism.

Mitochondria have other interesting characteristics which differentiate them from other structural parts of our cells. They have their own DNA, (known as mtDNA), which is separate the widely known DNA in the nucleus; (known as n-DNA. Mitochondrial DNA comes from your mother's line; that's why mitochondria is considered as our feminine life force.

If you have <u>ANY KIND OF INFLAMMATION</u> from anywhere in your body; you damage your mitochondria. (aka busted cells). The loss of function or death of mitochondria is present in most every disease. Dietary and environmental factors lead to oxidative stress; and finally to mitochondrial injury.

Autism, ADHD, Parkinson's disease, anxiety, depression, biopolar disease, brain-aging are all linked with mitochondrial dysfunction from oxidative stress. Mitochondrial dysfunction contributes to congestive heart failure, type 2 diabetes, autoimmune disorders, aging, cancer and other diseases.

NDNA provides the information your cells need to code for proteins that control metabolism, repair, and structural integrity of your body .It is the mDNA which directs the production and utilisation of your energy. A cell can still commit suicide (apoptosis); even if it has no nucleus or nDNA. Because of their energetic role, the cells of tissues and organs which require more energy to function are richer in their mitochondrial numbers. Cells in our brains, muscles, heart, kidney, and liver contain thousands of mitochondria;— <u>COMPRISING UP TO 40 PERCENT OF THE CELL'S MASS.</u>

MtDNA is less protected than nDNA because it has no "protein" coating,(histones). It is very vulnerable to neurotoxic chemicals, pesticides, herbicides, excitotoxins. This tips the balance of free radical production to the extreme—which then leads to oxidative stress which damages our mitochondria and its DNA. As a result, we get overexcitation of cells and inflammation which causes Parkinson's disease, mood and behavioural problems, etc.

<u>ENOUGH ENERGY MEANS A HAPPY AND HEALTHY LIFE.</u> It keeps our brains focused and energized; it provides razor-sharp thinking. Conversely—lack of energy means mood problems; dementia, slowed mental functions etc.

<u>MITOCHONDRIA ARE INTRICATELY LINKED TO THE ABILITY OF THE PREFRONTAL CORTEX- OUR BRAIN'S CAPTAIN!</u>

Brain cells are loaded with mitochondria that produce the necessary energy to learn, memorize, fire neurons harmoniously—and get our brain <u>ONLINE</u>. A family of genes, (Sirtuins) work by protecting and improving the health of our mitochondria.

These genes are positively influenced <u>BY THE PROPER DIET.</u> They work best when given a <u>NON-GLYCATING,</u> i.e. <u>LOW-CARB DIET VS.A HIGH CARB DIET. A HIGH-CARB</u> DIET INDUCES MITOCHONDRIAL DYSFUNCTION AND FORMATION OF REACTIVE OYGEN SPECIES.(ROS).

<u>HIGH CARBOHYDRATE DIETS INCREASE LEVELS OF MUSCLE CELL INFLAMMATION AND REDUCE PROTEIN SYNTHESIS;</u> (muscle-building). For some people, this leads to a catabolism (body eats muscle tissue). Obviously this is not conducive to building muscles-☺

A properly constructed Ketogenic diet maintains circulating branched chain amino acids (BCCA's). These BCCA's (leucine, isoleucine and valine) are essential for <u>PROTEIN AND MUSCLE SYNTHESIS IN THE BODY.</u>

<u>LEUCINE IS THE MOST POWERFUL REGULATOR OF MUSCLE PROTEIN SYNTHESIS. AS WE AGE- LEUCINE IS THE MOST IMPORTANT OF THESE</u>

3 AMINO ACIDS WE NEED MASSIVE AMOUNTS OF LEUCINE AS WE AGE. (Unless we weight train we lose muscle mass with age- aka sarcopenia.

Guess What?

BLOOD LEUCINE LEVELS INCREASE ON A KETOGENIC DIET!

Now- THAT'S COOL!

When you adopt a KETOGENIC DIET—what are other effects?

When you adopt a KETOGENIC DIET INSULIN LEVELS DECREASE AND MUSCLE INFLAMMATION DECREASES TOO! RESEARCH SHOWS THAT THE BODY ADAPTS TO KETONE METABOLISM AND IMPROVES THE EFFICIENCY OF THIS FUEL SOURCE OVER TIME. The specific liver hormone, FGF21 which is critical for the oxidation of the liver's fatty acids is UPREGULATED in individuals who are on a Ketogenic diet over time. This allows for a greater use of ketones as an energy source in the body.

When you adopt a KETOGENIC DIET- you're using your body as OUR CREATOR INTENDED. Our bodies were not just constructed willy-nilly in a haphazard way!

YOUR BODY IS A KETONE-FAT BURNING FURNACE. YOUR BODY AT THE CELLULAR LEVEL WAS PROGRAMMED AND HARD-WIRED TO BURN FAT- NOT SUGAR FOR FUEL!

YOU WILL BE ABLE TO BUILD MUSCLE BETTER AND EASIER ON A KETOGENIC DIET.

THE KETO-ADAPTED STATE IMPROVES THE EFFICIENCY OF PROTEIN UTILIZATION. YOU WILL CONSUME LESS PROTEIN, & STILL MAINTAIN SUPERIOR LEUCINE LEVELS.

YOU WILL BE BETTER ABLE TO BUILD MUSCLES—AND TO RECOVER BETTER FROM STRENUOUS WORKOUTS!

You need to ask yourself this question...

D.   ARE YOU A CARB-BURNER OR A FAT-BURNER?

In Diet and Metabolism studies conducted in the early 20th Century— CARBS were called the "ANTI-KETOGENIC FACTOR". EATING CARBS RAISES INSULIN LEVELS AND THE INCREASE IN INSULIN TURNS OFF THE PRODUCTION OF KETONES.

<u>How do you know if you are a carb-burner OR a fat-burner?</u>

<u>What is a carb-burner?</u>

It's someone whose broken metabolism forces them to eat <u>CONSTANTLY</u>; it's someone who has a carb addiction; it's someone who usually <u>CRAVES</u> starchy, carbs and/or sugar. Being a carb-burner robs you of energy; a carb-burner ages pre-maturely and has a mind dulled by carbohydrates.

<u>THE BIG PROBLEM IS THAT ALMOST EVERYONE EATING A MODERN WESTERN DIET IS: — A CARB-BURNER</u>- (insulin-resistant too).

This is largely because Big Government, Big Pharma, most conventional doctors and die-ticians have promoted a <u>DIET INSANELY HIGH IN CARBOHYDRATES- AND INSANELY LOW IN FATS! –THIS HAS BEEN A DOUBLE NUTRITIONAL NIGHTMARE!</u> They have promoted a diet consisting of 50 to 60 PERCENT of carbohydrate calories. Sadly- most people (including doctors) are brainwashed.

<u>ALMOST ALL NORTH AMERICANS ARE LITERALLY DESTROYING THEIR METABOLISMS!</u>

Throughout this book, "BUSTED CELLS" "DYSFUNCTIONAL MITOCHONDRIA," "BUSTED METABOLISM" are used interchangeably...because it's hard to say...

Which came first- the chicken or the egg?

<u>DO METABOLIC DISORDERS SPAWN INFLAMMATION- OR -DOES INFLAMMATION CAUSE METABOLIC ORDERS- OR BOTH?</u>

<u>ONE THING FOR SURE- THE MAIN CULPRIT IS CARBOHYDRATES!</u>

<u>So- how do you know if you are a CARB-BURNER?</u>

- IF you skip breakfast—you crash mid-morning;

- IF you don't snack (get a sugar fix); you get grumpy, hungry, irritable and/or angry;

- IF you don't consume <u>CARBS</u> every couple of hours... your thinking slows and you have no energy and

Come late afternoon; you crash- likely grab a caffeine fix on the way home; you barely have enough energy to drag yourself home from work; Then you flop on the couch.

Does this sound familiar? <u>NOT TO WORRY!</u> There is a simple fix for this.

There's a wonderful "**METABOLIC BIO-HACK** called a "**FAT-ADAPTED METABOLISM**"; aka **KETO-ADAPTED METABOLISM**.

THIS "SUPER-METABOLISM" allows you to tap into the body fat stored on your belly, hips, & butt –**FOR ENERGY**. Every day that jiggly fat just sits there— taunting you; mocking you; frustrating you;—as it swells bigger and bigger; -☺ **ENOUGH!**

Say good-bye to that ugly **BELLY FAT**! It's time to flip your metabolic switch and change your metabolism!

When you fix your busted metabolism- you will fix your weight problem. You can let the white-coated crowd sell their drugs to treat symptoms of disease. Once you fix your metabolism—you will **FIX YOUR HEALTH**!

This metabolic adaptation to "super metabolism" will allow YOU to:

- Skip breakfast without craving carbs; (It is an old wives tale that breakfast is necessary and that it is the most important meal of the day! This is a marketing ploy used by **BIG FOOD**! The necessity to eat breakfast has no biological scientific foundation.

- Skip breakfast without craving CARBS;

- **SNACK IF YOU WANT TO**- (not because you are forced to);

- **EAT TONS OF "FAT-LADEN" RICH, " PREVIOUSLY FORBIDDEN" FOODS!**

- **POWER** though your day with limitless **ENERGY**;

- **HAVE A FOCUSED MIND, & EXCEPTIONAL MENTAL CLARITY**;

- **ENJOY** a heightened exhilarated mental state and a positive mindset and mood;

How is ALL of this possible?

Well…as a **CARB-BURNER**- you have to rely on a very limited supply of **CARB ENERGY**.

You have about > 1,600 calories in your muscles (stored as glycogen);

- 4,000 calories in your liver;

- 100 calories stored in your blood.

BUT- those calories stored in your muscles are **OFF- LIMITS- UNLESS** you are exercising intensely; so that leaves you with only 500 calories or so for normal day-today activities before you are forced to <u>REFUEL</u> and eat more CARBS).

<u>NO WONDER YOU GET SO HUNGRY SO QUICKLY AFTER YOU SCARF DOWN YOUR FAVOURITE BAGEL OR YOUR 'HEALTHY' BRAN MUFFIN!</u>

<u>CONVERSELY—WHEN YOU TEACH YOUR BODY TO UTILIZE FAT FOR ENERGY—</u>

- <u>FAT</u> provides stable constant energy as opposed to the very unstable energy of a <u>CARB-BURNER</u> and

- <u>FAT</u> balances your hormones as opposed to a <u>CARB- BURNING DIET</u> that causes your hormones <u>TO BE TOTALLY OUT OF WHACK.</u>

What is it like on a daily basis when you are <u>KETO (fat) ADAPTED?</u>

It feels fantastic! Dr. Robert Atkins, <u>PIONEER OF A HIGH-FAT-LOW-CARB DIET</u> described <u>KETOSIS</u> this way:

"<u>It feels more energizing than sex</u>".

Dr. Atkins only made a couple of small errors with his dietary approach. But in the big picture of things- he had the right approach. His dietary approach helped hundreds of thousands of people. He was not popular with his medical colleagues partly because they thought he was a quack. It turns out <u>THEY WERE THE QUACKS</u>!

They thought he was a snake-oil salesman. The other reason his colleagues disliked him was that were jealous of his financial success.

The average person has about 135, 000 calories stored as fat. That's a lot of stored fat energy. That's about 270 times more "fat energy" than those 500 calories of stored "carb energy."

Guess what happens when you are able to tap into that <u>GIGANTIC RESERVOIR OF ENERGY</u> (belly fat-☺ that's conveniently stored (parked) on your belly, hips; thighs, arms, and butt? Your body sheds the belly flab that you've stored over the years from by eating too many carbs. When you learn to burn fat—your pancreas is able to take a well-deserved rest. As you teach your body to burn fat as your primary fuel—your liver becomes a <u>HUGE –FAT-BURNING MACHINE</u>! It now has its preferred fuel- <u>FAT</u>. It can then work more efficiently by converting protein and other fuels into <u>GLUCOSE</u>. Your new happy liver will send a happy/feel good message to your brain.

Once you become fat-adapted- you will likely never want to return to your previous diet.

I wake up each day <u>REFRESHED AFTER A DEEP RESTFUL SLEEP.</u>

I don't eat breakfast if I don't want to. Usually, I will have a cup of organic coffee. I will drink 3-4 litres of water w/organic lemon/ and/or a tbsp. of organic Apple Cider Vinegar (ACV). Most days, I'll have a <u>SUPER-CHARGED- HIGH-OCTANE KETOGENIC FAT COFFEE</u> -recipe infra).

For lunch, - I often <u>GORGE MYSELF OF SOME DELICIOUS FAT-RICH DELICIOUS</u> <u>FOODS.</u> <u>YUMMY!</u> I might have 3 pastured eggs, some happy bacon etc. or I may just have a piece of raw cheese and/or a delicious SMOOTHIE; maybe even another High Octane Coffee' it depends what I'm doing...and how I feel.

When late afternoon arrives, your mind (brain) is still <u>SHARP AS A RAZOR.</u> If you strength train (as I do about 4 p.m), you will find your energy levels very high and very stable. This works nicely for me because it's a good idea to refuel within two hours to promote muscle synthesis. (This is not carb-loading; I eat a ketogenic supper.)

<u>WHEN YOU BECOME KETO-APTED THERE ARE NO MORE AFTERNOON CRASHES AND DIPS.</u> Research is showing that it is healthy to take an afternoon nap but I'm pretty sure that the subjects in the study were carb burners- so who knows? Did our ancestors take a siesta or after- noon nap? Probably sometimes...

<u>AFTERNOON CRASHES AND DIPS ARE SIGNS OF A CARB-BASED BUSTED METABOLISM. ONCE YOU EXPERIENCE THIS KIND OF SUPER KETO METABOLISM—YOU WILL NEVER WANT TO RETURN TO BEING A CARB-BURNER AGAIN!</u>

The <u>SWEETEST PART</u> of becoming Keto-adapted? You will be pleas- antly surprised how that stubborn fat you thought would never go away— just steadily-effortlessly disappears. Day after day- the fat just melts off; (even if you do NOT exercise)!

After about 3 weeks, I RECOMMEND THAT you begin to <u>EXERCISE TO ACCELERATE FAT LOSS, METABOLIC CHANGES</u> <u>AND TO BUILD BRAIN CELLS AND STRENGTH.</u> For most people re-booting their metabolism is <u>STRESSFUL</u> on their body. Your body needs <u>TIME</u> to adjust and to build new metabolic pathways and new enzymes. When you <u>ADD</u> exercise into the equation <u>TOO SOON</u>—it could be a bit too stressful on the body. If you are already an exerciser- you may be able to con- tinue. There's no good reason to rush into a Ketogenic diet. Stress is partly responsible for your health condition. So- take your time. Go slowly. The Ketogenic Diet and Lifestyle will be the <u>EXACT OPPOSITE</u> dietary approach to what you have been told.

LISTEN TO YOUR BODY. ONCE YOU ARE KETO-ADAPTED AND ONCE YOU ENTER NUTRITIONAL KETOSIS—IT IS VERY LIKELY THAT YOU WILL REMAIN IN KETOSIS FOREVER!

Those frequent doctors' visits, medications and surgeries will only exist in a previous life. They will become a thing of the past. You will amaze yourself, your spouse, your family and friends.

Your biggest problem when you lose a lot of weight is that you will have to buy new clothes! If you eat pastured; butter-please be careful- YOUR PANTS MIGHT FALL DOWN! So- please don't blame me! I warned you. -☺

GUESS WHAT ELSE HAPPENS WHEN YOU BECOME KETO-ADAPTED?

YOUR GROCERY BILL WILL GET SLICED BY 30 PERCENT-OR A COUPLE OF HUNDRED DOLLARS A MONTH!

The take-home message

LOW-CARBOHYDRATE DIETS ARE THE HEALTHIEST, EASIEST AND MOST EFFECTIVE WAY TO LOSE WEIGHT AND REVERSE METABOLIC DISEASE.

MANY SCIENTIFIC STUDIES ARE REFERENCED IN APPENDIX A.

Are you ready to become KETO-ADAPTED? Are you ready to upgrade your metabolism? Are you ready to upgrade to a FAT-BURNING METABOLISM OF OUR ANCESTORS?

Please read on.

E.   THE HEALING KETOGENIC DIET

If you read a typical medical school biochemistry textbook, you will likely find a section devoted to what happens metabolically during starvation. What you'll learn is that:

THE METABOLISM OF CARB RESTRICTION=THE METABOLISM OF STARVATION"

Carb restriction was the norm for most of our existence as upright walking beings on this Planet. This is why biochemistry textbook authors call "STARVATION"-"THE NORMAL METABOLISM"

There are at least 4 types of fuel that your body can use as fuel. KETONES (fat bodies) are one of those types. A KETOGENIC DIET IS A LOW-CARBOHYRATE, HIGH-FAT-MODERATE PROTEIN DIET. A

Ketogenic Diet is one which put us in ketosis. Ketosis is an often misunderstood subject. Some people believe that ketosis is equal to starvation or a warning sign that something is going wrong with your metabolism. Nothing could be further from the truth. Ketones- contrary to popular belief and myth- are much needed essential healing fats for our bodies.

Our entire body uses ketones in a safer and more effective way than the energy source coming from <u>CARBOHYDRATES (aka SUGAR/ GLUCOSE)</u>. Our bodies produce ketones if we eat a diet between O and 50 CARBS per day (a la caveman)- we become <u>KETO-ADAPTED</u>. The range varies from person to person- but the general range is between 0 to 50 grams of carbs plus moderate intake of <u>PROTEIN</u>, between 0.8 and 1.5 grams of protein per Kg of ideal body weight. Protein intake should be calculated using <u>LEAN</u> body weight. (see also exercise chapter, infra) Pregnant women and children should not have their protein restricted. The latest research suggests that the appropriate <u>PROTEIN intake should be about one-half gram for each pound of lean muscle mass.</u>

The human body evolved burning mostly fats for energy; and a small amount of glucose. However, we are capable of burning protein; and a small amount of glucose. However, we are capable of burning protein if we are low on glucose (or glycogen- i.e. glucose that is stored in the liver and muscle). Protein can be converted into glucose by the liver- this is called <u>GLUCONEOGENESIS</u>; (supra.)

After a few weeks of restricting/reducing carbs, and ultimately insulin production, and INCREASING FAT in your diet; your genes will receive the message. They will be told that they should upregulate the biomechanical hardware needed to burn ketones effectively.

<u>THIS IS CALLED "FAT or KETO ADAPTED".</u> At this point the body relies primarily on <u>fat</u> for energy- instead of <u>glucose</u>. So, to put it more simply, ketosis is a state where the body burns fat for energy, instead of carbohydrates.

Our ancestors rarely had access to carbohydrates because they were simply not available like they are today. They were forced to go without them for weeks or even months at a time and <u>EXISTED PRIMARILY ON PROTEIN AND FAT</u>. Easy access to carbs did not occur <u>UNTIL</u> the agricultural revolution. The body can only store a little bit of glucose in the form of glycogen; which gets used up very quickly. Therefore, our genome and the circumstances demanded that we evolve a biochemical system that enabled the liver to take protein straight from our food or our muscles, and convert it to glucose- if we were going to remain alive! To repeat again- this process is called gluconeogenesis. This system enabled us to survive and thrive as a species during brief periods of starvation or when the only food source available was protein and fat.

IT ALSO ENABLED US TO DEVELOP BIGGER AND SMARTER BRAINS THAT BROUGHT US TO THE TOP OF THE FOOD CHAIN.

How are KETONES formed?

The body has two major energy sources. It burns glucose or ketone bodies. The majority of people burn glucose primarily because they are constantly supplying a steady form of sugar starches and proteins that can be turned into blood sugar; (carb-burners, supra). When one either FASTS- OR follows a low-carb-moderate protein—high fat diet; they switch their energy source to FAT.

In particular, the fatty acids are broken down into THREE MAJOR FORMS KETONES. THESE HEALING KETONES ARE:

- Acetoacetate, Acetone and Beta-hydroxybutyrate (BHB);

- Ketones are produced by the liver and released into the blood when insulin levels are low and hepatic liver metabolism is increased;

- Ketones can also be generated QUICKLY with the consumption of coconut fat, because coconut contains a particular type of fat. This fat is called MEDIUM- CHAIN TRIGLYCERIDES; which is converted into our primary BLOOD ketone- (BHB) by the liver.

When our bodies are running primarily on fats, large amounts of Acetyl-CoA are produced which exceed the capacity of the Krebs cycle, leading to the making of these three healing ketone bodies within the liver mitochondria. Our levels of ketone bodies in our blood go up and our brain readily uses them for energetic purposes.

KETONE BODIES READILY CROSS THE BLOOD BRAIN BARRIER (BBB). Their solubility makes them easily transportable by the blood to other organs and tissues. When ketone bodies are used as energy; they release Acety-CoA which then goes to the Krebs cycle AGAIN TO PRODUCE ENERGY. How cool is that!

Research has shown that a low-carbohydrate, ketogenic diet reduces oxidative stress in the body. This reduction in oxidative stress on the cell membrane allows for the formation of healthy insulin receptors and normalized blood sugar regulation. This improves insulin sensitivity which further reduces inflammation and fat storage in the body. The more sensitive the body is to insulin, the less stress it puts on the rest of the system. This makes it easier to build muscle and burn fat. A Ketogenic diet produces far fewer free radicals-aka (ROS) or reactive oxygen species.

A KETOGENIC DIET IS AN ANTI-INFLAMMATORY DIET!

A KETOGENIC DIET IS A PROTEIN- SPARING DIET TOO!

GLUCOSE/SUGAR BURNING DIETS ARE INFLAMMATORY DIETS!

HIGH –CARB DIETS INCREASE THE LEVEL OF MUSCLE INFLAMMATION AND REDUCE PROTEIN SYNTHESIS; (muscle-building). For many people high-carb diets are catabolic; (the body literally eats its muscle protein for fuel- a la cannibalistic-☺). The opposite of catabolic is anabolic (growing). Obviously, no one wants to lose muscle. A healthy body is not thin and weak. We don't need big muscles. We need strong, powerful muscles.

A properly constructed ketogenic diet maintains circulating branched chain amino acids (BCAA's). These BCAA's are <u>leucine</u>, <u>isoleucine</u> and <u>valine</u>. All of these amino acids are important but leucine is the most important for protein synthesis. Also, as we age, our body needs <u>MORE LEUCINE</u> than when we are younger.

The good news is: Blood leucine levels used for protein synthesis- (aka muscle-building) <u>INCREASE ON A KETOGENIC DIET!</u>

At the same time- <u>INSULIN LEVELS AND MUSCLE INFLAMMATIN DECREASE ON A KETOGENIC DIET!</u>

<u>THE KETO-ADAPTED STATE— IMPROVES THE EFFICIENCY OF PROTEIN UTILIZATION. THIS GREATER ECONOMY OF PROTEIN ALLOWS FOR LESS TO BE CONSUMED WHILE STILL MAINTAINING HEALTHY BLOOD LEUCINE LEVELS NECESSARY FOR MUSCLE DEVELOPMENT AND RECOVERY.</u>

This is why it is sometimes said that a ketogenic diet is a "<u>protein-sparing diet</u>".

<u>Popular Myth:</u>

There is a popular myth that for building muscle- the body needs carbohydrates and protein <u>IMMEDIATELY AFTER</u> exercising in order to properly recover. However, this is not necessarily true. With a properly- constructed ketogenic diet, keto-adapted people can often <u>FAST</u> for long periods; either before or even after high-intensity workouts and still make strength and muscle gains!

Traditional science looks at the liver as the only source of ketone production in human physiology. BUT- SCIENCE NOW SHOWS THAT OUR BRAIN CAN ALSO PRODUCE KETONES.

ASTROCYTES, a special type of GLIAL CELLS (which make up 90 percent of our brain cells) support and assist neurons. Astrocytes, (non-neuronal cells) can also produce KETONE BODIES with fatty acids, and the amino acid leucine, when glucose is scarce. These particular KETONES possess a powerful ability to protect the neuronal network (i.e. very neuro-protective) by increasing antioxidants and decreasing free radical production in the brain, increasing the formation of new mitochondria and preventing apoptosis (cell death).

Unlike fat and glucose—ketones cannot be stored in fat cells. They just travel freely throughout the bloodstream where they can easily be obtained for fat energy by any cell that wants or needs them.

"THE STATE OF KETOSIS" occurs when ketones that are in the bloodstream accumulate to a level that is higher than what is being used up by cells for energy. Thus, there is an ELEVATED LEVEL OF KETONES IN THE BODY.

IF YOU CONSUME A DIET TOO HIGH IN CARBOHYDRATES- THEN YOUR BODY IS NOT CAPABLE OF ACCESSING THOSE KETONES FOR ENERGY.

THIS IS BECAUSE YOUR GENES HAVE DOWN-REGULATED THE BIOCHEMICAL PATHWAYS USED IN THE PROCESS DUE TO THE PRESENCE OF "CARBOHYDRATES" IN YOUR BODY.

KETONES that are not used by the body are excreted in the urine, stool and breath. Until the body becomes keto-adapted; you may smell ketones on your breath (acetone smells like nail polish remover or ripened-apples) or you may have increased ketones in the urine.

You can do "oil-pulling" by swishing coconut oil in your mouth for 15- 20 minutes before SPITTING IT OUT. Do not swallow this used coconut oil—it is the best mouthwash in the world. It is anti-microbial, anti-bacterial and anti-viral. In short it will likely be contaminated with bad bacteria. You wouldn't put dirty engine oil back into your car would you?

ODD- SMELLING BREATH IS TEMPORARY! YOU HAVE NOTHING TO BE WORRIED ABOUT. THE BODY EXCRETES EXCESS KETONES!

WHEN YOU EAT TOO MANY CARBS- OUR BODY DOES THE EXACT OPPOSITE! YOUR BODY STORES CARBS AS BELLY FAT. This makes you fat, sick and disease prone.

Once you <u>DRASTICALLY REDUCE CARBS</u> in your diet, then it will probably take at least a few weeks for your genes to be reprogrammed. Your body will become capable of burning ketones for energy efficiently' accumulating and excreting <u>fewer ketones</u> and having a diminished need for glucose.

The entire ketogenic adaption process can take anywhere from <u>TWO</u> to <u>SEVERAL MONTHS.</u> Some people can jump into a Ketogenic diet with both feet-☺ Other people may have a metabolism which is <u>MORE BUSTED</u>—then the adaptation might take a few weeks longer. As you likely know, we all have a different metabolism. We all have a different health history. Our nutritional habits vary considerably so our metabolic machinery and pathways are all different. Some people will adapt <u>EASILY AND VERY QUICKLY.</u> Other people take longer to become keto-adapted.

<u>RESEARCH SHOWS THAT THERE IS A RANGE OF METABOLIC RESPONSES EVEN AMONG ULTRA-ELITE ATHLETES WHO ADOPT A KETOGENIC DIET!</u>

<u>IF YOU HAVE BEEN A CARB –BURNER YOUR WHOLE LIFE</u> (say 25 years or more— you're asking your body to <u>MAKE A HUGE METABOLIC CHANGE!</u>

<u>MY RECOMMENDATIONS ARE:</u>

1. <u>GET A FULL BLOOD LIPID PANEL DONE BEFORE STARTING ON THE KETOGENIC PLAN.</u>

   Why?

2. <u>SO YOU CAN COMPARE THE RESULTS OF YOUR BLOOD WORK- BEFORE AND AFTER.</u>

3. <u>PLEASE GO SLOWLY!</u>

   Try to cut your <u>CARB</u> intake in half- for the first week; i.e. drop down from 150 carbs/day down to 75 carbs/day. Then, it's a bit like <u>LIMBO</u>-☺- You need to go as low as you can go on the carbs...

1. <u>YOU CAN ADD BACK CARBS AT THE RATE OF ABOUT 5 GRAMS PER DAY.</u>

2. <u>ADAPTING TO A VERY LOW CARB KETOGENIC DIET IS A HUGE PHYSIOLOGICAL CHANGE FOR YOUR BODY!</u>

3. <u>IT COULD BE VERY STRESSFUL FOR SOME PEOPLE.—PLEASE GO SLOWLY.</u> (Remember Rome was not built overnight-☺

How <u>LOW</u> do you <u>NEED</u> to go to get into ketosis? Research shows that if you're diabetic and/or obese you should be aiming for a daily intake of 25 grams <u>OR LESS OF CARBS PER DAY</u>. Many clinical studies have used 10 to 20 grams of carbs per day…<u>SO</u>-

<u>PERHAPS YOU WILL BE ABLE TO JUMP WITH BOTH FEET RIGHT INTO A KETOGENIC DIET. OR-PERHAPS YOU WILL NEED TO TRANSITION MORE SLOWLY INTO A KETOGENIC DIET.</u>

You will immediately start to feel better. You will feel much better after 3 or 4 days of <u>CARB RESTRICTION WITH HIGH FAT INTAKE</u>. You will start to lose a few pounds. Your energy and vitality will increase. But- you need to be <u>PATIENT</u>. Be kind and gentle to your body. This is not a temporary diet. Short term <u>KETOGENIC DIETS are not effective</u>.

<u>THIS IS NOT A FAD DIET. A VLKD IS A SAFE THERAPEUTIC HEALING DIET.</u>

<u>THIS IS A PERMANENT LIFE CHANGING NUTRITIONAL APPROACH.</u>

<u>FUELLING YOUR BODY WITH FAT AS YOUR PRIMARY FUEL WILL CHANGE EVERY ASPECT OF YOUR HEALTH— & YOUR LIFE!</u> (The Chinese say: the road of a thousand miles begins with the first step. I promise you it will not take that long-☺

<u>MAJOR TIPS ON A KETOGENIC DIET</u>-

1. <u>YOU SHOULD DRINK A MINIMUM OF ONE-HALF OF YOUR BODY WEIGHT DAILY OF PURE CLEAN WATER</u>; (preferably before 1 p.m.

2. <u>YOU SHOULD TAKE AT LEAST A TEASPOON OF PINK HIMALYAN SALT EVERY AM</u>. (you may require more. This replaces electrolytes (80 or so) which will be flushed out in your urine;

3. <u>SODIUM AND POTASSIUM LEVELS SHOULD BE CLOSELY MONITORED.</u>

   Adequate hydration is important for everyone. People who follow a ketogenic diet should drink <u>EVEN MORE WATER THAN THEY DRANK AS SUGAR BURNERS</u>.

   <u>KETOMANIACS WILL FLUSH KETONES OUT THROUGH THEIR URINE</u>. On a ketogenic diet during the day, your kidneys will get a good workout. They will be called upon to clean toxic more toxic waste from your liver too.

4. <u>A KETOGENIC DIET IS SLIGHTLY ACIDIC BY NATURE</u>. Therefore, it's a good idea to put some organic <u>LEMONS /LIMES</u> (or lemon/lime juice) into your water. Lemons /limes taste acidic but in your body are <u>VERY ALKALINE</u>. They will help alkalize the pH of your blood.

You can drink lemon ice water or hot lemon water. If you are a coffee drinker you will find that drinking lemon water with coffee may make the coffee less acidic to your body.

5. <u>START DRINKING ACV</u> (Apple Cider Vinegar) a TBSP or two in morning andor before meals. A Tbsp. before bed will help you sleep too. Again, some people find ACV difficult to ingest; so start with a TSP if you have difficulty.

6. <u>ACV IS ONE OF THE MOST EFFECTIVE INEXPENSIVE BEST MEDICINES ON THE PLANET!</u>

In sum- by using a <u>slow transition</u> into a ketogenic diet you are giving your body the time it requires to adjust slowly until your genes start upregulating your software/hardware (metabolic pathways) for burning ketones effectively.

F. KETOACIDOSIS VERSUS KETOSIS

<u>ALLOPATHIC DOCTORS DO NOT KNOW THEIR ARSE FROM THEIR ELBOW.</u>

They are <u>completely confused about KETOSIS</u> vs. <u>KETOACIDOSIS.</u> They do not understand the difference between ketosis and ketoacidosis. They have received a very flawed education. They are taught ketones are bad. Just mentioning "ketosis" is likely to alarm your doctor as much as the word "death". -☺

Ketosis is an extremely desirable metabolic state. Ketoacidosis is a life-threatening condition that only affects Type 1 diabetics, or people who do not produce insulin from their pancreas. Type 1 can be potentially exposed to ketoacidosis if and when their bodies dump too many ketones into their blood and their blood sugar rises too much (not enough insulin) so the body <u>SIMULTANEOUSLY</u> is flooded with <u>TOO MANY NUTRIENTS;</u> which cannot be absorbed. In this isolated instance, ketones in the blood can rise over 20 mmol and in this one instance, ketoacidosis can be life-threatening.

Ketoacidosis is a serious, potentially life-threatening condition that affects insulin-dependent <u>TYPE 1 DIABETICS- ONLY.</u> BUT—this is a completely different state than ketosis. Diabetic Ketoacidosis happens in insulin-dependent type I diabetics when not enough insulin is available to metabolize glucose for fuel. The patient's body turns to <u>FAT</u> for fuel. The body produces ketones in dangerously high quantities in a completely out of control manner. These ketones become toxic as the body produces very high levels of elevated ketones. High levels can cause a serious imbalance in the pH level. At the same time, there is a big loss of bicarbonate which further lowers the pH (acidosis). Patients typically lose a lot of water, due to their elevated blood sugars. A medical emergency can develop with the patient going into a coma or death.

KETOSIS IS VERY SAFE AND DESIRABLE. YOUR DOCTOR IS THE DANGEROUS ONE! YOUR DOCTOR KILLS FAR MORE PEOPLE THAN ACIDOSIS KILLS TYPE ONE DIABETICS!

FOLLOWING A KETOGENIC DIET IS ALMOST IMPOSSIBLE TO GET YOUR KETONE LEVELS ABOVE 9 or 10 MMOL- unless you are a Type 1 Diabetic and has broken pancreas that produces NO INSULIN.

Guess what? It appears that the FDA recently issued a warning that some diabetic drugs can cause KETOACIDOSIS!

WHAT CAN BE VERY DANGEROUS IS: THE IMBALANCE IN pH THAT OCCURS IN THE CASE OF TYPE 1 DIABETICS.

Alcoholic ketoacidosis can also occur in chronic long-term alcoholism due to dehydration impairing gluconeogenesis and causing an imbalance in pH.

Generally speaking, when someone is in KETOSIS; KETONE LEVELS WILL NOT EXCEED A MAXIMUM OF 8 MILLIMOLAR (8(mM/L)

UNDER FASTING CONDITIONS- THE MEAN TOTAL CIRCULATING KETONE BODY CONCENTRATION IS IN THE RANGE OF 5.8 to 9.7 MILLIMOLARS (mM/L)

8 OR 9 MMOL IS FAR BELOW THE DANGEROUS LEVEL OF ABOUT 15-20 OR HIGHER REQUIRED TO ENTER KETOACIDOSIS.

AN INSULIN-RESISTANT DIABETIC IN KETOACIDOSIS WILL HAVE KETONE LEVELS AT A MINUMUM LEVEL OF 15 up to a MAXIMUM OF 25 MILLIMOLARS (25 mM/L)

ONCE YOU BECOME KETO-ADAPTED— IF YOUR BODY IS PRODUCING JUST A LITTLE BIT OF INSULIN- IT WILL BE IMPOSSIBLE TO ENTER A STATE OF KETOACIDOSIS.

KETONE LEVELS WILL NOT RISE TO THE DANGEROUS LEVEL—OF 20 OR SO mM/L

ONCE YOU BECOME KETO-ADAPTED—YOUR KETONE LEVELS WILL LIKELY BE ABOUT 0.5 TO 3 MILLIMOLARS (3mM/L) IF YOU ARE FORTUNATE ENOUGH TO GET INTO DEEP NUTRITIONAL KETOSIS OF ABOUT 6 OR 7 mmol—

YOU WILL KNOW IT BECAUSE YOU WILL FEEL FANTASTIC!

IN SHORT- UNLESS YOU ARE AN ACTIVE ALCOHOLIC OR HAVE INSULIN-DEPENDENT DIABETES, KETOSIS IS COMPLETELY SAFE.

DIABETIC KETOACIDOSIS WILL NEVER OCCUR BY EATING A KETOGENIC DIET. IF YOUR PANCREAS IS ABLE TO PRODUCE EVEN THE SLIGHTEST AMOUNT OF INSULIN—YOU CAN NEVER REACH THE DANGEROUS CONDITION CALLED 'KETOACIDOSIS".

YOU HAVE A PANCREAS THAT PRODUCES INSULIN TO REGULATE THE PROCESS AND YOU ARE RESTRICTING THE OUTPUT OF GLUCOSE (by your sugar factory).

NOTE BENE:

**There ARE anecdotal reports that the Ketogenic Diet has been successfully used by TYPE 1 DIABETICS. There do not appear to be any published studies-yet.

Dr. Richard Veech, a researcher at the United States National Institute of Health states that he would argue that:

"KETOSIS IS THE NORMAL STATE OF MAN"

The majority of ketogenic gurus go further and say:

> **"KETOSIS IS ARGUABLY NOT JUST A NATURAL CONDITION BUT EVEN A PARTICULARLY HEALTHY ONE".**

Dr. Phinney coined the term "NUTRITIONAL KETOSIS". This term is far more ELOQUENT AND ACCURATE to describe the state of ketosis.

You need to know: THERE ARE TWO TYPES of HYPOGLYCEMIA

The first type is Hypoglycemia. This normally happens when most people who have been eating a HIGH-CARB DIET DRASTICALLY REDUCE CARB INTAKE FOR THE FIRST TIME.

Hypoglycemia (reactive hypoglycemia) happens to MOST people when first beginning a low-carb Ketogenic Diet. It may be especially strong in people who have already developed INSULIN RESISTANCE (esp. diabetics, pre-diabetics). This type of hypoglycemia is due to a chronic excess of CARB INTAKE. This type often happens during the first several weeks of carb reduction; because the body has not had time to create the enzymes or metabolic pathways to burn internal fat stores for fuel. Basically, there is a gap in the amount of carbo-hydrate available for fuel, and the process of accessing fat stores for fuel. This "lack" of fuel sources results in transient/TEMPORARY low blood sugar.

As you now know, insulin is secreted from the pancreas in response to eating food; ESPECIALLY FOODS HIGH IN CARBS. Insulin's main job is to move the glucose that your body makes from the food you eat into your cells so that this excess sugar can be broken down/burned for energy- OR STORED AS FAT. Insulin, your powerful peptide hormone acts very quickly. The amount of insulin your body secretes is closely tied to how much blood sugar is being created from food. Eating a high-carb diet over a long period of time will cause a chronic elevation of your blood sugar, which results in a chronic elevation of your insulin levels.

INSULIN CAUSES INFLAMMATION AND OBESITY.

As you now know, elevated insulin levels cause increased FAT STORAGE. With high insulin levels-BURNING STORED FAT FOR FUEL IS INHIBITED. It's really a vicious cycle—the more CARBS EATEN- the higher the INSULIN—and the less stored FAT can be accessed to fuel the body- SO- MORE CARBS have to be eaten to provide fuel instead. That's why you have to shut down production of your inter-nal sugar factory. You need to re-wire the circuits of your brain/liver/pancreas so they learn to start burning high-octane- fuel aka FAT – aka KETONES.

One of the great benefits of eating a Ketogenic Diet is ITS ability to lower your average blood sugar and insulin levels. THIS ALLOWS YOUR BODY TO BURN STORED FAT.

However—when first starting this diet, your body will MOST LIKELY BE IN HIGH CARBOHYDRATE STATE and in HIGH INSULIN MODE. As you lower your carb intake, you begin a process of retraining your body to burn stored fat instead of carbs for fuel. Most often, it takes from 1 to 4 weeks for the body to ADJUST to the new lower level of carb intake; and to build enzymes needed to store burned fat. Some people may be able to jump into the Ketogenic diet with both feet.-☺). Some people may take a couple of months to make the metabolic adaptation necessary to burn fat as the primary fuel. Meanwhile, during this adjustment phase, your pancreas may continue secreting enough insulin for the OLDER, HIGHER LEVEL OF CARB CONSUMPTION. The pancreas is changing software pro-grams; because insulin levels are still high, the body is dependent on CARBS for fuel BECAUSE IT HAS NOT LEARNED to burn fat- stored or otherwise.

So- the body hums along with LESS CARB INTAKE for a couple of days because it can tap into stored carbs (GLYCOGEN) in your liver and muscles.

BUT— EVENTUALLY, GLYCOGEN STORES GET LOW—MORE INSULIN IS SECRETED. Can you guess what happens then?

A COUPLE OF HOURS LATER—YOU MAY HAVE A SLIGHT EPISODE OF REACTIVE HYPOGLYCEMIA! This is the second type of hypoglycemia- it's called "REACTIVE" hypoglycemia. Reactive hypoglycemia is a condition in which the body reacts to a "PERCEIVED" CATASTROPHIC DROP IN BLOOD SUGAR.

I say "perceived" because during an "episode" the BLOOD SUGAR READINGS may be in the NORMAL RANGE— BUT STILL FEEL LIKE LOW- BLOOD SUGAR TO THE PERSON HAVING THE REACTION.

YOUR BODY "PERCEIVES" YOUR BLOOD GLUCOSE IS TOO LOW.

YOUR BODY STARTS TO PANIC LIKE AN ALCOHOLIC WHO NEEDS A DRINK BUT CANNOT GET ONE! THE BRAIN TELLS THE ADRENALS TO PUMP OUT SOME ADRENALIN TO TELL THE LIVER TO FIND/ BREAKDOWN SOME PROTEIN INTO GLUCOSE—FAST!—AND TO DUMP IT INTO THE BLOODSTREAM FAST!

A stressed out body then pumps out MORE CORTISOL TO GO ALONG WITH the additional adrenaline. These two stress hormones produce the FOLLOWING "SYMPTOMS" ASSOCIATED WITH REACTIVE HYPOGLYCEMIA:

- Heart palpitations/fibrillations; dizziness; light-headedness;
- Sweaty; irritability, shaking& tremors headaches nervousness'
- Craving for sweets; flushing, intense hunger;
- Panic attack; feeling nauseous;
- Numbness/coldness in the extremities;
- Fatigue and shakiness for a few hours afterwards;

ALL OF THESE "SYMPTOMS" ARE SIGNS OF CARBOHYDRATE ADDICTION AND WITHDRAWL REACTIONS BY YOUR BODY.

The slang term for "THESE CONDITIONS" is called "THE CARB FLU". What should .

You could EAT ONE OF MY HIGH-CARB DESSERTS ;(see infra).

HOW DO "ALMOND FUDGE BARS" OR" CHOCOLATE BROWNIES" SOUND?

AND/OR- YOU CAN HAVE A HEALTHY- STEVIA SWEETENED SNACK.

YOU CAN HAVE YOUR FAVORITE BEVERAGE SWEETENED WITH SOME STEVIA. A few drops of Stevia will be perceived AS A SUGAR FIX BY YOUR BRAIN.

YOU WILL FIND THAT YOUR EPISODE OF REACTIVE HYPOGLYCEMIA WILL DISSIPATE AND YOUR SYMPTOMS WILL ABATE. Some people who experience chronic carb flu symptoms find that waiting 5-6 hours after quickly feeding their carb addiction becomes possible. My advice is: LISTEN TO YOUR BODY! Some people can quit smoking cold turkey. Some people cannot. Kicking the sugar addiction is the same. Our metabolisms are all different. Our carb/glucose tolerances vary enormously also. How long it takes for you to stop being a carb(sugar) burner and become a fat- burning beast is a personal matter.

How should you avoid the "Carb Flu" aka reactive hypoglycaemia?

PERMANENTLY REDUCING YOUR CARBS IS THE BEST WAY.

This will eventually lower your daily blood sugar and circulating insulin. Once insulin levels return to normal levels, your body can start to develop its love affair with FAT. Your body can quickly switch over to burning fats and can access its fat stores.

DURING THE FIRST PHASE OF EATING A LOW-CARB KETOGENIC DIET- it's a good idea to wean yourself off of your heavy CARB LOAD—GRADUALLY. You should be patient with yourself and gradually reduce your carb intake. Gradually extend your timing between meals- to say 4-5 hours. One of the BEST ways to kick off a Ketogenic diet is to try a 24 FAST—(intermittent fasting, infra).

NOTE BENE (1)

Be aware that mainstream doctors are clueless about the "carb flu" (reactive hypoglycemia). THIS CONDITION IS ROOTED IN NUTRITIONAL CAUSES. Conventional doctors and dieticians are not taught about the POWER OF NUTRITION and they may pooh-pooh your concerns about it. There is no pill or needle for the carb flu. The solution is healthy nutritious food.

If you have any of these symptoms- this might indicate that you are on the path of INSULIN RESISTANCE- OR PRE-DIABETES- EVEN IF YOUR BLOOD GLUCOSE IS NORMAL. You may have to reduce your carb consumption slowly over a longer period of time to minimize any of the above symptoms.

EVENTUALLY- BY IMPROVING YOUR DIET BY CONSUMING FEWER HIGH-CARB FOODS—YOU WILL AVOID THE CARB FLU COMPLETELY!

YOU SHOULD HAVE CONFIDENCE THAT YOUR SUGAR/CARB CRAVINGS WILL ABATE AND EVENTUALLY DISAPPEAR FOREVER.

NOTE BENE (2):

IT IS BETTER TO USE THE EXPRESSION "NUTRITIONAL KETOSIS". This term is more descriptive, more accurate than "ketosis". It also helps obviate confusion between nutritional ketosis and the medical term "ketoacidosis".

G. THERAPEUTIC BENEFITS OF THE KETOGENIC DIET

The amount and variety of mitochondrial dysfunction today is staggering.

THE KEY TO SUPERHEALTH IS TO HAVE SUPER MITOCHONDRIAL HEALTH.

The terms- mitochondrial dysfunction, mitochondrial impairment, busted mitochondria and busted cells have been used interchangeably to describe different kinds of mitochondrial dysfunction. These modern day "maladies" are all related to how our bodies metabolize food. Optimal energy sources are essential if we are to HEAL FROM CHRONIC AILMENTS. At the cellular level, it is our mitochondria that lie at the junction between our fuel from foods that come from our environment and our bodies' energy demands. Mitochondrial and cellular health are the key players in the production of our ENERGY. The process of converting food into energy is the process of metabolism. Most often, if mitochondrial function exists-it will mean that the process becomes a dysfunctional metabolism (aka busted metabolism). In reality, carb metabolism is a busted metabolism.

Our bodies are designed to run on FAT- NOT GLUCOSE-(CARBS). A CARB-BASED METABOLISM IS A BUSTED METABOLISM.

THE KETOGENIC DIET IS A METABOLISM BASED ON FAT FUEL or a KETONE METABOLISM. THIS METABOLISM SIGNALS EPIGENETIC CHANGES THAT MAXIMIZES ENERGETIC OUTPUT WITHIN OUR MITOCHONDRIA.

WHEN WE PROVIDE OUR BODY WITH PROPER NUTRITION—OUR BODY WILL HEAL ITSELF.

OUR BODIES HAVE BEEN DESIGNED TO HEAL THEMSELVES.

HEALING KETONES— contrary to popular belief and myth are a much needed and essential healing energy source for our cells that comes from the normal metabolism of FAT. The entire body uses ketones in a safer more effective way than the energy coming from CARBS (aka SUGAR aka GLUCOSE). Our bodies will produce ketones if we eat a diet devoid of CARBS, or a low- carb diet-(less than 50 grams) By eating this "caveman- type diet" we can enter NUTRITIONAL KETOSIS AND BECOME KETO-ADAPTED.

Paradoxically, what is known today as the "ketogenic diet" was the NUMBER ONE TREATMENT FOR EPILEPSY CIRCA 1920!

Conventional doctors were taught to FEAR KETOACIDOSIS- as being lethal for Type 1 diabetics. When Big Pharma arrived with its boat-load of dangerous- anti-epileptic drugs— the Ketogenic diet as a viable treatment for EPILEPSY WAS SUPPRESSED!

Here is a short history lesson.

Starvation, with attendant ketosis has been used as a treatment for refractory epilepsy since the early 20th Century. Pierre Marie pro-posed this treatment on the theory that epilepsy resulted from intes-tinal intoxication. On this assumption, a diet consisting of water only, for 30 days was used to successfully treat some refractory epileptics by Hugh Conklin- an Osteopath from Wisconsin.

The inference that ketone bodies themselves were the effective agent—led Russell Wilder at the Mayo Clinic to propose a high-fat, low carbohydrate diet for the treatment of EPILEPSY. HFLC diets were first used in medicine as a treatment for refractory epilepsy.

Studies of diabetic patients with insulin-induced HYPOGLYCEMIA messed up RATHER THAN CLARIFIED THE SCIENCE OF HUMAN METABOLISM. A PROPER UNDERSTANDING OF THE NORMAL METABOLISM OF THE BRAIN WAS OBSCURED.

THE" TREATMENT" FOR DIABETES BECAME AVAILABLE WITH THE DISCOVERY OF INSULIN AT THE UNIVERSITY OF TORONTO in 1921-22.

This scientific breakthrough was a dramatic event for the manage-ment of any disease. By lowering the blood glucose, insulin's impact on a diabetic patient was sensational and seemly miraculous. There was only one little problem. This was an erroneous hypothesis.

Initial research on BRAIN METABOLISM was hindered by the wide-spread, yet ERRONEOUS HYPOTHESIS THAT DEVELOPED AS A CONSEQUENCE OF TREATING DIABETIC PATIENTS WITH INSULIN. THIS WAS ANOTHER MAJOR ALLOPATHIC GAFFE.

As you now know, the most severe form of Diabetes Mellitus is manifested during "Diabetic Ketoacidosis". This is a state of CATASTROPHIC TISSUE BREAKDOWN, in which all of the fuels used by the body for energy production are SIMULTANEOUSLY DUMPED INTO THE BLOODSTREAM. This diseased state floods the blood with an overabundance of mostly USABLE FUEL. Thirst develops and profuse urination occurs even as the body becomes progressively dehydrated. The body literally melts away and IS DRAINED OUT OF THE BODY IN THE URINE AS GLUCOSE AND KETONE BODIES. Fortunately, insulin reverses this devastating tissue breakdown. The presence of ketone bodies in the blood and urine of insulin-deficient diabetic patients was recognized in the 1880's and was associated with severe disease states.

In the 1920's, it became evident that insulin lowered the content of glucose in the blood and urine of diabetic humans; AND IT ALSO REMOVED KETONE BODIES!

NEVERTHELESS— the idea that insulin controlled ONLY glucose metabolism and that TOO LITTLE GLUCOSE IN THE BLOOD LED TO BRAIN DYSFUNCTION LED TO THE WIDELY HELD (ERRONEOUS) CONCEPT THAT GLUCOSE WAS THE ONLY FUEL USED BY THE BRAIN.

Unfortunately, this research was suppressed by you know who. THIS RESEARCH DID NOT CORRECT THE WIDELY HELD MISCONCEPTION THAT KETONE BODIES WERE UNHEALTHY AND THAT GLUCOSE WAS THE ONLY SOURCE OF FUEL FOR THE BRAIN.

In the 1950-60's researchers learned that INSULIN LOWERED NOT ONLY THE CONCENTRATION OF GLUCOSE AND KETONE BODIES IN THE BLOOD AND URINE- BUT ALSO A HOST OF OTHER FUELS, INCLUDING FREE FATTY ACIDS!

The fact that our BRAIN can derive 2/3 of ITS ENERGY FROM KETONE BODIES synthesized mostly from FAT- ALLOWS HUMANS TO SURVIVE FOR 60 TO 90 DAYS WITHOUT STARVNG! Who knew?

THE INTERNET AND HEALTHY FOOD WILL SOON BANKRUPT BIG PHARMA. People are now able to read scientific literature. This fact alone could be the death knell for Big Pharma's God like control over the health of Western society.

Guess what?

THE HEALING KETOFENIC DIET AS EPILEPTIC THERAPY HAS RECENTLY RE-SURFACED AFTER ALMOST 100 YEARS!

BIG PHARMA MAY BE ABLE TO DELAY MOTHER NATURE— BUT BIG PHARMA WILL NEVER CONQUER HER! Good will always trump Evil-☺

The ketogenic diet for epilepsy was recently RE-DISCOVERED by a parent who demanded it for his 20-month old baby boy who had severe seizures. The boy's father was desperate to learn out about the ketogenic diet. A resourceful father was able to save his young son's life when the boy's doctors were medically impotent.

THE NEUROLOGISTS WHO TREATED HIS SON WERE CLUELESS ABOUT HOW TO TREAT HIS SON'S EPILEPTIC SEIZURES.

THE BOY'S FATHER WENT TO THE LOCAL LIBRARY AND LEARNED ABOUT THE KETOGENIC DIET. THE BOY'S NEUROLOGISTS WERE DUMBFOUNDED.

AFTER ONLY 4 DAYS ON THE KETOGENIC DIET—THE LITTLE BOY'S SEIZURES STOPPED AND NEVER RETURNED! THE CHARLIE FOUNDATION was born after the baby's name and his successful recovery. Just Google it up!

NOWADAYS— THE KETOGENIC DIET IS AVAILABLE TO THE ENTIRE WORLD AND IT'S SPREADING BY WORD OF MOUTH THANKS TO ITS HEALING EFFECTS.

IT IS WITH GREAT JOY THAT I TELL YOU ABOUT THE THERAPEUTIC WONDERS OF THE HEALING KETOGENIC DIET!

Most people will do almost anything to drop a few pounds of belly flab.

OBESITY IS A UNIVERSAL GLOBAL PROBLEM. THE SCIENCE IS CLEAR.

THE SCIENCE IS SHOUTING THAT THE KETOGENIC DIET IS THE BEST DIET TO MAKE YOU LEAN, HEALTHY AND HAPPY!-☺

EAT FAT TO LOSE FAT! Who knew? EAT FAT TO GET LEAN! Who knew?

NUMEROUS SCIENTIFIC STUDIES PROVING THE WONDROUS THERAPEUTIC HEALING BENEFITS OF THE KETOGENIC DIET are reproduced in the References, infra. Here's a typical study.

One OBESITY /Ketogenic study from Kuwait in 2004 studied effects of a ketogenic diet on 83 obese subjects. Previous short term studies of ketogenic diets showed good fat loss. In the Kuwait study, the 83 obese subjects (39 men and 44 women) followed a ketogenic diet (30 grams/carbs/daily) for 24 WEEKS.

Results: All of the usual health biomarkers, cholesterol, triglycerides etc. improved.

Moreover— THE SUBJECTS LOST AN AVERAGE OF 33 LBS IN 24 WEEKS!

THE HEALING KETOGENIC DIET IS NOT ONLY USED AS A PRESCRIPTION FOR A HEALTHY LIFESTYLE—

IT ALSO USED TO HEAL ALL OF THE FOLLOWING CONDITIONS:

- INFANTILE SPASMS; DIABETES, AUTISM, BRAIN TUMORS. AL-ZHEIMER'S DISEASE, LOU GEHRIGS DISEASE, MULTIPLE SCLEROSIS, DEPRESSION, STROKE, HEAD TRAUMA, PARKINSONS' DISEASE, POLYSYSTIC OVARIAN DISEASE, CANCER, SCHIZOPHRENIA, ADHD, CARDIOVASCULAR DISEASE, STROKE, IBS (IRRITABLE BOWEL DISEASE), PSORIASIS, SLEEP DISORDERS, MIGRAINES, ANXI-ETY, GASTROINTESTINAL PROBLESM, RESPIRATORY FAILURE!

HOW AMAZING IS THAT? (APPENDIX A)

THE KETOGENIC DIET ACTS ON MULTIPLE LEVELS AT ONCE!

THERE'S NOT A DRUG IN THE WORLD THAT CAN DO THAT!

Douglas C. Wallace, PhD, Director of the Center for Mitochondrial and Epigenomic Medicine says:

> "The Ketogenic Diet may act at multiple levels. It may decrease excitatory neuronal activity, increase the expression of bioenergetics genes, increase mito-chondrial biogenesis and oxidative energy production, and increase mitochondrial NADPH production, thus decreasing mitochondrial oxidative stress."

OUR MITOCHONDRIA (organelles) ARE SPECIFICALLY DESIGNED TO BURN FAT USE/ FOR ENERGY. When our cells burn fat as an energy source; the cellular toxic load is decreased. Genes produce epigene-tic effects; energetic output is increased; and fat is a cleaner burning fuel. Fewer inflammatory -(AGES etc- end- products are produced.

NUTRITIONAL KETOSIS cleans our cells from proteins that act like "debris" (cellular waste), which contribute to aging by disrupting the proper functioning of a cell. It does this through a process called "autophagy" which preserves the health of our cells and tissues by replacing outdated, damaged cell tissue with new ones. This process prevents <u>DEGENERATIVE DISEASES, AGING; CANCER</u>, and protects you against <u>MICROBIAL INFECTIONS AND VIRUSES TOO!</u>

Ketone-enhanced autophagy is very important because it can target intracellular viruses and bacteria. These can lead to <u>BIG-TIME MITOCHRIAL DYSFUNCTIONS</u> (busted cells). Ketosis is our best chance against mitochondrial dysfunction. It seems logical to replace/repair cells with fat.

<u>AFTER ALL— OUR CELL MEM-BRANES ARE MADE FROM FAT!</u>

Our cells are mostly <u>FAT</u>; so it makes sense <u>TO USE FAT TO FIX BUSTED FAT CELLS-AND TO MAKE NEW CELLS TOO!</u>

<u>NUTRITIONAL KETOSIS</u> solves multiple problems caused by a <u>HIGH-CARB DIET</u>. This latter "sad" diet is recommended by main-stream science; it's a diet that leads to <u>ANXIETY, FOOD CRAVINGS, DEPRESSION, IRRITABILITY, TREMORS, MOOD PROBLEMS; PLUS A WHOLE SPECTRUM OF METABOLIC DISEASES SUCH AS DIABETES, CANCER, ALZHEIMERS, CVD DISEASE ETC. ETC.</u>

<u>CONSIDERING THE VAST ARRAY OF MIRACULOUS, HEALING EFFECTS PRODUCED BY A SMART BRAIN- KETOGENIC DIET—</u>

> <u>"IT'S A CRIME TO DISCOURAGE EATING A NEUROPROTECTIVE HIGH-FAT DIET".</u>

<u>IT IS INDISPUTABLE</u> that a Ketogenic Diet <u>PRODUCES POWERFUL NEUROPROTECTIVE EFFECTS FOR OUR BRAINS</u>. It can be employed by all of us living in an extremely stressful and toxic environment. Ketone bodies are <u>HEALING BODIES</u> that helped our ancestors thrive and evolve. Nowadays, our besieged mitochondria are always busted in some way or another. We are constantly bombarded by our toxins in our environment. There will be some people whose cells are so busted that a Ketogenic diet will at best serve to slow down further damage. Our ancestors ate a ketogenic diet; so they ate optimally.

<u>THE LEAST WE CAN DO IS:</u>

- <u>EAT TO RESPECT OUR GENOME & EAT OP-TIMALLY FOR OUR PHYSIOLOGY.</u>

<u>THE INTERNET IS RIFE WITH EXAMPLES OF PEOPLE REVERSING CANCER USING A KETOGENIC DIET:</u>

- Dr. Fred Hatfield, World Record holder for Squat (1, 087 lbs) recently <u>CURED</u> himself of cancer- with a Ketogenic Diet. He was diagnosed with widespread metatastic skel-etal <u>CANCER</u>. His 3 doctors gave him 3 months to <u>LIVE!</u> He stopped eating <u>CARBS</u>; which turn into glucose inside your body. <u>CANCER CELLS LOVE GLUCOSE (SUGAR/CARBS)</u>!

- Dr. Otto Warburg won the NOBEL PRIZE FOR MEDICINE IN 1930 when he discovered that <u>CANCER CELLS THRIVE ON SUGAR. IT'S THEIR PREFERRED FUEL. CANCER CELLS CANNOT BURN FAT (KETONES)</u>.

- After one year on a Ketogenic Diet- Dr. Hatfield <u>HAD NO TRACE OF CANCER! HE HAD USED A KETOGENIC DIET TO STARVE OUT HIS CANCER CELLS</u>!

- Dr. Dominic D'Agostino, a scientist who researches "metabolic therapy" at University of South Florida was not surprised by his recovery. He stated "we have dramatically increased survival with "metabolic therapy." Dr. D'agostino has seen <u>SIMILAR RESULTS WITH LOTS OF PEOPLE</u>.

- Dr Terry Wahl and Butch Machan BOTH REVERSED ALS (Lou Gehrig's Disease) (ALLEGEDLY NO KNOWN CURE) BY USING A KETOGENIC DIET.

<u>ALL CANCER CELLS ARE FUELED BY GLUCOSE.</u>

But if you deprive healthy cells of glucose- they switch to using <u>FAT- (KETONES FOR FUEL)</u>.

<u>EXCEPT CANCER CELLS</u>—a metabolic defect prevents them for making the switch to using ketone bodies as <u>FUEL</u>. Therefore, <u>CANCER CELLS</u> can only survive on <u>GLUCOSE. ALL OTHER CELLS CAN USE GLUCOSE OR KETONE BODIES.</u>

Your normal cells have the metabolic "<u>FLEXIBILITY</u>" to adapt from using glucose to using ketone bodies. But cancer cells lack this metabolic flexibility. It's quite simple. You cut off the fuel source of cancer cells—<u>AND CANCER CELLS DIE. THEY DIE! THEY STARVE TO DEATH!</u> When you eat sugar- you are feeding cancer cells!

Bet your doctor never told you <u>THAT</u>!

<u>CARBS ARE NOT NUTRIENTS.</u>

<u>THEY ARE TURNED INTO SUGAR/GLUCOSE AND CAUSE DIABETES, CANCER OR ALZHEIMERS.</u> Dr. Rosedale says: the more <u>SUGAR THAT YOU BURN</u>- the sooner you die. The more <u>FAT</u> you burn- the longer that you will live.

Can a Ketogenic Diet <u>PREVENT AND REVERSE ALZHEIMER'S DISEASE</u>?

ABSOLUTELY!

You can Google up- Dr. Mary Vernon. She reversed her husband's ALZHEIMER'S DISEASE WITH A KETOGENIC DIET. She administered a THERAPEUTICDOSE OF COCONUT OIL TO HER HUSBAND. She gave him: 3 TBSPS OF COCONUT OIL EVERY DAY. She has since introduced her own MCT oil product on the market.

H.   FASTING AND INTERMITTENT FASTING

"Fasting is the Greatest Remedy-The Physician Within" Paracelsus, 15th Century, Swiss German Renaissance Physician, Botanist.

Our ancestors consumed food much less frequently and often had to subsist on one large meal per day, and thus from an evolutionary perspective, human beings were adapted to intermittent feeding, rather than to grazing. (Mattson, PhD, Lancet (2005) 1978-80.

FASTING

Fasting has been used therapeutically for thousands of years. It has also played an integral part of many of the world's major religions. Hippocrates, the Father of Western Medicine, advocated its use and taught his disciples FASTING ACTIVATED THE BODY'S ABILITY TO HEAL ITSELF.

Fasting vs. Feasting

In North America most people are overfed and undernourished. We tend to overeat and this constant feasting puts a continual strain on our digestive system. Our organs are spending most of their time and efforts breaking down this often "questionable food." This puts undue stress on our immune system. With this constant feasting, our digestive and immune systems are "chewing" up a large part of our available energy to perform this arduous task. This means less energy is available to the body to detoxify and to repair cells, tissue, and organs.

What happens when we fast?

When the body is not directing its energy towards digestion, it uses that extra power to clean our internal insides. When fasting, whether it's water or liquids, the body starts to use stored fat as a source of energy. In the beginning, it will rid itself of diseased tissues, excess nutrients, accumulated wastes, and toxins. This internal cleansing process creates an environment for the body to begin its healing.

It starts to repair and regenerate different organs by repairing and regenerating different areas of the body, including the digestive and immune system.

A published study in November 2014 from University of California showed that: EXTENDED FASTING NOT ONLY PROTECTS AGAINST IMMUNE SYSTEM DAMAGE—BUT IT ALSO INDUCES COMPLETE IMMUNE SYSTEM REGENERATION!

Yes -you read that correctly!

In a clinical trial involving patients who were receiving chemotherapy, scientists found that when patients didn't eat for an extended period of time- THEIR WHITE BLOOD CELL COUNT WENT DOWN. This induces changes that trigger stem cell based regeneration of new immune cells

THUS- CYCLES OF FASTING HELP GENERATE A NEW IMMUNE SYSTEM.

In this instance, the cancer cells are trying to find all of the sugar and diseased, injured cells. The cancer cells STARVE. The cancer cells commit cellular suicide.

The researchers also stated: FASTING FLIPS A REGENERATIVE SWITCH; WHICH PROMPTS STEM CELLS TO CREATE NEW WHITE BLOOD CELLS AND BEGIN REGENERATING THE ENTIRE IMMUNE SYSTEM.

Not only that, but they found that prolonged fasting also reduces the enzyme PKA, which is linked to a hormone which increases cancer risk and tumor growth.

In response to criticism that fasting could cause issues in cancer patients, Professor Longo stated:

> "...there is no evidence at all that fasting would be dangerous while there is strong evidence that it is beneficial. Thus far the great majority have reported doing very well and only a few reported some side effects including fainting and a temporary increase in liver markers."

Dr. Longo also mentioned that he had received dozens of e-mails from cancer patient telling how beneficial fasting was. He added:

> "When you starve, the system tries to save energy, and one of the things it can do to save energy is to recycle a lot of the immune cells that are not needed especially those that may be damaged."

Dr. Longo added:

"With a system heavily damaged by chemotherapy or aging, fasting can regenerate, literally a new immune system."

YOU CAN HAVE A NEW IMMUNE SYSTEM IN 3 DAYS BY NOT EATING! ZOWIE! ...OUR BODY CAN CREATE A NEW IMMUNE SYSTEM IN 3 DAYS BY STARVING!

How cool is that!

Tech Times reported: " Whether for 2 or 4 days, the fasting drives the body into "survival mode in which it begins using up stores of SUGAR AND FAT, and also breaks down old cells."

The Times of India came out with an artic entitled" Fast 8 days a year to boost immunity." It also reported the same California study that "fasting forced the body to initiate stem cells" to regenerate and rebuild an entire immune system"/

FASTING IS AN ANCIENT MEDICAL PRACTICE.

Medical fasting is the practice of abstaining from solid food for a specific and predetermined period of time in order to obtain a variety of therapeutic benefits, both preventative and curative. All 3 Fathers of Western Medicine have fasted and have prescribed fasting. Hippocrates, Galen and Paracelsus, who 500 years ago founded the Western Discipline of Toxicology proclaimed that" Fasting is the greatest remedy, the physician within."

Throughout history the world's greatest philosophers and sages, including Socrates, Plato, Buddha and Gandhi have enjoyed fasting and preached its benefits. Ayurveda, the 5,000-year-old healing system from India has long advocated fasting and its therapeutic benefits. In Europe, medically supervised fasting has been traditionally used to heal and restore patients' health. German healing spa experts estimate that most Americans store between 5 and 10 pounds of toxic substances in their bodies. (We actually detox more through our breath than we do through our urine or stool.)

Fasting has never been taught in America's 127 medical schools. Allopathic doctors never have known or have forgotten about their "Fathers of Medicine." Fasting is with any doubt, the most effective biological method of treatment...

FASTING IS "AN OPERATION WITHOUT SURGERY". It is a cure involving exudation, reatunement, redirection, loosening up and purified relaxation. Prolonged scientific fasting has proven itself over several thousand years.

FASTING IS HUMANITY'S OLDEST, QUICKEST AND MOST EFFECTIVE WEIGHT-LOSS, DETOXIFICATION, HEALING AND LONGEVITY-ENHANCING MODALITY KNOWN TO MANKIND—BOTH CURATIVE AS WELL AS PREVENTATIVE.

THERE ARE SEVERAL TYPES OF FASTING- including **NO FOOD OR DRINK— JUST WATER AND JUST LIQUIDS.**

INTERMITTENT FASTING CAN BE AS LITTLE AS 16 HOURS OR AS MUCH AS 30 DAYS OR MORE.

INTERMITTENT FASTING IS AN ESSENTIAL COMPONENT OF A WELL-CONSTRUCTED KETOGENIC DIET.

AN ESSENTIAL KETOGENIC STRATEGY IS:

"TO INCORPORATE INTERMITTENT FASTING AS AN INTEGRAL PART OF YOUR KETOGENIC DIET."

Unlike other mammals, our brain can burn fat during starvation or fasting. During times of starvation (or fasting) we can break down fat into ketone bodies, or ketones. The main one ketone (already discussed) is beta-hydroxybutyrate (BHB)-which is the brain's **SUPERFUEL.** Ordinarily, our daily food consumption supplies our brain and our body with glucose for fuel. In between meals, our brain is continually supplied with glucose coming from the glycogen in our liver and muscles. But glycogen supplies can only provide so much glucose. When our reserves are depleted, our metabolism changes so that we can take amino acids from muscle protein—(aka gluconeo-genesis). But this catabolic process sacrifices our muscles. Needless to say- muscle breakdown is not a good thing for a **STARVING HUNTER/GATHERER. -☺)**

Fortunately we have an amazing body. After 3 days without food, our liver begins to use stored body fat to make ketones for fuel (BHB). For our ketogenic purposes, we need only adopt **INTERMITTENT FASTING.**

THERE ARE SEVERAL KINDS OF INTERMITTENT FASTING.

Ideally, we should fast 3 or 4 times each year for 3 days. This is a great detox and rebuilds our immune system. BUT- the intermittent fasting protocol that I recommend is 16 to 18 hours every day. Intermittent fasting of course is counter to conventional "wisdom" that says that fasting lowers the metabolism and forces the body to hold onto fat in a so-called starvation mode. This is nonsense.

THE AMAZING BENEFITS OF INTERMITTENT FASTING:

- **It's one of the most effective ways to normal-**

ize your INSULIN AND LEPTIN SENSITIVITY;

- It GREATLY REDUCES INFLAMMATION;

- It turns on the genetic machinery so that your brain can function better; it protects brain cells and generally helps to protect your neuro-muscular system from degradation;

- It also improves your brain function by boosting production of the protein 'BDNF (Brain-derived neurotrophic factor). This activates brain stem cells to convert into new neurons and triggers other chemicals that promote neural health; this protein also protects your brain cells from Alzheimer's disease and Parkinson's disease.

- It powers up your Nrf2 pathway which leads to superior detoxification;

- It turns you into an EFFICIENT FAT BURNER. It causes your brain to shift away from burning glucose to burning ketones for fuel;

- It boosts your production of HUMAN GROWTH HORMONE (HGH)

- It reduces cell apoptosis (cell death); turns on genes to leading to replication of mitochondria;

- It enhances energy production leading to better brain function and GREATER MENTAL CLARITY;

- Fasting and ketogenic diets increase the permeability of the blood-brain barrier (BBB) TO KETONES;

- UNDER FASTING CONDITIONS, the mean total circulating KETONE BODY CONCENTRATION IS IN THE RANGE OF 5.8 to 9.7 mmol./L Both (BHB) and Acetoacetate are converted to Acetyl-CoA in the cytosol as well as in the mitochondrial matrix;

Sidebar:

The normal count of white blood cells in the human body is 4,000 to 11, 000. New findings are important for people with BUSTED CELLS (damaged immune cells). Old immune cells become weaker. When you starve, the immune system tries to save energy; and one of the things it can do to save energy is to RECYCLE a lot of the immune cells that are not needed; (especially those that are busted(damaged). Starving the body boosts stem cells which in turn start producing NEW WHITE BLOOD CELLS – called "EUKOCYTES". THESE IMMUNE CELLS DEFEND AND PROTECT YOUR BODY AGAINST BOTH INFECTIOUS DISEASE AND FOREIGN INVADERS.

<u>The take-home message</u>:

<u>OUR BODIES KNOW HOW TO HEAL THEMSELVES. WE JUST NEED TO GIVE THEM THE TIME AND OPPORTUNITY TO DO SO.</u>

<u>WHEN WE FAST- WATER OR LIQUIDS- OUR BODY STARTS USING ITS STORED FAT AS A SOURCE OF ENERGY.</u> When you are sick, your appetite decreases. Animals often lie down and don't eat or drink. In both instances, the bodies' energy is used to <u>HEAL— INSTEAD OF DIGESTING FOOD!</u>

<u>THE INTERMITTENT FASTING PROTOCOL-SKIP BREAKFAST!</u> (Break-the -fast).

<u>Hey—THERE'S NO LAW THAT SAYS YOU MUST EAT BREAKFAST!</u>-☺

<u>IF YOU CAN- TRY TO BEGIN A KETOGENIC DIET IS WITH A 24 HOUR FAST.</u>

For example, you would eat dinner on Sunday evening at say 6 p.m. and then not eat until Monday at 6pm.Unless directed by your physician –you should continue taking your meds. Weaning off drugs is a difficult responsibility. You know your body better than anyone else-so you know what's best for you.

<u>YOU SHOULD DRINK AT LEAST A GALLON OF PURE SPRING WATER.</u> <u>YOU SHOULD TAKE A TBSP OF PINK SALT TO REPLACE ELECTROLYTES.</u>

<u>ALSO, YOU SHOULD DRINK THE JUICE FROM AN ORGANIC LEMON OR TWO.</u>

You will likely be pleasantly surprised how good you feel before you eat on Monday at 6.P.M. If you believe that 24 hours is too long- start with a 16 hour fast. Monday (in my opinion) is the best day to start a new nutritional program.

On Tuesday, <u>TRY</u> not to eat before 12 A.M. That would mean an intermittent fast for 18 hours. If you can only last until 10 or 11 A.M, before you MUST eat—no problem. Your goal will be <u>EVENTUALLY – TO EAT ONLY IN A WINDOW OF 6 HOURS.</u> (eg. 12 to 6 for example). After a few weeks, you will likely find that you are comfortable eating only <u>ONE OR 2 MEALS A DAY.</u> This is the way you will reprogram your body to get into <u>NUTRITIONAL KETOSIS.</u> Always remember- Rome wasn't built overnight. Neither was your metabolic software and hardware.-☺

On February 16th 2015, in a study published on line in the Journal "Nature Medicine" researchers at Yale School of Medicine, discovered the ANTI-INFLAMMATORY MECHANISM INVOLVED IN DIETING AND FASTING.

In essence, the researchers confirmed that the Ketone (BHB) can block a part of the immune system involved in several inflammatory disorders such as AUTOIMMUNE DISEASES; TYPE-2 DIABETES, ATHEROSCLEROSIS, ALZHEIMER'S DISEASE AND AUTOINFLAMATORY DISORDERS.

It was found that (BHB) directly inhibits NLRP3, which is part of a complex set of proteins called the "Inflammasome." The Inflammasome causes INFLAMMATION IN ALL OF THESE DISEASES.

THIS STUDY ILLUSTRATES THE POWER OF THE KETOGENIC DIET!

RECENT SCIENCE HAS AGAIN PROVEN THE AWESOME POWER OF FAT!

THE KETONE (BHB) HAS NOW EMERGED AS THE KING OF FAT! -☺ Professor Dixit, lead author said:

> "It is well-known that fasting and caloric restriction reduce inflammation in the body...

He added these brilliant words:

> "(BHB) is a metabolite PRODUCED in the body in response to:
>
> FASTING, HIIT (high-intensity exercise), CALORIC RESTRICTION, OR CONSUMPTION OF THE LOW-CARBOHYDRATE KETOGENIC DIET"
>
> (author's caps and underline)

THIS STUDY IS ONE OF THE MOST IMPORTANT SCIENTIFIC STUDIES OF THE 21st CENTURY!

THIS STUDY LINKS TOGETHER THE SYNERGISTIC THERAPEUTIC BENEFITS OF THE KETOGENIC DIET –and-THE MASTER KETONE- (BHB)!

THIS STUDY ILLUSTRATES THE IMPORTANCE OF 3 LIFESTYLE STRATEGIES:

FASTING- HIIT- CALORIC RESTRICTION!

HIIT benefits are examined; (infra). It's important to mention some of the amazing health benefits OF CALORIC RESTRICTION. The subject of caloric restriction has caused a lot of ink to flow.

Please remember- on a Ketogenic Diet-

YOU DO NOT NEED TO COUNT CALORIES-BUT YOU NEED TO USE CARB EYEGLASSES-☺

YOU EAT UNTIL YOU ARE SATISFIED/FULL. AUTOMATICALLY- YOU WILL FIND THAT YOU EAT LESS AND FEWER CALORIES.

THE KETOGENIC DIET IS SELF-REGULATING.

All you need to do is become Keto-adapted and then **STAY IN NUTRITIONAL KETOSIS.** Some people cycle in and out of ketosis-

BUT- I DO NOT RECOMMEND IT! Some people can eat a **VERY HIGH-CARB MEAL AND THEN EAT/FAST TO RETURN TO KETOSIS.**

I know several people (myself included) who had ONE high-carb dinner. I paid the price. I got a mild case of the 'carb flu'. For an entire day, I felt "rum-dumb"; in a mental fog. I will never do that again. We're all different so you may be one of those people who can successfully do a cyclical ketogenic diet.

If you have converted your body to burn high-octane rocket fuel (**FAT**)- why would you want to **RETURN TO BE A SUGAR BURNER?** I have included a low-carb dessert or two in my recipe section.

PLEASE DO NOT OVEREAT CARBS! YOU DO NOT WANT TO FIRE UP YOUR SUGAR FACTORY AGAIN! -☺

HERE ARE THE BENEFITS OF CALORIC RESTRICTION:

- A calorie-reduced diet (say 30 percent) boosts brain production of BDNF- which shows dramatic improvement in memory and cognitive function;
- A side-effect of increasing **BDNF IS REDUCED APPETITE;**
- It was first effectively used to treat epileptic seizures;
- It confers profound neuro-protection; increases neurogenesis (grows new brain cells- and helps with neuroplasticity of brain;
- It decreases (ROS) free radical production and enhances mitochondrial chemical energy (ATP)supra;
- It reduces cell apoptosis;
- It boosts natural antioxidant enzymes;
- It **REDUCES INFLAMMATON**- (supra);
- Caloric restriction and the ketogenic diet share two characteris-

tics- reduced carb intake & a compensatory rise in ketone bodies;

- Caloric restriction, (according to a Sept. 2014 study at University of Wisconsin)CAN PROLONG LIFE AND LEAD TO MORE ROBUST HEALTH THROUGHOUT THE AGING PROCESS. A CALORIE-CONTROLLED DIET AND CHOOSING NUTRIENT-DENSE FOODS CAN HELP AVOID COMMON AND SERIOUS DISEASES OF AGING- including, Cancer; cardiovascular disease, diabetes, and Alzheimer's disease; The latest scientific research suggests that activation of the so-called "longevity cell signals" is the critical factor for slowing the AGING PROCESS;

I. KETOGENIC FOODS

The ancestral Ketogenic Diet consists of AT LEAST 75-80 PERCENT FAT; 15-20 PERCENT PROTEIN, AND 5 PERCENT CARBOHYDRATES.

For your 'carbohydrate eyeglasses"—Here are the (22) lowest carb vegetables.

LOW CARB VEGETABLES

In order to compose a well-constructed Ketogenic Diet, you will need to scrutinize the number of carbohydrates that you eat on a DAILY BASIS. Here is a brief synopsis of the carb values.

1. **Arugula**

   - 1 cup= one gram of carbs

2. **Cucumber**

   - ½ cup= two grams of carbs

   - Good source of Vitamin C & caffeic acid (good for skin)

   - Skin has fiber, magnesium & potassium, (good combo to lower blood pressure

3. **Broccoli**

   - ½ cup cooked= three grams of carbs

   - Boosts immune system

   - Rich source of lutein and zeaxanthin (goof for vision)

   - Rich source of calcium, potassium, Vitamin C & bone-building Vitamin K

4. **Sugar Snap Peas**

   - ½ cup of raw sugar peas= 1 gram of carbs

   - Vitamins C,E, and zinc, O-3 fatty acids

5. **Iceberg Lettuce**

   - 1 cup shredded= two grams of carbs

   - Excellent source of potassium, (good for blood pressure)

     Excellent source of manganese (good for bone health & regulating blood sugar)

   - Good source of iron, calcium, magnesium and phosphorous

6. **Celery**

   - 2 med stalks of celery= 2.5 grams of carbs

7. **White mushrooms**

   - ½ cup raw sliced= two grams of carbs

   - Rich in selenium, rich in antioxidants, anti-inflammatory

8. **Radishes**

   - ½ cup of raw radishes= 2 grams of carbs

   - Rich in Vitamin C, calcium, fiber,

9. **Kale**

   - ½ cup of chopped cooked Kale=4 grams of carbs

   - Rich in nutrients, powerful phytochemicals (e.g. indoles)

   - Loaded with calcium, iron, beta-carotene, Vitamins, A, C, & K lutein& zeaxanthin; high in PROTEIN ("The new beef")

10. **Turnizps**

    - ½ cup of cooked turnips= 4 grams of carbs

    - Rich in antioxidants, glucosinolates, Vitamins C, E, Beta-carotene & manganese

    - God source of Vitamin K and O-3 fatty acids

11. **Romaine Lettuce**

    - 1 cup of shredded romaine lettuece= one + ½ carbs

    - Excellent source of Vitamin C & beta-carotene; rich in potassium

12. **Asparagus**

   - ½ cup cooked= 3.5 grams of carbs

   - Rich in antioxidants, phytonutrients, vitamin C, beta-carotene, zinc, manganese and selenium, B vitamins.

13. **Green Pepper**

   - ½ cup sliced green peppers= 2 grams of carbs

   - Great source of Vitamins A, C, K, folic acid,

14. **Okra**

   - ½ cup of cooked sliced Okra= 3.5 grams of carbs

   - Contains glutathione, high in fiber;

15. **Cauliflower**

   - 1 cup of cooked cauliflower= 5 grams of carb

   - Potent nutrients to detox, antioxidants and anti- inflammatory

16. **Yellow Pepper**

   - ½ cup of sliced yellow pepper= 3 grams of carbs

   - Good source of Vitamins A, and C, K,

   - Rich in folic acid

17. **Cabbage**

   - 1 cup of cooked cabbage= 8.5 grams of carbs

   - Rich in glucosinates, anti-oxidants , anti-inflammatory

18. **Red Bell Pepper**

   - ½ cup of sliced red peppers= 3 grams of carbs

   - Good source of vitamins C,A, K, B-6 and folic acid

19. **BROCCOLI**

   1 cup of cooked broccoli= 11 grams of carbs?

20. **Spinach (Popeye's Food)**

   - ½ cup of cooked spinach= 3.5 grams of carbs

   - One of best sources of Vitamin K (bones)

   - Contains more than a 12 flavonoids, lutein& zeaxanthin

21. **Green Beans**

- ½ cup of cooked green beans=5 grams of carbs

- Good source of folate, B Vitamins, manganese;

22. Carrots

- ½ cup= 6 grams of carbs

- Richest vegetable source of Vitamin A carotenes;

BERRIES on a Keto Diet

Many of our ancestors had very little access to fruit. Usually it was seasonal berries. There are not too many fruits growing on the Artic tundra. -☺ One serving of the following is permitted per day of:

- Blue (brain) berries

- Raspberries

- Black berries

- Strawberries,

- Lemons & limes;

  Eat other high-fructose fruits in very modest amounts; you don't want to fire up your sugar factory- ☺

KETO CLEAN PROTEIN

- Wild-caught fish, (salmon(Alaskan or sock-eye), cod, sole, mackerel, trout)

- Shellfish(wild- not farmed)- (sardines, clams, oysters, lobster, shrimp; crab, scallops, mussels, squid);

- Whole eggs (pastured-free range);

- Meat- pastured- grass-fed beef, lamb, goat, bison, elk, buffalo, venison, and other w/game; (organ meats from these animals especially nutritious);

- Bacon & sausage- organic no nitrate/additives;

- Pork- organic grass-fed loin, pork ribs; chops, ham (watch sugar;

- Poultry- organic- free- range chicken, duck, quail, turkey, Cornish hen, pheasant;

HEALTHY FATS

- All fats are not created equal. Only some are beneficial. Most conventionally-trained die-ticians warn that saturated fats and trans- fats are unhealthy; and can raise levels of harmful LDL cholesterol. Of course, trans-fats or highly processed (heated) vegetable oils should be avoided like the plague. The truth is: you can get HEALTHY FATS from flaxseed, olive, coconut and hemp oil. Flaxseed and hemp oil contain optimal balances of Polyunsaturated fats (PUFA's) BOTH OF THESE feature and Omega-3 fatty acid called ALPHA-LINOLENIC ACID OR ALA. A University of Maryland Medical Centre study showed that ALA reduced the incidence of fatal heart attacks and other CVD problems.

- Avocadoes (82.5 % fat)

- Butter (100 % Saturated Fat)

- Whole Eggs (61% Fat)

- Coconut Oil (100% Saturated Fat)

- Coconut (88 %Fat) & all coconut products

- Extra-virgin Olive oil

- Sour cream (88.5% Fat)

- Full-Fat Cheddar Cheese (74%Fat)

- Cream cheese (88%Fat)

- Bacon (69.5% Fat)

- Ground Beef (59.5 % Fat)

- Dark Chocolate (65 % Fat)

- Beef tallow, lard(non-hydrogenated), chicken fat, goose fat;

- Ghee (organic- great for people who have ca-sein or lactose intolerance)

- Red palm oil

- Coconut butter,

- Cacao butter,

- KRILL OIL IS THE BEST SOURCE OF OMEGA -3 FATTY ACIDS;

Coconut Oil is the King of Healthy Oils.

NUMEROUS studies show that Coconut Oil (MCT's) -Medium-chain fatty acids destroy cancer cells; reverse Alzheimer's disease and reverse a plethora of metabolic diseases. It is called "The Cure for all Diseases"/ Healthy populations around the world (about 1/3 of the earth's population) eat massive amounts of saturated fat- especially coconut oil. There do not appear to be any "bad brands of coconut oil.

Olive Oil is the Queen of Healthy Oils.

A study published from Rutgers University in February 2015 in the journal "Molecular & Cellular Oncology PROVED that Olive Oil (Oleocanthal 2015 compound in olive oil) KILLED CANCER CELLS IN 30 MINUTES!

A staple of the (heart-healthy) Mediterranean Diet), Oil), olive oil contains generous amounts of POLYUNSATURATED FATS and MONOUNSATURATED FATS. ** A word of caution- not all Olive Oil is created the same. Many brands contain additives, fillers and other oils. Scrutinize the Quality very carefully.

Here in Canada, I use Acropolis brand Organic EV Olive Oil made on the island of Crete; Its quality and taste is superlative. (I have no financial ties whatsoever to any supplements and/or products in this book which I recommend.)

NOTE BENE: Up to 70 PERCENT OF OLIVE OIL EITHER IS RANCID AND/ OR CONTAINS UNHEALTHY FILLERS! So- Caveat Emptor!

Nuts & seeds

Macadamia nuts are best, followed by walnuts & almonds. Many kinds of nuts are high in CARBS and many contain too many Omega 6 fats. You must keep a healthy ratio of about 1 to 1- of O-3's to O-6's. Excessive Omega 6 fatty acids can be inflammatory.

Pumpkin seeds, sesame seeds, sunflower seeds are fine- but watch the carbs. One of the potential boo-boos on a Keto Diet is to eat too many nuts and or seeds. You can eat saturated fats like coconut oil and butter until its coming out of your ears. Watch out that your pants don't fall down though. -☺

J.   20 AMAZING BENEFITS OF A KETOGENIC DIET

1. Lower blood pressure

Los carb diets are excellent at reducing blood pressure. If you are taking any blood pressure meds- be warned that you might start feeling dizzy for too much medication while on a keto diet. You SHOULD be able to wean yourself off...see infra)

2. <u>Good changes in cholesterol</u>

Cholesterol can be made from excess glucose in the diet. As you eat less sugar creating foods (CARBS), you do less damage to your arterial system. INFLAMMATION drops; your cholesterol may drop as your body has less glucose from which to make it- and less need for repairing the damage inflicted by inflammatory chemicals. Also, the particle size of your LDL will increase- and become safer- fluffier- not small dense particles which can more easily penetrate your heart/brain.

3. <u>Increase in HDL cholesterol</u>

The more saturated fat you eat- the <u>HIGHER IT WILL GO!</u> This is very healthy. It improves the ratio of HDL/LDL. Higher HDL indicates a healthier heart. Above 39mg/dL is good. (Research shows that more saturated fat that you eat- the less remains in your bloodstream!

4. <u>Drop in triglycerides</u>

Carb consumption is closely tied to triglycerides levels- (one of most well-known benefits of a Keto diet). The few carbs that you eat the lower your triglycerides will go. The ratio of triglycerides t HDL is the best biomarker (indicator) of heart attack risk. It is one of the blood test results you should really pay attention to. The closer this ratio is to 1:1- the healthier you are.

5. <u>Drop in fasting blood sugar and fasting insulin levels</u>

Less sugar coming in- less firing up your sugar factory/driving up your blood sugar; & less wearing out your insulin pump, and raising insulin levels.

<u>WHEN YOU HAVE NO INSULIN RESISTANCE, LOW INSULIN LEVELS, LOW-STABLE BLOOD SUGAR- YOU WILL FEEL GREAT AND YOU WILL HAVE REACHED YOUR GOAL OF SUPERHEALTH!</u>

6. <u>Lower Levels of "C" Reactive Protein (CRP) and Hlc proteins will decrease.</u> These are both markers of <u>INFLAMMATION</u> and heart disease risk.

7. <u>MORE ENERGY!</u> You'll be amazed at how much energy you have !Any chronic fatigue symptoms should get better.

8. <u>Decrease in stiffness</u>

Elimination of grains (and gluten/bad carbs) on a Keto-genic Diet will improve joint pain and muscle stiffness.

9. <u>Clearer, razor-sharp thinking</u>

The mental "fogginess" that is caused by a high-carb diet will disappear.

10. <u>Improved sleep patterns and sleep quality</u>

You will sleep better and you will not find yourself falling asleep at your desk every afternoon.

11. <u>Weight loss</u>

The pounds will melt off. When you exercise and use some good whey protein shakes this will help ramp up your metabolism to lose weight faster.

12. <u>Lack of hunger</u>

Ketone bodies dampen the appetite because <u>FAT</u> is very <u>SAT-ISFYING</u>. You'll notice that you may at times <u>FORGET TO EAT!</u>

13. <u>Food cravings and Addictions will MAGICALLY disappear!</u>

14. <u>Heartburn relief</u>

If you suffer heartburn issues/acid reflux, (Gerd), will gradu-ally lessen and disappear; (unless you have a food allergy;

15. <u>Gum disease & tooth decay</u>

Sugar changes the pH of your mouth and contrib-utes to tooth decay. After about 3 months on a Keto diet- any oral issues should disappear.

16. <u>Better Digestion & Gut Health</u>

You'll see a decrease in any digestive is-sues such as gas, bloating etc.

17. <u>Mood stabilization</u>

Ketones have been shown to be beneficial in stabilizing neurotransmitters such as serotonin dopamine etc.

18. <u>LESS STRESS IN YOUR LIFE!</u>

You will likely find that you pump out less cortisol; your brain becomes calmer and you become more relaxed.

Thoughts of food will not occupy so much of your precious time. Food is information. You will be eating better food. You will be getting better information

19. **Changed DNA gene expression**

    You can experiment with your Ketogenic Coffee by adding MCT oil, Grass-fed Butter, Coconut Oil, cacao butter, coconut butter, almond butter, eggs, etc… SO THE POSSIBILITIES ARE LIMITLESS!

20. **A BETTER SEX LIFE**

    You will find that your sex life is better with your significant other. You will have more energy; your self-esteem will increase; testosterone and other hormones will be better balanced. As you eat more good fats, your libido will increase- so will the quality of your sexual relations.

    Aren't those amazing benefits? Another amazing benefit will be the richness of the foods that you will eat on a Ketogenic diet. Below, I have provided SEVERAL of my own favorite recipes. There are dozens more available from Dr. Google too.-☺

K.   MY FAVOURITE KETOGENIC RECIPES

There are DOZENS OF GREAT KETOGENIC RECIPES available from Dr. Internet. Here are my nine personal favourite recipes. I know that you will **LOVE THESE!**

1. Ketogenic Coffee

   Cook organic coffee in a stovetop coffee maker (French press-or other). Add organic heavy whipped cream and top with cinnamon/organic red pepper. Add organic vanilla and several drops of chocolate Stevia to whipped cream before whipping. (This recipe is my version of Dave Asprey's Bulletproof Coffee)

   You can vary your Keto Coffee by adding MCT oil, GRASS-, COCONUT OIL AND FED BUTTER…SO THE POSSIBILITIES ARE LIMITLESS!

2. World's Healthiest Best-tasting Pizza

   Ingredients for pizza pie crust

• 3 pastured eggs; ¼ cup/melted grass-fed butter/ghee or melted coconut oil;

- 2/3 cup of coconut flour + 2 TBSP of coconut flour;

- 2 TBSP of organic psyllium husk;

- 1 clove (or minced garlic)

- 1 Tsp Alum-free baking powder;

- 1 Tsp dried oregano (optional)

- ¼ Tsp pink salt

Instructions: Mix wet ingredients together in bowl. Add to dry ingredients in separate bowl. Mix well. Let stand 5 min. Use your hands to make into ball. Use rolling pin to roll between 2 sheets of parchment paper. Quickly flop pizza pie into a lightly greased aluminum foil 14 inch pizza pie plate. Knead pizza dough with hands until about ¼ inch thick. Bake pizza pie shell in oven at 300/325 F 15-20 minutes. Remove from oven. Brush on organic hot salsa (o sugar content-best).

ADD

PIZZA TOPPINGS- small slices of pastured bacon or nitrate free pastured salami, ¼ cup finely diced onions. ¼ cup finely chopped organic shitaki mushrooms, ½ cup finely chopped orange organic pepper; Cover the pizza with raw mozzarella cheese   s l i c e s and raw (unpasteurized) grated Parmesan cheese. -Bake for another 15 or 20 minutes until cheese is nicely melted together in a gooey sticky mass-☺ Yum...

Remove from oven- poke holes in pizza pie and drizzle with organic extra virgin oil oil. Serves 4 people. Wash down pizza with a glass of organic red wine (optional- but best!- ☺

This pizza uses psyllium husk- THE WORLD'S BEST SOLUBLE FIBER-And GREAT PREBIOTIC. This pizza is loaded with healthy FATS! The toppings are loaded with nutrients. The orange pepper will give you laser vision!

This pizza (one slice will fill you up) it will feed those wonderful critters in your gut. This pizza will make you lean, strong, healthy ...and SMART TOO! THIS WILL BE THE BEST PIZZA THAT YOU HAVE EVER TASTED OR EATEN! (I personally guarantee it-☺)...and the next morning when you wake up you will feel GREAT!

3. Almond Butter FUDGE Bars:

Ingredients:

- 11/4 cups of almond butter

- ¼ cup of coconut oil

- ¼ cup of grass-fed butter

- 2-3 TBSP of chia seeds

- 1 Tsp of cinnamon

- a pinch of pink salt

- 1 TBSP or raw honey —(or sweeten with Stevia to avoid raising blood sugar and turning on your insulin pump)

Mix ingredients in a food processor or by hand. Transfer to glass 8 X 8 container. Freeze one hour. Refrigerate. Fudge will last 5-6 days in fridge. You will find that a piece of FUDGE will satisfy any residual symptoms of reactive hypoglycaemia- or carb/sugar cravings)

4. COMFORT Coconut Cake

   Ingredients:

- 1 cup of cashew or almond butter

- ½ cup of coconut flour

- ¾ cup of almond flour

- ½ -3/4 cup of grass-fed butter (or melted coco oil/ghee)

- 6 pastured eggs

- ½ tsp of alum-free baking powder

- ½ tsp of baking soda

- ½ tsp of pink salt

- 2 Tsp of Apple Cider Vinegar

- 2 TBSP of raw honey (or Stevia to sweeten)

Blend ingredients together well. Pour batter into loaf pan

Bake at 300 F for 20 minutes and 350 F for additional 30-35 minutes.

A slice of this "Cake" will help protect your brain against the ravages of sugar-induced mental diseases…

5. Ketogenic Fudge Brownies

Ingredients:

- 6 TBSP of coconut flour
- ½ cup grass-fed butter
- 2 TBSP of coconut oil
- 3 pastured eggs
- 1 Tsp of vanilla
- a pinch of pink salt
- ½ cup of organic chocolate chips
- Sweeten with ½ of raw honey or 10 drops of Chocolate Stevia)

Instructions: Mix ingredients well. Pour batter in 8 X 8 glass loaf pan. Bake 300 F for 30-35 minutes.

6. Ketogenic Blue (Brain) Berry Muffins

Ingredients:

- 3 pastured eggs
- ½ cup of melted coconut oil (or grass-fed butter/ghee)
- 1.5 cups of almond flour
- ¼ cup of coconut water (or water
- ½ tsp of pink salt
- ½ cup of coconut flour
- 2 TBSP (organic psyllium husk-(optional)
- 1/2 tsp of alum-free baking powder
- 1 cup of blueberries (fresh or frozen/thawed)
- Sweeten with 2 TBSP of raw honey or few drops of Stevia

Instructions: Add blueberries last. Mix well. Let batter stand for 5 minutes. Bake in muffin tins for 20-25 minutes at 325 F. Makes 6-8 muffins

These "brain" berry muffins are neuroprotective; These muffins are loaded with healthy FATS to protect your brain make you smart, strong and healthy.

7. **Ketogenic Kale LASER-VISION BREAD**

Ingredients:

- 2 cups of packed kale (de-stemmed)
- ½ large onion
- 1 cup of sunflower seeds
- 1 cup of walnuts
- 2 pastured eggs
- 2 TBSP of grass-fed butter or coco oil
- ½ tsp of lemon juice
- 1 tsp of pink salt

Instructions: Blend together well in food processor until smooth. Spread batter on well-greased cookie sheet; bake 325 F for 50 to 60 minutesm. KALE IS THE NEW BEEF. It has tons of nutrients…it will give you LASER-LIKE VISION. It contains high amounts of two eye nutrients- lutein and zeaxanthin.

8. **Gold Dollar Pancakes**

Ingredients:

- 5-6 pastured eggs
- ½ cup of almond/meal
- ½ cup of coconut flour
- ¼ cup grass-fed butter (or melted coco oil)
- 1 tsp vanilla extract
- 11/2 tsp alum-free baking powder
- a pinch of pink salt
- ½ cup pumpkin puree;

Fry pancakes on well –greased cast-iron pan preferably in bacon fat or lard. Slather with grass-fed butter. Lightly drizzle with organic maple syrup.

9. **Ketogenic Nova Scotia Blueberry GRUNT**

it's called 'grunt" because blueberries are so popular with black bears...who like to grunt when they chow down on blueberries- to show their enjoyment and to warn off greedy blueberry humans-☺

This recipe has been adapted from the traditional blueberry grunt which used sugar and flour. Blueberry grunt is so nutritious it has been eaten as a primary meal by "Bluenosers" for hundreds of years. Who doesn't like warm sweet blueberries in a sauce?

Ingredients:

- 4 to 6 cups of fresh Nova Scotian wild blueberries-

- 2 tsp of cinnamon

- 12- 15 drops of Stevia

- 2 Tsp of lemon juice

- 1 cup of water

This is a two-part recipe. The above part consists in putting the above ingredients in a large pot or Dutch oven. Bring the blueberries to a boil.

Drop in the "cooked doughboys".

- 1 TBSP of Psyllium

- 1 -2 TBSP of almond flour/meal

- 1 pasteured egg

- 1 tsp of alum-free baking powder

- 1 TBSP of melted grass-fed butter

- a pinch of pink salt

- a few drops of Stevia

Instructions: Mix dry ingredients in one bowl- add wet ingredients. Make into small balls. Drop spoonful (small balls of batter) into boiling water. The doughboys should be cooked in a 2-3 minutes.

NB**Making the doughboys is a bit tricky. You will have to play with the mixture of the ingredients- once or twice.

Add your doughboys to your hot blueberry mixture.

ENJOY THE TASTE AND YOUR ADDED BRAIN POWER!- ☺

L. THE KETOGENIC WRAP UP

We all have unique metabolisms and unique biochemistry mechanisms; based on our life experiences. Every minute 300 million cells in your body die—and 10 to 50 trillion cells are repaired and/or created in your body every day! Your body is a chemistry set. Thousands of chemical reactions take place your body at any given second,

Whatever you eat- you must ensure that your body has all vital nutrients- in the correct ratios- otherwise your chemistry set suffers. Example: without the presence of 3 vital nutrients-(vitamin C, D and magnesium) in sufficient amounts and ratios—your body's biochemistry suffers.

Transitioning from a carb/sugar- burning metabolism will be easy for some people but difficult for others. The more mitochondrial damage to your metabolism and/or insulin resistance that you have—the greater will be your challenge to repair your busted mitochondria, busted cells and busted carb metabolism.

Dieting is a lonely business. You should anticipate possible scepticism from some family members and friends. You can use their reaction to your decision to change your food/eating habits as your litmus test. Avoid people with fragile egos that are not supportive of you and your efforts to become healthier. It's highly likely that these are negative and/or pessimistic people that have their own personal emotional issues to resolve.

Remember- you are the average of the 5 people who are closest to you in your life.

Choose your friends wisely. Research says that if you associate with fat people—it's highly likely that you will be fat. The opposite is also true. If your friends are lean, strong and smart—chances are much greater that you will be the same.

You may prefer to start your Ketogenic Journey with a close friend or loved one so that both of you can become fat-burning beasts together. After a few days or a week on a Ketogenic diet—most people start to feel GREAT. Feeling good is what life is all about. You may decide to fire your doctor as soon as you become keto-adapted—or before- that's your personal decision. You are the doctor; you are the patient—you are your own health advocate! You are the master of your own health destiny.

By way of synthesis for the Ketogenic Diet- I really admire what Jimmy Moore says. He uses the word KETO as an acronym:

K .....KEEP CARBS LOW

E......EAT MORE FAT

T......TEST KETONES OFTEN

O......OVEREATING PROTEIN IS BAD.

I would add to the O—OVEREATING ON FERMENTED FOODS IS GOOD-☺-

What is your personal "Goldilocks Carb Zone". It could be 10 carbs/day or it could be 50 carbs or more per day.

YOU ARE THE ONLY PERSON WHO CAN FIGURE OUT YOUR GOLDILOCKS CARB ZONE-☺ YOU ARE THE MASTER OF YOUR HEALTH DESTINY.

YOU'RE THE ONLY PERSON THAT LIVES INSIDE OF YOUR BODY

YOU ARE THE ONLY PERSON WHO KNOWS HOW YOU FEEL AFTER YOU EAT VARIOUS FOODS.

OUR CREATOR HAS PROVIDED US WITH THE BEST SET OF CARBOHYDRATE EYEGLASSES. You need to do your carb homework-☺

PLEASE REMEMBER- our bodies require time to build the new enzymes needed to burn fat efficiently and to induce ketosis. Your body needs time to build new metabolic machinery and to establish new metabolic pathways. Dr. Ketosis is your best doctor...probably your best friend too-☺

All of the clinical therapeutic research focused on the correct ratio of fats, protein and carbs. Most often the therapeutic ratio was 3:1 or 4:1- (3 or 4 fats to I protein/carbs). In many of the studies—most patients were able immediately reduce their "meds" by 50 percent or more. As long as you closely monitor your blood sugar/ ketone levels- you should be able to SAFELY WEAN YOURSELF OFF horrific synthetic chemicals called drugs.

In many clinical studies, patients were given a "good supplemental Multivitamin." Also the clinicians conducting the ketogenic trials made sure that patients drank PLENTY OF PURE CLEAN WATER (courtesy of Dr. Clean Water).

The biggest potential pitfall is to make sure you have SUFFICIENT ELECTROLYTES- especially POTASSIUM AND SALT (pink). In all of the studies I reviewed- I found only one patient who had a slight problem...He forgot to EAT!... but he did not require hospitalization for that.

MANY CLINICAL KETOGENIC TRIALS BEGIN WITH A 24 HOUR FAST.

If you can do that- it is the fastest way to kick start your metabolism towards becoming keto-adapted.

Actually—you must <u>BE CAREFUL AND DO NOT FORGET TO EAT!</u>

It's also a good idea to eat to about 80 percent fullness. Healthy good fats have a way of filling you up more than you think!

Finally be patient with yourself and Listen to your body.

Listen with your Ketogenic heart.

Personally, I stick with a raw and liquid nutrition during the daytime on most days. I usually eat my cooked solid food in the early evening (5 to 6 P.M.) This keeps my energy high during day when I am doing my most stressful and demanding activities. Liquid nutrition is easier and doesn't strain my digestive system while I am engaged in mentally and physically strenuous activities.

So actually- I keep my eating window between 1 P.M and 6 P.M

GOOD LUCK WITH DR. KETOSIS!

Are you helping or hurting your brain and your health? Are you eating junk food and hanging around with the wrong people? Are you one of the smart people who eats wholesome, organic food and has positive, smart, friends? Do you waste hours on Facebook or do you enjoy personal social FACE TO FACE talking with friends and colleagues?

Do your friends support and honour you? Research tells us that you are the average of the 5 people closest to you. If these people are obese/fat or couch-potatoes- you will most likely be the same. Conversely if you are lean, healthy have an active lifestyle you are more likely to hang out with like -minded friends.

CHAPTER EIGHT

DR. SUNSHINE —
SUPER MEDICINE

20 Minutes of Sunshine a day- will keep the doctor away...

A. INTRODUCTION

As previously stated, supra; -if doctors tested and prescribed Vitamin D- doctors waiting rooms would be <u>EMPTY</u>!

There is a lot of truth in the old adage the best things in life are free. It certainly is true when it comes to sunshine and sunlight.

<u>MOTHER NATURE DOES IT AGAIN</u>! The sun is the most important thing for Planet Earth and all living things- even the micro-organisms living in our water and soil.

Humans are not programmed nor designed to spend their waking hours indoors. Everybody knows that humans are not designed to stay indoors or to sit on our butts for 8 or 10 hours every day. We are <u>OUTDOOR</u> mammals. Theoretically, man is programmed to spend his life outside- except when he requires protection from predators and the elements.

A sedentary lifestyle has accelerated in the last 300 years throughout industrialized countries.

Everything on planet earth needs sunshine. All plants and animals would die without the nourishment provided by our sun. Sunshine and water nourish all plants and animals. Man shares the same requirements. "O' Solo Mio" is what keeps us alive. Moreover, when we do not get enough sun exposure, like plants, we wither up and die. Plants absorb goodness via photosynthesis. They transfer this solar energy to us.

Research shows that too little sun exposure is likely worse for our health than too much. We are deprived of the good solar energy. WE ARE ELECTRICAL BEINGS. Energy from the sun goes through our bodies to the earth. We absorb negative electrons from the earth when we walk barefooted on grass or bare ground.

Even common sense tells us that either too much or too little sun exposure is bad for our health. Avoiding the sun and getting burnt to a crisp by over-exposure at one time makes no sense. Staying indoors for fear of getting skin cancer is equally silly.

WITHOUT THE NOURISHMENT, SUSTENANCE AND ENERGY SUPPLIED BY DR. CLEAN WATER AND DR. SUNSHINE- HUMANS BEINGS WOULD PERISH-PERIOD.

It is important to ensure that we GET OPTIMUM QUALITY SUN EXPOSURE.

We must get the PROPER KIND AND THE OPTIMAL AMOUNT of sun-shine. Optimal sun exposure will help make us strong and healthy. Staying indoors and keeping totally covered up from head to toe when exposed to sun is absolute nonsense!

This flies in the face of logic and common sense.

LACK OF OPTIMUM SUN EXPOSURE WILL MAKE US SICK.

Our bodies cannot make enough Vitamin D-3, aka The Sunshine Vitamin. Chronic diseases from A to Z will be the result.

VITAMIN D DEFICIENCY CAUSES PREMATURE DEATH.

Your number one option to get Vitamin D FREE is from MOTHER NATURE!

Never let anyone tell you that SUNSHINE is not good for you— even if that person is wearing a white coat-☺) Remember the 99 percent Rule? You guessed it.

Doctors have got it 99 PERCENT WRONG- AGAIN!

LACK OF SUNSHINE WILL MAKE YOU SICK AND KILL YOU PREMATURELY!

SUNSCREENS CAUSE CANCER!

MOTHER NATURE WORKS WITH DR. SUNSHINE AND DR. EARTH TO MAKE YOU STRONG AND HEALTHY!

Your dermatologist (skin doctor) does not know his arse from his elbow-☺

IT IS IMPOSSIBLE TO GET ADEQUATE AMOUNTS OF VITAMIN D FROM OUR DIET. Some foods and supplements will help a bit.

BUT— THERE IS NO SUBSTITUTE FOR THE HEALTH BENEFITS BESTOWED UPON US BY DR. SUNSHINE!

MOTHER NATURE got it right the first time. Her sunshine medicine will make us healthy and strong. LACK of her sunshine medicine will cause us to be sick and die. It's as simple as that.

Mother Nature provides us with her beautiful sunshine. We are designed to spend a reasonable portion of our time outdoors bathing in Mother Nature's Medicine.

No matter what our skin-colour— we are designed by our Creator to spend large amounts of time outside in the sun. Our hunter/gather forbears spent almost all of their waking hours outside. And we have provided with the best protection in the world from the elements. It's called our skin. It is our largest organ and protects the contents of our bodies.

Do you honestly believe that our Creator would create our Sun to warm us and then not provide our bodies with good skin protection from reasonable sunshine exposure?

Why would anyone recommend staying indoors?

Why would anyone recommend slathering on sunscreen to protect us from absorbing Vitamin D?

Is it true that BIG PHARMA, dermatologists, and doctors are lying to you to separate you from your hard-earned cash? Are dermatologists and drug manufacturers lying to us about the benefits of Dr. Sunshine? Absolutely! This is another Big Pharma scam that is killing thousands of naïve brainwashed people.

Could anyone be that dishonest? Unfortunately, there are many dishonest people who profit by fear-mongering so that that they can sell their poisonous products to the uneducated masses.

There is a widespread rumour that humans began to wear clothes— not to cover their privates— but rather to keep warm from the elements-☺ This might explain why early European explorers were often shocked when the dark-skinned peoples encountered were most often naked. Sun-burned skin- and SKIN CANCER has never been a problem in the tropics. Mother Nature did provide a sunscreen remedy- just in case.

It's called the aloe plant. Why does this plant only grow in very warm climates?

Hmm...Do you think this was done to allow sunscreen manufacturers (drug companies) to be able to sell their poisonous sunscreen products to North Americans?

Five hundred years ago, even among the fair-skinned European sailors, cancer was not a problem. The word cancer was not even in any language. These sailors spent every waking minute in the sunshine and open air. Sunburn was not problematic. They simply covered their heads, kept in the shade and worn light colored clothing to shield themselves from the hot tropic sun.

Our sun is similar to fire. We are designed to feel the warmth of the heat of both. Fire cooks our meat and provides us warmth. Obviously, it's not a good idea to burn our bodies- nor should we be foolish enough to burn our meat to a crisp. This would be sheer insanity.

Research shows that when we eat a piece of char-broiled meat—we increase our RISK OF CANCER BY 462 PERCENT!

It is unhealthy to eat char-grilled meat. It is also unhealthy to char-broil our skin.

We should eat our meat lightly cooked. We should also spend 10 or 15 minutes in the sunshine EVERYDAY—IF we are fortunate to live in a warm part of the world.

If we live in colder climes, we need to do whatever we can to get enough sunshine exposure.

Our sun- like fire—warms our bodies. Tanned skin is Nature's Way to protect us. The darker our skin, the less protection we need from the sun and the greater our sun tolerance. African and peoples with very dark skin have developed a sun tolerance for many generations. The have "sun-tolerant" genes.

With the advent of shelters made from wood and concrete, humans started to spend more time indoors. More time inside obviously meant less time feeling the glorious sun warming our bodies. To compensate for the lack of sunshine, modern man began to build houses with bigger windows and patio doors.

Unfortunately research shows that <u>more people develop SKIN CANCER by sun exposure through the glass than when outside</u>!

Even many people who live in cooler climates spend a lot of time outside. The Inuit peoples (Eskimos) are good examples. Before the advent of modern housing, Eskimos had to spend a good portion of their waking time huddled in their igloos wrapped in furs. But—their food was outside; so to eat their main diet (whale and seals); they had to go outside to hunt.

Most Eskimos have dark-tanned skin. This dark tan is largely due to spending most of their life in the sunshine—even on days when the temperature is minus 20 degrees! When Eskimos adopted the western lifestyle they stopped spending time in the sunshine and eating healthy food. Eskimos started spending more time inside watching T.V and less time using their harpoon outside. Let's not forget that most never covered their faces outside in the sunshine.

Do you ever hear of an Eskimo having a cancerous melanoma tumor on his face?

<u>RECENT RESEARCH SHOWS THAT NORTHERN AMERICAN CITIES HAVE MUCH HIGER RATES OF CANCER (including SKIN CANCER) AND ALL OTHER CHRONIC DISEASES</u>!

<u>WHY DO SOUTHERN CITIES HAVE LOWER RATES OF CANCERS?</u>

Is it because people in warmer southern climates wear less clothing? Is the incidence of SKIN CANCER higher in warmer climates because people are smarter and AVOID spending lots of time in the sun?

<u>THE TRUTH IS:</u>

<u>THERE ARE HIGHER RATES OF CANCERS (AND CHRONIC DISEASES)</u> in cities such as Boston, New York, Chicago and Cleveland—<u>VERSUS LOWER RATES OF CANCERS AND DISEASES</u> in cities like Miami, San Diego and Honolulu.

Is this because these southern people are just smarter and put on <u>TONS</u> of sunscreen and spend all of their waking hours indoors? <u>ABSOLUTELY NOT!</u>

<u>SKIN CANCER</u> (and most other cancers) ARE <u>MAN-MADE DISEASES</u>.

<u>BAD CHEMICALS IN OUR ENVIRONMENT CAUSE MOST SKIN AND OTHER CANCERS.</u>

MOTHER NATURE IS OUR BEST FRIEND. MOTHER NATURE IS HERE TO PROTECT US FROM BAD CHEMICALS SOLD BY BAD CHEMISTS AND DRUG COMPANIES.

Skin cancer caused by "too much sun exposure" never existed among native North American Indians. These native peoples lived in tee-pees and spent most of their waking hours in the sunshine. That's why they were referred to pejoratively as "redskins". These native Americans, like the Innuit (Eskimo) peoples spent virtually all of their waking hours outside—in the healing sunshine. History does not report any skin cancers in these peoples.

Is skin cancer <u>CAUSED</u> because people are not putting on enough <u>SUNSCREEN</u> when they sunbathe?

In the last 10 years the <u>SALES OF SUNSCREENS</u> (both OTC and pre-scribed) have steadily climbed as has the rates of skin melanoma (cancer) has increased.

What's going on? Is this a coincidence? Are people NOT following the advice of their doctors and dermatologists?

There lies the problem.

MOST PEOPLE ARE FOLLOWING THE ADVICE OF DOCTORS AND DERMATOLOGISTS.

MOST SKIN CANCER IS CAUSED BY A LACK OF SUNSHINE.

MOST SKIN CANCER IS ALSO CAUSED BY POISONOUS SUNSCREENS.

Once again conventional medicine and Big Pharma are killing you with the <u>WRONG ADVICE!</u> More proof that doctors do not know their arse from their elbow-☺

HOW DO SUNSCREEN PRODUCTS CAUSE CANCER?

1. <u>SUNSCREENS plug up the pores in your skin. THEY STOP YOUR BODY FROM ABSORBING THE GOOD UVB RAYS THROUGH YOUR SKIN. They prevent your body from being able to manufacture Vitamin D.</u>

2. Poisonous chemicals indirectly <u>ROB</u> your body from <u>OBTAINING THE RAYS IT REQUIRES TO MANUFACTURE LIFE GIVING VITAMIN D.</u>

   <u>THE ABSENCE OR DEFICIENCY OF THIS ESSENTIAL NU-TRIENT CAUSES YOUR BODY TO GET SICK.</u>

   <u>CANCER OR OTHER CHRONIC DISEASE IS CAUSED BY A LACK OF VITAMIN D.</u>

3. When you apply a chemical topically on your skin, it's <u>ABSORBED</u> into the bloodstream better and faster than if you EAT it. Most substances that you eat usually pass through your digestive system and your gastrointestinal tract. When you place poisonous chemicals on your skin, they pass through your skin and most chemicals pass directly into your bloodstream. Your poor immune system caught by surprise is overwhelmed by the toxic chemicals.

THERE ARE CHEMICAL POISONS IN SUNSCREEN PRODUCTS?

Many sunscreen products contain toxic chemicals and prevent the good (UVB) rays from penetrating through the skin in order to allow the production of VITAL VITAMIN D. These chemicals cause damage on a cellular level—which is how cancerous cells are formed—once they are absorbed through the skin and enter the bloodstream.

The most toxic sunscreen products contain:

- OXYBENZONE, which is a "hormone disruptor."(also sometimes referred to as "a gender-bender). It causes cancerous cells to grow. Oxybenzone is in 56 PERCENT OF SUNSCREENS according to the Environmental Working Group (EWG);

- BENZOPHENE, PABA, AVOBENZONE, HOMO-SALATE and ETHOXYCINNMATE;

- VITAMIN A used in sunscreens may speed up the development of skin tumors or skin lesions;

- A HIGHER SPF LEVEL which has not been proven to be effective and could actually cause more exposure to UV radiation;

- FRAGRANCE(S) which are linked to allergies and other serious health problems;

- PARABENS which are hormone disruptors;

  (Source: http://www.FoodBabe.com

As Dr. Parselsus said:

"THE DOSE DETERMINES THE POISON"

The more sunscreen that you slather on—the bigger the dose of <u>CHEMICALS</u> that you are eating—the faster you will get cancer; skin infections. Skin lesions and/ or some other type of serious illnesses/ health conditions.

The jury is in.

LISTEN TO CONVENTIONAL MEDICINE — GET SICKER, AND DIE.

IF YOU APPLY THAT POISONOUS DRUG THAT YOUR DERMATOLOGIST RECOMMENDS; IT MAY REMOVE THAT WART—BUT IT MIGHT GIVE YOU SKIN CANCER TOO!

DO YOU REALLY WANT TO TAKE THAT RISK!

If Mother Nature didn't make it –you don't need it.

Again, better to — fire your doctor or dermatologist; and hire yourself.

Why do we need sunshine?

SUNSHINE PROVIDES US WITH THE PROPER NUTRIENTS TO MAKE VITAMIN D-3 – aka THE" SUNSHINE VITAMIN" Vitamin D is made mostly from sun exposure.

What is Vitamin D-3?

Vitamin D-3 is NOT A VITAMIN.

Vitamin D-3 is actually a STEROID HORMONE!

The clinical term for Vitamin D-3 is "25-hydroyvitmaminD."

How is Vitamin D-3 made in our body?

Here is the Coles" Notes explanation of the biological process of creating this steroid hormone called Vitamin D-3.

Cholesterol sulfate is essential for healthy cells and making vitamin D.

It is widely known that red blood cells produce cholesterol sulfate and that this molecule protects our red blood cells from falling apart. If our red blood cells are unable to produce enough cholesterol sulfate; they fall apart and spill their contents into the bloodstream. (This condition is called 'hemolysis").

Red blood cells need cholesterol sulphate to stay healthy and to function properly. Discussing red blood cells, world- renowned scientist, Dr. Stephanie Seneff (infra) says:

> "It's a very elegant concept that they need sunlight to make sulfate. I came upon this as an idea when thinking about the skin. The skin makes a huge amount of cholesterol sulfate. It's the main producer. Your skin is exposed to sunlight and produces both cholesterol

sulfate and Vitamin D sulfate at the same time. The Vitamin D that's produced in the skin is transported in the sulfated form...

Dr. Seneff adds: The cholesterol sulfate serves the really important role of distributing both cholesterol and sulfate to all tissues. I think that's one of the really important things that it does. It's incredibly important because the cholesterol and the sulfate are absolutely essential to the well-being of all the cells."

The learned scientist tells us that when the walls of arteries are depleted in sulfate they don't work properly. That's when you get cascades that end up producing things like cardiovascular plaque because there's not enough sulfate in the artery walls. That's what causes the plaque to build up...

If you are not getting enough sunshine exposure; you are building plaque on your artery walls. Not only will you not produce enough Vitamin D—the downstream result is likely to be cardiovascular disease. YUK!

How does the body use Vitamin D?

MAGNESIUM IS ESSENTIAL FOR VITAMIN D ACTIVITY.

Magnesium is another important player for the activity of Vitamin D. It CONVERTS Vitamin D into its ACTIVE FORM- VITAMIN D-3.

Magnesium activates enzyme activity that helps your body use the Vitamin D. In fact, all enzymes that metabolize Vitamin D require magnesium to work.

Magnesium also plays an important part in Vitamin D's IMMUNE-BOOSTING EFFECTS. As noted by MAGNESIUM EXPERT, Dr. Carolyn Dean, MD. ND.

"The effectiveness and benefits of Vitamin D are greatly undermined in the absence of adequate levels of mag-nesium in the body. Magnesium acts with and is essen-tial to the activity of Vitamin D, and yet most Americans do not get their recommended daily allowance, (RDA) of this important mineral." (Authors underline).

SIDEBAR-

VITAMIN K-2 REQUIRED TOO!

Magnesium has been described as the "Lamp of Life".

AN ADEQUATE AMOUNT OF MAGNESIUM IS REQUIRED BY OUR
BODIES TO DO A PLETHORA OF BODILY FUNCTIONS. Good dietary
sources of magnesium include sea veggies,(kelp, dulse nori) and
many other veggies.

(The best magnesium supplements appear to be magnesium citrate
& magnesium threonate). Bathing in Epsom salts (magnesium
sulfate) helps too.

IF OUR MAGNESIUM LEVELS ARE TOO LOW—SICKNESS AND DISEASE
WILL OCCUR SOONER OR LATER!

When we get sunshine exposure our bodies make Vitamin D-3. But
our bodies react by scavenging for VITAMIN K-2 Fortunately we can
get THIS essential vitamin from a few food sources. Good dietary
sources of K-2 are inter alia- Gouda and Brie cheeses.

As with Vitamin D and K-2, magnesium deficiency is also common as
Dr. Dean notes. But beware- if are magnesium deficient and you take
a CALCIUM SUPPLEMENT—you could be worsening your health!

Vitamin   K-2,   magnesium,   calcium,   and   Vitamin   D—   ALL
WORK TOGETHER.

IT'S VITALLY IMPORTANT TO MAKE SURE THAT THE RATIOS OF EACH
ARE APPROPRIATE. Other co-factors that work with Vitamin D are
Vitamin A, Zinc and Boron.

WHEN   TAKING   SUPPLEMENTS   BE   CAREFUL   NOT   TO   CREATE
IMPROPER RATIOS OF VARIOUS NUTRIENTS!

IT'S ALWAYS PREFERABLE TO GET YOUR NUTRIENTS FORM ORGANIC
WHOLE FOODS!

B.   30 MINUTES OF SUN EACH DAY-
KEEPS THE DOCTOR AWAY

The reality is that the vast majority of people, including doctors,
have been duped into believing the myth that the sun is toxic, car-
cogenic— a DEADLY health hazard. That explains why most people
lavishly slather toxic sunscreens all over their bodies.

In fact—most conventional sunscreens are CANCER-CAUSING
BIOHAZARDS. (source: www.faim.org) (Biohazards could also be
considered as neurotoxins.)

OMG! And you thought we were finished talking about NEUROTOXINS!-☺

The multi-billion dollar Cancer Industry and the Billion Dollar Toxic Sunscreen Industry are duping you out of your hard-earned cash, while making you sick. They are laughing their way to the bank as you become sicker and sicker.

That is quite scandalous and borderline criminal. That is one of the reasons that I am writing this book. You need to wake up to all of these hoaxes before it's too late for you and your loved ones.

Dr. Dave Mihalovic, ND (source: www. preventdisease.com) states it clearly:

> "Those who have attempted to convince the world that the Sun, the Earth's Primary source of energy and Life causes cancer, have done so with malicious intent to deceive the masses into retreating from the one thing that can prevent disease."

THE COLD TRUTH IS THAT YOU HAVE BEEN LIED TO ABOUT THE SUN CAUSING SKIN CANCER FOR DECADES.

Statistics show that the dreaded Malignant MELANOMA SKIN CANCER IS ON THE RISE. (Source: www.institutefornaturalhealing. com)

DID YOU KNOW THAT THERE IS NO DEFINITVE PROOF THAN THE SUN ALONE CAUSES SKIN CANCER?

In his book, The Healing Sun, Dr. Richard Hobday documents a wide array of studies which show that the sun protects against cancer of the breast, colon, ovaries, and prostate. It can also prevent diabetes, multiple sclerosis, heart disease, high blood pressure, osteoporosis, psoriasis s and seasonal affective disorder; (SAD).

According to Dr. Bernarr Zouluck:

> "Cancer is helped by Sunbathing."

> Dr. Zane R. Kime writes:

> "...those who get more sunlight have less cancer. Sun-bathing heals cancer by building up the immune system and increasing the oxygen in the tissues." (source: www. curezone.org)

We are less acclimated to the natural heat and light giving power of the sun. Our skin can easily lack vital antioxidants too. The sun's rays are not always used effectively anymore, especially when we age and or skin and body is not acclimated to absorb the sun's energy. Poor ability to absorb the suns; rays may burn more easily; cause our skin to peel more easily which causes us to fear the sun. We become more vulnerable to believe that the sun can cause cancer.

Some fraudulent medical authorities claim that the sun is the evil that causes cancer. Fortunately some experts tell the truth:

According to studies conducted by Professor Rachel Neale from QIMR Borghofer Medical Research Institute in Brisbane, Australia—'

> "CANCER RISK CAN ACTUALLY BE SLASHED IN HALF (BY 50 PERCENT)- when people are exposed to more time in the sun.
>
> In her studies, she found that those who lived in areas receiving higher levels of UV rays had a 30 to 40 PERCENT lower chance of being diagnosed with pancreatic cancer. Some epidemiology studies showed how excess sun exposure can cut the risk of certain cancers by 50 PERCENT."

The Cancer Council proposes that everyone obtain at least 30 minutes of sun exposure in the middle of the day—TO KEEP THE DOCTOR AWAY.

DR. SUNSHINE IS THE FREEST OF ALL MEDICINES. —AVAILABLE TO ALL.

UTILIZING THIS ENERGY AND HARNESSING ITS TIMELESS POWER ULTIMATELY INCREASES LEVELS OF CIRCULATING VITAMIN D, EMPOWERING THE IMMUNE SYSTEM, WHICH IS ULTIMATELY THE VESSEL THAT CURES A BODY'S CANCEROUS STATE.

Professor Neale believes that everyone should be getting sun exposure every day.

> "Even if it's only 2-3 minutes each day, it will be enough to get that source of Vitamin D" Professor Neale said.
>
> Author's note: This would appear to be enough for people living below the equator—but may NOT be enough for people living in more northern climes.

Exposing more skin in a short period of time is better than less skin in the long run. You should go outside and lift up your pants and/or

your shirt, showing your tummy and legs. This is even more important for naturally dark-skinned people, expectant mothers or those
who work indoors. Children who don't have enough sun exposure
and Vitamin D can develop <u>RICKETS</u>, which may lead to soft bones in
adulthood.

C.   HOW MUCH VITAMIN D IS NECESSARY?

<u>A ROBUST AND GROWING BODY OF RESEARCH</u> clearly shows
that Vitamin D is absolutely CRITICAL for good health and
disease prevention.

Vitamin D affects your DNA through Vitamin D receptors (VDRS)
which bind to specific locations of the human genome. Vitamin D
receptors have been found throughout the body.

One recent study at the Tulane University, (source: <u>www.tulane.edu</u>)
found that Vitamin D is a vital nutrient that plays an important role
in the prevention of osteoporosis. This is what the researchers said:

> " <u>A large body of evidence is accumulating to support</u>
> <u>the profound effects of Vitamin D in reducing the risk of</u>
> <u>other major disorders, including cancers, autoimmune</u>
> <u>diseases, heart disease, high blood pressure, muscle</u>
> <u>weakness, and depression. Vitamin D is not a simple</u>
> <u>nutrient. Its metabolic product is a steroid hormone</u>
> <u>regulating over 3000 genes in the human genome.</u>"

<u>SCIENTISTS SAY THAT 3,000 GENES THAT ARE INFLUENCED BY</u>
<u>VITAMIN D LEVELS! WOW!</u>

<u>THE SCIENTIFIC STUDIES ARE ABUNDANT AND PRESENT</u>
<u>COMPELLING EVIDENCE.</u>

Let's examine what the most recent studies conclude about the
importance of Vitamin D.

1. On April 13, 2014 in a block-buster study published in the Journal
   of Public Health (source: <u>www.ajph.nphapublications.org</u>), researchers analyzed 32 studies over a 40 year period of time; the
   authors concluded that the risk of <u>PRE-MATURE DEATH IS SIGNIFI-</u>
   <u>CANTLY HIGHER IF YOUR VITAMIN D LEVEL IS BELOW</u> 30ng.ml.

Dr. Frank Garland & his brother Cedric, pioneers in Vitamin D
research stated:

"Over 600, 000 cases of colorectal and breast cancer could be prevented each year if Vitamin D levels (worldwide) were increased.

That while overexposure of sunlight is certainly harmful, under exposure of helpful UVB light can significantly lead to a lack of Vitamin D in the body."

(author underline)

According to William B. Grant Phd. Director, Sunlight, Nutrition and Health Research Center: " There are now about 100 conditions and diseases linked to low serum 25 hydroxy vitamin D concentrations."

On August 6th, 2014 in a study published in Science Daily (www.sciencedaily.com),

covering Vitamin D deficiency and mental diseases, researchers found that

Adults in the study who were moderately deficient in Vitamin D had a 53 PERCENT INCREASED RISK of developing dementia of any kind.

The risk increased to a whopping 125 PERCENT in those who were severely deficient.

Similar results were recorded for Alzheimer's disease, with the moderately deficient group 69 PERCENT more likely to develop this type of dementia, jumping to a whopping 122 PERCENT increased risk for those severely deficient.

SIDEBAR-

A wide variety of BRAIN tissue contains Vitamin D receptors. When they are activated by Vitamin D, this facilitates the growth of nerve tissue. Researchers also believe that optimal Vitamin D levels boosts levels of important BRAIN CHEMICALS, and protects brain cells by increasing the effectiveness of GLIAL cells in nursing damaged brain cells back to health.

VITAMIN D's ANTI-INFLAMMATORY EFFECTS AND IMMUNE-BOOSTING PROPERTIES HAVE BEEN WELL-ESTABLISHED.

DEMENTIA is one of the greatest challenges of our time.

Presently there are 44 MILLION CASES WORLDWIDE. That number is expected to TRIPLE by 2050—due to the rapid aging of the world's population.

According to Harvard School of Public Health—

1 BILLION PEOPLE WORLDWIDE HAVE LOW VITAMIN D LEVELS.

IT IS ESTIMATED that more than 66 PERCENT of North Americans have blood 25 (OH) D levels lower than the acceptable level (75 nmo/L).

HOWEVER, IT IS MORE LIKELY THAT THE ACTUAL LEVEL OF LOW VITAMIN D IS ABOUT 90 PERCENT OF NORTH AMERICANS.

Older people are at a GREATER RISK because their skin and bodies are less efficient at absorbing sunlight and converting it to Vitamin D-3.

3. In a study conducted by researchers from the Peninsula Medical School of Cambridge University published in 2009 in the Journal of Geriatric Psychology, elderly adults with lower Vitamin D blood levels scored lower on tests of memory, attention and orientation.

4. A 2008 study on Vitamin D and health published in the Journal Advances in Experimental Medicine and Biology found that Vitamin D deficiency causes growth retardation and rickets in children and will precipitate and exacerbate osteopenia, osteoporosis and increase risk of fracture in adults.

5. A study of severely obese people published in the April 2014 issue of the Journal of Clinical Endocrinology and Metabolism, researchers found that Vitamin D-deficient participants walked slower, were more sedentary than people with normal levels. Conversely the participants with the highest levels of Vitamin D walked the fastest, and reported getting the most exercise.

6. In a study published on October 18, 2014 conducted by Dr. Jin Wi, found that Vitamin D deficiency increased the risk of poor neurological outcome after sudden cardiac arrest by 7 FOLD! Nearly one-third of the patients who were deficient I Vitamin D had died 6 months after their cardiac arrest. Conversely, all patients with sufficient levels of Vitamin D levels were still alive. (source: http://www.escardio.org)

7. In a study published in Los Angeles Times on June 12, 2006, the L,A. Times called Vitamin D "THE ULTIMATE WONDER DRUG". The paper showcased a study that found that seniors with the lowest levels of Vitamin D are 11 TIMES MORE DEPRESSED than those who had normal levels. Numerous studies have shown that Vitamin D deficiency can predispose you to depression. That depression can be restored by optimizing Vitamin D levels.

8. In a study published in OnLine, on May 9th, 2014, the authors concluded that people with Vitamin D levels below 20ng/m: had an 85 PERCENT INCREASED RISK OF DEPRESSION compared to

those people whose Vitamin D levels are greater than 30 ng/mL.

9. A study reported in 2013 in PUBMED no 23744412 reported in Pharmcol. Rep. examined the relationship between Vitamin D and the central nervous system. (CNS).

This is what the abstract stated:

"Vitamin D is formed in human epithelial cells via photochemical synthesis and is also acquired from dietary sources.

The so-called classical effect of this vitamin involves the regulation of calcium homeostasis and bone metabolism. Apart from this, the non-classical effects of Vitamin D have recently gained renewed attention.

One important little known effect of the numerous functions of Vitamin D is the regulation of the nervous system development and function. The neuro-protective effect of Vitamin D is associated with the influence on neuro-trophic production and release neuro-mediator synthesis, intracellular calcium homeostasis, and prevention of oxidative damage to nervous tissue. Clinical studies suggest that Vitamin D deficiency may lead to increased risk of disease of the central nervous system (CNS), particularly schizophrenia and multiple sclerosis. (author underline.)

10. In the Journal, Nervenaret, published in 2013 Pubmed study no. 23052893, the researchers studied Vitamin D and Multiple Scelerosis: The Role of Disease and Treatment; they stated:

"Because of its suggested immune-modulatory capacity, Vitamin D deficiency or disturbance in the Vitamin D metabolism might be a risk factor for the development of autoimmune diseases such as multiple sclerosis—but supplementation with Vitamin D might also be a therapeutic option.

Substantial epidemiologic evidence indicates an association between Vitamin D levels and risk of multiple sclerosis, suggesting Vitamin D to be one of the long searched environmental factors for the development of this most common chronic inflammatory disease of the central nervous system.

11. In an article published in October 2013, in the Journal Breast Cancer Research & Treatment, Pamella J. Goodwin, and colleagues from the University of Toronto selected 8 studies involving 5,69l

women diagnosed with breast cancer. Blood samples showed deficient levels of Vitamin D in <u>36.8 PERCENT</u> of the subjects. When the lowest versus highest categories of Vitamin D were compared in a pooled analysis, women whose levels were low had a risk of recurrence that was <u>MORE THAN DOUBLE</u> than that of those whose levels were high; and the <u>RISK OF DEATH WAS 76 PERCENT HIGHER.</u>

<u>The authors remarked:</u>

<u>"Vitamin D when activated can alter the transcription and expression of specific genes, resulting in growth arrest, apoptosis, aromatase suppression, decreased inflammation, and inhibition of angiogenesis, invasion and metastasis, all of which help combat cancer. "</u> (authors underline)

12. In a study dated September 25th, 2014 in the BMC Nephrology Journal, the authors published their results. It showed that Vitamin D therapy was associated with a lower risk of mortality among kidney disease patients.

13. For this MEGA- ANALYSIS researchers selected 17 studies involving a total of 489,254 end stage renal disease patients receiving dialysis and 3 studies that included 2,603 chronic kidney patients NOT on dialysis. Subjects were treated with active Vitamin D sterols that included alfacalcidol, doxerclciferol, calcitrol, maracalcitrol, falecalcitriol or paricalcitol. Follow up periods ranged from 12 to 140 months. In comparison with no treatment—subjects who received Vitamin D compounds had up to <u>39 PERCENT LOWER RISK OF DYING FROM ALL CAUSES</u> over follow up. Pooled analysis of dialysis patients associated active vitamin therapy with a <u>20 PERCENT LOWER RISK OF DYING</u>; and among those patients NOT on dialysis, the <u>RISK WAS 41 PERCENT LOWER.</u>

   **ed. Note: When cardiovascular mortality was examined active Vitamin D was associated with a 41 Percent lower adjusted risk of death over follow up.

14. In a recent <u>META-ANALYSIS</u> which included a study of 280,000 people. This study published in the March issue of the European Journal of Epidemiology, had the researchers examine the connection between high blood pressure, hypertension and low levels of Vitamin D. Some studies looked at Vitamin D intake from diet and the others looked at blood serum or plasma levels of Vitamin D. 55,000 of the subjects developed hypertension. The upper <u>THIRD</u> of the subjects showed a 30 percent LOWER risk for developing hypertension compared to the lowest group.

This study showed that with EACH 10 ng/mL INCREASE IN Vitamin D, there appeared to be a 12 percent REDUCTION in the risk for hypertension at some point in the subjects' lifetime.

Also the study suggested that DIETARY INTAKE of Vitamin D may not be a valid way to assess Vitamin D levels; but it might be inaccurate because SUNLIGHT EXPOSURE is the major source of Vitamin D.

SIDEBAR:

So called "normal blood pressure" is said to be 120/80. Blood pressure refers to the pressure exerted on the walls of your arteries as blood flows through them. The 2 blood readings are systolic (when your heart contracts); and diastolic (when your heart relaxes and refills with blood between beats). Then of course you have your pulse or the number of heart beats per minute.)

If EITHER top (systolic) or bottom (diastolic) number is higher than normal that's when you get into "hypertension". Hypertension sometimes leads to arteries hardening; heart problems etc.

Most allopathic doctors will whip out their prescription pad as soon as either blood pressure number is up 5 points. In real life you should know that there is a phenomenon known as" white coat syndrome." This means that evidence shows that just the sight of a white coat or a blood pressure cuff can send your blood pressure soaring. The result—often your blood pressure is only temporarily elevated. You can check this yourself.

You should monitor your own blood pressure. Buy an automated blood cuff for $50.00 or you can go to most pharmacies and check it yourself for free. You will usually find that your blood pressure is near normal because you are relaxed. Also, blood pressure fluctuates with blood glucose levels, time of day etc.

Take your own blood pressure after you have fired your doctor-☺

15. A recent study published in PLoS Medicine suggested that OBESITY itself can actually be a cause of Vitamin D deficiency. That means fatter people have poorer mobility get less D-3; get fatter…a truly VICIOUS CYCLE!

16. Researchers from the D-CarDio collaboration are the first to associate high BMI with low Vitamin D levels. This finding suggests that as obesity increases, Vitamin D levels are reduced.

A report by Medical News Today stated:

"For each 10% increase in BMI there was a 4.2 % drop Vitamin D."

17. In a 2012 study published in the Journal of Clinical Nutrition, researchers from Purdue University found that supplementing a resistance training regime with Vitamin D appears to improve muscle power and help shed inches from the waistline of overweight and obese people. According to the researchers— "Therefore, the greater decrease in waist circumference associated with higher vitamin D intake represents a potential reduction in risk for metabolic disease and cardiovascular risk."

18. Recent studies published in The American Journal of Clinical Nutrition (http://ajcnnutrition.org) have linked weight gain to Vitamin D deficiency;

19. Multiple studies have shown that the risk of fractures especially among older people is significantly when vitamin D levels are low. Evidence in 12 studies researchers determined that taking Vitamin D supplements reduced hip and other non-spinal fractures y 20 percent. Another study found that among older populations, vitamin's D muscle-strengthening powers helped decrease the risk of falls- a common cause of disability and death—by nearly 20 PERCENT. (source: www.bmj.com)

20. In a Chinese study published on October 30th, 2014 in a paper presented to the American Thyroid Association, Dr. Guofang Chen found that low Vitamin D levels are associated with Autoimmune Thyroid Disease.(source: http://www.healio.com)

21. In a study published on October 31st, 2014 presented to the American Association of Neuromuscular & Electro Diagnostic Medicine (AAREM), researchers found that people with neuromuscular disease were most often Vitamin D deficient. The also suggested that falls in frail, elderly patients were likely due to low Vitamin D levels, and NOT weak muscles.

22. In an Israeli study published on October 3rd, 2014, in PUBMED no. 25139052 in the Journal Asthma, researchers studied 308,000 patients! They concluded that there was a 25 PERCENT greater exacerbation of ASTHMA problems which were due to low Vitamin D levels or Vitamin D deficiency.

23. A recent study conducted by researchers at Harvard found that people who had low levels of Vitamin D were TWICE as likely to have a heart attack as those who had adequate levels of the vitamin;

24. A recent study in Utah examined Vitamin D levels and heart

disease in nearly 30,000 men and women. The researchers found that those with lower levels of Vitamin D were
more likely to have cardiovascular disease than those
with adequate levels. (source: www.eurekalert.org)

25. Researchers at Orthopaedic Hospital in Vienna, Austria
published a study in the January issue of the medical journal "Pain" which showed that 30 women had their fibromyalgia helped by taking Vitamin D supplements. The
subjects reported less chronic morning fatigue.

26. In a 3 year study published in Saudi Medical Journal, research-
ers found that out of 100 women with fibromyalgia- 61 PER-
CENT were deficient in Vitamin D. With increased doses of
Vitamin D the women showed significant improvement.

THE FOREGOING STUDIES ARE CONCLUSIVE.

BOOSTING YOUR BLOOD LEVELS OF VITAMIN D (serum 25 (OH) D)
LEVELS IS A SUPER WAY TO BOOST YOUR IMMUNE SYSTEM !

THIS GREATLY PROTECTS YOU FROM THE FLU AND COLDS BY
ACTIVATING YOUR IMMUNE SYSTEM. IT CAUSES YOUR IMMUNE
SYSTEM TO ATTACK AND DESTROY BACTERIA AND VIRUSES.

How much Vitamin D-3 is needed?

Dr. Robert P. Heaney (www.cjasn.asnjournals.org) found that outdoor
workers in the tropics typically have-

"serum 25 (OH)D levels ranging from " 120 to 200 nmol/L"

WOW!

WE SEE THAT EVIDENCE ABOUT "APPARENTLY" HEALTHY
INDIVIDUALS WHO ARE OSTENSIBLY HEALTHY TODAY...

NEVERTHELESS MAY BE DEFICIENT IN VITAMIN D!

Most experts suggest a range of at least 50 – 70ng.ml – or 1235-
175 nmol/L

There does not appear to be a toxicity level for Vitamin D.

THIS EXPLAINS WHY SOME HEALTH CARE PROVIDERS ARE
PRESCRIBING HIGH THERAPEUTIC DOSES TO PATIENTS WITH HEALTH
PROBLEMS. (Daily doses of 10,000 I.U. are common).

Dr. Holick, renowned Vitamin D scientist in 2002 in American Clinical
Nutrition Journal stated:

"It is reasonable for everyone to have his or her blood 25 (OH) D concentration measured once a year to achieve the optimum Vitamin D level".

IF —ALLOPATHIC PHYSICIANS TESTED FOR AND PRESCRIBED VITAMIN D TO THEIR PATIENTS THEIR WAITING ROOMS WOULD BE EMPTY!

BIG PHARMA CAN'T GET THE PATENT ON SUNSHINE-AND ALLOPATHIC DOCTORS DO NOT TEST FOR VITAMIN D.

DOCTORS CANNOT MAKE ANY MONEY PRESCRIBING SUNSHINE-☺

SHOCKINGLY—A study dated October 20, 2014, found that:

ONLY SEVEN (7) PERCENT OF PHYSICIANS COULD IDENTIFY THE MONTHS OF THE YEAR WHEN IT IS DIFFICULT TO GET ENOUGH SUNSHINE EXPOSURE TO PRODUCE ADEQUATE VITAMIN D!! (source: http:www.dailymail.co.uk)

Would you guess Nov. Dec. Jan. Feb & Mar?

OMG! Another reason to fire your doctor—Your doctor does not EVEN know the warm sunshine months of the year! -☺) OMG!

Do you need any BETTER proof that-

Your doctor does not know his arse from his elbow? Lol.

THE TAKE-HOME MESSAGE:

The levels of D-3 in your body could mean the difference between LIFE and DEATH...LITERALLY!

ENSURE THAT YOUR BODY CONTAINS AN APPROPRIATE LEVEL OF VITAMIN D-3 BY PROVIDING IT WITH GOOD SUNSHINE RAYS—

YOU CAN USE DR. SUNSHINE TO BULLETPROOF YOUR IMMUNE SYSTEM!

GET YOURSELF TESTED! Better yet- DO-IT YOURSELF!

IDEAL LEVEL OF VITAMIN D IN YOUR BLOOD IS 80ng/dL.

CHAPTER NINE
DR. EXERCISE-
ESSENTIAL MEDICINE

"Give me a can of WD 40 and a roll of duct tape and I
will fix the problems of the world."

-Gray Cook,

A. INTRODUCTION

The above statement was made by Mr. Gray Cook- world renown
Orthopedic Physical Therapist and Strength and Conditioning
Specialist. Gray is the creator of the Functional Movement Screen
(aka FMS).

FMS has spread from the USA throughout Europe and is rapidly
spreading eastward to the Orient. FMS is composed of 7 Fitness
tests that evaluate your movement patterns to determine your
"weakest link". (see FMS below).

I personally heard Gray make the above statement to one of his
friends. Actually— I was eavesdropping his conversation at the
time...-☺. Gray's analogy was pure genius.

Gray did NOT mean this statement LITERALLY. He was using
an analogy.

I believe Gray meant that MOVEMENT DIFFICULTIES OF OUR
BODIES can be resolved by ADDRESSING MOBILITY AND STABILITY
ISSUES.

Hence—his analogy about WD oil, (mobility) and duct tape (stability).

B. YOUR CHAIR IS KILLING YOU!

Whether you are an attorney, or any kind of DESK PROFESSIONAL—

YOUR DESK JOB IS LITERALLY KILLING YOU!

YOUR CHAIR IS YOUR MORTAL ENEMY!

IF YOU'RE LIKE 99.9 PERCENT OF ALL DESK PROFESSIONALS—

YOU LIKELY HAVE "THE SITTING DISEASE."

WHO (The World Health Organization) lists INACTIVITY as the 4th BIGGEST KILLER OF ADULTS WORLDWIDE!

SITTING ADVERSELY AFFECTS THE HEALTH OF MILLIONS OF PEOPLE WORLDWIDE.

THE SOLUTION IS SIMPLE.

STAND-UP OFTEN-AND AVOID SITTING

For 10 years now, Dr. James Levine, Director at the Mayo Clinic has been shouting:

THE CHAIR IS A KILLER!

Dr. Levine says there are at least 24 different chronic diseases and conditions associated with excess (chronic) sitting.

NOTE BENE: (There could be even more than 24...)

SITTING IS THE "NEW SMOKING" OF THE MODERN AGE.

The average American adult spends 35.5 hours/week watching T.V. (computer time NOT included). People know they should be more active and should exercise more often. A recent study published in JAMA (Journal of American Medical Association) found that 2 HOURS IN FRONT OF THE TV INCREASES YOUR RISK OF DEVELOPING DIABETES AND HEART DISEASE BY 20 PERCENT!

EVEN IF YOU GO TO THE GYM 3 TIMES PER WEEK—YOU ARE NOT GOING TO UNDO THE EFFECTS OF 6 HOURS OF SITTING!!

HERE'S THE GOOD NEWS –DOING JUST ONE SIMPLE THING-

STANDING UP OFTEN —WILL DO MORE TO KEEP YOU HEALTHY THAN EXERCISING AND GOING TO THE GYM 3 TIMES PER WEEK! Who knew?

Everyone understands that a sedentary lifestyle is unhealthy.

BUT— BIG DIFFERENCE BETWEEN SITTING TOO MUCH—versus-

EXERCISING TOO LITTLE.

WHILE BOTH BEHAVIOURS ARE LETHAL— SITTING TOO MUCH IS FAR WORSE!

Sitting too much is known as "THE SITTING DISEASE."

We have been designed as humans to MOVE. We must move OFTEN and we MUST MOVE WELL. WE MUST MOVE SAFELY AND EFFICIENTLY.

THE EVIDENCE IS OVERWHELMING. 10,000,00 STUDIES AND GROWING—ALL PROVING THAT PROLONGED CONTINUOUS SITTING IS BAD FOR YOUR HEALTH.

For example:

After 24 hours of sitting- INSULIN LOSES 40 PERCENT OF ITS ABILITY TO UPTAKE GLUCOSE INTO OUR CELLS!

THE SCIENCE SHOWS THAT IF YOU DO ANYTHING—EVEN STAND IN PLACE FOR 20 MINUTES—YOU WILL BE HEALTHIER.

A recent study says that STANDING 6 HOURS A DAY REDUCES OBESITY BY 1/3rd.

CHRONIC SITTING ACTIVELY PROMOTES DOZENS OF CHRONIC DISEASES, INCLUDING OBESITY AND TYPE 2 DIABETES...EVEN IF YOU'RE VERY FIT AND EXERCISE REGULARLY!

SITTING IS AN INDEPENDENT RISK FACTOR FOR AN EARLY DEATH—WITH A MORTALITY RATE SIMILAR TO SMOKING.

MEN CAN REDUCE THEIR RISK OF OBESITY BY 59 PERCENT BY STANDING 12 HOURS PER DAY i.e. ½ of the day).

RESEARCH ALSO SHOWS YOUR RISK OF ANXIETY AND DEPRESSION RISES RIGHT ALONG (commensurate with) THE NUMBER OF HOURS SPENT IN YOUR CHAIR.

ONE HOUR OF EXERCISE CANNOT UNDO THE HARM CAUSED BY SITTING FOR 10 TO 12 HOURS PER DAY.

When you sit down—

YOUR METABOLISM PLUMMETS—YOUR BODY SHUTS DOWN—

YOUR BODY STARTS TO PREPARE FOR DEATH☺

BUT TAKE HEART!

Dr. EXERCISE PROVIDES YOU WITH BRILLIANT HEALTHCARE PRESCRIPTIONS— PROFESSIONAL ADVICE—AND HEALTH SOLUTIONS!

Here's what more published science says.

1. In a study published on March 31st, 2014, in the American Heart Association's Journal, "Circulation" researchers studied 82,000 men aged 45 to 69 for 10 years. The researchers found that the risk of heart failure was more than <u>DOUBLE</u> for men who sat at least 5 <u>HOURS</u> a day outside of work an didn't exercise compared with men who were physically active and sat for less than 2 <u>HOURS</u> a day.

   <u>N.B. "heart failure" is when the heart pump doesn't work properly but it does not mean that the heart stops beating)</u> (Source: http://www.usatoday.com)

2. In a study published in May 2010 in Journal of Medicine & Science in Sports & Exercise, the researchers found that men who were sedentary for more than <u>27 HOURS</u> a week had a <u>64 PERCENT GREATER RISK OF DYING FROM HEART DISEASE</u> than those who were sedentary less than 11 hours per week. (source: http;//journals.lww.com)

3. In a study of more than 17,000 Canadians published on May 4, 2009 found that the mortality risk from <u>ALL CAUSES</u> was 1.54 <u>TIMES HIGHER</u> among people who spent most of their day sitting compared to those who sat infrequently. (source Med. Sports Science Exercise)

4. In a <u>MEGA-STUDY</u> of more than 220,000 Australians aged 45 & up, published in the Arch. Of Internal Medicine on March 26th, 2012, researchers concluded that people who sat for more than <u>11 HOURS A DAY</u> had a <u>40 PERCENT GREATER CHANCE OF DYING</u>. (One could easily imagine 8 hrs desk, 1 hr commute, & 2 hrs evening computer/TV.

5. In a study published on July 9th, 2012 in Journal BMJ Open, researchers found that <u>REDUCING</u> the average time you spend sitting down to <u>LESS THAN 3 HOURS PER DAY</u> <u>COULD INCREASE</u> your life expectancy by 2 YEARS.

Here's what lead researcher Peter Katzmarzyk from Biomedical Research Centre in Baton Rouge, La. Said:

   "<u>The research elevates sedentary behavior as an important risk factor, similar to smoking and obesity</u>."...

Other studies have found our culture of sitting may be responsible for about 173,000 cases of cancer each year." (source :NBC Report http;//vitals.nbcnews.com)

(author underline-)

6. In a study published in the British Journal of Sports Medicine in October 2012, researchers studied 12,000 Australians and they concluded that EACH HOUR spent watching TV after the age of 25 reduces your life expectancy by 22 minutes. (Each cigarette reduces your life by 11 minutes). Adults who spend 6 HOURS in front of TV reduce their life expectancy by about 5 YEARS.

7. In a MEGA-STUDY of 794,577 participants published on August 19th, 2012, in journal Diabetologia; researchers concluded that those who sat the longest periods of time on a daily basis were TWICE AS LIKELY TO HAVE DIABETES OR HEART DISEASE. Moreover, these people had a 50 PERCENT INCREASE IN MORTALITY FROM ALL CAUSES.

8. In a study published in the online edition of Mayo Clinic Proceedings, in August 2014, researchers found that 6 HOURS OF UNINTERRUPTED SITTING WAS FOUND TO COUNTERACT THE POSITIVE HEALTH BENEFITS OF ONE HOUR OF EXERCISE! Researchers also scaled it down to say that 2 hours of sitting can nullify 20 minutes of daily exercise. ((source: PUBMED 25012770).

SITTING IS DEPRESSING AND WREAKS HAVOC ON YOUR MENTAL HEALTH.

9. A study of 9,000 women,(in their 50's) published in the Amer. J. Prev. Medicine in September 2013 found that those who sat for 7 HOURS per day-and who were physically inactive—were 3 times as likely to have symptoms of depression than individuals who sat for fewer than 4 hours per day. (source: PUBMED no 23953353) (*note: Depression saps people's energy and motivation to move; and sitting a lot just makes the depression worse.)

What about sitting and emotional health?

A handful of recent studies have looked at the damage caused by sitting to emotional health- or psychological STRESS.

10. In a study published in June 2013 (source: http://sciencedirect.com) researchers studied more than 3, 000 government workers in Australia. It was found that those who spent more than 6 hours of a typical workday sitting were likely to score in the moderate to high range on a test of psychological distress, than those who sat less than 3 hours.

AND— THIS WAS TRUE— NO MATTER HOW MUCH LEISURE EXERCISE TIME THEY GOT!

1. Another study published this year compared those who ex-
    ercise <u>often</u> and are <u>hardly sedentary</u> to those who <u>rarely ex-
    ercise</u> and are <u>very sedentary</u> i.e. spend many hours sitting
    have <u>8 TIMES INCREASED RISK OF DYING PREMATURELY</u>.

In sum-

Sitting is the new smoking. Sitting increases your risk of lung cancer by 50 Percent. Sitting is far more dangerous than second hand smoke. Sitting was found to increase your risk of death for virtually all health problems, from T2D and CVD to cancer and all cause mortality. Sitting for more than 8 hours per day was associated with a 90 Percent increased rate of Type 2 Diabetes. All cause mortality is also increased by 50 Percent. Chronic sitting has a mortality rate similar to smoking. The less you exercise the more pronounced the detrimental effects of sitting.

Those who sit the most have a <u>112 PERCENT INCREASED RELATIVE RISK</u> of diabetes and a <u>147 PERCENT INCREASED RELATIVE</u> of cardiovascular disease.

Our body is designed to move. When we don't move, our brain function shuts down. When you sit down there are shocking effects on our body. Electrical activity in our body drops; our metabolism shuts down; and <u>WE BURN ONLY ONE CALORIE PER MINUTE</u>.

After 24 hours of sitting our body's insulin loses 40 percent of its ability to push sugar into cells.

After 2 weeks of prolonged sitting our LDL cholesterol <u>INCREASES DRAMATICALLY</u>. Other important effects of sitting include:

- Fat burning enzymes begin to breakdown;

- Muscles begin to breakdown;

- blood and oxygen flow to the heart and brain is im-
  peded (caused by lack of physical movement);

- production of neurotransmitters produced
  by physical movement decreases;

After 3 hours of sitting our <u>ARTERIES CONSTRICT BY 50 PERCENT</u>.

When you've been sitting for a period of time and then stand up—a number of BENEFICIAL MOLECULAR CASCADES TAKE PLACE INSIDE OF YOUR BODY.

Within 90 SECONDS OF STANDING UP- the muscular and cellular systems that process blood sugar, triglycerides, and cholesterol that are mediated BY INSULIN-ARE ACTIVATED.

ALL OF THESE MOLECULAR EFFECTS ARE ACTIVATED SIMPLY BY CARRYING YOUR OWN BODY WEIGHT; i.e. BY OVERCOMING THE EFFECTS OF GRAVITY.

THESE CELLULAR MECHANISMS ARE ALSO RESPONSIBLE FOR PUSHING FUELS INTO YOUR CELLS.—AND IF DONE REGULARLY- WILL RADICALLY DECREASE YOUR RISK OF OBESITY AND TYPE 2 DIABETES.

Dr. EXERCISE HAS A SURPRISE FOR YOU!

GRAVITY IS YOUR FRIEND!

Dr. EXERCISE HAS TEAMED UP WITH Dr. EARTH!

In her book, "Sitting Kills, Moving Heals" Dr. Joan Vernikos, former director of NASA presents a scientific explanation for WHY SITTING has such a devastating effect on our health. For many years Dr. Vernikos' job was to work with the top astronauts to keep their bodies from deterioration due to the effects of flying in a rocket ship.

You might think that you are a gym rat who has a phenomenal exercise program. You might think that because you are an active lawyer/ desk professional—you have no reason to be concerned about SITTING.

THINK AGAIN!

What Dr. Vernikos tells us ABOUT THE EFFECTS OF GRAVITY IS ABSOLUTELY ASTONISHING!

STANDING UP IS EXERCISE!

STANDING IS MORE EFFECTIVE THAN WALKING!

AND EVERYONE KNOWS THAT "WALKING IS A SUPERFOOD!"

IT IS THE SHEER ACT OF STANDING UP—i.e. OVERCOMING GRAVITY BY CHANGING OUR POSTURE THAT PREVENTS MANY DISEASES!

STANDING UP FREQUENTLY IS THE MOST POWERFUL SIMPLE BENEFICIAL THING THAT YOU CAN DO FOR YOUR HEALTH!

AND IT'S FREE! -☺)

THIS FREE EXERCISE COULD BE MORE VALUABLE THAN A GYM MEMBERSHIP TO OLDER PEOPLE. When patients are confined to bed for long periods of time, bedsores are not the worst part of LYING DOWN.

THE WORST PART OF LYING DOWN IS THAT YOU ARE LOSING OUT ON THE BENEFITS PROVIDED BY GRAVITY.

YOU MUST TAKE ADVANTAGE OF DR. EARTH.

YOU MUST SIT OR LIE AS LITTLE AS POSSIBLE.

THE BEST THINGS IN LIFE REALLY ARE FREE!

DR. HAPPY, DR. SUNSHINE, DR. EARTH, DR. EXERCISE, DR. FRESH AIR, DR. SLEEP AND DR. CLEAN WATER ARE ALL FREE.

DR. KETOSIS WILL CHARGE YOU FOR HIS MEDICINE (FOOD)—BUT YOU HAVE TO EAT NO MATTER WHAT... MOREOVER— WHEN YOU EAT ACCORDING TO DR. KETO's PRESCRIPTION YOU WILL SAVE SOME MONEY!

AND BEST OF ALL- You can fire your doctor- and be your own doctor.

OUR CREATOR PROVIDED EVERY LIVING CREATURE ON THIS PLANET WITH MOTHER NATURE'S FARMACY.

OUR CREATOR PROVIDED US WITH FREE HEALTH CARE TO MAKE US HEALTHY AND HAPPY!

EVERYTHING HUMANS REQUIRE TO BE HEALTHY, PROSPEROUS AND HAPPY HAS BEEN PROVIDED BY OUR CREATOR.

HUMANS DO NOT NEED A "DOCTOR" TO PRESCRIBE PETROCHEMICAL POISONS.

WE HAVE BEEN PLACED ON THIS PLANET TO BE OUR OWN DOCTOR.

Your doctor does not know that he is killing himself by sitting on his chair! Big Pharma never taught your doctor anything about HEALTH. That's why doctors do not know their arse from their elbow.

As humans, we are designed to be in constant perpetual movement. Our modern lives, office work, and home environment make this is difficult.

PLEASE UNDERSTAND—ALL ACTIVITY AND HABITUAL DAILY MOVEMENT COUNTS— EVEN FIDGETING! - tell that one to your boss!..-☺

The bottom line-

DR. EARTH WAS CREATED TO HELP US GET AND REMAIN HEALTHY!

A BIG KEY IS— TO OVERCOME GRAVITY—

AS OFTEN AS POSSIBLE!

Even for bed-ridden patients, just the act of standing up frequently makes patients healthier. We all need to stand up as much as possible.

Dr. Vernikos says:

THE MOST IMPORTANT THING WE CAN DO IS TO OVERCOME THE EFFECTS OF GRAVITY. This is conclusively supported by the clinical studies.

HERE'S A GOLDEN HEALTH NUGGET— Dr. Vernikos states:

> **"The key to lifelong health is more than just traditional gym exercise once a day, three to five times a week, she says …the answer is to rediscover a lifestyle of constant natural low-intensity non-exercise movement that uses the gravity vector throughout the day.**

Even if people meet the current recommendations of 30 minutes of physical activity on most days each week there may be significant adverse metabolic and health effects from prolonged sitting—the activity that dominates most people's remaining 'non-exercise' waking hours.

This applies to people who spend long hours doing computer work; couch potatoes and inactive seniors too. When you make inactivity a way of life- the fundamental fueling systems in your body are switched off and your blood sugar levels, blood pressure, cholesterol and toxic build up all rise.

Last year a Swedish study concluded that those who live a generally active life have better heart health and live longer than those who remain sedentary for most of the day. This held true even for those who didn't engage in a regular exercise routine. If you're older you'd be wise to make a concerted effort to spend more time doing low-intensity, everyday activities—**ANYTHING- REALLY- TO CUT DOWN ON THE TIME YOU SPEND IN A SEATED POSITION.**

If you spend a lot of time sitting—YOU SHOULD REALIZE THAT THE ACT OF STANDING UP FROM YOUR CHAIR CAN BE A POWERFUL TOOL TO IMPROVE YOUR HEALTH.

IT IS THE CHANGE IN POSTURE THAT ACTS AGAINST GRAVITY THAT IS THE MOST POWERFUL IN TERMS OF HAVING A BENEFICIAL IMPACT ON YOUR HEALTH.

REGULARLY STANDING UP FROM A SEATED POSITION HAS BEEN FOUND TO BE MORE EFFECTIVE THAN WALKING!

IN AN "ANTI-GRAVITY" SITUATION YOUR BODY DETERIORATES AT A FAR MORE RAPID PACE; BECAUSE SITTING FOR AN EXTENDED PERIOD OF TIME SIMULATES A LOW-GRAVITY TYPE ENVIRONMENT FOR YOUR BODY.

ANY AND ALL ACTIVITIES SUCH AS HOUSECLEANING, ROLLING DOUGH, GARDENING, HANGING CLOTHES TO DRY, BENDING OVER TO TIE YOUR SHOES, OR SEARCHING FOR AN ITEM ON A HIGH SHELF... ALL OF THESE FALL WITHIN THE SPECTRUM OF MOVEMENTS YOU WOULD IDEALLY ENGAGE IN MORE OR LESS CONTINUOUSLY DURING DAILY LIFE FROM MORNING UNTIL NIGHT.

Dr. Vernikos calls all of these types of activities as 'G HABITS'. The reason why these kinds of activities are so critical for your health is that WHEN YOU MOVE YOU INCREASE THE FORCE OF GRAVITY ON YOUR BODY.

AN ANT-GRAVITY ENVIRONMENT SPEEDS UP CELLULAR DETERIORATION- SO- THE KEY IS TO DISENGAGE FROM THE GRAVITY VECTOR—THIS LOW ANTI-GRAVITY SITUATION AS MUCH AS POSSIBLE.

It turns out that the best technique is quite different from the common method of exercising in a gym once a day or several times a week; rather a multitude of frequent low intensity stimuli through-out the day, 365 days a year is the OPTIMAL APPROACH.

IN OTHER WORDS—

THE SECRET TO GOOD HEALTH ON EARTH THAT SPACE EXPLORATION REVEALED IS THE NEED FOR PERPETUAL MOTION!

THERE IS NOT A DRUG ON PLANET EARTH THAT CAN RIVAL OR COMPETE WITH DR. EXERCISE!

HERE ARE SOME PRACTICAL RECOMMENDATIONS:

- Ditch your traditional office desk and chair- BEFORE THEY KILL YOU!

- Consider replacing these killers with either a STAND-UP DESK (my personal favorite). You can start with a barstool or a highchair for brief rest periods. There are also treadmill desks which are available.

- Buy a timer and set it for 12-15 minutes. When it goes off you stand up for 90 seconds. (90 SECONDS IS THE MINIMUM TIME TO RE-START YOUR METABOLISM).

- ADOPT THE 35 STAND-UPS RULE— Stand-up (for 90 seconds) FOUR TIMES PER HOUR plus a 3 extra ones…

- Have one or more tables to place your water/coffee so that you are forced to get out of your chair.

- When talking on your phone, make it a point to stand while talking. You will find that you will be more relaxed and think better. (You will keep the blood flowing to your brain-☺)

- If you can change work places often; from office to conference rooms; take frequent breaks; research shows that 8 minute tasks give better results.

- Try to use walking meetings with clients; schedule short 30 MINUTE standing conferences; you may find that these are more productive because people will want to get moving…rather than slouch in a chair.

- If you are a hard-nosed litigation attorney—make it a point to get up on your hind legs AS OFTEN AS YOU CAN—to make sure the JUDGE is not falling asleep.

If the judge queries you—just reply that you were going to object to a question but that you changed your mind. You can say that you have leg cramps or that you have sore hips. Suggest frequent pee /coffee breaks to judges; sometimes they are reluctant to do this " proprio motu",

If you ask politely for a pee break often—you can justify it by saying that you have a weak bladder or drank too much coffee. (In practice, I found that most Judges are WAIT-ING and hoping that one of the attorneys ask…-☺)

Then too, some judges like to doze through long-winded testimony of expert witnesses…because they get bored-☺

In addition to the above recommendations, there is a <u>PLETHORA</u> of little movements that you can add and/or add to your daily office/home habits. These little movements appear small but together, they all add up.

I'm confident that you can find a boatload of ways to:

<u>STAND UP MORE FREQUENTLY; GET MORE LOW INTENSITY MOVEMENT AND GET MORE EXERCISE INTO YOUR LIFE.</u>

<u>NOTE BENE:</u>

<u>STANDING UP IN COURT OR IN YOUR OFFICE—</u>

<u>IS A RADICAL STRESS-BUSTER!</u>

You have likely discovered that being healthy helps if you remain relaxed, cool, calm and collected- in any situation. Attorneys and desk professionals are prone to <u>GREAT</u> amounts of <u>STRESS</u>. Anything that reduces your stress level will support your immune system.

<u>SITTING CAN BE VERY STRESSFUL FOR MODERN MAN.</u>

Sitting —for our ancestors was likely the exact opposite. Sitting in a tree after sprinting to escape being lunch for a tiger was likely calming …-☺

The Centre for Disease Control (CDC) says that <u>85 PERCENT OF ALL DISEASE IS CAUSED BY STRESS.</u>

<u>STRESS COMES IN (at least) TWO VARIETIES—GOOD AND BAD.</u>

<u>TOO MUCH BAD OR TOO MUCH GOOD STRESS IS UNHEALTHY.</u>

In my last chapter—"Think with Your Ketogenic Heart", Dr. Happy provides his best <u>"STRESS-BUSTING" TECHNIQUES AND RECOMMENDATIONS.</u>

<u>NUMBER ONE RECOMMENDATION IS:</u>

<u>DO EVERYTHING POSSIBLE TO ELIMINATE ALL STRESS AND THE VARIOUS STRESSORS IN YOUR LIFE.</u>

<u>DR. EXERCISE IS ONE OF THE BIGGEST STRESS BUSTERS OUT THERE!</u>

B.   HEALTH CARE SCREENING

We have examined the science behind the dangers of a sedentary lifestyle and especially the disease of sitting. Now we shall examine the good or beneficial side of an active lifestyle and THE AMAZING BENEFITS OF EXERCISE.

AS YOU PROBABLY KNOW- DR. EXERCISE HAS A BOATLOAD OF TRICKS UP HIS SLEEVE TO MAKE YOU STRONG AND HEALTHY-☺

You may be surprised to learn about some of the amazing benefits of exercise. You have likely heard of most of these. But—I am confident that you will be pleasantly surprised to learn about some of the recent discoveries about the amazing benefits of exercise- BOTH FOR OUR BODIES AND FOR OUR BRAINS!

Sooner—but more often later— most people come to realize that:

DR. EXERCISE IS GREAT MEDICINE.

DR. EXERCISE IS THE FOUNTAIN OF YOUTH!

Most people spend a lifetime trying to get wealthy. Then they take that money and try to get healthy. The red warning light goes on; then they learn that they need to take care of their body! The word exercise becomes synonymous with HEALTH AND WELL-BEING. Muscle/body building to look like Arnold Schwartznagger is not what motivates most people to start an exercise program.

In the USA—75 PERCENT OF THE POPULATION NEVER ENGAGE IN ANY VIGOROUS ACTIVITY LASTING MORE THAN 10 MINUTES PER WEEK!

There are two main types of exercisers. The first type is the VOLUNTARY exerciser. This group comprises the sports-minded competitive jocks (professionals and amateurs) that enjoy playing their favorite sport as long as they can. When an injury occurs, they often end up buying a rocking chair prematurely.

It is well known that professional athletes are not known for LONGEVITY. Our bodies are not totally bulletproof; they can withstand just so much HIGH-IMPACT AND STRESS.

The remaining part of the first type are the people that LOVE to exercise whether it be working out at the gym or simply walking, yoga, tai chi or other kinds of gentle exercise. These people enjoy exercise. They view exercise as an enjoyable activity. They like how it makes them feel —so they build it into their lives. This kind of exerciser explicitly or implicitly understands that exercise is therapeutic in nature. Exercise becomes medicine.

The SECOND kind of exercisers is the INVOLUNTARY exerciser. These are people who are badgered by friends, family (or possibly even a doctor-☺) to start an exercise program to lose some weight/ lower blood pressure etc. Sometimes people visit an honest health care provider who bluntly asks you—

> "What fits your busy schedule better—exercising one hour a day –OR BEING DEAD 24 HOURS A DAY! (Randy Glasbergen)

This quickly inspires FEAR! Given a choice between the treadmill at the local gym and the local funeral parlor most people choose the former...☺

NOW YOU KNOW ABOUT THE DANGERS OF YOUR KILLER CHAIR/COUCH.

YOU HAVE LEARNED ABOUT THE DANGERS OF CHRONIC SITTING.

Dr. Exercise provides you with a blueprint to deal with this challenging issue. I am sure that if you use your imagination- you can come up with some of your own strategies to combat sitting. Sitting behind a desk is such a huge part of the life of a desk professional.

So, if you are stuck at your desk for a while, shift positions frequently; get up and stretch in the middle of a thought; pace while on a phone call, or even fidget.

Take the stairs instead of the elevator. Park further away from your office. Just find a way to get more MOVEMENT, WALKING AND EXERCISE INTO YOUR LIFE.

YOU MUST EMPLOY YOUR OWN STRATEGIES TO STAND UP MORE OFTEN.

YOU MUST FIND ANY WAY YOU CAN TO MOVE AND WALK MORE OFTEN.

OVERCOMING THE EFFECTS OF GRAVITY IS ONE OF DR. EXERCISE'S BEST HEALTH CARE STRATEGIES-☺

OVERCOME GRAVITY FOR AT LEAST 90 SECONDS- AS OFTEN AS YOU CAN.

YOU WILL FEEL BETTER. YOUR ENERGY WILLS WILL SKYROCKET!

Your mood will be elevated- TOO! Your adrenal glands will not be exhausted. You may find that you even become more optimistic. Your productivity and professional skills will improve- that means that you will maximize your time spent as a desk professional.

If you are not interested to exercise for yourself...why not exercise for them?

How 'bout living long enough to enjoy playing with your grandchildren? Imagine being able to tell your grandchildren that you are <u>DRUG-FREE</u>! You must be role model for your grandkids. You must tell them " Just say "<u>NO TO DRUGS</u>!"

Imagine the look on their faces when you tell them Grandpa is his own doctor". You can play sports with them and teach your grandchildren the joys of being healthy, happy and <u>DRUG FREE</u>. If you are fat, sick and confined to a hospital; you will be sending the wrong message to them.

You must be the classic grandparent that existed 100 years ago. Grandparents used to know how to stay healthy and strong. Parents and grandparents knew that they needed to eat healthy food—to be <u>HEALTHY</u>.

100 years ago, people in Western society knew that they had to rely on themselves to heal themselves. Quack western doctors pushing pills were not an option.

<u>ARE YOU READY TO ADOPT DR. EXERCISE AS ONE OF YOUR DOCTORS</u>?

<u>YOU SHOULD NOT FEAR EXERCISE.</u>

Exercise is a critical part of an active lifestyle. You can do as little or as much as you like. You can choose to look at exercise as a chore. You can also choose to learn to <u>LOVE </u>exercise. Any exercise is good. Any exercise is better than none

<u>IT'S NEVER TOO LATE TO START AN EXERCISE PROGRAM</u>!

You can quietly rejoice knowing that by standing up 35 times a day and doing the everyday active things in life—<u>YOU ALREADY HAVE AN IMPORTANT</u> "<u>LEG UP</u>" on most people-☺)

<u>GETTING OFF OF YOUR CHAIR OR COUCH IS SIMPLE GOOD EXERCISE</u>!

<u>STANDING IS EXERCISE</u>!

The best exercise is the one that you like to do. Hey- even getting up from the couch during TV commercials is better than sitting!-☺

<u>DR. EXERCISE PROVIDES MORE THAN MEDICINE.</u>

DR. EXERCISE PROVIDES THE FOUNTAIN OF YOUTH!

BUT LIKE ANY "LEGITIMATE MEDICINE"-YOU NEED TO TAKE THE RIGHT KIND—AND THE PROPER DOSE.-☺)

YOU SHOULD NOT "OVER-EXERCISE" AND YOU SHOULD NOT DO THE WRONG KIND OF EXERCISE! SAFETY FIRST- ALWAYS!

YOU ARE FOREWARNED!

YOU CAN'T EXERCISE YOUR WAY OUT OF A CRAPPY DIET!

You should forget everything you thought you knew or heard about exercise.

MOST EXERCISE INFORMATION IN THE MEDIA IS ERRONEOUS.

FEW PEOPLE KNOW ABOUT EXERCISE OR WHAT KINDS OF EXERCISE ARE MOST BENEFICIAL.

Just because some doctor has given you the "OK" to exercise—

THIS DOES NOT MEAN THAT YOU ARE READY TO EXERCISE!

EXERCISE WILL TRANSFORM YOUR BODY AND YOUR LIFE.

What should be your next step?

YOUR NEXT STEP SHOULD BE TO GET AN APPROPRIATE FITNESS EVALUTATION.

In the fitness industry, we advise prospective exercisers "**TO GET**"**SCREENED" OR TESTED.** You should get tested or evaluated by an appropriate **FITNESS PROFESSIONAL.** "If you're not testing— you're only guessing".

The correct term for a fitness evaluation is called "**HEALTH CARE SCREENING.**"

Why perform Health Care Screening?

One size does not fit all. Everyone is an individual and has a unique body; with a unique medical and injury history. Almost everyone has some physical issues that limits and affect our ability to move safely and effectively.

How can you discover what physiological difficulties you might have which prevent you from **MOVING SAFELY AND EFFECTIVELY?**

How are you going to know which exercises are safe and beneficial for YOU- UNLESS YOU ARE EVALUATED (SCREENED)? Are you going to ask some petrochemical salesman?

PHYSICIANS KNOW NOTHING ABOUT MUSCLES, MUSCLE PHYSIOLOGY OR EXERCISE.

Your doctor likely learned anything he knows about muscles and exercise from the same fitness magazine as you.

Remember- your doctor does not know his arse from his elbow- literally-☺

Often new exercisers fall into the TRAP of listening to some conventionally trained doctor who gives them the "ok to exercise". Most incompetent doctors or other medical "professionals" are not QUALIFIED to prescribe exercises the "patient" should do-or refrain from doing.

YOUR DOCTOR IS NOT QUALIFIED TO PROVIDE ANY ADVICE REGARDING EXERCISE.

YOUR DOCTOR HAS NO TRAINING IN MUSCLES OR MUSCLE PHYSIOLOGY.

YOUR DOCTOR IS CLUELESS ABOUT WHICH EXERCISES ARE SAFE AND APPROPRIATE FOR YOU- NOR ANYONE ELSE.

YOUR DOCTOR IS CLUELESS ABOUT EXERCISE.

TAKING EXERCISE ADVICE FROM YOUR DOCTOR IS A PRESCRIPTION FOR INJURY OR POSSIBLY DEATH.

When it comes to EXERCISE ADVICE- don't listen to some self-proclaimed expert wearing a white, green or blue frock. For example- most cardiologists warn their by-pass survivors to avoid doing any strenuous exercise to improve their heart.

THIS IS "DEAD" WRONG!

Most cardiologists are clueless about exercise or how to train your cardiovascular system. Most cardiologists are clueless about how to make your heart healthy and strong. Cardiologists are pill pushers, and cutters that sell stents and other products to place into your body. Exercise is exactly what patients recovering from bypasses MOST need. Unfortunately, doctors do not learn about muscle physiology in medical school.

Most allopathic doctors tell their overweight clients to start losing weight by pounding a treadmill.

THIS ADVICE IS DEAD WRONG AGAIN!

Pounding a treadmill is the last thing that most overweight people should do. Most people desirous to lose a few pounds should first address their nutritional intake. You can't exercise your way out of a crappy diet.

Also, most overweight desk professionals that are overweight are usually STRESSED OUT OF THEIR MINDS! Exercise can be stressful too.

A radical change in dietary habits IS VERY STRESSFUL TO YOUR BODY! That's why I recommend that when you adopt a Ketogenic Diet- you should wait at least TWO TO THREE WEEKS before starting a vigorous exercise program. You must give your body a chance to adapt to an entirely new nutritional program. Your body needs time to build new metabolic pathways.

Dr. Exercise and Dr. Keto work together to help you build a new metabolism- beginning at the cellular level. Both of these "doctors" understand the importance of building strong MITOCHONDRIA.

THESE "SUPERDOCTORS" BUILD SUPER BODIES AND SUPERHEALTH!

AS A GENERAL RULE—BE VERY SKEPTICAL ABOUT ANY ADVICE THAT YOU RECEIVE FROM ANY WHITE-COATED INDIVIDUAL—BECAUSE—

NINETY-NINE PERCENT (99) OF THE TIME THIS "UNEDUCATED ADVICE" IS SIMPLY WRONG!

IF YOU FOLLOW YOUR OWN COMMON SENSE AND DISREGARD THE EXERCISE ADVICE RECOMMENDED BY IGNORANT DOCTORS—

99 PERCENT OF THE TIME YOU WILL BE RIGHT!

You must think for yourself; use your judgment and your God-given common sense. Do your own due diligence in ALL HEALTH MATTERS! This is especially important when it comes to risking your life by doing some dangerous exercise.

Using treadmills and any other MACHINES FOUND IN GYMS CAN BE VERY DANGEROUS! Doctors will unknowingly advise you to add strength or fitness to a dysfunctional platform. Don't be suckered by your doctor. Doing exercises beyond your physical capacity or beyond your physical capacity is A PRESCRIPTION FOR INJURY!

Orthopedic surgeons also know very little about <u>muscles or</u> exercise. Most surgeons are butchers who make money by slicing off pieces of flesh/tissue and body parts.

These people are trained to cut off body parts for money. Your local meat market guy likely knows more than your orthopedic surgeon about muscles and how they work. Your butcher knows his muscle physiology better than most surgeons.

The average person has great reverence for someone with the letters M.D after their name. Just remember- these letters allegedly stand for "medical doctor",—BUT in real life better acronym for M.D. is "More Dinero"-☺

With that in mind- you should ignore the following insane advice:

"Consult your physician before doing any exercise."

This terrible advice was invented by the Medical Profession and/or Big Pharma to protect their monopoly...<u>AND TO SCARE THE "BEE-GEEBERS" OUT OF YOU!</u>- ☺

<u>FEAR IS A VERY POWERFUL MOTIVATOR!</u>

Most allopathic doctors are experts when it comes to scaring patients.

<u>ALLOPATHIC DOCTORS ARE "THE BIGGEST FEAR-MONGERS" IN THE WORLD!</u>

Are you going to let some pill pusher scare you into exercise that is unsafe and/or too difficult for you? When you are injured by exercise, your doctor will be able to sell you a boatload of NSAID's or other opiates/pain-killers.

Are you going to let some pill pusher scare you into taking some petrochemical product to help you get healthy? You know more about what is best for your health and well- being.

Do you believe an allopathic physician knows anything about body mechanics? Do you believe that your doctor knows anything about kinesiology? Is your doctor a certified personal trainer? Is your doctor qualified as a strength or sports coach?

Does your doctor know anything about Sports Medicine?

The only exercise your doctor probably gets is when he scribbles an illegible note on a prescription pad. Your doctor gets his information about drugs from drug salesmen.

YOUR DOCTOR RECEIVES MISINFORMATION ABOUT EXERCISE FROM TELEVISION AND MAINSTREAM NEWS.

YOU ARE FOOLISH IF YOU FOLLOW EXERCISE ADVICE FROM YOUR DOCTOR.

The cold hard <u>truth</u> is that your doctor (surgeon, cardiologist or other doctor) knows 'squat' about "<u>SQUAT</u>" (pun intended)! As previously mentioned that your doctor has no education about nutrition. Unfortunately your doctor knows <u>even less</u> about exercise.

MOST ALLOPATHIC DOCTORS ARE ARROGANT FEAR-MONGERS.

DOCTORS SCARE PATIENTS INTO BUYING TOXIC CHEMICALS THAT ARE CALLED 'MEDICATIONS".

Your doctor is a very frightening person. Your doctor makes money by <u>FRIGHTENING </u>people into buying <u>POISONOUS CHEMICAL PILLS</u>.

YOUR DOCTOR'S FAVOURITE SURGERY IS VACCINES.

WE MUST PUT AN END TO THE BARBARIC PRACTICE OF VACCINE SURGERY.

VACCINE SURGEONS SHOULD BE PROSECUTED FOR CRIMES AGAINST HUMANITY.

You can do yourself a big favour and fire your doctor. You can spread the message across the Internet. Let's help people get healthy by convincing them to sack their <u>FEAR-MONGERING PILL-PUSHER</u>.

Often a doctor "prescribes" exercise to a client to whom he has also prescribed a statin drug- such as Lipitor. Most allopathic doctors do not warn their patients about <u>THE DANGERS OF THIS DEADLY COMBO OF DRUGS AND EXERCISE.</u>

EXERCISE AND DRUGS DO NOT MIX!

MIXING STATING DRUGS WITH EXERCISE IS A PRESCRIPTION FOR DEATH BY KIDNEY FAILURE!

Mixing statin drugs and exercise will often cause "Rhabdomyolsis". This is a deadly condition whereby your kidneys are destroyed by an overload of toxic chemicals and dump your bodily fluids into your bloodstream-followed by an agonizing death.

Chances are that your doctor has never even stepped foot in a gym! You may notice that his/her belly is bigger than yours. Oops—another reason to fire your doctor-☺

Your doctor has no knowledge to make an <u>EXERCISE/ FITNESS EVALUATION OF ANY KIND</u>. You can take your own blood pressure. Your mirror can tell you more about your body than a visit to your doctor. You don't need to listen to some chowder- headed pill pusher who has been brainwashed by Big Pharma. Big Pharma sucks bazillions of dollars out of unsuspecting naïve medical students.

How smart is it to take medical advice from a doctor who'll commit suicide at the age of 56?

<u>BEFORE HITTING THE GYM OR THE WEIGHTS- YOU SHOULD OBTAIN AN APPROPRIATE FITNESS EVALUATION FROM AN APPROPRIATE KNOWLEDGEABLE FITNESS PROFESIONAL.</u>

<u>YOU SHOULD NEVER ASSUME BECAUSE YOUR DOCTOR GIVES YOU THE OK TO EXERCISE THAT IT'S SAFE FOR YOU TO START AN EXERCISE PROGRAM.</u>

Your personal trainer/or coach could be right around the corner at your local gym.

There are <u>MANY</u> kinds of fitness evaluations in the marketplace.

<u>IN MY HUMBLE OPINION -THE MERCEDES OF FITNESS EVALUATIONS IS</u>:

> <u>"FUNCTION MOVEMENT SCREENING" OR "FMS"- for short.</u>

You can search the website at www.functionalmovement.com FMS is the brainchild of Mr. Gray Cook. There are <u>TWO PARTS</u> to this Healthcare Screening.

The first part is FMS for Fitness professionals. You can go on-line and locate a Fitness Professional in your part of the World. This individual who is a <u>CERTIFIED FMS SPECIALIST</u> will perform 7 fitness Tests or "Evaluations" which comprise the FMS evaluation or FMS "Screen". The results of this evaluation will then identify your "<u>WEAKEST LINKS</u>."

The FMS generates the Functional Movement Score, which is used to target existing movement problems and track progress. Should <u>PAIN</u> be identified by <u>ANY</u> of these 7 tests, you will then be referred to a <u>CLINICIAN</u> who will address your <u>PAIN</u>. The pain specialist/clinician is known as an" SFMA" specialist. This is a clinician trained in the "Selectional Functional Movement Assessment" which is the <u>SECOND PART</u> of the functional movement paradigm. <u>A CERTIFIED SFMA</u> clinician then uses corrective exercises to address your pain.

If <u>NO PAIN</u> is identified during the FMS evaluation; you will be provided with an exercise program. This program provides specific exercises to address your weakest mobility/stability issues. You are given corrective exercises (often by a computerized program) to address your weakest links.

Experience shows that the best indicators of future injuries are past injuries. The FMS is able to" flush out" and identify and correct weak or bad movement patterns <u>BEFORE INJURY</u>. It is preventative in nature.

<u>FMS is used by serious athletes and serious exercisers— WORLDWIDE.</u>

<u>IT IS SIMPLY THE BEST—PERIOD.</u>

<u>YOU ARE STRONGLY RECOMMENDED TO CHECK OUT FMS BEFORE YOU DO ANY EXERCISE!</u>

<u>RESEARCH SHOWS THAT 20 PERCENT OF ALL PEOPLE –YOUNG AND OLD- ATHLETES AND NON-ATHLETES SCREENED BY FMS WILL BE IDENTIFIED WITH PAIN—</u>

<u>AFTER THEY HAVE BEEN CLEARED FOR EXERCISE BY A PHYSICIAN!</u>

OMG! How amazing is that?

<u>FMS IDENTIFIES UNDIAGNOSED PAIN IN 20 PERCENT OF PEOPLE WHO HAVE BEEN TOLD BY THEIR DOCTORS THAT THESE SAME "EXAMINED" PATIENTS ARE SAFE TO DO EXERCISE!</u>

OMG!

<u>YOUR DOCTOR CANNOT EVEN DIAGNOSE PAIN!</u>

<u>YOUR DOCTOR FAILS TO DIAGNOSE PAIN IN ONE OUT OF FIVE PATIENTS!</u>

Can there be a better reason to fire your doctor!

<u>Bottom line:</u>

If you are serious about injury prevention and you want to identify <u>YOUR WEAKEST LINKS IN YOUR BODY—</u>

<u>FMS evaluation/protocol is the best way to do it- PERIOD.</u>

<u>Once your movement patterns are corrected TO A SAFE LEVEL—YOU CAN PROGRESS TO AN APPROPRIATE STRENGTH AND CONDITIONING PROGRAM.</u>

FMS IS FOR PEOPLE WHO DESIRE TO PREVENT INJURY FIRST- AND TO PROCEED TO PERFORMANCE SECOND. Don't add strength and/or fitness to a dysfunctional platform! That's what most chowder-headed doctors recommend! When you take advice from a doctor about which exercises are appropriate for you—that's the equivalent of putting a list of exercises on a dartboard and choosing exercises by throwing darts!

TO BE STRONG AND MOVE WELL— GET FMS'd.

IT'S THE BEST HEALTH-CARE SCREENING TOOL IN THE WORLD.

WHETHER OR NOT YOU DECIDE TO EXERCISE-

THIS ASSESSMENT WILL TELL YOU MORE ABOUT YOUR BODY'S MECHANICS AND INJURY POTENTIAL THAN ANY OTHER TEST OUT THERE!

YOU MAY BE ONE IN FIVE PEOPLE WHO ARE WALKING AROUND WITH UNIDENTIFIED PAIN!

ARE YOU INJURED AND DO NOT KNOW IT YET?

FMS will provide you with the fitness evaluation you **NEED TO BE ABLE TO GET OUT OF BED AND WALK SAFELY.**

YOUR FIRST GOAL IS TO PREVENT INJURY.

YOUR SECOND GOAL IS PERFORMANCE.

YOUR FIRST STEP ONCE YOU HAVE MADE THAT CRITICAL DECISION TO START AN EXERCISE PROGRAM IS TO -Fire Your Doctor and Get FMS Screened).

Congrats on your decision!

C. TRADITIONAL CARDIO IS A LIE

"Continuous aerobic work is basically exercise- induced castration."

Coach Charles Poliquin

"If your personal trainer uses the word "cardio"—change trainers"

– Gary W. Pitts

What is aerobic training?

Aerobic training is low to moderate intensity exercise where your heart rate is maintained throughout the duration of the workout. More than likely it is what most people are doing on the exercise machines at your local gym. It is considered aerobic because your body is utilizing oxygen throughout the workout because of the LOW INTENSITY AND THE DURATION – GREATER THAN 2 MINUTES.

Aerobic training has more NEGATIVE effects than positive effects. Just look at all of the people on the "cardio machines- e.g. treadmills, elliptical and stationary bikes at your local gym. How many of them do the same routine, year after year? Other than when they first started to exercise, they will see very few changes to their physiques. They often sweat a lot and then go to the local hamburger joint to celebrate how many calories they have supposedly burned. In all likelihood they get fatter over time.

What about those exercisers who run in races from 5 K's to full marathon races? Have you ever closely examined their bodies? Most have one foot in the grave. Check out the number of runners who literally die in races. It turns out that most runners cause themselves heart problems- especially in the right ventricle.

On the other hand, look at gymnasts and sprinters. Gymnasts never do aerobics. Like sprinters- they do high-intensity burst training. Sprinters have less body fat than marathoners. Marathoners do an insane amount of running.

Which kind of body would you rather have? Do you want a gaunt thin weak marathoner's body? Would you rather be lean- muscled and powerful like a sprinter or gymnast?

"Cardio" is short for cardiovascular endurance training. It's the idea that you have to raise your heart rate for a long duration—at least 20 minutes, and usually much more. It's when you spend 45 minutes pounding a treadmill, or run or bike miles every day— or take an hour -long aerobics class.

CARDIO DOES NOT MEAN going for a brisk walk, or spending a few minutes on a treadmill or bike.

TRADITIONAL CARDIO IS A LIE.

It is a dangerous lie that will ruin your health in the long term. You should become anti-cardio. The concept of cardiovascular endurance exercise-like marathon running or aerobics goes against our entire body's design. Humans were designed to move often in short bursts.

As we have seen in the preceding section; our bodies are designed to AVOID SITTING!

Our ancestors didn't jog for miles at a time. They didn't jump around in an aerobics class wearing spandex pants sucking cool-aid through a straw- ☺)They had to move- OFTEN AND OFTEN VERY FAST. THEY HAD TO SPRINT TO CATCH FOOD- OR BEING EATEN AS FOOD-☺ That's how our human ancestors were able to stay lean and strong.

Jogging is an activity which was invented by the manufacturers of running shoes. Our ancestors did not need SUPER-PADDED -CUSHIONED, ULTRA- PADDED PIECES OF RUBBER on the bottom of their feet.

Do you really think that it is healthy to pound your joints by spending hours doing "cardio" on treadmills and other man-made machines? Cardio can damage joints (excessive pounding); alter your posture and negatively affect your body composition.

Treadmills may be more dangerous than cars. Even brakes in cars are safer than brakes on many treadmills. On some of these machines— YOU are the brake! That's one BIG PROBLEM WITH MOST KINDS OF MACHINES that you will find in gyms. Machines in gyms are like allopathic doctors.

Often they both can hurt you— if you are not careful...-☺ At least machines are not arrogant or priest-like...

You should not follow some of the modern fitness advice from "experts" who tell you to do cardio so that you can get into the "fat-melting zone."

THE TRUTH IS: TRADITIONAL CARDIO MAKES YOU FAT, OLD AND UGLY!-☺

CARDIO ACTUALLY MAKES YOUR BODY STORE FAT! YUK-☹ (I'll bet your doctor doesn't know that-☺ In medical school, your doctor was not taught about traditional cardio, aerobic OR anaerobic EXERCISE. Your doctor was never introduced to Dr. Exercise-☺ You doctor was only taught drugs and how to use a scalpel to slice off tissue.

Cardio drains your body of energy. It wears you out. When people stop doing it- they often have more energy and they feel better. LISTEN TO YOUR BODY!

CARDIO BURNS MUSCLE- NOT FAT!

Cardio trashes your immune system; it wears out your joints. It causes inflammation. It shrinks your lungs. It reduces your heart's pumping ability.

Here are 6 reasons to ditch traditional cardio that is bad for your health.

SIX REASONS TO DITCH CARDIO

1. Aerobic Training increases STRESS and raises CORTISOL.

Aerobic training increases adrenal STRESS which will likely make you fatter. According to Dr. James Wilson, author of Adrenal Fatigue-The 21st Century Stress Syndrome,) "normally functioning adrenal glands secrete minute, yet precise and balanced, amounts of steroid hormones".

When one does too much continuous aerobic exercise, the adrenal glands are stressed in a way that can upset this delicate balance which could lead to adrenal fatigue. Adrenal fatigue s associated with such symptoms as tiredness, fearfulness, allergies, frequent influenza, arthritis, anxiety, depression, reduced memory, and difficulties in concentrating, insomnia, feeling worn-out, and most importantly- the INABILITY TO LOSE WEIGHT despite extensive efforts.

Aerobic training raises CORTISOL levels and accelerates aging. Cortisol is one of "fight or flight" stress hormones. If your cortisol levels are chronically elevated, your body WILL STORE FAT instead of burning it. High cortisol also leads to VISCERAL BELLY FAT GAIN.

If your cortisol levels are chronically elevated, your body will store fat instead of burning it. High cortisol levels also leads to more visceral fat gain. This increases fat accumulation and inflammation.

High cortisol also makes you age faster because it increases oxidative substances in the body that produce inflammation all over. This includes the brain, heart, gastrointestinal tract and reproductive organs. It is common knowledge that exercise raises cortisol because exercise stresses the body, which for strength training is a good thing, because it forces the body to adapt and to grow and get stronger.

But with strength training, cortisol increases BUT so do anabolic hormones that build muscle that overrides any negative effects of increased cortisol.

Aerobic training, in contrast, stresses the body without the boosting anabolic hormones, which results in an overall, catabolic, inflammatory response in the body.

Research has shown evidence of long-term high cortisol levels in aerobic endurance athletes. These high cortisol levels suggest that repeated physical stress of intensive training and competitive races among endurance athletes is associated with elevated cortisol exposure over prolonged periods of time.

Chronic high levels of cortisol put the body at a greater risk for a host of psychiatric problems, including depression, anxiety, or worse. Studies show that people who suffer from personality and mood disorders have abnormally high cortisol levels.

HIGH CORTISOL PRODUCES INSULIN RE-
SISTANCE—DIABETES FOLLOWS.

What is Visceral Fat?

Visceral fat sits deep behind the abdominal wall and surrounds the organs within the peritoneal cavity. Visceral fat is a very dangerous type of fat. It negatively affects health by increasing inflammation in the organs. It releases substances called adipokines, which are cell-to-cell signalling proteins that increase blood pressure and interfere with insulin health. Adipokines are released by visceral fat. They include IL-6 and TNF-a, which raise blood pressure, decrease insulin sensitivity and cause inflammation. Fat builds fat especially visceral fat; visceral fat causes catabolic degrading of muscle, which leads to more fat. YUK!

Visceral fat also decreases the amount of ADIPONECTIN in the body. "Adiponectin" is an essential fat-burning hormone that helps speed up metabolism that means that there are more triglycerides getting into the bloodstream. The combination of decreased insulin sensitivity, hypertension, and elevated triglycerides often results in atherosclerosis, higher LDL levels- which can lead to diabetes.

Adiponectin is secreted from adipose or subcutaneous fat and it helps with glucose uptake and insulin sensitivity. It has anti-inflammatory effects that support healthy blood pressure and heart function. Diabetics and obese people have lower levels of adiponectin, which means that THE MORE FAT THAT YOU HAVE—THE MORE FAT THAT YOU WILL HAVE! YUK! MORE FAT!

More visceral fat leads to LOWER TESTOSTERONE levels in men. Studies have found a link between greater visceral fat and lower total and free testosterone, and lower sex-hormone-binding-globulin, (SHBG). Also, insulin levels and C-peptide levels that are elevated usually means a "pre-diabetic" state. Again, lower testosterone in men leads to diabetes, muscle mass loss, less bone mineral density. Men tend to have more visceral fat than women.

What is subcutaneous fat?

This is the fat that is just under the outermost layer of skin. This is the fat you can pinch with your fingers—without using skin calipers. Women tend to have more jiggly subcutaneous fat than men. When women reach menopause, however, they start to develop more visceral fat due to lower estrogen levels.

Your thumb and forefinger will tell you how much subcutaneous fat you have. This is the fat covering that covers your abdominal muscles (ABS). In order to get a "6 pack-abs" you need to eliminate/reduce this fat so that your rectus abdominus is visible.

Sidebar-

What is the best exercise for getting 6 Pack ABS?

The best exercise for building a 6- pack ABS is called a "Table Push-away"-☺

The fastest way to get a 6 pack is to take the 6 pack out of your fridge=☺)

2. **Aerobic training increases oxidative stress which can accelerate aging.**

It is well established that aerobic exercise causes OXIDATIVE STRESS. This was evidenced in a study in June 1997 in the Journal of Sports Science. It was found that strenuous aerobic exercise causes oxidative stress which can overwhelm antioxidants.

According to Endocrinologist Dr. Diana Schwartzbein, (author of The Schwartzbein Principle) "oxidation" is a process that forms free radicals in the body. Normally the body can neutralize free radicals with substances known as antioxidants. It is only when there is an excessive build-up of free radicals that the body cannot neutralize all of the free radicals. This leads to changes in your metabolism which accelerates aging.

There is widespread evidence and accepted evidence of chronic inflammation from aerobic exercise as seen from increase in free radicals, damage to lipids and DNA, and decreased measurements of antioxidant such as glutathione.

GLUTATHIONE HAS BEEN CALLED THE "MASTER ANTIOXIDANT".

Studies have shown that marathon runners had inflammatory markers TWICE AS HIGH AS SPRINTERS. The cells of the marathoners were overwhelmed by the need to detox cells which caused chronic oxidative stress.

3. Long- term aerobic exercise compromises the immune system

There is lots of evidence that aerobic endurance athletes suffer more frequent and greater upper respiratory problems. Aerobic training leads to immune system suppression. Endurance athletes are at greater risk of infections. Evidence shows that aerobic work plateaus after 8 weeks. Moreover, power actually starts to diminish. Lower body aerobic work weakens your vertical jumps. Upper body aerobic work weakens your medicine ball throws. Etc.

The worst kind of aerobic exercise that leads to the worst immune dysfunction is when the exercise session is long (e.g. 90 minutes). Overreaching or intensified aerobic training leads to greater risk of illness and disease.

4. Aerobic training negatively affects testosterone/reproductive system

Aerobic training has been shown to increase cortisol levels and decrease testosterone levels in rats. In a study reported in April 2004, in the Canadian Journal of Applied Physiology, rats doing intensive aerobic swimming suffered oxidative stress. This stress caused numerous reproductive problems- such as decreased reproductive size and function... hmm...

Gentlemen—do you really want a smaller p*** and accessory reproductive organs? Do you really need THAT increased STRESS? -☺

Cardio can be used for short intervals- such as to rehab from car accidents etc. but then is best used for only a few weeks or so. It can be used as a bridge from rehab to full mobility exercise.

5. Aerobic training, low-intensity cardio will make your heart and lungs smaller!

When you exercise for long periods at a low to medium intensity, you train your heart and lungs to get <u>SMALLER</u>! If you only exercise within your current aerobic limits, you don't improve your aerobic capacity. This kind of exercise produces smaller muscles a smaller heart and smaller lungs. What's even worse- it wipes out your reserve capacity. Your reserve capacity is what your heart and your lungs use to deal with stress. Injuries or physical trauma, a shocking emotional blow, a particularly intense session in the bedroom with your partner...-☺- these all demand reserve energy. Reserve capacity means that your heart has the ability to pump out more oxygen- faster in times of physical STRESS. Without reserve capacity, you are much more likely to drop dead from a heart attack or pneumonia when faced with stress.

HIIT builds up reserve capacity for your lungs and ramps up oxygen delivery to your cells.

6. <u>HERE ARE TWO TYPES OF EXERCISE THAT ARE SUPERIOR TO CARDIO.</u>

   <u>These 2 TYPES ARE:</u>

   1. HIIT or High-Intensity Interval Training

   2. RESISTANCE aka STRENGTH Training.

Here's a summary of traditional cardio:

- Requires a lot of time, 20 to 60 minutes need- ed to burn calories for fat loss;

- Will not build muscular or bone strength, in fact can cause loss of both;

- Increases inflammation- may further complicate condi- tions associated with chronic inflammatory disease;

- Only improves one cardiovascular system (aerobic), both aerobic and anaerobic are needed for health;

- Overproduces free radicals causing stress on the immune system;

As to Hormones-

- Glucagon is lowered; HGH (Human Growth Hormone is lowered);

- Cortisol is increased;

- Insulin is increased

- Leptin is increased

D.   (HIIT) TRAINING

Now you know about the negative effects of continuous aerobic exercise. I like to call this LSD- like the drug or "Long slow distance"-☺

Does this mean that you have been LIED TO in the last 20 years? Yes!

Traditional Cardio is a big fat lie …a myth that has been propagated to sell treadmills and aerobic machines.

THE WHOLE AEROBIC CRAZE IS ANOTHER HUGE SCAM!

Long aerobic training is popular because it is SO EASY TO IMPLEMENT.

THE MEDIA HAS GLORIFIED IT.

THE CARDIO CRAZE SELLS GYM MEMBERSHIPS TOO!

Many people been suckered by celebrity stars who used some fantastic aerobic program to lose weight and get in shape. In reality, if most of these fake exercise types out there ever did any REAL exercise- they would likely vomit.

Getting as six-pack is about 80 percent diet and only about 20 percent Exercise.

INTERVAL   TRAINING   IS   HARD.   INTERVAL   TRAINING IS UNCOMFORTABLE.

HIGH-INTENSITY INTERVAL TRAINING (HIIT) IS FAR SUPERIOR!

HEY—IF HIIT training were easy—everyone would be doing it!

Our ancestral roots prove that our bodies are designed and programmed to thrive on HIGH-INTENSITY INTERVAL TRAINING. The acronym is HIIT. Sometimes this is shortened to HIT. We are designed and programmed to do burst training. Very quick sprints were necessary to escape predators…but nowadays you don't find too many tigers around…

The human body evolved performing very high-intensity activities for brief periods of time; and this kind of activity appears to be part and parcel of our GENOME. Today, when re-creating this kind of ancestral activity, you have plenty of options.

In evolutionary terms, HIIT is like being on a hunt an intermittently-SPRINTING FOR YOUR LIFE FOR A SHORT SPAN OF TIME.

In evolutionary terms, our ancestors needed to be strong. To carry an animal that weighed 1.5 times more than your body weight- you needed to be able to deep squat to safely lift that amount to carry it... if need be.

INTERVAL TRAINING DEVELOPS AEROBIC CAPACITY BETTER THAN AEROBIC TRAINING.

THE QUICKEST WAY TO VO2 MAX—THE ACCEPTED STANDARD MEASURE OF AEROBIC FITNESS —IS THROUGH INTERVAL TRAINING.

Another principal benefit of Interval Training is in regards to BODY COMPOSITION. Interval training causes positive changes in the body. Sprinters have leaner bodies with less body fat; their bodies are more aesthetically pleasing too-☺ Most people who engage in interval sports usually have a stronger more athletic body.

People who do LSD or steady-state aerobics are not as attractive and often look sickly and pale. Look at your average skinny marathon runner- or endurance athlete.

WHY WOULD ANYONE DO AEROBIC TRAINING?

Who knows? It does produce "a runner's HIGH—but unfortunately wrecks your metabolism, your joints...and your heart!

What is HIIT?

IT IS SHORT HIGH-INTENSITY BURST TRAINING- WITH SHORT INTERVALS.

TWO IMPORTANT FACTORS ABOUT FITNESS TRAINING ARE:

1. HIGH-INTENSITY

2. DURATION.

The higher the level of INTENSITY that you do during HIIT, the MORE EFFECTIVE that it will be. Also, the DURATION of this high intensity can be increased as you progress.

BIG SURPRISE! If you go to your local gym and do the opposite exercises from what everyone is doing—you will probably be correct.

YOU ONLY NEED 12 MINUTES OF EXERCISE PER WEEK TO BECOME A SUPERB ATHLETE!

FOUR- MINUTE WORKOUTS- 3 TIMES PER WEEK ARE ALL YOU NEED TO BE STRONG AND HEALTHY! ... Sounds like an infomercial...☺

YES- IT'S ABSOLUTELY TRUE!

There are several ways to do HIIT in the 12 minutes per week. My personal favorite HIIT program is called <u>TABATA.</u> Just Google it up!

The Tabata protocol study works like this. Dr. Izumi Tabata compared moderate intensity endurance training; (at about 70 percent of VO2 Max), with high-intensity intervals done at 170 PERCENT VO2 max.

Dr. Tabata used a unique <u>TRAINING PROTOCOL OF TWENTY (20) SECONDS WORK to 10 SECONDS REST.</u> He did <u>7 or 8 INTERVALS</u>-OR BOUTS OR BURSTS OF TRAINING.

<u>TOTAL AMOUNT OF EXERCISE- 140 to 160 SECONDS!</u>

<u>THE RESULTS OF TABATA WERE NOTHING SHORT OF AMAZING!</u>

The 20/10 <u>PROTOCOL</u> improved the VO2 Max and <u>ANAEROBIC CAPABILITIES MORE THAN THE STEADY-STATE PROGRAM.</u>

We have two major energy systems is our bodies. There is our aerobic system and our anaerobic system. For example, if you sprint for 30 seconds. you are using your anaerobic system. If you go for a walk or slow jog you use mostly your aerobic system. The beauty of HIIT, or burst training is that it <u>TRAINS BOTH AEROBIC AND ANAEROBIC SYSTEMS AT THE SAME TIME!</u>

<u>THERE ARE DOZENS OF STUDIES THAT PROVE THE SUPERIOR BENEFITS OF HIIT TRAINING.</u>

Canadian researcher and sport scientist Martin Gibala, Professor of Kinesiology at McMaster University published a study in the Journal Physiology. The study was conducted over a two-week period. The study compared a 20 minute interval program versus a steady-state aerobic program (ranging from 90 to 120 minutes).What was the result?

The 20 minute program <u>COMPRISED ONLY TWO MINUTES AND THIRTY SECONDS OF ACTUAL EXERCISE (WORK) BUT SHOWED THE SAME IMPROVEMENT IN OXYGEN UTILIZATION AS THE STEADY-STATE GROUP.</u>

Each group exercised <u>3 TIMES PER WEEK.</u>

The interval group exercised for a <u>TOTAL ELAPSED TIME OF ONE HOUR PER WEEK- BUT WITH ONLY 6 TO 7.5 MINUTES OF INTENSE EXERCISE DURING THAT HOUR.</u>

The steady-state group exercised <u>BETWEEN 4.5 AND 6 HOURS EACH WEEK- BUT THE AEROBIC BENEFITS WERE THE SAME!</u>

Would you rather do 2.5 minutes a day of exercise for 3 days a week? Or would your prefer to do 5 or 6 hours of weekly exercise for the same result? That's kind of a no-brainer-☺

There are studies which show that if you do HIIT training of 3 times a week for 4 minutes per session- for a total exercise time of 12 minutes each week – and you do that HIIT for 12 weeks-YOU WILL DOUBLE YOUR CARDIOVASCULAR CAPACITY!

OMG!

YOU CAN DOUBLE YOUR CARDIOVASCULAR WITH 144 MINUTES OF EXERCISE!

One HIIT study showed that 3 minutes of HIIT per week for 4 weeks IMPROVED INSULIN SENSITIVITY BY 24 PERCENT! HIIT increases HGH (the "Fitness the

It was reported at the Canadian Cardiovascular Congress in 2010 in Montreal that regular exercise reduces cardiovascular heart disease risk by a factor of 3- BUT extended vigorous exercise performed during a marathon raises your cardiac risk SEVEN FOLD!

HIIT has been proven to produce greater health benefits than conventional aerobic training—such as increased insulin sensitivity, and glucose-tolerance, both of which are critical components of optimal health .

HIIT increases the insulin sensitivity of your muscles thereby decreasing your fasting insulin and helps you lose weight.

30 Seconds is all it takes!

Researchers at Karolinska Institute in Sweden recently investigated what happens in muscle cells during bouts of short, high-intensity exercise. They had 30 subjects perform 30 seconds of maximum effort exertion cycling followed by a brief period of rest. The subjects repeated this 6 TIMES; and had their muscle tissue examined for the effects.

The results were astounding...!

A mere 6 short bursts of exercise followed by rest were enough TO TRIGGER A NOTICEABLE GENERATION OF HEALTHY NEW MITOCHONDRIA IN ALL OF THE SUBJECTS!

The study also revealed the why. Biochemical analysis showed that short, intense bouts of exercise breakdown CALCIUM CHANNELS IN YOUR MUSCLE CELLS AND SIGNALS THOSE CELLS

TO INCREASE THE NUMBER OF NEW MITOCHONDRIA TO IMPROVE MUSCULAR ENDURANCE.

The take-home message:

The key to staying young is creating more mitochondria that are healthy enough to produce this energy and endurance.

Also, studies using the HIIT protocol show faster fat loss; lower tri-glycerides and many other improved biomarkers for HIIT exercisers.

You can see that there really is **NO EXCUSE NOT TO EXERCISE** a few minutes 3 times per week! You should not feel intimidated if you are a couch potato who is carrying around a few extra pounds-☺

IT IS NEVER TOO LATE TO START AN EXERCISE PROGAM!

DR. EXERCISE REALLY IS THE FOUNTAIN OF YOUTH!

DR. EXERCISE HELPS YOU LOSE FAT BY DOING THE RIGHT KIND OF EXERCISE.

HIIT IS THE BEST EXERCISE AND THE QUICKEST FOR FAT LOSS.

THE SCIENCE SHOWS THAT IF YOU DO JUST ANYTHING- EVEN STAND IN PLACE FOR 20 MINUTES- YOU WILL BE HEALTHIER!

There is no need to jump into an exercise program and try to exercise **TOO LONG AND TOO VIGOROUSLY!** That is just a prescription for INJURY. The best approach is to start slowly…and within a few weeks you will build a new body at the cellular level-☺

You can start with the **35 STAND-UPS PER DAY.**

Perhaps you can take public transit or walk or bike to your office. You can even park one or two blocks from your office. Take the stairs instead of the elevator. These good little habits all add up.

Any little thing you can do (even fidgeting) will help you be healthier-☺)

ANY MOVEMENT IS BETTER THAN NONE!—even if that movement is getting off of the couch- or up from your chair-☺

When you start exercising— you may just decide to go for a brisk walk with your spouse. You will feel a difference within a few days. Some people buy a dog as a way to get a bit of regular exercise. Also, a few minutes of exercise on a grass surface is much more beneficial than the same exercise indoors.

This exercise is a form of "GROUNDING OR EARTHING" (supra). This is a super health strategy—which few people know about.

THE MOST IMPORTANT THING IS TO START AN FITNESS/EXERCISE PROGRAM NOW!

IT IS NEVER TOO LATE!

Recently a lady athlete named Ms Olga Kotelko passed away at the age of 95. This lady had started training at the tender age of 77 years young. She established more than 30 track and field records in her age category. After her death, they scanned her brain. The white of her brain was healthier and contained more neurons. Moreover, her hippocampus of her brain (memory center) was also LARGER!

Here's a summary of HIIT benefits:

- Only requires 4 to 8 minutes to burn need-ed calories for effective fat loss;

- Helps increase muscle and bone strength as well as mass;

- Reduces inflammation-helps reduce chron-ic inflammatory conditions;

- It trains both aerobic and anaerobic systems at the same time. It can actually improve aerobic sys-tem better than traditional aerobic training;

- Increases fuel for the immune system.

An old Chinese adage says "The journey of a thousand miles starts with the first step."

F.   RESISTANCE OR STRENGTH TRAINING

HIIT training and cardiovascular training is very beneficial. Some people (the present author included) prefer resistance or strength training. Strength training should start with bodyweight training. You may never wish to progress beyond that. That is fine.

Did you ever see the late actor Jack Palance (as a senior) do a one-arm push-up on stage at the Academy awards in front of millions of people? Now THAT takes strength!

YOU CAN GET VERY STRONG AND FIT— WITHOUT EVER SETTING FOOT INTO A GYM!

Designing a strength program can be simple or it can be very complicated.

That's what coaches and trainers do. You can design your own. You can learn from the best coaches and trainers in the world.

HERE'S A SIMPLE PROGRAM FROM MIKE BOYLE- THE WORLD'S BEST!

Coach Michael Boyle, also known as The Godfather of Strength & Conditioning suggests the following FULL BODY WORKOUT.

(You can also subscribe to his website: www.strengthcoach.com for a nominal fee). You do not have to be a coach or a trainer to subscribe. On this site you will find a boatload of world-class coaches who are more than pleased to answer your questions. You will find hundreds of articles AND DOZENS OF VIDEOS DEMONSTRATING EXERCISES. This website is simply the best out there if you want serious exercise information. You do not need to hire a personal trainer. You may wish to find

HERE'S FIVE BASIC EXERCISES THAT MIKE BOYLE SUGGESTS:

Exercise number one: A PUSH-UP

Exercise number two: A SPLIT- SQUAT(misnamed stationary lunge)

Exercise number three: A SINGLE-LEG-DEADLIFT

Exercise number four: A DUMBELL ROW

Exercise number five: A SIDE PLANK (Both sides)

THIS IS A COMPLETE PROGRAM.

PUSH-PULL-HIP- KNEE- CORE EXERCISES.

THIS IS A SIMPLE FULL-BODY COMPLETE WORKOUT!

YOU can use the HIIT format- mix and match, as much or as little as you can.

Always remember- it's preferable to get FMS'd or SCREENED BEFORE YOU START YOUR EXERCISE PROGRAM!   There is a good chance that you are unable to perform one or more of these exercises OR THAT YOU HAVE UNDIAGNOSED/ UNIDENTIFIED PAIN.

Mike Boyle also uses FMS-AND A JOINT BY JOINT FUNCTIONAL APPROACH TO PERSONAL TRAINING.

THERE'S A BOATLOAD OF EXERCISE INFORMATION ON LINE.

BUT— MUCH OF THE ON-LINE EXERCISE INFORMATION IS NOT SAFE INFORMATION!

If you are serious about learning about exercise and designing your own exercise program, <u>here are the best 3 EXERCISE books</u> (in my humble opinion).

- Michael Boyle's book " Advances in Functional Training";

- "Core Performance" by Mark Verstegen.

- "Movement" by Gray Cook.

Without an exhaustive exercise discussion- I would like to briefly mention a few valuable training techniques/ strategies that I strongly recommend.

THE MOST IMPORTANT TRAINING TOOL MOST EXERCISERS DO NOT KNOW ABOUT IS:

> <u>IT'S A FOAM ROLLER; —or the portable version—</u> "The Tiger-Tail"

Foam rollers are 3 foot long , 6 inch compressed rollers. They are made in very hard density or in softer density –for beginners. The Tiger-Tail is a rubber -coated rolling pin.

I call the Tiger-tail- the 15th club in a golfers bag!

Our bodies are covered in a thin gauze- like substance called" fascia". We are born with a kind of a "Spiderman Suit" which covers our bodies from head to toe. You will NOT find pictures of this anywhere in anatomy books—YET!

Thomas Myers, in his book—"Anatomy Trains" explains our myo-fascial slings that cover our bodies from head to toe.

When we bend over- what limits our movement and prevents us from touching our toes is that our fascia is tight. When we are young –our Spiderman suit is flexible and we move well easily. As we get older, our Spiderman suit dries out and becomes like "beef jerky"-☺

That prevents us from moving.

PERSONAL TRAINING AND EXERCISE IS ALL ABOUT TRAINING OUR FASCIA!

Personal training is largely about making our fascia more supple soft and capable of stretching. When we stretch we actually stretch our fascia much more than our muscles. The older we get the more difficult for us to move...the old beef jerky gets harder to move...- ☺What is the solution? The SOLUTION IS "A FOAM ROLLER".

A FOAM ROLLER IS USED TO ROLL ALL PARTS OF YOUR BODY ON! In essence, the foam roller has been called the "poor man's massager". We just have to iron out all of our fascia, muscles and connective tissue. Roll every part of our body...except our face and neck...

What does the rolling on the foam roller do?

It effects what is known as "self-myofascial release.

A FOAM ROLLER (and a TigerTail)DOES IMPORTANT THINGS FOR OUR BODIES.

FOAM ROLLERS ALLOW US TO CONDITION AND REPAIR OUR MUSCLES, FASCIA AND CONNECTIVE TISSUES.

FOAM ROLLERS ALLOW US TO MOVE!

FOAM ROLLERS ARE GREAT TOOLS FOR CORRECTIVE EXERCISE.

YOU CAN FOAM ROLL ANY PART OF YOUR BODY (except face, neck and throat). YOU CAN GOOGLE UP MIKE BOYLE TO SEE HOW FOAM ROLLING IS DONE- or go to his website: www.strengthcoach.com

YOU SHOULD FOAM ROLL ONE DAY PER WEEK FOR EVERY DECADE... so if you are 40- you would foam roll 4 times per week.

FOAM ROLLING IS A GREAT EXERCISE—BE CAREFUL- IT'S TOUGH! But it is worth the GREAT BENEFITS!

G. THE LYMPHATIC SYSTEM

"Every degenerative disease involves blockages to the circulation. Whether these blockages precede or follow an insult to the tissues, the result is the same. The name of the disease may only serve to tell us where the block-ages are located."

-Dr. C. Samuel,

Like natural death, degenerative diseases are simply states of local-ized morbidity. Discoveries that reveal how the body recovers from a morbid state ARE NOT TAUGHT IN ANY MEDICAL SCHOOLS. Not many people know much about the lymphatic system. It's complicated. It runs throughout the body. It works side by side with the circulatory system spanning various nodes, organs, vessels and tissues in the body.

The keys to enabling the body to <u>HEAL ITSELF ARE SIMPLE</u>- yet they are as advanced as nature itself.

The basic life and <u>HEALING PROCESS</u> in any tissues of the body is made possible by many essential services being performed by <u>OUR BLOOD AND OUR LYMPHATIC SYSTEMS</u>. Every day there are numerous things, mental, nutritional, and physical we do that influence the intimate relationship between these two systems.

Most natural healing processes work by helping the lymphatic system <u>ELIMINATE BLOCKAGES</u>. If your lymphatic system isn't working properly, it is unable to drain excess <u>TOXINS AND FLUIDS FROM THE BODY</u>. This causes problems such as swollen limbs, tonsillitis, lymphatic cancer and other conditions.

A working lymphatic system balances the body's fluids; absorbs fat into your system, and helps your body's immunological defense. Obviously, it is important to keep it in tip-top shape. When your blood travels throughout your body it releases fluids from the capillaries. This fluid is called interstitial fluid; it provides nutrients and oxygen for the tissues as it flows throughout the body.

In response to this generosity, the cells throw their garbage and waste products out for the interstitial fluid to pick up on its way back to the bloodstream. Luckily, the interstitial fluid doesn't mind this treatment.-☺ The interstitial fluid carries that waste back to the capillaries where 90 <u>PERCENT OF IT IS RE-ABSORBED</u>. The remaining 10 percent contains particles too large to pass through the capillary walls—so the <u>LYMPH SYSTEM</u> swoops in and <u>SUCKS IT UP!</u>

With the transfer to a new system in the body, this interstitial fluid also gets a name change. It's now called "<u>LYMPH</u>". This fluid filters through the lymph nodes and finishes its odyssey back where it started- in the bloodstream. This process is critical as the pile up of waste in the cells can <u>KILL</u> them!

Without a flowing lymph system fluid and waste would build up and bad things would happen. Think of what happens when your toilet backs up...-☺

Your lymphatic system is an important ally for boosting your immune system. Your spleen removes dead cells and foreign invaders from the body. Your tonsils (strategically placed lymph nodes- provide a line of defence against throat infections. Adenoids are lymph nodes in the nasal cavity minimize the effect of harmful pathogens entering the body. Lymph nodes' best protection to your immune system is their command of lymphocytes aka- <u>THE ALMIGHTY WHITE BLOOD CELLS</u>. These cells originate in the bone marrow. They control (modulate) immune reactions. They fight viruses and cancer cells.

When lymph fluid builds up, if your body is unable to get rid of the fluid and waste; the build-up can cause tissues in the body to swell; this can lead to cancer painfully enlarged organs or infections throughout the body. A properly working lymphatic system relies on these cells to clean out toxins.

<u>YOUR LYMPHATIC SYSTEM LACKS A BUILT-IN PUMP (your cardiovascular system has a pump- it's called your heart-</u>☺

<u>IN THE CASE OF YOUR LYMPHATIC SYSTEM—YOU MUST PROVIDE THE PUMP. YOU MUST SUPPLY THE PUMP!</u>

<u>YOU MUST SUPPLY THE PUMP FURNISHED BY DR. EXERCISE!</u>

<u>TO KEEP YOUR LYMPH FROM ACHIEVING THE CONSISTENCY OF COTTAGE CHEESE AND CAUSING YOUR FINGERS FROM LOOKING LIKE SWELLED SAUSAGES...</u>

<u>YOU MUST GET MOVING!</u>

A lifestyle of transferring your butt from the car to the office chair-to the sofa in front of the T.V. —

<u>DECREASES THE FLOW OF LYMPH FLUID BY 90 PERCENT!</u>

<u>THE BEST WAY TO CIRCULATE LYMPH IS EXERCISE.</u>

<u>THE BEST EXERCISES TO MOVE YOUR LYMPH ARE:</u>

- Jump rope; bounce on a trampoline (be careful- trampoline's are dangerous). If your baby cries... try bouncing your baby on your knee...chances are his/her lymph needs moving and he/she will stop crying-☺

- Simple movements like walking, stretching, bending over, toe-touching et.

- <u>MASSAGE FROM A FOAM ROLLER IS SUPER!</u>

- Drink a gallon of pure, clean water will help you get your lymph flowing;

- Doing a detox/cleanse or dry-brush rubbing;

- Eating an organic diet of fresh veggies and fruits will do wonders for your lymph and propel you on your way to SUPERHEALTH;

H. METABOLIC EFFECTS OF EXERCISE.

Exercise is one of one of the "magic bullets" to prevent disease and slow the aging process; besides helping you regain your insulin and leptin sensitivity that is the root cause of most chronic diseases.

HIIT boosts your body's production of HGH- a biochemical referred to as the "Fitness Hormone" for its invigorating, age-defying effects. It not only promotes muscle growth and effectively burns excessive fat- it also promotes longevity. Once you turn 30- you enter what's called "somatopause" at which point your levels of HGH begin to drop off dramatically. This decline of HGH is part of what drives your aging process- so maintaining your HGH levels high gets increasingly important with age.

Exercise also induces changes in mitochondrial enzyme content and activity; which increases cellular energy production and TRIGGERS MITOCHONDRIAL BIOGENESIS. (The process by which new mitochondria are formed in your cells.)

This reverses significant age-associated declines in mitochondrial mass- (repairs busted mitochondria); and in effect stops aging in its tracks. HIIT specifically BOOSTS TESTOSTERONE LEVELS NATURALLY; unlike aerobics or prolonged moderate exercise which has been shown to have an unhealthy or no effect on testosterone levels.

40 it's especially important to either start or increase your exercise program. This is the time when your physical strength, stamina, balance and flexibility start to decline and exercise can help counter-act most age-related decline.

Increasing age leads to a decline in cell functionality, generally termed "AGING". All tissue and organs of the body are involved in the phenomenon of aging; but the extent of the cellular impairment is greatly variable; since post mitotic tissues are the most sensitive targets of the aging process. Skeletal muscle tissue is profoundly affected during aging- but the extent of the cellular impairment and its functional decline is characterized by a progressive atrophy, that becomes most severe with advancing age and that from a certain point onwards can lead to mobility impairment, increased risk of falls and physical frailty.

The loss of function in skeletal muscle is also responsible for the development of AGE- DISTURBANCES.(Busted cells). For these reasons, understanding the mechanisms underlying aging in skeletal muscle is fundamental for the promotion of health and mobility in the elderly. Loss of skeletal muscle protein mass during aging partially explains the decline in muscle performance.

MITOCHONDRIA PLAY AN EXTREMELY IMPORTANT ROLE IN THE AGING PROCESS. HERE IS A SCIENCE BASED EXPLANATION OF THE MITOCHONDRIAL CHANGES THAT EXPLAIN THE AGING PROCESS.

MITOCHONDRIA PLAY A MAJOR ROLE IN ENERGETIC HOMEOSTASIS BY DETERMINING ATP AVAILABILITY IN THE CELLS. A decrease in mitochondrial function causes an inability to meet ATP cellular demands (busted mitochondria) so that skeletal muscle cells lose their ability to adapt to physiological stress imposed across the entire lifespan.

DYSFUNCTIONAL MITOCHONDRIA (busted mitochondria) contribute to the development of age-induced insulin resistance since mitochondrial oxidative capacity has been considered a good predictor of insulin sensitivity. When studying mitochondria in skeletal muscle-the mitochondrial population is heterogeneous—composed of TWO TYPES OF MITOCHONDRIA—

Located either beneath the SARCOLEMMAL MEMBRANE (SUB-SARCOLEMMAL) aka "SS" — OR—between the MYOFIBERS (INTERMYOFIBRILLAR aka "IMF".

These two mitochondrial populations exhibit different energetic characteristics and are differently affected by physiological stimuli. The mitochondrial performance depends on organelle number, organelle activity, and energetic efficiency of the mitochondrial machinery in the synthesizing of ATP from the oxidation of fuels. Consensus among experts, aging skeletal muscle has a blunted capacity for generation of new mitochondria. In response to both endurance exercise training and chronic electrical stimulation, it has been found that in SS and IMF mitochondria the capacity for ATP production was reduced as a result of diminished mitochondrial content per gram of muscle. There are different aging effects on these two mitochondrial populations.(SS & IMF). It is well-known that the amount of fuels oxidized by the cell is dictated mainly by ATP turnover—rather than by mitochondrial oxidative capacity and therefore a decrease in mitochondrial capacity and/or number becomes more important when cells increase their metabolic activity; i.e. during contraction.

The efficiency with which dietary calories are converted to ATP is determined by the degree of COUPLING OF OXIDATIVE PHOSPHORYLATION. If the respiratory chain is highly efficient at pumping protons out of the mitochondrial inner membrane, and the ATP synthesis is highly efficient at converting the proton flow through its pro ton channel into ATP (from ADP), then the mitochondria will generate maximum ATP and minimum heat per calorie.

In contrast- if the efficiency of the proton pumping is reduced and/or more protons are required to make each ATP molecule—then each calorie will yield less ATP. The main point of regulation of oxidative phosphorylation efficiency is represented by the degree of COUPLING between oxygen consumption and ATP synthesis- which is always lower than 1 and can vary according to the metabolic needs of the cell.

Among the factors that affect mitochondrial degree of COUPLING-an important role is played by the permeability of the mitochondrial inner membrane to H+ions (Leak).

It is now well known that mitochondrial inner membrane exhibit a basal PROTEIN LEAK PATHWAY, whose contribution to the basal metabolic rate has been estimated to be 20 to 25 %. Also- it is well known that FATTY ACIDS can act as NATURAL UNCOUPLERS of oxidative phosphorylation—generating a fatty-acid dependent proton leak pathway which is a function of the amount of unbound fatty acids in the cell.

A decreased mitochondrial mass has been found in senescent rats – thus suggesting that an IMPAIRMENT OF MITOCHONDRIAL BIOGENESIS OCCURS IN LATE-AGING and/or it takes place SELECTIVELY IN SPECIFIC MUSCLES-SUCH AS MITOCHONDRIAL MASS HAS BEEN FOUND DECREASED IN OLD RATS. Therefore, the decreased proton leak found in SS and IMF mitochondria is physiologically relevant. When mitochondria are mitochondria are more efficient—less substrates are oxidized to obtain ATP. Therefore- the increased MITOCHONDRIAL COUPLING in skeletal muscle could contribute to the decreased energy expenditure that is evident even after the decrease in lean mass has been taken into account; AND THIS IS THE BASIS OF AGE-INDUCED OBESITY.

SKELETAL MUSCLE ENERGY ACCOUNTS FOR ABOUT 30 PERCENT OF WHOLE BODY ENERGY EXPENDITURE IN RESTING CONDITIONS.

When mitochondria are more COUPLED- ATP is produced at a slower rate that could be unable to meet cellular energy demands—especially during skeletal muscle contraction.

In fact, it has been found in elderly people that –LOWER speed of ATP production is associated with a HIGHER FATIGABILITY.

METABOLIC CHANGES.

Exercise reverses metabolic diseases, T2D, osteoporosis and cardio-vascular disease. Strength training is especially important for seniors.

EXERCISE PREVENTS HEART FAILURE BY FORMING NEW MITOCHONDRIA. Your skeletal muscle derives its energy from your mitochondria-(the energy batteries of your cells) responsible for the utilization of energy for all metabolic functions.

Mitochondria make up on average- about 1 to 2 PERCENT OF YOUR SKELETAL MUSCLE BY VOLUME—BUT—this is usually enough to provide the needed energy for your daily movements. Your CARDIAC MUSCLES are similar to your skeletal muscles in that they are striated (banded) but there is an important difference.

YOUR CARDIAC MUSCLE CONTAINS UP TO 35 PERCENT MITOCHONDRIA. This large volume of mitochondria supplies a steady source of energy right to your heart—and this explains why your heart rarely needs to rest

What is exercise metabolism?

Exercise metabolism is the regulation of metabolic processes during exercise. The rate of exercise metabolism depends on the energy available to the skeletal muscles. The muscles store ATP (adenosine triphosphates) and burn it when the muscle is in use. Your body provides the correct amount of ATP that each muscle needs.

When you exercise, you increase the need for ATP by the muscles; which in turn creates more conversion of food to ATP for the muscles to use. This is why one of the best ways to increase your metabolism and to lose weight (fat) is by adding exercise/weight training to your daily regime.

Metabolic Effects of Exercise include:

EXERCISE REGULATES INSULIN AND LEPTIN LEVELS.

EXERCISE UPREGULATES DYSFUNCTIONAL MITOCHONDRIA- or in technical terms: Exercise fixes "busted cells-☺

EXERCISE TRIGGERS MITOCHONDRIAL BIOGENESIS- or in technical terms: "Exercise grows new mitochondria and grows new cells"-☺

It has been known for 4 decades that exercise serves as a mediator of systemic mitochondrial biogenesis. Exercise causes increases in skeletal muscle enzyme content and activity; i.e. mitochondrial biogenesis.

Increasing evidence confirms that exercise induces mitochondrial biogenesis in a <u>WIDE</u> range of tissues—not normally associated with the demands of exercise.

<u>PERTURBATIONS</u> in mitochondrial content or function have been linked to a wide variety of diseases, in multiple tissues.

EXERCISE SERVES AS A <u>POTENT APPROACH BY WHICH TO PREVENT AND/OR TO TREAT PATHOLOGIES AND DISEASE.</u>

<u>WHEN YOU EXERCISE- YOU EXERCISE YOUR GENES!</u>

<u>ZOWIE!</u> Who knew?

Exercise increases the messenger RNA (or RHA) expression and protein levels of a <u>PLETHORA</u> of genes regulating mitochondrial function and fuel usage.

A recent study in the Journal Cell Metabolism showed that when healthy, inactive people exercise intensely (even if brief)- it produces <u>AN IMMEDIATE CHANGE IN THEIR DNA!</u>

Exercise causes important <u>STRUCTURAL AND CHEMICAL CHANGES TO THE DNA</u> molecules within your muscles. This contraction-induced <u>GENE ACTIVATION</u> appears to be early events leading to the reprogramming of muscle for strength; and to the <u>STRUCTURAL AND METABOLIC BENEFITS OF EXERCISE</u>. Several genes affected by acute exercise are genes involved in fat metabolism.

Research proves that when you exercise, your body almost <u>IMMEDIATELY</u> experiences genetic activation that increases the pro-duction of fat busting exercise proteins.

Muscle biopsies show that when a sedentary person does strength training for the first 3 weeks- <u>THERE IS NO PHYSICAL CHANGE IN THE SIZE OF THE MUSCLE.</u>

What changes?

Answer: <u>BRAIN STRUCTURE CHANGES!</u>

<u>EXERCISE MAKES YOUR BRAIN LARGER BEFORE IT MAKES OTHER MUSCLES LARGER!</u>

<u>EXERCISE MAKES YOU SMARTER!</u>

- Exercise promotes the growth and builds <u>NEW BRAIN CELLS</u> through a process known as '<u>NEUROGENESIS OR NEUROPLAS-TICITY</u>'. Exercise releases hormones from the muscles that grow new brain cells. Exercise isn't just to make you look good naked-☺ Exercise will provide you with a strong heart. "

- The emerging scientific view of human evolution and role of physical activity gives a whole new meaning to the phrase "Jog Your Memory"-☺ Physical including aerobic exercise targets the "BDNF GENE"- which is: "<u>BRAIN'S GROWTH HORMONE</u>".

- Exercise increases serum levels of BDNF (Brain-derived Neurotrophic Factor) Humans have triumphed over long distances because we could outwalk, outrun and outthink most any other animal. Increasing the size of our brains ultimately helped make us the clever human beings that we are today.-☺

- Exercise boosts brain performance. The hippocampus belongs to the ancient part or your brain known as the "limbic system". The hippocampus consolidates short-term information into long-term memory. Your brain's hippocampus i.e. your memory center is particularly adaptable and capable of <u>GROWING NEW CELLS UNTIL YOU DIE- EVEN IN YOUR 90's</u>! One study proved that adults enlarged their brain's memory center by 1 to 2 <u>PERCENT PER YEAR</u>. Older lose 2 <u>PERCENT OF THEIR HIPPOCAMPAL VOLUME EACH YEAR</u>.

- Exercise training increases size of hippocampus and improves memory. Medial temporal lobe volumes are larger in higher-fit adults. Physiological activity training increases hippocampal perfusion. Training increases the size of anterior hippocampus leading to improvements in spatial memory. Increased hippocampal volume is associated with greater serum levels of BDNF- a mediator of neurogenesis in dentate gyrus.

- Exercise helps protect and improve your brain function by:

  - Improves and increases blood flow to the brain;

  - Increases production of nerve-protecting compounds;

  - Improves/builds brain cells and neurons;

  - Reduces damaging plaques e.g. amyloid proteins, Tau proteins and cellular waste products etc.

  - Alters the way that these damaging brain proteins reside in your brain...prevents brain fog-☺

  - Helps your glymphatic (brain waste system) take out the brain garbage at night-☺

- Exercise triggers an anti-aging process. <u>WALKING IS A SUPERFOOD</u>.

- **WALKING ADDS 3 TO 7 YEARS TO YOUR LIFES-PAN.** (Walking is a very creative brain process- you will get very good ideas when you walk),

- When you strengthen your body- you strengthen your **BRAIN;**

- Research shows that 20 minutes of strength training improves/enhances your long term memory by 10 **PERCENT**! Move iron and build your brain.

- **CANCER CELLS HATE DR. EXERCISE!** Dr. Exercise provides a very hostile and unpleasant environment for cancer cells. Dr. Exercise kills cancer cells by making them commit cellular suicide (apoptosis)-☺ Dr. Exercise is your best friend.

- Sidebar:

STRETCHING:

Static stretching is okay after exercise. But active stretching is superior...before, during or after exercise. See **www.stretchingusa.com** (Aaron Mattes).

FAVOURITE PRE-WORKOUT FUEL: Black organic coffee.

DR. EXERCISE'S TAKE-HOME MESSAGE:

AVOID SITTING AS MUCH AS YOU CAN.

STAND AS OFTEN AS YOU CAN.

WALK AS MUCH AS POSSIBLE.

FOAM ROLL AS OFTEN AS POSSIBLE.

DO AS MANY MINUTES OF HITT OR OTHER EXERCISE AS YOU CAN SQUEEZE INTO YOUR LIFE,

AND FINALLY- SQUEEZE IN AS MUCH MOVEMENT AS YOU CAN INTO YOUR LIFE!

CHAPTER TEN

DR. SLEEP

"Without enough sleep, we all become tall two year olds."

— JoJo Jensen

A. INTRODUCTION

According to the US Centers for Disease Control and Prevention, (CDC) <u>INSUFFICIENT SLEEP IS CLASSIFIED AS A PUBLIC HEALTH EPIDEMIC!</u>

<u>25 PERCENT OF AMERICANS SLEEP LESS THAN 6 HOURS PER NIGHT.</u>

If you could do <u>ONE THING</u> to increase your brain power, build muscle, lose fat, look better, and live longer—

<u>Would you do it?</u>

There can be little doubt that <u>QUALITY SLEEP</u> is one of the most important variables to improve your brain function, longevity and performance in all aspects of life.

You may say: "Who has time to sleep?"...you can sleep when you're dead- right?-☺ That's true—what if more sleep actually means better performance and greater longevity? A majority of Americans are not getting enough sleep, and modern technology is in large part to blame.

According to the 2014 Sleep in America poll, <u>53 percent</u> of respondents who turn electronics off while sleeping rate their sleep as excellent, compared to <u>27 percent</u> wo leave their devices on.

Even children are becoming sleep deprived. The poll shows that 58 percent of teens aged 15-17 get only seven hours of sleep per night. Between 7 and 9 hours may be optimal for the average adult, but common sense dictates that children need more sleep than adults. Proper physiological growth and developmental learning requires quality sleep. Lack of proper sleep will negatively impact their education .It appears that the male brain, for example is not fully developed until age 25.

THE WORLD OF ELECTRONICS IS LITERALLY KILLING THE PRESENT GENERATION—BOTH CHILDREN— AND YOUNG ADULTS.

We are living in an era of electronic revolution. The health care problems caused by electronics will only become evident in the next 10 or 15 years. The present generation is being killed both by the electromagnetic fields (EMF's) <u>directly</u> by the harmful rays which are causing cancer. Computers, iPads, I Phones, tablets are also killing our children (and many people too) by keeping them up late at night playing video games and surfing the Internet. Many kids have their electronic devices on their bodies all day. Then- they take them to bed to play with them… Electronic radiation and its addictive effects may replace sugar as the king of neurotoxins.

If your child is overweight and/or exhausted most of the time— chances are high that <u>POOR SLEEP PATTERNS likely resulting from too many LIGHT-EMITTING ELECTRONIC GADGETS ARE THE REAL CULPRITS.</u>

The exposure to excessive amounts of light at night, from T.V. electric light bulbs and ALL KINDS OF ELECTRONIC GADGETS make it very difficult for kids to wind down and get proper quality sleep. Their brains are constantly inflamed 24/7 with bad rays and blue light. How can anyone sleep when their brain is on fire? A brain MRI after exposure to EMF's for a few hours would likely shock most people.

B. THE PHYSIOLOGY OF SLEEP

Humans are hard-wired to sleep in a normal— automatic fashion. Our caveman ancestors had no sleep problems. He went to sleep in his cave when darkness came and he simply got up when the sun came up. He didn't need to fight bright lights, TV or computer screens. Our ancestors did not have problems with good sleep hygiene. They had daylight and darkness—period. Humans have bodies and brains that manufacture sleep and other hormones automatically.

Humans are creatures of light and darkness. We are programmed to get sleepy when darkness comes and to wake up when daylight comes. It's really quite simple.

One key to optimum human health is our ability to produce the appropriate hormones in synchronization with the time of the day or night. This whole process means that humans function according to the "Circadian Rhythm" The circadian rhythm really means that our 24 hour daily existence is broken up into two parts. We are programmed to sleep for about 8 hours (about one-third) of the day. The other 16 hours (about two-thirds) of the day we are supposed to forage for food, and enjoy our daily activities. Darkness signalled the end of the daylight part. Darkness usually meant a big feast; a glowing fire followed by nourishing restorative sleep.

Our brains are hard-wired to work outside in the (sunlight) daylight cycle. They don't call it the "graveyard shift for no reason! Shift workers are often unhealthy and short-lived. Their circadian rhythms are wrecked; hormone cycles and hormone production often are "out of whack".

Our brain chemistry identifies when it is daylight and when it is dark. That's our internal software— our circadian rhythm.

Inside of our brain is a walnut-sized gland known as the pineal gland. The key function of this gland is to synthesize and secrete melatonin, which controls OUR SLEEP/WAKE CYCLE.

According to Dr. Stepahnie Seneff, the pineal gland is a neuroendocrine organ of the brain that resides in close proximity to the ventricles.

The key role of the pineal gland is to produce melatonin to deliver sulfate to the neurons (brain cells) at night during sleep. In her words, melatonin is a sulfate delivery system. She says that this intricate delivery system operates as follows:

1. With sunlight exposure serving as a catalyst, the pineal gland builds up supplies of sulfate by day— storing it in heparin sulfate molecules.

2. The pineal gland produces melatonin in the evening, transporting it a melatonin sulfate into the CSF.

In healthy individuals, melatonin plays an important part in inducing REM sleep, which may be the most important stage of sleep. When

461

the pineal gland's ability to make sulfate is impaired, this, in turn, reduces the production of melatonin, which is <u>ALL IMPORTANT</u> <u>FOR ADEQUATE HEALTHY SLEEP</u>.

The endothelial and neuronal nitric oxide synthase-both of which are present in the pineal gland- produce sulfate from reduced sulfur sources catalyzed by the sunlight.

<u>THIS PROCESS IS IMPAIRED THROUGH LACK OF SUNLIGHT EXPOSURE</u>. The bad result is a sulfate deficiency and then a melatonin deficiency. No sunlight exposure means inadequate melatonin production; and lack of sleep also disturbs the production of melatonin. Lack of daylight exposure (due to staying indoors) completely messes up our circadian rhythm!

The result is poor sleep coupled with attendant negative health consequences. Thus, we see that sleep is a physiological process. We are supposed to get enough sunshine ;(<u>OR AT</u> <u>LEAST ENOUGH DAYLIGHT EXPOSURE</u>) in order to absorb rays to activate and signal our brain that it is daylight. If we stay indoors in artificial lights, our brain is messed up.

Thereafter, when outside darkness comes; INSIDE darkness only comes a few hours later. We injure our brains further. We <u>BOMBARD OUR BRAINS</u> with artificial blue light.

Our poor brain believes that it's still <u>DAYTIME—NOT NIGHT TIME</u>— so it does not make melatonin. The electronic and artificial light bombardment really messes up our brain. Then we go to bed when we're still all jacked up—and our brain is inflamed!

To repeat— our sleep/wake cycle, our Circadian rhythm is thus badly disrupted. The lack of proper melatonin production and <u>TOO MUCH CORTISOL PRODUCTION</u> becomes A <u>DEADLY PRESCRIPTION</u>!

When light, (natural daylight- or artificial light), enters our eye's rods & cones; a visual signal is sent to our visual system. The light goes to our "<u>MASTERCLOCK</u>" brain and a signal goes to <u>ALL</u> parts our body to synchronize our sleep cycle. Unfortunately, repeated constant artificial light signals confuse our brain. They damage our brain too.

Artificial lights disrupt our brain and our neuroendocrine functions. Artificial lights in our lives <u>HAVE SKYROCKETED IN THE LAST DECADE</u>.

Could the huge proliferation in electronic devices, neon overhead lights, street lights and the the plethora of different kinds of artificial light be the cause of many of our man-made modern diseases? What do you think? Does this sound plausible? Are we suffering from too much artificial light in our lives? Are we becoming like the proverbial "deer in the headlights"?

Maintaining a natural rhythm of exposure to sunlight during the day and darkness at night is <u>THE CRUCIAL FOUNDATIONAL COMPONENT OF PROPER QUALITY SLEEP.</u>

Exposure to bright sunlight serves as the major synchronizer of your MasterClock or special group of brain cells called Suprachismatic nuclei (SCN). These nuclei synchronize to the light/dark cycle of your environment when light enters your eye.

You also have biological clocks throughout your body and those clocks subsequently synchronize to your MasterClock. One major reason why so many people get so little sleep or such poor quality sleep can be traced back to a MasterClock disruption.

In sum, most people spend their days indoors shielded from bright sunlight. On top of that, most people spend their evenings in <u>TOO BRIGHT ARTIFICIAL LIGHT.</u> This behaviour has serious health consequences.

<u>ARE YOU BOMBARDING YOUR MASTERCLOCK WITH ARTIFICIAL LIGHT?</u>

<u>IS THIS ARTIFICIAL LIGHT RUINING YOUR SLEEP AND YOUR HEALTH?</u>

The science is clear.

<u>LACK OF QUALITY SLEEP HAS SERIOUS HEALTH CONSEQUENCES— FOR EVERYONE!</u>

C.   NEGATIVE CONSEQUENCES OF LACK OF SLEEP

Good sleep is one of the foundations of good health. Sleep can even be a <u>PERFORMANCE ENHANCEMENT TOOL.</u>

Sleep deprivation is such an insidious chronic condition today; you may not even realize that you suffer from it!

Science has now shown that a sleep deficit can have serious, far-reaching permanent effects on your health. In colloquial terms, lack of quality sleep will make you sick, fat and ugly.-☺ Here is a more scientific explanation.

<u>IMPAIRED OR INTERRUPTED SLEEP CAN HAVE THE FOLLOWING ADVERSE EFFECTS ON YOUR HEALTH:</u>

- It can seriously weaken your immune system;

- It can accelerate tumour growth—tumours grow 2 to 3 times faster in lab animals with severe sleep dysfunctions;

- It can cause obesity problems, pre-diabetic state, diabetes and generally wreak havoc with your metabolism;

- It can cause cognitive problems; memory issues, brain fog;

- It can impair your performance on physical or mental tasks and decrease your problem solving abilities;

- It can cause disruption of the production of hormones such a s melatonin and serotonin and various other neurotransmitters;

- It can cause stomach ulcers, constipation

- It can cause depression, mood disorders, anger and irritability;

- It (chronic sleep disturbance) is an environmental risk factor for Alzheimer's disease;

- It can cause heart disease and cardiovascular disease;

- It can lead to cancer because of hormone regulation problems and because the body is unable to fight off free radicals;

- It can cause premature aging by interfering with hormone production (including HGH or human growth hormone;

- One study showed that people suffering chronic sleep deprivation/insomnia HAVE A THREE TIMES GREATER RISK OF DEATH FROM ANY CAUSE.

Artificial light from electronic devices such as cell phones, computers, and the like have devastating effects on sleep health.

Checking your e-mails at night not only exposes you to WORK-RELATED STRESS; it exposes you to artificial light. The quality of your sleep has a lot to do with all kinds of light- both indoor and outdoor lighting—because it serves as the major synchronizer of your Masterclock.

Exposure to even minute amounts of light from your computer, tablet or smartphone can interfere with your body's production of melatonin. As mentioned; melatonin production problems destroy your sleep/wake cycle.

The research clearly shows that people who use their computer, tablet or smartphones near bedtime are more likely to report symptoms of insomnia. PLUS- when you are connected to the internet; your phone or computer is communicating with nearby cell towers, which means that they're also emitting low levels of radiation. (EMF's).

The National Sleep Foundation polls show approximately 95 percent of Americans use an electronic device within a hour of going to sleep. In 2013, the foundation found that 89% of adults and 75 percent of kids have at least one electronic device in their bedroom.

Research shows that children with electronic devices in their bedrooms sleep less and experience lower quality of sleep than children without gadgets.

A 2008 study showed that people exposed to radiation from cell phones for 3 hours before bedtime had more trouble falling asleep and staying in a deep sleep.

In a very recent study published on September 2, 2014 in the Journal Behav. Sleep Med. Reported at PUBMED no.24156294 the researchers studied 532 students aged 18 to 39. The study investigated whether the use of a television, computer, gaming console, tablet, mobile phone or an audio player before going to bed was associated with insomnia; daytime sleepiness, morningness or chrono type. Average time of media usage per night was 46.6 minutes. The results showed that computer usage for playing/surfing/texting was POSITIVELY associated with insomnia and chrono time, and negatively associated with morningness. The use of the other media showed no daytime sleepiness.

The take-home message: the new electronic devices are wrecking your sleep health.

Does late evening exercise interfere with sleep?

The research is scant. It is well known that exercise during the day is beneficial to sleep and to health generally. Here's what some of the studies say.

In a small sleep study (11 young fit adults), published on March 20th, 2011 in J. Sleep Res. – the effects of vigorous late-night exercise on sleep quality were studied. The authors stated: "In sleep hygiene recommendation, intensive exercising is not suggested within the last 3 hours before bedtime, but this recommendation has not been adequately tested experimentally." The authors stated: "The results indicate that vigorous late night exercise does not disturb sleep quality. However, it may have effects on the autonomic control of the heart during the first sleeping hours."

In a study published in March 2012 in Eur. J. App. Physiol. In PUBMED no. 21667290, the researchers studied the effects of high-intensity exercise on 14 healthy young males. The subjects exercised from 6 P.M. Some exercised 30 minutes, some exercised for 60 minutes and one group finished at 7:30 P.M. The researchers stated that increased exercise intensity or duration does not seem to disrupt sleep quality.

In a study published in September 2014 in www.sleep.journal.com 52 regular exercisers were tested. The researchers concluded:

"Against expectations and general recommendations for sleep hygiene, high-perceived exercise exertion before bedtime was associated with better sleep patterns in a sample of healthy young adults.

Thus we see that the studies are somewhat inconclusive. That said;

THE GOOD NEWS IS— YOU CAN RESTORE YOUR SLEEP HEALTH—FAST!

So—What are the positive benefits of quality sleep?

D. POSITIVE BENEFITS OF QUALITY SLEEP

Mental Benefits

- One good night's sleep can improve your ability to learn a new motor skills

- By 20 PERCENT;

- 8 hours of quality sleep increases your ability to gain new insights into complex problems by 50 PERCENT!

Physical Benefits

- Quality sleep is one of the most important variables to improve your BRAIN FUNCTION, LONGEVITY AND PERFORMANCE;

- sleep promotes skin health and a youthful appearance;

- sleep increases testosterone levels;

- sleep controls optimum insulin secretion and maximum production of human growth hormone (HGH);

- sleep encourages healthy cell division (and helps prevent cancer)

- sleep protects and supports the immune system;

- sleep promotes healthy weight loss and proper weight maintenance;

- sleep is neuro-protective; allows the brain to better operate the brain's waste system (aka the glymphatic system), and build new brain cells;

- SLEEP AUGMENTS ATHLETIC PERFORMANCE.

Here are 2 interesting studies:

- In a 2011 study at Stanford University. Basketball players were asked to aim for 10 hours of sleep per night. Most of the participants in the study added 90 minutes or more to their sleep. Their athletic performance improved. They increased their free throw and 3pt shooting by an average of 9%. They also shaved more than a second from 282 feet sprints; (2X the length of the basketball court.

- In a sleep study published in the Journal of Athletic Training in December 2012, female Chinese basketball players took 30 minutes of irradiation from a red-light therapy instrument for 14 nights. The researchers concluded that their sleep was improved; due to improved serum melatonin levels.

- AFTERNOON EXERCISE HELPS REGULATE YOUR CIRCADIAN RHYTHM!

  In a study published in the Journal of Physiology on December 1st, 2012 reported at PUBMED no> 22988175, researchers found that exercise helps regulate your circadian rhythm—and the effect may be most profound if done in the middle of the day! The authors commented:

  "The circadian system co-ordinates the temporal patterning of behavior and many underlying biological processes. In some cases, the regulated outputs of the circadian system such as activity, may be able to feed back to alter core clock process."

E. A MID-AFTERNOON NAP?

Taking a mid-afternoon is not a good idea.

TAKING A MID-AFTERNOON IS A <u>GREAT</u> IDEA!

In a ground- breaking study published in **February 2010** at (<u>www. erekaerert.org</u>) researchers made an **<u>ASTONISHING DISCOVERY</u>!**

The researchers found THAT A <u>MID-AFTERNOON NAP</u>—

1. <u>TOTALLY REFRESHES YOUR MIND AND YOUR BODY</u>. &

2. <u>IT MAKES YOU SMARTER</u>!

This sounds incredible but the science is conclusive.

F. KEY TIPS FOR GETTING QUALITY SLEEP

- **REFRAIN FROM EATING FOR 3 HOURS PRIOR TO BEDTIME;**

- **PLACE BLACK SHADES ON YOUR BEDROOM WINDOW- (You do not even want the slightest bit of light in your bedroom! Remove everything such as clocks, digital devices etc. A sleep mask will help but is not the best- because you have 'mini-clocks in every cell in your body which detect light-☺**

- **AVOID TV AND ALL ELECTRONIC DEVICES FOR AT LEAST ONE HOUR BEFORE PUTTING YOUR HEAD ON YOUR PILLOW.**

- **HAVE A WARM BATH AND/OR READ SOME-THING HAPPY AND RELAXING.**

- **SLEEP IN YOUR BODY'S RECOVERY FETAL PO-SITION ON YOUR RIGHT SIDE.**

- **SMELL SOME VANILLA OR LAVENDER…AND THINK OF DO-ING WHATEVER BRINGS YOU JOY—Not your work!**

- **DREAM BIG—BIG DREAMS COST THE SAME AS LITTLE DREAMS-☺**

<u>The take-home message</u>:

DR. SLEEP DOES HIS BEST WORK AT NIGHT-☺

YOU SLEEP AT NIGHT—BUT OTHER PARTS OF YOUR BRAIN ARE ACTIVE AND HELP TAKE OUT THE "toxic stuff" that has built up during the daytime-☺

ENSURE THAT YOU GET AT LEAST 8 HOURS OF QUALITY SLEEP.

PROPER REST IS ESSENTIAL TO KEEP YOU AND YOUR BRAIN HEALTHY!

CHAPTER ELEVEN
THE DISEASE YOUR DOCTOR CAN'T DIAGNOSE

"All disease begins in the gut"
— Hippocrates, The Father of Medicine

A. INTRODUCTION

Almost 2,500 years ago, Hippocrates made this brilliant observation about our health. Today, scientists and researchers have confirmed that he was absolutely right.

What you eat can make or break your gut health.

On June 17th, 2014, in the Nutrition Journal the authors stated:

"The notion that diet, stress and environment can, for better or worse imprint upon the bowel has been around since the ancient Egyptian pharaohs. However, only recent focus and technological advances have allowed accurate elucidation of the mechanisms by which our lifestyle impacts our microbiome and leads to dysbiosis."

In the gut (and on the skin) there is an optimal, albeit not yet fully elucidated, balance of bacterial species. Some strains of bacteria are needed to digest dietary fibers while others produce valuable nutrients like Vitamin K.

> Beneficial bacteria aide their hosts by occupying space and/or modifying the microenvironment in ways that prevent harmful bacteria from gaining a foothold. More importantly, the commensal flora provides a type of training to the immune system. Like a sparring partner in boxing— the immune system interacts with the normal commensal flora providing an education that is indispensable when a pathogenic opponent is encountered. "

The old adage-"YOU ARE WHAT YOU EAT"—has taken on a new meaning!

Scientists have recently learned a lot more about how our diet influences the gut bacteria (microbes) in our gut. They have found that Dr. Hippocrates was far ahead of his time in his understanding of the gut/bacteria/brain connection.

Our diet and our gut bacteria play a HUGE role in regulating our metabolism—as well as our weight loss/gain mechanisms.

What we eat is the greatest determiner of VARIETY AND KIND OF BACTERIA THAT LIVE IN OUR GUT. The guts of Japanese people, for example, contain specialized bacteria, or bugs, that aid in the digestion of seaweed.

There is a growing body of evidence that increased intestinal PERMEABILITY plays a PATHOGENIC role in a BOATLOAD of autoimmune diseases; including Celiac disease and Type 1 diabetes. In addition to genetic and environmental factors, the concept of "LEAKY GUT" used to be confined to the outer fringes of medicine. This concept was employed by "alternative practitioners"e.g. D.C. and N.D. after their names. Truth be told—these are the "real doctors"—not the allopathic crowd.

Most conventional allopathic doctors (as we have seen) have traditionally scoffed at Mother Nature's powers. They have scoffed at the idea that a LEAKY GUT plays a foundational role in the development and progression of autoimmune diseases—not to mention a BOATLOAD of other adverse health conditions.

Recent research has demonstrated unequivocally that different species of gut bacteria exert POWERFUL INFLUENCES on our metabolism.

The gut bacteria in a lean person usually are quite different than the bacteria in an obese person. Moreover, science demonstrates that each individual has his own UNIQUE personal gut ECOSYSTEM. That personalized ecosystem acts like a personalized fingerprint— unique to each person.

<u>YOUR MICROBIOME IS ONE OF MOST COMPLEX ECOSYSYSTEMS IN THE WORLD.</u>

The concept of a leaky gut as a foundational cause of poor health has shocked and rocked the world of conventional Western Medicine. <u>Conventional allopathic doctors, formerly in denial— are now being forced to "eat their words."</u> (pun intended-☺)

<u>THE TAKE HOME MESSAGE IS—</u>

<u>THE DISEASE THAT YOUR DOCTOR CAN'T DIAGNOSE IS CALLED "LEAKY GUT SYNDROME" OR (LGS)</u> for short.

- <u>Some important facts:</u>

- The average human body contains AT LEAST 37.2 TRILLION CELLS;

- Humans possess about 23,000 TO 30,000 genes;

- The commensal gut genome (microbiome) is 150 times LARGER than the human genome;

- Our gut houses 10 TIMES the number of cells in the form of <u>LIVING BACTERIA</u>, <u>BACTERIOPHAGES</u>, and PRO-TOZOA; (source: www.smithonianinstitute.com).

  Yes, our body, (our gut) is the home of more than <u>100 TRILLION BACTERIA OR</u> 100,000,000,000,000…That is a number that is even difficult for us to appreciate!

- Our body also houses <u>ONE QUADRILLION VIRUSES</u> called "BAC-TERIOPHAGES". That's a huge number which hard to imagine!

- <u>ALL OF THESE MICRO ORGANISMS</u> perform a multitude of es-sential biological functions in the various systems of our bodies.

- <u>ALL OF THESE MICROORGANISMS</u> must be properly balanced and maintained in order for the human body to be healthy;

- <u>OUR GASTROINTESTINAL TRACT</u> (or GI tract) is home to <u>90 PERCENT OF</u> <u>OUR ENTIRE IMMUNE SYSTEM</u>;

- Our gastrointestinal tract (GI tract) is MUCH MORE than a digestive centre;

- The weight of our brain is about 2 pounds;

- The weight of our gut microbiome (all living bacteria & other bugs in our gut) is between 2 and 6 POUNDS!

- Our gut contains about 95 percent of the body's hormone SEROTONIN;

- The bacteria in our gut do more than aid in our digestive tract—they support and influence our immune responses, our CNS (Central Nervous System) and our (ENS) Enteric Nervous System; as well as the interaction between these two systems;

- These "bugs" support our immune system- in that:

    - They protect the body from invading organisms;

    - they create hormones and neurotransmitters;

    - they create and synthesize vitamins;

    - they have an complex SYMBIOTIC relationship with our brain;

    - they exert a powerful influence on our mood and temperament; (Have you ever found yourself saying " My initial gut reaction was…?"

AND PERHAPS THE MOST SURPRISIING FACT OF ALL—FOOD IS INFORMATION;

THE FOOD THAT YOU EAT CAN TURN" ON—OR –"OFF" GENETIC EXPRESSION.

PUT ANOTHER WAY—FOOD CHOICES DICTATE OUR DNA GENETIC EXPRESSION!

ZOWIE!

WE LITERALLY HAVE THE POWER TO CONTROL OUR DESTINY WITH FOOD! Who knew?

World- re-known neurologist Dr. David Perlmutter (author of "Grain Brain" and others doctors have gone so far as to suggest that: "OUR GUT MAY BE OUR FIRST BRAIN! Some pretty heavy stuff, isn't it?

Our GI tract is really a long hollow tube; comprised of a large and a small intestine, (about 20-25 feet long) which starts in our mouth and ends in our anus. Our digestive tracts are really passageways from one end of the body to the other— that for the most part provide a barrier between the outside world and our insides. It's only through the digestive process involving specialized cells that the nutrients from food actually enter the body.

Any disruption in the health, function, or interaction of these cells with each other or with their environment can SIGNIFICANTLY COMPROMISE OUR ABSORPTION OF NUTRIENTS—AND CAN MAKE US VERY SICK!

That said, our digestive tract is loaded with TRILLIONS of microorganisms. They form an entire NATURAL ECOSYSTEM commonly called the "gut flora"; or "gut microbiota". This ecosystem is SYMBIOTIC in that it benefits both the individual and the microbes. It also acts in synergy with our brain. Everyone knows that our gut and brain work intimately together. An illustrative example is when athletes and performers sometimes suffer nausea before public performances.

Sometimes lifestyle stressors, (toxins or different kinds of stress) upset this natural symbiosis and cause the production of pathogenic microbes; (aka" bad bugs"). These bad bugs cause chronic gut inflammation which then damage the gut lining.

The digestive tract is a dark, moist environment that provides a steady stream of fluid and nutrition so it is an optimal breeding ground for microbes for a wide species of bacteria. Apparently, there are 500 to 1000 different species of microorganisms in the gut. The vast majority of these bacteria are beneficial or good bacteria. These good bacteria help breakdown and metabolize food particles and form highly absorbable nutrients for us to digest. These bacteria are the "good immune soldiers" of our body. They fight off the bad guys/bugs who attack our immune system. This symbiotic relationship between gut-brain and host (us) is a good one—PROVIDED THAT THE HOST FEEDS THE BACTERIA THE RIGHT FOODS!

We often hear about "good bacteria"; or "bad bacteria". The good bacteria, (also known as PROBIOTICS); are "progenic"— which means they support life.

What are "Probiotics"?

Probiotics are "live micro-organisms which when administered in adequate amounts, confer a health benefit on the host, beyond the common nutritional effects". (Source: FAO/WHO 2001).

Probiotics facilitate digestion, boost the immune system and prevent or treat diarrhea. Today, dozens of bifidobacteria and lactobacilli are marketed in certain foods (such as yogurts and fermented milk products). We have been consuming these probiotics since the Neolithic Era; (ABOUT 12, 000 YEARS AGO).

These bacteria provide a protective barrier that guards the intestinal wall against bad or "pathogenic" bacteria, parasites, fungi; viruses and environmental toxins. The good bacteria also create anti-microbial substances that destroy pathogenic organisms.

They are Mother Nature's powerful natural antibiotics, antivirals and antifungals!

Humans would be unable to survive without a rich and diverse array of good bacteria. These good bugs—our good immune soldiers protect our immune system. The main species which pre-dominate the small intestine are the" lactobacteria". The "bifidobacteria" predominate the large intestine. Humans depend on these microorganisms to absorb nutrients and to fight against infection. They also support the mucous membranes of the reproductive tract, respiratory system and sinus cavities.

In short—these "immune soldiers" comprise what is estimated to be 83 percent of the body's immune system.

TAKE-HOME MESSAGE:

MAINTAINING THE IDEAL RATIO OF "GOOD BACTERIA" OR "PROBIOTICS" TO BAD BACTERIA IS NOW RECOGNIZED AS THE SINGLE MOST IMPORTANT STEP YOU CAN TAKE TO PROTECT YOUR HEALTH (and to burn off some belly fat too1 ☺)

THE IDEAL RATIO OF GOOD TO BAD BACTERIA IS SAID TO BE ABOUT 9 TO 1 or 85 PERCENT GOOD TO 15 PERCENT "BAD".

Studies performed on obese people analyzing gut bacteria found higher amounts of bad bacteria and lower levels of good bacteria within these people.

1. In a recent study published on November 6th, 2014 in the Journal "Cell" at Cornell University; it was found that people with a higher amount of the most heritable gut microbe- "Christensenell Acae minuta" tend to be leaner. When added to germ-free mice without bacteria—the mice got leaner.

Thus, we can see the presence of lower levels of good bacteria within obese individuals could be a big reason why these people struggle with losing stubborn abdominal fat. Bad bugs could be sabotaging your efforts to slim down. You need to cultivate more good critters and fewer bad ones.

THE SOLUTION IS TO DITCH THE PROCESSED JUNK FOOD.

Trust me—when you clean out your INTESTINES AND YOUR COLON— you not only will LOOK better—you will FEEL better!

2. A recent double blind study in the European Journal of Clini-cal Nutrition found that obese test subjects who took pro-biotics daily for 12 weeks to RE-BALANCE their gut bacteria ratio were able to REDUCE THEIR ABDOMINAL FAT by nearly 5 (FIVE PERCENT! (source: Eur. J. Clin. Nutr.2010 June)

CORRECTING THE BALANCE between good and bad bacteria can have an IMMEDIATE EFFECT on losing belly flab!

B. THE DISEASE THAT YOUR DOCTOR CAN'T DIAGNOSE

WHAT IS LEAKY-GUT SYNDROME?

"Leaky Gut Syndrome" (LGS) for short; is also known as "Hyper-permeable Intestine" (source: www.scdlifestyle.com—)

Leaky Gut Syndrome is a fancy medical term that means the intes-tinal lining has become more POROUS— with more holes that are developing; these gaps are larger in size and the screening out process is no longer functioning properly.

Leaky gut is a condition that causes a BOATLOAD of health problems. This condition is rarely discussed in mainstream media. Most people do not have a clue that they have LGS!

THE UNKNOWN TRUTH IS THAT LGS IS A CHRONIC HIDDEN EPIDEMIC!

LGS AFFECTS MILLIONS OF PEOPLE IN INDUSTRIALIZED COUNTRIES!

Who knew?

LGS is also rarely discussed in doctors' offices—mostly because they CAN'T DIAGNOSE IT and don't recognize it. Ladies and gentlemen—it is MY DUTY to tell you—

LEAKY GUT SYNDROME IS THE DISEASE THAT YOR DOCTOR CAN'T DIAGNOSE. Oops—another reason to fire your doctor.

Later in this chapter, and throughout this book, you will be provided some LIFE SAVING HEALTH STRATEGIES.

DIETARY/DIGESTIVE STRATEGIES provided will show you how to REDUCE INFLAMMATION in your body— by choosing REAL WHOLE FOODS THAT "HEAL AND SEAL" YOUR GUT.

YOU CAN LEARN HOW TO FIX YOUR GUT TO FIX YOUR HEALTH

THIS WILL ALLOW YOU TO AVOID UNPLEASANT DOCTOR'S OFFICES!

Leaky gut begins in your small intestine. The small intestine is important because that's where most of your vitamins, minerals and other nutrients are absorbed. The small intestine contains microscopic pores so that nutrients can be absorbed into the bloodstream. When they are transferred to the bloodstream, these nutrients are then shuttled and deposited throughout the body by the blood.

The intestinal wall of the intestine is ULTRA –THIN. IT IS A ONE CELL-THICK WALL ONLY! Who knew? Think about that the next time you eat processed junk food. Do you ever consider where that slice of pizza really ended up? -☺)

The gut -lining is considered to be "semi-permeable". This means that the pores only allow certain SMALL things to enter the bloodstream and block other things from entering from the bloodstream. For example, specific molecules and nutrients are allowed to pass through but TOXINS and LARGE undigested food particles are BLOCKED.

Leaky gut causes the pores in your intestine to widen. GAPS are thus formed in the gut lining. When this happens, the undigested food particles and toxins that are SUPPOSED to be blocked— are allowed to make their way into the bloodstream. Because these "things" are not supposed to be in the blood, they USUALLY cause serious health problems.

When the gut is DAMAGED by environmental toxins, such as antibiotics, chlorinated water, industrial meat, processed food & drinks —ANY OF THOSE NEUROTOXINS allows these pathogenic organisms to take control.

These pathogenic organisms or bad bugs include Staphylococci, Straptococci, Bacilli, Clostrida, Candida Albicans, Enterobacteria, other parasites AND GOD KNOWS WHAT ELSE!

THESE PATHOGENIC TOXINS EAT THROUGH THE INTESTINAL WALL AND CAUSE GAPS IN THE GUT 'MUCOSAL' LINING.

THESE GAPS THEN ALLOW LARGE FOOD PARTICLES, YEASTS, BACTERIA AND ENVIRONMENTAL TOXINS TO CROSS INTO THE BLOODSTREAM.

From there, these "things" or pathogenic items travel THROUGH the bloodstream. They often cross the blood/brain barrier and lodge into

NEURAL TISSUE. (e.g. brain tissue, as well as the liver, other major organs, joints etc.

What happens next?

For example—let's say that undigested particles pass through the large pores or gaps in your gut lining. Your immune system says "Hey—! These foreign particles/toxins should not be here!

The immune system perceives this as an ATTACK by foreign invaders.

The immune system immediately mounts AN IMMUNE SYSTEM RESPONSE!

The immune response is to build up antibodies and create INFLAMMATION. Inflammation is the body's way of dealing with many diverse health issues- ranging from a sprained ankle to leady gut.

IT IS KNOWN THAT INFLAMMATION IS THE CORNERSTONE OF ALL DISEASES.

The real culprit underlying cardiovascular disease is inflammation— rather than cholesterol issues. (Statin drugs are not the answer; they inhibit your immune soldiers from protecting your immune castle-☺

As mentioned, because of the wider gaps in the gut lining, the toxins continue to POUR into the bloodstream and lodge in the body. The immune system builds MORE ANTIBOIDES— (healthy cells are attacked too.) The inflammation then becomes chronic—this starts a vicious cycle. This whole process destroys brain, organs, cells and joint tissues. This sets off the production of all kinds of "free radicals". Free radicals are those pesky "oxidants" which cause premature aging. Antioxidants are nutrients that are found in foods and supplements. They are kind of like our bodies "anti-rust" solution.

The net result of this vicious cycle is that your immune soldiers can't defend your immune castle. The bad bugs/bacteria wreak havoc on your health.

How does Leaky Gut happen?

There are several ways that LGS can develop. For example, if you are chronically constipated, over time the toxins in your stool will irritate the lining of your intestines. This irritation will eventually cause inflammation. This inflammation causes GAPS in the small intestine. The gaps widen; irritation and inflammation increases. Chronic inflammation then leads to IBS or IBD, Crohn's disease or colitis- or other digestive/autoimmune health problems.

ANOTHER MAJOR CAUSE OF LGS IS AN IMBALANCE IN THE RATIO BETWEEN GOOD AND BAD GUT BACTERIA.

This often shows up as leaky gut—or one of a <u>PLETHORA OF CONDITIONS</u> which either <u>CAUSES LEAKY GUT OR IS ASSOCIATED WITH LEAKY GUT</u>. Antacids and lozenges will not fix leaky gut— despite what the white coat crowd may tell you.

C.   THE REAL CULPRITS BEHIND GUT PROBLEMS

The real culprits behind LGS are <u>POOR DIET AND BAD LIFESTYLE CHOICES</u>.

<u>What are some of the symptoms of LGS?</u>

- Bloating, gas, constipation, diarrhea, acid-re-flux and/or digestive problems;

- Chronic fatigue and adrenal exhaustion;

- Food allergies and/or sensitivities;

- Skin rashes, acne, rosacea and other skin problems;

- Headaches and depression;

- Trouble sleeping'

- Inability to lose weight;

- Cravings for sugar/heavily refined carbohydrate "foods";

- Irritability, hostility, anger and belligerent behaviour;

This list is not <u>EXHAUSTIVE</u>—only <u>ILLUSTRATIVE</u>.

These symptoms may indeed be an indication that you have LGS. The problem is that these symptoms are also often intimately related and/or associated with <u>OTHER AUTOIMMUNE DISEASES</u>! They become mixed together as general symptoms of feeling miserable— a general sense that you are not feeling well.

Dr. Alessio Fasano suggests that you <u>CANNOT HAVE AUTOIMMUNE DISEASES WITHOUT</u> <u>LGS</u>! Thus—often identifying many gut/health issues is like asking which came first—the chicken or the egg?

Is a particular disease masquerading as LGS or is LGS only a symptom of such autoimmune diseases as Celiac disease, Multiple Sclerosis, Grave's, Hashimoto's etc.?

EITHER WAY—SCIENCE confirms Dr. Hippocrate's statement.. <u>All disease does begin in the gut</u>. Science tells us that 83 PERCENT of our immune system is in our gut.-

Who can argue with modern science? Who can argue with the Father of Medicine? His logic is unassailable.

On his website, <u>www.drperlmutter.com</u> , Dr. Perlmutter, appears to agree with Dr. Fasano, when the former states:

> <u>"Like these diseases, MS is a condition of increased inflammation with autoimmunity. It is known that the blood-brain barrier is broken down in Multiple Sclerosis. It is now becoming clear, however that like other auto-immune conditions, there is evidence to suggest that there is increased permeability in multiple sclerosis as well."</u>

If you have any doubts about <u>ALL OF THIS</u>—

<u>YOU CAN CONSULT "Dr. GOOGLE" (aka the WWW.)- ABOUT GUT HEALTH, DIGESTIVE HEALTH ISSUES AUTOIMMUNITY.</u>

<u>THERE YOU WILL FIND MORE THAN 11,000 SCIENTIFIC STUDIES THAT MODERN HEALTHCARE HAS OVERLOOKED!</u>

<u>TO FIND THE ANSWER TO YOUR HEALTH QUERIES—YOU WILL FIND THE EVIDENCE AND THE ANSWERS HIDDEN IN PLAIN SIGHT—VERY OFTEN IN PUBMED CLINICAL STUDIES!</u>

You will discover the strong association between poor health, linked with chronic diseases, such as Asthma, diabetes, rheumatoid arthritis, irritable bowel syndrome (IBS), psoriasis, chronic fatigue, heart failure, etc.—AND LGS. Later herein we will examine some of the scientific studies <u>CONNECTED WITH HEALTH ISSUES/DISEASES and BACTERIA.</u>

<u>What are the MAIN dietary triggers and lifestyle factors LINKED TO / CAUSING LGS?</u>

<u>THE 3 WORST CULPRITS CAUSING 'LGS' ARE:</u>

1. <u>ALL PROCESSED FOOD</u> (including GMO foods-
   or other "Franken-foods"-☺)

If Mother Nature didn't make it—YOU SHOULD N'T EAT IT!

2. **CHRONIC STRESS—**

   - **REDUCES BLOOD FLOW TO THE GUT!!**

3. **TOXIC ENVIRONMENTS- INCLUDING TOXIC NEGATIVE PEOPLE IN OUR LIVES.** (It really is true— a negative thought can kill you faster than a germ...-☺)

4. **SO—ENSURE THAT YOU HANGOUT WITH POSITIVE UPLIFTING PEOPLE!**

   Don't stay around negative people who suck your energy.

   "The greatest expression of strength is the up-lifting of others."

SIDEBAR—

According to the CDC (Center for Disease Control), **STRESS IS RESPONSIBLE FOR 85 PERCENT OF ALL CHRONIC DISEASES.**

It only makes sense that **STRESS** is a **HUGE LIFESTYLE FACTOR** in the development of **LGS and MOST DIGESTIVE AILMENTS/DISORDERS AND CHRONIC DISEASES.**

My last chapter- "Listen with your Ketogenic Heart" examines emotional health.

THE OTHER WORST CULPRITS (and DIETARY TRIGGERS ARE:

   - **DRUGS and ALL KIND OF MEDICATONS— (VACCINES TOO!)** — both prescribed and OTC e.g. antacids, laxatives, NSAIDS, CORTICOSTEROIDS and birth-control drugs;

     Sidebar—Vaccines, drugs and other toxic poisons;

   - **ANTIBIOTICS** — prescribed medications and/or antibiotics found in factory farmed MEAT and POULTRY;

   - **PASTEURIZED DAIRY**—besides possible other contaminants the component which will most damage your gut is A1 CASEIN;

   - **GLUTEN, GMO'S GRAINS, MANY FLOURS AND SUGARS ARE NEUROTOXINS WHICH EAT A HOLE IN YOUR GUT AND CAUSE "LEAKY GUT SYNDROME**

   - **SUGAR- aka-"The king of Neurotoxins"- in all of its EVIL FORMS;**

   - Artificial sweeteners, & additives most often found in sodas;

- ALCOHOLIC beverages;

- Chlorinated and/or fluoridated water is PARTICULARLY DAMGEROUS BECAUSE IT STERILIZES OUR GUT and repeated exposure DESTROYS THE PROGENIC BACTERIA IN OUR GUT;

- 80 THOUSAND TOXIC CHEMICALS AND OTH-ER POLLUTANTS— such AS:

    Pesticides/herbicides and poisons sprayed on plants and/or found in most soils. (Glyphosate is PURE evil.)

    PBA and PBS plastic that has leached into your gut;

- DENTAL FLUORIDE, and FLOURIDE-BASED TOOTHPASTES,

- AND THE EVIL NEUROTOXIN- TRICLOSAN- FOUND IN SOME ANTI-BACTERIAL SOAPS AND TOOTHPASTE;

- MERCURY FROM FOOD, WATER AND THE ENVIRON-MENT (ESPECIALLY FROM DENTAL WORK;

ANY TOXIC CHEMICAL THAT DOES NOT COME FROM MOTHER NATURE'S FARMACY WILL LIKELY CAUSE YOU TO SUFFER FROM A LEAKY GUT SYNDROME.

You will need to adopt an Elimination Diet to find out what culprit (s) are to blame for your gut health problems.

Recent scientific studies-

There is new research that clarifies how inflammatory bowel diseases (IBD) conditions that include ulcerative colitis and Crohn's disease are triggered and develop.

1. A study at Emory University published on September 13, 2012 in the online Journal "Immunity" (source: www.science-daily.com), studied LGS in Inflammatory Bowel Disease (IBD) Susceptibility. Lead author, Dr. Charles Parkos stated:

    Our results suggest that when there is a chroni-cally leaky intestine, defects in the immune system need to be present for the development of IBD.

    Breakdown of the intestinal barrier can occur as a result of in-testinal infections or STRESS. The normal response involves several components of the immune system that help to heal the injury while controlling invading bacteria. When this nor-mal responsive is defective and there is a leaky barrier, the risk of developing IBD is increased. (author's cap and underline)

2. A study from Yale University published in the Journal "Cell" on August 28th, 2014, (source" www.sciencedaily.com) looked at the effect of a handful of bacterial culprits that may cause inflammatory bowel diseases such as Chrohn's Disease and Ulcerative Colitis.

   I t is known that trillions of bacteria exist within the human intestinal microbiota. These bacteria play a critical role in the development and progression of IBD; yet it's thought that only a small number of bacterial species affect a person's susceptibility to IBD and is potential severity.

Professor Flavel from Yale stated:

> "A handful of bad bacteria are able to attain access to the immune system and get right at the gut...If you look at the bacteria to which we have made an immune response, you can begin to find those factors/"

Dr. Flavel's team focused on antibody coatings on the surface of bacteria. In particular his Yale researchers looked at bacteria with high concentrations of an antibody coating called "Immunoglobulin A (IgA).

> "The coating is our body's attempt to neutralize the bacteria, It binds to the bad bacteria." We only make those IgA responses to a limited number of organisms."

His team confirmed a correlation between high levels of IgA coating and inflammatory responses in the human intestine. To do this, his team collected "good" and "bad" bacteria from a small group of patients and transplanted them into mice. In HEALTHY mice, there was no influence on intestinal inflammation. In mice with induced colitis those with suspected "bad" bacteria showed signs of excessive inflammation.

The study's result indicates that anti-bacterial therapies for IBD ARE POSSIBLE. It was strongly suggested that such anti-bacterial approaches might include highly specific antibiotics, vaccines and probiotics. Dr. Flavel stated" We believe an anti-bacterial strategy has a place in treating IBD"

author's comment: -

Many doctors/researchers are afraid to ADMIT that Mother Nature knows best. It's the old story— most conventional doctors are afraid to think outside of the pill...-☺)

3. Fortunately Belgium researchers are not so close-minded. In their studies, they found that people with either CHRONIC

FATIGUE SYNDROME OR MAJOR DEPRESSIVE DISORDER
showed laboratory evidence of Leaky Gut Syndrome (LGS).

They compared a LGS group with a normal healthy group. They clearly demonstrated that treatment with DIET AND SPE-CIFIC NUTRIENTS NOT ONLY REVERSED LABORATORY SIGNS OF LGS—BUT ALSO IMMPROVED SYMPTOMS OF FATIGUE, MALAISE AND DEPRESSION. (Sources: J. Affect. Disord. April 2007; Neuro Endocrinol. Lett. June, Feb and Dec. 2008

D.   STRATEGIES TO "HEAL AND SEAL" YOUR GUT

Now that you know what LGS is and how it occurs, you need to take the appropriate strategies to "heal" and "seal" your gut. BTW, do not feel intimidated by LGS.

IN TODAY'S MODERN WESTERN WORLD—MOST PEOPLE HAVE A SYMPTOM OR TWO OF LGS—

EVEN IF THEY DO NOT HAVE GUT PROBLEMS THEY CONSIDER AS SERIOUS.

If you have headaches and keep POPPING aspirin, ibuprofen, Tylenol etc…How would you feel if you go blind? Btw: Never, ever take Tylenol after a bout of drinking at the local bar. It may be the last pill that you ever take. This is only one of thousands of examples where taken together –2 drugs have a much greater death RISK than either one taken alone. If you have that grilled factory farmed steak, followed by a few drinks and take Tylenol –- you had better be prepared to meet your Maker!

Most serious health issues like cancer often take years to develop. You should not wait until the gaps in your gut lining become large enough to send us to emergency room. Please take a proactive position. No one can fix your gut—but YOU.

ONLY YOU ARE IN CONTROL OF YOUR FOOD INTAKE.

You need to pay attention; LISTEN to what your body is telling you. If you take the pill approach—sooner or later have you will have to pay the piper. It's like the old commercial where the mechanic used to say—"you can pay me now or pay me later".

Don't wait until you're too sick before you find out what is going on with your health. I think that's why they call it a "Check-up?" There's a lot of wisdom in the old adage—"A stitch in time, saves nine". Many people take better care of their car than their bodies. It's easy to buy a new car;—not so easy to get a new body.

Gentlemen—if there is a lady in your life—discuss your health issues with her. Research shows that the members of the distaff generally are smarter about taking care of their health. Mother Nature likely provided them with more common sense because they are usually the parent who plays a bigger part in the health decisions affecting their children.

If you have pain or don't feel well, you should take active measures to address the problem <u>FORTHWITH—THE DAY BEFORE YESTERDAY AS WE LAWYERS SAY!</u> Fortunately if you are reading this book—you have already decided to take control of your health.

<u>YOU WILL BE GLAD THAT YOU MADE THE DECISION TO TAKE CONTROL OF YOUR HEALTH.</u> Don't be one of those people who are so busy making millions of dollars only to wake up and find that that nagging little pain has turned into a very serious health issue.

If you neglect your health—what about your spouse, children and family members?

What happens to them?

If you choose to be negligent about getting in shape—are you being fair to the rest of your family? Have you thought about what it would be like to say that you've been diagnosed with diabetes or heart disease? If you keep your cell phone next to your cheek for 10 years, research suggests that that is the average time required for cancer of the cheek.

Will you be diagnosed with diabetes because you felt that being overweight was only a normal part of growing old?

<u>YOU HAVE TO DO YOUR OWN DUE DILIGENCE!</u>

If you spend 10 minutes each day researching a particular health issue or potential health issue which interests you—after a few months you will discover that you can and you need to be YOU OWN DOCTOR. You need to find health solutions for yourself. I am convinced that I have given you some excellent tools and resources in the present book. You can always consult www.greenmed.info.com or dr. Google... Thanks to the internet, you can get the health information that you need. If you do decide to keep your doctor, you must go to him armed with knowledge. You will likely be able to educate him! If he is too busy taking his own rectal temperature to read the scientific literature—you can read and understand the case studies in the medical literature.

LGS and all of the related health issues are pivotal in your quest for SUPERHEALTH. With the dietary strategies that are provided below— you will be in a positon to understand the dietary solutions to gut problems. Once your gut is restored then you can verify whether the KETOGENIC DIET is right for you.

(As you might guess- it's my favourite… that's one of the reasons that I'm writing this health book-☺) I want you to have the BEST-LEADING EDGE HEALTH INFORMATION available. This book will be a good reference book for the rest of your days.

Obviously, because the entire notion of LGS is largely unknown to most conventional doctors—you will have to DIY;

Indeed—the central theme in this book is that if you want something done—do it yourself. Of all things in life—there are no better examples than taking care of your health. Food is information. Food is Medicine. Medicine is food.

You have the power to re-program your genes by eating a healthy diet!

How awesome is that?

Step Number one.

Dr. Robert Rountree, a reputed expert in Autoimmune diseases, including LGS —points out that poor gut health develops in the CONTEXT OF AN INFLAMMATORY GUT.

From my research it appears that all of the notable health care providers in the gut/brain/health area agree that IMPROVING A PATIENT/ CLIENT'S DIET IS THE NUMBER ONE STEP.

Many experts suggest an ELIMINATION DIET (you can Google up that). This kind of diet is used to identify food(s) that are or could be causing INFLAMMATION. During an Elimination Diet, you remove common inflammatory triggers from your diet for about 2 weeks. Then you add back one at a time, while gauging your symptoms.

If you feel better when you avoid one food, but your symptoms return when you add it back in, you continue to avoid that food.

YOU CAN START BY ELIMINATING THE BIG FOUR TOXIC TRIGGERS:

- Conventional Dairy

- Gluten- Sugar- <u>AND ALL OF THE NEUROTOXINS!</u>

- **Excessive Alcohol**

You can also check out THE GAPS DIET (Gut and Psychology Syndrome) advocated by Dr. Natasha Campbell-McBride.

If the toxic food(s) is identified- you can proceed to step number two. If not, then you need some expertise to have some serious blood and body fluids analyzed for some of the bad things mentioned above. All to say, if dietary factors are not identified as the culprits, it is likely that the culprit is one or more of the other toxic chemicals or toxic environmental factors.

You may have an undiagnosed problem of <u>STRESS</u>. Btw—<u>EVEN TOO MUCH GOOD</u> STRESS YOUR LIFE CAN CAUSE PROBLEMS!

<u>YOU MUST REDUCE YOUR STRESS!</u>

<u>Step number Two</u>

<u>EAT A VARIETY OF ORGANIC WHOLE FOODS.</u> Your body needs the proper nutrients to heal. Eat a "rainbow" often- richly colored veggies – organic (of course!) Try to add one new green veggie (e.g. broccoli, kale, spinach etc.)

<u>YOUR BODY KNOWS HOW TO RECOVER AND HEAL-</u>

<u>ONCE YOU GIVE IT THE RIGHT THINGS!</u>

Dr. Jeffrey Smith reminds us that you should avoid the dangerous potential of GMO foods and eat only organic.

<u>YOU CAN REMIND YOURSELF— TO STOP PUTTING GASOLINE ON THE FIRE!</u>

<u>Step number three</u>

TAKE CARE OF YOUR GUT MICROBIOME!

The Health of your Gut is fundamentally important for the Health of your entire body. You gut is your <u>FIRST BRAIN.</u> It is a theme of this health book that you need to care for both of your BRAINS- first and foremost.

As stated supra, ONE HUGE STEP you can take to prevent or reverse autoimmune disease is to care for your Microbiome. If you take care of the trillions of microscopic critters living in your gut—THEY WILL TAKE CARE OF YOU! It's that simple.

In the remaining subsections of this chapter, we will examine some amazing new research involving your microbiota. You will see how powerful these microorganisms really are.

Dr. David Perlmutter says that you've got to focus on <u>THE RESTORATION OF YOUR GUT BACTERIA</u>. Dr. Perlmutter will be the Chief Editor of a very prestigious new journal called the Gut and Brain Journal. It will be accessible to the public.

You are also advised to consult his website at <u>www.drperlmutter.com</u> He is also on Facebook. He is THE MAN in this entire area of Gut/Brain Health. If you have any gut heath issues and or want to learn more- highly recommend checking him out.

<u>Step number four</u>

<u>REPAIR YOUR GUT WITH HEALING FOODS, PREBIOTICS AND PROBIOTICS</u>

<u>AND EAT AN ANTI-INFLAMMATORY DIET</u> (A HEALING KETOGENIC DIET).

The research is now clear that "Supplementing with Probiotics every single day is <u>even more important to your health than taking a daily multi-vitamin!</u>

<u>OVEREAT A VARIETY OF FERMENTED FOODS</u> (Probiotics):

- **Quality Sauerkraut, Kombucha, Coconut Water Kefir, Kimchi,**

- **Lassi (Indian yogurt drink)**

- **Tempeh,**

- **Organic Good Quality Probiotic Yogurt**

- **Fermented veggies such as pickles, beets, eggplant, on- ions, squash, cucumbers (actually a fruit), carrots**

<u>OTHER GREAT ANTI-INFLAMMATORY FOODS:</u>

- **Coconut products, avocadoes, olive oil, ber- ries, grass-fed beef; wild game, wild salmon, or- ganic pastured poultry and eggs), raw cheese,**

- **Apple cider vinegar**

- **Chia seeds – <u>ARE ONE OF THE BEST FOODS ON THE PLANET.</u>**

- **<u>BONE BROTH and MORE BONE BROTH!</u>**

- Garlic (Far more effective than Pharmaceutical Antibiotics in fighting common bacteria known as " tcampylactobacter bacterium" which currently affects more than 2.4 million Americans every year- source: Washington State University study.)

SUPPLEMENT WITH A QUALITY PROBIOTIC such as L-Glutamine, Quercetin, Licorice Root, Tumeric, D-3 etc.

This sums up my best gut-healing strategies.

E. OUR GUT IS OUR FIRST BRAIN!

WOW— it's true! Many researchers in the scientific community profess "your gut is your second brain."

Now— researchers/scientists/neurologists now suggest that that our gut MAY BE OUR FIRST BRAIN!

This is an EXCITING NEW AREA of active, fascinating research. The relationship between our gut and our brain is so complex and intricate.

They really work as ONE COMPLEX NEURAL/GUT SYSTEM. Who knew?

Actually, there is one gentleman who had a darn good idea about the gut-brain connection. That man was named Dr. Hippocrates. He had this figured out 2, 500 years ago.

Our brain and gut work together on so many of the same neural and other pathways. Our gut and our brain are constantly taking to each other and exchanging information. The gut-brain is one complex loop of nerves/bacteria and all sorts of chemical messengers.

Above, we mentioned that about 95 percent of our serotonin (our "feel good hormone') is manufactured in our gut. Many of our neurotransmitters travel back and forth via our CNS, central nervous system and our ENS, or enteral nervous system. The information processed by the gut and sent up to the brain has everything to do with our sense of well-being. Our gut—and its trillions of bacteria play a huge role in our health and well-being.

THIS IS A ' THE' STARTING POINT FOR ANYONE WHO WANTS TO BE HEALTHY

TO HAVE SUPERHEALTH —you should FIRST AND FOREMOST LOOK TO YOUR GUT—from the outside AND FROM THE INSIDE! -☺)

An recent gut microbe study was titled: The way to a man's heart is through his gut- MICROBIOTA! Incredible but true!

MOST cravings originate with the gut-brain connection. Fermented foods (probiotics) for example, play an extremely important role; they not only fix LGS—but also tell our brain that good bacteria will repair that indigestion. As we have seen, gut health is all about the trillions of good bacteria that support and nourish our immune system. Now research shows that these good bacteria also have a HUGE INFLUENCE ON OUR BRAIN HEALTH.

4 ways our MICROBIOME affects brain health and behavior.

- It activates a large nerve called the VAGUS nerve. This nerve connects the gut and the brain. Our vagus nerve connects 100 million nerve cells from the digestive tract to the base of our brain. Research shows that when this nerve is cut in rats—it causes big behavioral and other health problems;

- Our microbiome and our brain act together to activate our immune system—our gut/brain especially activates and regulates special cells called "T-cells";

- The brain activates the gut's endocrine system—which produces many kinds of different neurotransmitters (SPECIAL BACTERIA PRODUCE NEUROENDOCRINAL HORMONES);

- Micro-based therapy allows the inoculation of the gut with good bacteria to "fix" problems like autism, depression and some bad behaviors;

This is a thumbnail sketch of some very complex physiological gut/brain connection mechanism. The gut /brain/ microbial relationship is SO COMPLEX — it has been dubbed a new science.

This science is called "MICROBIAL ENDOCRINOLOGY".

What is microbial endocrinology?

It's a form of signalling which is based on bidirectional neurochemical interactions between our neurophysiological system and our microbiome. It was introduced two decades ago. It has been termed microbial endocrinology.

An abstract from a scientific study published in the Journal Adv. Exp Med Biol. 2014, reported at PUBMED no. 24997027 describes it:

"Microbial endocrinology is defined as the study of the ability of organisms to both produce and recognize neurochemicals that originate either within the micro-organisms themselves or with the host they inhabit. As such microbial endocrinology represents the intersection of the fields of microbiology and neurobiology. The acquisition of neurochemical –based cell-to-cell signalling mechanisms in eukaryotic organisms is believed to have been acquired due the case horizontal gene transfer from prokaryotic microorganisms. When considered in the contest of the macrobiotics ability to influence host behavior, microbial endocrinology with its theoretical basis rooted in shared neuroendocrine signalling mechanisms provides for testable experiments with which to understand the role of microbiota in host behavior and as importantly the ability of the host to influence the microbiotic through neuro-endocrine-based mechanisms."

Pretty complicated eh? Not to worry. All you need to remember is that we're all in the same boat. This new science is new to the world. Here is some fancy technical explanations but you'll get it.

Many of the neuroendocrine hormone biosynthetic pathways are more commonly associated with eukaryotic cells are found in prokaryotic cells. The acquisition of such neurochemical-based synthesis pathways by eukaryotic systems is believed to be due to lateral gene transfer from bacteria. This leads to treatment or specific mental illness or by modulation of the microbiome-gut-brain-axis. THIS IS A SCIENTIFIC explanation showing the intimate interaction of gut/brain.

Some individuals suffering from inflammatory bowel diseases, which are characterized by altered microbial diversity, have demonstrated poorer EMOTIONAL FUNCTIONS SUCH AS ANXIETY AND DEPRESSION.

Many studies demonstrate the ability of a specific pathogen or altered microbiome to influence (HOST) BEHAVIOR. These studies all produce immune-related sequelae that result in the release of host immune factors—such as cytokines and inflammatory mediators, that have known NEURONAL TARGETS, both within the CNS (Central Nervous System) and the (ENS), the Enteric Nervous System.

Since the 1990's this microbial-gut-brain-axis (connection) has been the subject of growing investigation. It has even created the use of the expression 'MIND-ALTERING BUGS". Most of the studies have focused on the ability of bacteria (commensal, pathogenic or probiotic) to make a plethora of neural substrates in the ENS and CNS. Little attention had been focused on the evolutionary properties that suggest that the microbiome is in <u>CONSTANT COMMUNICATION</u> with the host (our) neurophysiological system. The ability of bacteria to recognize the very same neurotransmitters that are found in host suggests a <u>BIODIRECTIONAL ENVIRONMENT</u> where the microbiome can influence the host and the host can influence the microbiome. This complex level of interconnection by a shared evolutionary pathway signalling mechanism suggests that:

"THEY MONITOR US...AND WE MONITOR THEM!"

How cool is that?

<u>WE ARE ONLY BEGINNING TO SCRATCH THE SURFACE OF THE IMPORTANCE OF THE MICROBIOME FOR HUMAN HEALTH!</u>

<u>THE KEY TO SUPERHEALTH IS TO BUILD BRAIN HEALTH.</u>

<u>TO OBTAIN SUPERHEALTH WE MUST FEED BOTH OF OUR BRAINS- THE BRAIN IN OUR HEAD AND THE OTHER BRAIN IN OUR GUT!</u>

In the next subsection, we examine some recent case studies that really help to explain the practical health implications of the gut/brain connection. A brief review of these studies will provide you with a much clearer understanding of the gut/brain relationship.

You will gain a new respect for bacteria, phages and other microorganism. You will come to appreciate the pivotal role that bugs play not only in our gut health—but in our <u>ENTIRE HEALTH</u>. So—let's get started with a review of some recent scientific studies.

F. PROBIOTICS 101

What we eat is the <u>GREATEST DETERMINER</u> of what kinds of bacteria live in our guts. For example, the guts of people living in Japan, for example, contain specialized bacteria that aid in the digestion of seaweed.

Studies have shown that we can change the composition of our gut flora within <u>AS LITTLE AS 24 HOURS AFTER CHANGING OUR DIET!</u>

How cool is that?

Ditch the ANTIBIOTICS, tums, antacids, lozenges and poison pills!

<u>FEED YOUR BODY SOME REAL MEDICINE.</u>

Feed your body some good probiotics—from Mother Nature's Farmacy.

You remember that microorganisms (probiotics) when administered in adequate amounts, confer A HUGE HEALTH BENEFIT on the host (US) beyond the common nutritional effects.

They facilitate fiber digestion, boost the immune system and prevent or treat diarrhea. Today, dozens of bifidobacteria and lactobacilli are marketed in certain foods (such as yogurts or fermented milk products).

Unless you have been living under a rock, you know that fermented foods—especially yogurts—contain larger amounts of live bacteria. (You have no doubt seen the commercials by yogurt companies.) We have been consuming these kinds of fermented foods since the Neolithic Era (12,000 years ago—give or take a few hundred years.). But—our understanding of the REAL IMPACT of these kinds of foods ON OUR DIGESTIVE TRACT has remained largely unknown.

Great news—the Jury is in!

THE GREAT NEWS IS THAT THE PLAINTIFFS—THE TRILLIONS OF BACTERIA/MICROSCOPIC CRITTERS— HAVE WON THEIR CASE!—☺)

1. In a study published in the Journal Scientific Reports on September 11th, 2014, researchers from INRA, The French National Institute for Agricultural Research has made a major breakthrough in this field. (source: www.press.inra.fr) This breakthrough has expanded the scientific knowledge on the role of this microbiota and resulted in the discovery of many bacterial species hitherto unknown. In this study, researchers studied the effect of the ingestion of fermented milk on individuals afflicted with Irritable Bowel Syndrome (IBS).

SIDEBAR-

IBS IS A PATHOLOGY AFFECTING 20 PERCENT OF THE ADULT POPULATION IN INDUSTRIALIZED COUNTRIES.

The researchers found that the fermented milk product (probiotic) increased the abundance of certain bacteria naturally producing "butyrate"; but—the global composition of the gut flora remained unchanged. Butyrate is known for its beneficial effects on gut health. Previous studies had shown a DECREASE in butyrate producing bacteria in IBS individuals. Moreover, the scientists observed a DECREASE of "Biophila wadsworthia bacteria—which is thought to be involved in the development of intestinal diseases.

The lead author of the study, Dusko Ehrlich stated:

"Up until now, it was impossible to study the impact of probiotics n gut microbiota at a bacteria species level. From now on we will have a much more detailed view of the dynamics of this ecosystem".

2. In a study published in the European Journal of Clinical Nutrition in 2010, researchers studied the effects of supplementing with a fermented dairy (strawberry-flavoured) probiotic for 90 consecutive days. The drink contained the bacteria lactobacillus casei and was administered to 638 children—(3 to 6 years old) in Washington D.C.

   The researchers found the incidence rate of CIDS (Common Infectious Diseases) was 19 PERCENT LOWER.

3. In a study published on March 5th, 2014, in the European Journal of Clinical Nutrition 425 hay fever sufferers took probiotics for 5 weeks. The probiotics contained Lactobacillus paracases, and subp.paracasei LP33.

   What were the results? The sufferers showed significant improvements—especially in OCULAR SYMPTOMS.

SIDEBAR—

THIS IS THE FIRST STUDY TO SHOW THAT A PROBIOTIC IS EFFECTIVE IN ALLERGIC RHINITIS… The researchers suggested that a probiotic is effective in allergic rhinitis as an ADD ON THERAPY "to recommended medicinal treatment".

Do you have any drug-related questions?

SIDEBAR 2-

HAY FEVER is an allergic reaction to POLLEN or fungal spores, most commonly—grass pollen. According to the American Academy of ALERGY ASTHMA AND IMMUNOLOGY—about 60 MILLION PEOPLE IN the USA ARE AFFECTED BY "ALLERGIC RHINITIS"

The immune system mistakes the spores for harmful invaders and white blood cells- T helper type 2 (Th 2) Lymphocytes which produce protein-like cytokines, such as interleukin- 4 (iL-4, IL-5, and iL-6 which in turn promote the synthesis of the immune chemicals immunoglobulins (IS) to bind to the pollen and fight them off.

Would you rather take Mother Nature's probiotics and get relief?

Would you prefer to suffer the effects of some poisonous drug?

Are you prepared to suffer physically and financially for the rest of your life!

Do **PROBIOTICS** help with the prevention of URT'S? (URT'S are another fancy medical term for Upper Respiratory Infections). What do you think? Do you think that the right kind of good bugs can kill these bad bugs—and/or prevent them from making us sick?

Many studies have proven **A "POSITIVE CORRELATION" BETWEEN PROBIOTIC SUPPLEMENTATION AND IMMUNITY.**

BUT –ONCE AGAIN- THOSE FRIENDLY LITTLE CRITTERS HAVE SHOWN US THEIR POWER AS MEDICINE!

4. A study published on September 23, 2014 in the European Journal of Clinical **NUTRITION LEAVES NO DOUBT ABOUT THE EFFECTIVENESS OF PROBIOTICS FOR PREVENTING THE COMMON COLD.**

   The study gave fifty-seven kids aged 3 to 5 years) some PROBIOTICS CALLED Lactobacillus acidophilus, bifidobacterium and bifidobacterium lactis strains coupled with Vitamin C.

Can you guess what happened?

The kids who received the **PROBIOTICS HAD 33 PERCENT FEWER URTS-!**

Moreover all kids were less reliant on 'medicine"; spent less time was spent on antibiotics; pain-killers, cough medicines, harmful drugs etc. Oops—less money for Big Pharma and your doctor.

OMG! If you give your kids the proper nutrients/probiotics—**FEWER SICK DAYS MEANS MORE TIME FOR YOU**- less money to pay for doctor's bills, baby-sitters etc.

In MANY OF THESE STUDIES you can read the exact words of the researchers. They are often very cautious not to bite the pharmaceutical hand that feeds them. They often use qualifying words to **DOWNPLAY THE EFFECTIVENESS OF NATURAL REMEDIES.**

5. Another study used strains of these 3 bacteria—Lactobacillus Acidophilis Rosell-52, Bifodobacterium infantis Rosell-33 and Bifidobacterium Rosell 71 in a trial of 135 children. This combination of probiotic and prebiotic significantly reduced the risk of URTs and GASTOINTESTINAL INFECTIONS BY 25 PERCENT over a 3 month period.

Another recent study published in 2014 in Nutritional Reviews, analysed 5 notable studies investigating the effects of prebiotics and their impact on infant immunity. The researchers concluded that there was significant evidence to suggest that prebiotics can play a preventative role to DECREASE INFECTIONS in children—AS WELL AS REDUCE THE PRESCRIPTION OF ANTIBIOTIC TREATMENTS TO CHILDREN.

6. Studies in adults also report a positive correlation between probiotics and immunity. Bifidobacterium Lactis B1-04 was found to reduce the incidence of URTs in a group of 465 by 27 PERCENT! The scientific evidence is showing that PROBIOTICS PLAY A SIGNIFICANT ROLE IN PREVENTING URT INFECTIONS in both children and adults. Further research will identify exactly which specific strains are most effective..

THE EVIDENCE SHOWS THAT PROBIOTICS COULD CUT HEALTH CARE COSTS AND ANTIBIOTIC USE AND MAKE US MUCH HEALTHIER!

7. A recent study published by Medical News on September 2014 reported on a study suggesting that "Granny Smith Apples" could protect against OBESITY by balancing out the proportions of "good gut bacteria," Researchers from Washington State University found that the fibers and polyphenols in these apples are unscathed when they reach the colon, even after they are exposed to stomach acid and digestive enzymes. The bacteria in the colon then ferment these compounds producing butyric acid that triggers the growth of good bacteria. The result is protection against obesity.

   Once again, Mother Nature flexes her bacterial muscles.

8. A study reported in July 2014 detailed the creation of a probiotic that researchers say could prevent OBESITY. Dr. Sean Davies of Vanderbuilt University in Nashville, TN genetically modified a strain of bacteria that colonizes the gut. "Eschenicia cociNisssle 1917 was used to produce a compound called "N-acyl-phosphatdyleethanolamine (NAPE) which can reduce food intake. On giving this bacteria to mice fed a high-fat diet for 8 weeks, the team found that it significantly reduced their food intake, body fat and the incidence of hepatosteatosis, (fatty liver) compared with control mice.

9. Another recent study published in the Journal of Clinical Investigation found that certain bacteria can produce a therapeutic compound in the gut which stopped weight gain; insulin resistance and other health complications on a high-fat diet.

10. A 2012 study reported by Medical News Today suggested that bacteria residing in the large intestine can slow down the activity of ener-

gy-burning BROWN FAT, contributing to the development of obesity.

EXTENSIVE RESEARCH PROVES THAT NATURAL GUT BACTERIA PLAY AN IMPORTANT ROLE IN THE DEVELOPMENT OF OBESITY, DIABETES AND CARDIOVASCULAR DISEASE.

11. A recent Japanese study published in the Journal of Functional Foods on November 2012 found that people who consumed yogurt containing <u>TWO</u> novel strains of probiotics experienced small losses in <u>BODY FAT</u> (13.3 percent reduction in subcutaneous fat)— but no changes in bodyweight. The Japanese study extends previous findings from Kyushu University researchers which showed "LG205- Lactobacillus gasseri) may reduce fat levels (adiposity) and fat cells in animals.

    The bacteria "BACILLUS SUBTILIS" is an important part of the fermented food called" NATTO". The consumption of this traditional Japanese Food has been linked to several health benefits. Various strains of this fermented food have been shown to be beneficial in humans. A comprehensive clinical review showed that probiotic supplementation with bacillus subtilis improves symptoms of IBS (Irritable Bowel Syndrome); suppress the growth of harmful pathogens and enhances the growth of lactobacillus. (source: Thompkins, T.A. et al. (2008 and Thompkins et al. (20100" A comprehensive review of Post market clinical studies performed in adults with an Asian Probiotic Formulation")

12. In a study published in 2012 in the British Journal of Nutrition found that certain probiotic strains boost measures of immune response. A 2001 Cochrane review concluded that probiotics may prevent colds, flu and upper respiratory infections.

13. A 2010 Review of the scientific controlled studies published in the World Journal of Gastroenterology found that certain strains of B. lactis and L casei improved stool consistency and frequency of bowel movements in people with constipation.

These clinical studies show <u>COMPELLING EVIDENCE</u> of the importance of the variety of good bacteria or probiotics.

<u>BUILDING A HEALTHY MICROBIOME IS STEP ONE ON YOUR JOURNEY TO SUPERHEALTH</u>. -after firing your doctor of course—☺)

<u>YOU CAN SEE HOW INTIMATE IS THE GUT/BRAIN CONNECTION!</u> You can really appreciate why the gut is considered by many to be our first brain.

At the outset of this chapter, we mentioned how our microbiome or gut flora is composed of millions bacterial bugs. Above, we mentioned that our gut houses 1 QUADRILLION VIRUSES CALLED "BACTERIOPHAGES".

Let/s now examine how these microscopic critters affect our gut health.

G.   SNOT CAN BE YOUR FRIEND

What is a "bacteriophage'? or "phage" for short.

According to (http://phages.org)

> "A bacteriophage is kind of virus that can infect and rep-licate itself inside bacterial cells. The virus has a protein-encapsulated DNA or RNA genome and can have simple or complex anatomies. There are many types of phages including M13, T phage, lambda page, MS2 64 and Phix 174.
>
> Viruses cannot multiply through the division of cells because they are acellular—(they do not have cells). Instead they seek a host cell in which they replicate and assemble themselves using the metabolism and machinery of the host cell.
>
> Different species of viral populations undergo viral life cycles, but for temperate phages they must choose between "lystic and lysogeny"..." (author underline)

In essence—phages are viruses created by BACTERIA—THAT TARGET AND DESTROY OTHER BACTERIA.

They are of great interest to scientists, because if they could be CONTROLLED- they could provide THE ULTIMATE ANTIBACTERIAL AGENT! Unfortunately, despite a lot of research since this observa-tion, nearly a century ago, very little is known about how phages function—particularly in the human gut.

An exciting new discovery has been made by accident. Scientists discovered something that HAD NEVER BEEN SEEN BEFORE. They discovered a strain of bacteria that create a phage for the express purpose of KILLING OFF OTHER BACTERIA that are competing for the same resources.

Researchers are calling it "A FORM OF BACTERIAL WARFARE!

In this study published by the University of Texas on October 9th, 2012 at http//phys.org, researchers found that a certain type of bacteria that lives in the mammalian gut creates a virus to kill of competitors.

As studied above, we know that the gut is home to trillions of bacteria. Some provide benefits to the host (US), such as helping to digest certain foods. But—others are bad and they cause digestive problems.

One bug in particular—the plentiful ENTEROCOCCUS FAECALIS appears to live benignly without causing problems in the gut. BUT— it causes a LOT of problems when it gets into the BLOODSTREAM.

THIS BUG ACCOUNTS FOR A BOATLOAD OF HOSPITAL ACQUIRED INFECTIONS.

In looking at a particular STRAIN of Enterrococcus Faecalis known as U583, the researchers found that when it was introduced ALONE in a germ-free mouse gut—IT BEGAN CHURNING OUT PHAGES; which seemed counter-productive, because it takes a lot of energy to do that. Upon a closer look, here is what they discovered.

V583 DID HAVE A PURPOSE— TO KILL OFF OTHER STRAINS OF E. FAECALIS that might show up gobbling resources.

How cool is that—Bacterial Warfare! Researchers were excited about the future possibilities to create phages to use as targeted weapons. Let the bug wars begin! -☺)

Another recent study also revealed some surprises about viruses. We know that BACTERIA can be friends or foes. The can cause infection and disease. But the can also help us lose weight and get healthy.

This study published on May 20th, 2013 in the online Journal of The Proceedings of National Academy of Science found that VIRUSES HAVE A DUAL NATURE TOO.

FOR THE FIRST TIME RESEARCHERS HAVE SHOWN THAT VIRUSES CAN HELP OUR BODIES FIGHT OFF INVADING MICROBES.

One of our most important lines of defence against bacterial invaders is MUCUS.

You guessed it— SNOT CAN BE OUR FRIEND! -☺)

Mucus is a slimy substance that coats the inside of the mouth, nose, eyelids, and digestive tract, to name just a few places; creating a barrier to the outside world.

According to Jeremy Barr, a microbiologist at San Diego State University in California-

" Mucus is actually a really cool and complex substance"

Its gel-like consistency I thanks to mucins— large bottled- brushed shaped molecules made up of a protein backbone surrounded by strings of sugars. In between the mucins is a soup of nutrients and chemicals adapted to keep germs close, but not too close. Microbes such as bacteria live near the surface of the layer, whereas he mucus at the bottom, near the cells that produce it , is almost sterile.

Mucus is home to phages, viruses that infect and kill bacteria. They can be found wherever bacteria reside. Mr. Barr notices that there were even MORE PHAGES IN MUCUS- THAN IN MUCUS-FREE AREAS JUST MILLIMETERS AWAY.

For example, the saliva surrounding human gums had about 5 phages to every bacterial cell (5 to 1)—whereas the ration at the mucosal surface of the gum itself was closer to 40 to 1.

What are these phages doing?

To find out, Mr. Barr grew human lung tissue in his lab. (Lungs are one of the body's surfaces that are protected by mucus.) Researchers took some lung cells—WITHOUT MUCUS and CELLS WITHOUT MUCUS- MAKING ABILITY.

When incubated overnight with the bacterium Escherichia coli, about 50 PERCENT of the cells in each culture died. The mucus made no difference to their survival.

BUT- when the researchers added a phage that targets E. coli to the cultures—SURVIVAL RATES SKYROCKETED FOR THE MUCUS – PRODUCING CELLS.

How cool is that?

This disparity shows that phages can kill harmful bacteria. Barr says: "It's not clear whether they help or hurt beneficial bacteria—that may depend on which types of phages are present.

In a related series of experiments, the team found that the phages are studded with antibody-like molecules that grab onto the sugar chains in mucins. This keeps the phages in the mucus—where they have access to bacteria and suggests that the viruses and the mucus-producing tissue have adapted to be compatible with each other.

Mucus-covered surfaces are not unique to humans. This kind of slime can be found throughout the animal kingdom. Protective phages seem to be equally widespread and dense populations were in every species that the scientists sampled.

Added Mr. Barr:

> " It's a novel immune system that we think is applicable to all mucosal surfaces, and it's one of the first examples of a direct symbiosis between phages and an animal host. "

Mother Nature makes no mistakes. Snot is our friend.

H. THE POWER OF POO! OMG!

What does "Poo" (a slang word for fecal matter or stool) have to do with BACTERIA?

Fecal matter is a gray area (actually more brown-☺), neither DRUG NOR DEVICE NOR TISSUE. Actually, FECAL MATTER IS ABOUT 50 PERCENT BACTERIA.

We are in the age of do-it-yourself- DIY .

CONVENTIONAL MEDICINE HAS FAILED. If you want something done RIGHT—YOU MUST DO IT YOURSELF. You must take control of your health—no one else will or can. It's entirely up to you.

In the last few years a forward-thinking healthcare providers have started using "FMT" which stands for "FECAL MICROBIOTA THERAPY". This treatment also goes by the names of —

- "FECAL BACTERIOTHERAPY

- " STOOL TRANSPLANT"

- " HUMAN PROBIOTIC INFUSION

Apparently FMT is approved and widely available—but NOT USED-AND DIFFICULT TO OBTAIN!

There ae a set of guidelines, battery of tests for donors, blood tests for diseases like HIV, stool screening for parasites, etc. The price for donor testing is $ 500-to $ 1,500.00 depending...

Does FMT work? ABSOLUTELY!

It's a BRAND-NEW THERAPY. HISTORY TELLS US THAT THE YELLOW EMPEROR SUCCESSFULLY USED FMT IN THE 4TH CENTURY B.C!

It has been successfully used by the Mayo Clinic.

IN A RECENT TRIAL, FMT THERAPY (an infusion of feces) WENT HEAD TO HEAD AGAINST A DRUG CALLED VANCOMYCIN. ALL OF THE PATIENTS HAD THE DEADLY INFECTION OF C.DIFFICLE.

Guess what?

MOTHER NATURE'S BACTERIA WON HANDS DOWN!

THE PATIENTS WHO RECEIVED A FECAL TRANSPLANT HAD A 94 PERCENT CURE RATE!

THE DRUG VICTIMS ONLY HAD A 27 PERCENT CURE RATE.

THE RESULTS WERE SO DRAMATIC THAT THE TRIAL WAS STOPPED!

IT WAS CONSIDERED UNETHICAL TO KEEP HALF OF THE PATIENTS ON ANTIBIOTICS WHEN A BETTER, SAFER CURE WAS AVAILABLE.

There are no man-made drugs that can work better than Mother Nature!

HALLELUJAH FOR MOTHER NATURE!

Gastroenterologists agree: FMT is not just EFFECTIVE- it's extremely SAFE. There more money to be made selling drugs. There's not much money to be made from selling poo-☺

The American College of Gastroenterology writes in their C. diffi- cile treatment guidelines that "no adverse effects or complications directly attributable to the procedure have yet been described in the literature."

The FDA requires an Investigative New Drug Permit that is now required. The FDA denies or approves applications within 30 days without explaining criteria used.

IT APPEARS THAT BY TRYING TO MAKE FECAL TRANSPLANTS SAFER, THE FDA IS ACTUALLY PUSHING THEM UNDERGROUND...(no pun intended).

DO IT YOURSELF IS THE WAY TO GO!

Check out Dr. Google and the power of poo website) If you find that you have a life-threatening infection such as C. difficile—YOU SHOULD DEFINITELY CONSIDER A FECAL TRANSPLANT.

Australia is much more progressive. The Center for Digestive Diseases gives patients instructions on doing the procedure at home. So— DIY instructions fit right in.

PARADOXICALLY—if you have Crohn's, C. difficile, or ulcerative colitis, fecal transplants mean dealing with LESS POOP- LESS OFTEN! It appears that the medical crowd haven't figured out that one yet.

<u>MANY DIGESTIVE/GUT HEALTH PROBLEMS CAN BE SOLVED BY A POO TRANSPLANT-</u>☺

The medical crowd is clueless about FMT. Now you know the power of POO- and DIY- DO IT YOURSELF!

I.   VITAMIN B12 DEFICIENCY

What does Vitamin B-12 deficiency have to do with bacteria?

I'll get to that.

<u>40 PERCENT OF PEOPLE HAVE A VITAMIN B12 DEFICIENCY.</u>

<u>Vitamin B12 is like an energy vitamin. It is essential to prevent "megaloblastic anemia" (severe fatigue...as in no energy. Vitamin B12 helps the body's nerve and blood cells to be healthy; all the while it helps to make DNA—the genetic material in ALL of our cells.</u>

Common symptoms of B12 deficiency include:

- Fatigue/tiredness

- Weakness

- Constipation

- Loss of appetite/weight loss

- Megaloblastic anemia

Vitamin B 12 deficiency varies from country to country. Younger people are just as deficient in this vital nutrient as older people. Why is that?

For the record, animals don't make it. But neither do plants either! Animals get their vitamin B12 from eating foods "<u>CONTAMINATED</u>" with Vitamin B12. Thus animals are an indirect source of the vitamin. Yes, you read that correctly—I said "contaminated". The truth is that

NO FOODS- animal or plant- naturally CONTAIN Vitamin B12. (source: Nov. 9th, 2014 www.collective-evolution.com)

Microorganisms, primary bacteria and fungi are the ONLY ORGANISMS that can produce Vitamin B12. Some people use the term "residue Bacteria"-according to a recent study from Tufts University.

The big problem is that technological and chemical processes have depleted it from our soils. Our society is on of pesticides and artificiality, filled with toxic cleansers, antibiotics and over-sanitation; ALL of which remove the richness from Mother Nature's good earth.

VEGETABLES AND SOIL THAT ONCE HARBORED HELPFUL MICRO-ORGANISMS THAT GAVE US GOOD LEVELS OF VITAMIN B12 ARE HARD TO COME BY.

That's why our levels are so low.

VITAMIN B-12 is a MICROBE—A BACTERIA—IT IS PRODUCED BY MICROORGANISMS.

Who knew? It is the only vitamin that contains a trace element, Cobalt. How certain animal meats manage to become a source of B12 is that the animal tissue stores the bacteria—synthesized B12 in that which they also consume.

Historically, most people living on farms would receive a sufficient amount of B12 just by being in close contact with farm animals. Since cow, chicken, sheep and many other animal feces all contain large amounts of active B12, since these feces are regularly used as manure to grow crops; B12 would be consumed as a "residue bacteria" living on un-sanitized vegetables.

Interestingly, research studies have shown that bacteria capable of producing B12 can live inside of our intestinal tract. One example known to produce B12 and also able to colonize parts of our digestive tract is "proprionibacterium shermanii" which inhabits the terminal ileum which is in part of our small intestine. It appears that this is the primary site for B12 absorption.

It appears that B12 is excreted into the bile and is effectively re-absorbed by the body. This is known as "enterohepatic circulation". The amount excreted varies. People on diets low in B12 including vegans and some vegetarians may be obtaining more B12 from re-absorption than from dietary sources.

Re-absorption may be the reason it can take 15 or 20 years for a "deficiency" disease to develop.

If B12 deficiency is due to a failure in absorption, I can take only three years for a deficiency disease to occur. B12 is the <u>ONLY VITAMIN</u> that contains a trace element- <u>COBALT</u>. At the centre of its molecular structure is its chemical name Cobalamin. Humans require Cobalt but it is assimilated only in the form of B12.

<u>Three ways to get Vitamin B12 in your diet</u>

1. Eat Nutritional Yeast

2. Go <u>ORGANIC</u>.

3. Crimini mushrooms (According to World's Healthiest Foods website, these mushrooms are the <u>ONLY NON-ANIMAL</u> derived food source for Vitamin B12).

J.   <u>MICROBES FEAST ON DARK CHOCO-LATE & RED WINE- TOO!</u>

<u>YES!</u>

<u>THIS IS ABSOLUTELY TRUE! THERE IS ABUNDANT SCIENTIFIC EVIDENCE PROVING THAT DARK CHOCOLATE AND RED WINE ARE SUPERFOODS THAT CONTAIN A LOT OF POLYPHENOLS.</u>

<u>THE BIGGEST SURPRISE IS THAT DARK CHOCOLATE AND RED WINE BOTH ARE PREBIOTICS TOO!</u>

<u>THIS MEANS THAT CHOCOLATE AND WINE FEED OUR GOOD BACTERIA AND THESE GOOD BACTERIA FEED US! WE FEED THEM AND THEN THEY FEED US!</u>

<u>How cool is that!</u>

K.   YOU LITERALLY ARE WHAT YOU EAT

While your genome or assembly of your DNA does not change, your epigenome does— in response to a variety of factors, not the least of which is your diet. The epigenome is made up of chemical compounds and proteins that can attach to DNA and can turn genes ON AND OFF controlling the production of proteins in cells. This is called "marking the genome". These marks are sometimes passed on from one cell to another.

WHAT IS MOST AMAZING IS YOUR POWER TO INFLUENCE AND MODIFY YOUR GENOME ON A DAILY BASIS WITH YOUR DIET— DIRECTLY BY THE NUTRIENTS THAT YOU EAT!

CELLULAR METABOLISM PLAYS A FAR MORE DYNAMIC ROLE IN OUR CELLS THAN WE EVER THOUGHT!

NEARLY ALL OF A CELL'S GENES ARE INFLUENCED BY CHANGES IN THE NUTRIENTS THEY ARE PROVIDED.

Example; You can eat cruciferous veggies such as broccoli—and—

YOU CAN SWITCH ON AND ACTIVATE YOUR CANCER FIGHTING GENES!

YOU REALLY DO HAVE THE POWER TO CHANGE YOUR GENES AND CHANGE YOUR HEALTH…TO SUPERHEALTH!

YOUR HEALTH DESTINY IS IN YOUR HANDS!

YOU CAN NOURISH BOTH BRAINS WITH FOOD.

YOU SHOULD START WITH FEEDING AND BUILDING YOUR GUT MICROBIOTA- WHICH ARE YOUR FIRST BRAIN!

YOU LITERALLY ARE WHAT YOU EAT!

CHAPTER TWELVE
LISTEN WITH YOUR KETOGENIC HEART (Dr. HAPPY)

"Fear less, hope more, eat less, chew more, whine less,
breathe more, talk less, say more, hate less and LOVE
more, and all good things will be yours."
–Swedish proverb

"The secret of happiness, you see is not found in seeking
more, but in developing the capacity to enjoy less."
- Socrates

These quotes really are a prescription for <u>SUPERHEALTH AND HAPPINESS</u>. Socrates lived 400 years before Christ. He was the original Dr. Happy!

According to recent research- ANXIETY (characterized by constant and overwhelming worry and fear) is exploding in the USA. Anxiety now eclipses cancer by 800 PERCENT! 13 million adults have struggled with anxiety in the last year. 4.3 million of these people were full-time employees; and 6 million people were unemployed.

A 2010 research study published in the American Journal of Psychiatry concluded that the modern (SAD) American or Western diet leads to high rates of depression and anxiety. A "traditional" dietary pattern characterized by vegetables, fruit, fish etc. was associated with lower odds for major depression or dysthymia and for anxiety disorders. A "Western" diet of processed or fried foods, refined grains, sugary products and beer was associated with a higher GHQ-12 (depression/anxiety score).

In December 2012 review study in the Journal of Medicine and Life titled "Nutrition and Depression at the forefront of Progress"; the authors wrote:

> "Depression is undeniably linked to nutrition, as suggested by the mounting evidence by research in neuropsychiatry. An adequate intake of good calories, healthy proteins, omega 3-fatty acids and all essential minerals is of utmost importance in maintaining mental health. In addition, the link between fast food and depression has recently been confirmed."

A Ketogenic diet is an anti-inflammatory- anti-anxiety diet. As the old adage goes: the proof of the pudding- is in the eating A ketognic diet is very satisfying; very calming.

A Ketogenic diet is euphoric. It will not only chase away the blues...it will uplift your spirits!

Talking about your concerns can also be a great way to vent and release anxiety. "Just getting the problem out" can help you feel better. Not only does it feel great—but it can also give you new insights into what's happening in your life.

You don't have to confront your problems alone. There are benefits of talking to someone about how you feel. You can find a loved one or friend to listen. When that person listens with a Ketogenic heart –both of you will reap the benefits of the experience and positive changes that it brings.

Depression has swiftly become the leading cause of disability- WORLDWIDE. In the USA alone, one in four people suffer from a diagnosable mental disorder.

Many people walk into their doctor's offices- describe the symptoms in 5 minutes- or less- and walk out with a powerful PSYCHIATRIC DRUG like Prozac, Paxil, Wellbuttron, Effexor or the like.

THAT'S 30 MILLION PEOPLE ON AT LEAST ONE TOXIC POISONOUS PSYCHIATRIC DRUG.

Big Pharma wants you to believe that HAPPINESS COMES IN A PILL BOTTLE.

CHASING HAPPINESS IS BIG BUSINESS FOR THE SALE OF ANTI-DEPRESSANT DRUGS. THE STATS ARE BOTH ALARMING AND HEARTBREAKING.

Antidepressant drugs most often lead to suicide. The news is full of horror stories of some drugged up person committing murders; and acts of violence.

Antidepressant drugs and alcohol are actually depressants. Like almost all drugs—they mask symptoms and ultimately cause great illness or death.

You must just say no to all of Big Pharma's poisonous drugs.

You cannot buy happiness in a bottle.

A (2014) study published in the Journal Health Behavior and Policy Review found that optimistic people are twice as likely to remain in optimal cardiovascular health –than those with negative perceptions of reality. The study followed 5, 000 adults for more than 11 years. The study showed a positive correlation between cardiovascular disease and pessimism.

A (2012) MEGA- study from Harvard University came to similar conclusions. Researchers looked at 200 studies comparing cardiovascular risks and emotional states.

THEY FOUND THAT BEING HOPEFUL, HAPPY AND OPTIMISTIC GOES A LONG WAY IN REDUCING THE RISK OF HEART DISEASE AND STROKE.

Another study showed a lower risk of heart disease in folks who reported being happy in their families, careers, sex lives and other relationships. Having constant depression or anxiety on the other hand was linked to higher disease risk—and lower survival- if sick.

Research finds that PPWB (Positive Psychological Well-being) protects consistently against CVD independently of traditional risk factors and ill being.

A study published in 2011 in the European Heart Journal found that STRESS and DEPRESSION are both associated with an increased risk of CHD (coronary heart disease). The study followed 8,000 participants and looked at the risk of CHD in association with 4 primary life domains—1. One's job 2. Family 3. Sex-life and 4 Self -Satisfaction. Most of these were associated with a reduced CHD risk.

RESEARCH FINDS THAT SATISFACTION WITH LIFE PROMOTES HEART HEALTH.

The Science of Healing Thoughts

YOUR MIND CAN HEAL YOUR BODY.

511

Research proves that our mental perception of the world constantly informs and guides our immune system, in a way that makes us better able to respond to future threats.

BEING HAPPY IS A CHOICE YOU NEED TO MAKE.

Your state of mind influences the state of your immune system. Your mind wields incredible POWER over the health of your immune system. STRESS- for example- has a major NEGATIVE influence on the function of your immune system; which is why you have likely noticed that you're more likely to catch a cold-when you're under a lot of stress.

STRESS IS ACKNOWLEDGED BY THE CDC AS A MAJOR CONTRIBUTOR TO DIS-EASE. 85 PERCENT OF DIS-EASE IS DRIVEN BY EMOTIONAL FACTORS.

INFLAMMATION is partly regulated by the hormone CORTISOL. When cortisol is not allowed to serve this function- inflammation can get out of control. The immune system's ability to regulate inflammation predicts who will develop a cold-but more importantly it provides and explanation of how stress can promote disease.

When we are under STRESS- cells of our immune system are unable to respond to hormonal control; and consequently, they produce levels of inflammation that promote disease. As oft repeated herein- inflammation plays a key role in many diseases such as cardiovascular, asthma and autoimmune disorders.

The opposite is also true.

POSITIVE THOUGHTS AND ATTITUDES ARE ABLE TO PROMPT CHANGES IN YOUR BODY THAT STRENGTHEN YOUR IMMUNE SYSTEM; BOOST POSITIVE EMOTIONS; DECREASE PAIN AND CHRONIC DISEASES—AND- PROVIDE STRESS RELIEF.

"The Greatest Weapon against Stress is our ability to choose one thought over another."-(William James)

Research shows that Happiness, Optimism, Life Satisfaction and other POSITIVE psychological attitudes are associated with a lower risk of heart disease.

IT HAS BEEN SCIENTIFICALLY SHOWN THAT HAPPINESS CAN ALTER YOUR GENES! OMG!

A team of researchers at UCLA showed that people with a deep sense of HAPPINESS AND WELL-BEING HAD LOWER LEVELS OF

INFLAMMATORY GENE EXPRESSION AND STRONGER ANTIVIRAL AND ANTIBODY RESPONSES.

Thoughts mould our lives. Thoughts are things. We become our thoughts. Not only do you become your thoughts- your thoughts also attract people, places and things into your life according to thought patterns.

THINK NEGATIVE—AND- NEGATIVITY YOU WILL RECEIVE.

THINK POSITIVE- AND-POSITIVITY YOU WILL RECEIVE!

THIS IS PRECISELY WHY THE ANCIENTS ALWAYS WARNED US TO GUARD AGAINST OUR THOUGHTS—THOUGHTS BECOME THINGS!

Research in Quantum physics shows that human intention and directed thought- CAN ACTUALLY HEAL- EVEN AT A DISTANCE OF THOUSANDS OF MILES!

OMG! How powerful is that!

We control our genes through our thinking; through our intentions and through our CHOICES. WE GET TO CHOOSE!

OUR CELLS AND OUR GENES ARE RE-PROGRAMMABLE!

YOU CAN SWITCH ON YOUR "HAPPY GENES"! Bruce Lipton PhD states:

" The implication is that this basic idea we have that we are controlled by our genes is false. It's an idea that turns us into victims. I'm saying we are the creators of our situation. The genes are merely the blue-prints. We are the contractors; and we can adjust these blueprints. And we can even rewrite them".

A person's health isn't generally a reflection of genes, but how their environment is influencing them. Genes are the direct cause of less than ONE PERCENT OF DISEASE.

99 PERCENT IS HOW WE RESPOND TO THE WORLD.

"OUR GENES LOAD THE GUN- ENVIRONMENT PULLS THE TRIGGER".

How amazing is all of this new science!

In a universe made out of ENERGY, everything is entangled; everything is one. When we're not in harmony with the environment, we're destroying the environment that supports us. There's a theory that says that life is based on a competition and the struggle and fight for survival; and it's interesting because when you look at the fractal character of evolution, it's totally different. It's based on cooperation among the elements of geometry- and not competition.

When we look at human bodies, we look at our body as a singular entity, It turns out that if I could reduce us to a small size- the size of a cell and put you inside of your body- rather than seeing a single entity, what you would see is a metropolis of 50 to 60 trillion citizens.

NATURE is based on harmony. So –it says- if we want to survive and become more like nature, then we have to understand that it's cooperation versus competition. We are made in the image of God our creator. We need to put Spirit back into the equation- when we want to improve our physical and mental health. Our planet's hope of salvation lies in the adoption of revolutionary new knowledge being revealed at the frontiers of science.

A human being is a community of 50 or 60 trillion cells. When you understand that, you realize they're all living entities. They have their own little world inside of us. All cells have jobs and they all live in a community; and they exchange energy like we exchange money and they have the same requirements in their world that we have in our world.

PROTECT YOUR MENTAL FORTRESS FROM NEGATIVE TALK.

You must change your <u>MINDSET</u>. You must carefully monitor yourself. You must monitor everything you say or think! One negative thought can start a cascade of chemical reactions in your body. Russian researchers have shown that they can re-program DNA in <u>TWO MINUTES</u>!

<u>YOU HAVE IMMENSE POWERS WITH YOUR WORDS AND YOUR THOUGHTS!</u>

You must watch your language and be <u>POSITIVE</u>. Don't THINK OR SPEAK negatives. The word "no" can switch off thousands of genes!

Conversely- the word <u>"YES" IS ONE OF THE MOST POWERFUL WORDS IN THE ENGLISH LANGUAGE</u>! Could this be the reason I have used many 'caps' and underlines in this book?-☺

When a person adopts a positive mindset of health self-reliance— they no longer allow a medical doctor to diagnose them with some kind of psychological condition. By shrugging off diagnoses and seasonal sickness mindsets, one learns to correct the imbalance in their body-holistically-

YOU NEED TO AVOID A MEDICAL SYSTEM THAT PERPETUATES HEALTH PROBLEMS WITH PATCHWORK DRUG WITH HORRENDOUS DIRECT EFFECTS THAT ONLY MAKE THINGS WORSE.

You must stop accepting depression as a label. This only gives the problem authority over you- effectively thrusting a new negative pattern of victim mentality onto the future reality.

Illness is perpetuated by bringing attention to it and its label. Claiming "depression" makes a person feel comforted by the attention of a "diagnosis". This is how a person becomes trapped- victimizing themselves- mentally.

A person may not be aware of the POWER OF HIS OWN WORDS— AND HOW THE NEGATIVE CONNOTATION OF HIS LANGUAGE FEEDS THE PROBLEMS.

YOUR ATTITUDE TOWARD SICKNESS EITHER PERPETUATES ITS EXISTENCE OR DIMINISHES ITS STRONG HOLD.

Albert Einstein reputedly said: Disease avoids me because I am too much an inhospitable host."

YOU MUST BECOME A BEING OF POWERFUL POSITIVE THOUGHTS!

YOU MUST ADOPT A POWERFUL POSITIVE MINDSET!

YOU MUST MAKE POSITIVE AFFIRMATIONS SUCH AS: "Great things are coming my way!"

YOU SHOULD FOCUS ON LOVE- GRATITUDE AND HAPPINESS IN YOUR LIFE.

How do you increase HAPPINESS?

According to Harvard researcher Shawn Anchor, your brain actually works 31 PERCENT BETTER AT POSITIVE, THAN AT NEUTRAL OR STRESSED STATES.

When your brain is positive- you actually are more creative, more productive and HAVE MORE ENERGY! With looming deadlines, a super busy work schedule, family commitments and a business to run-so it can be hard to stay positive.

YOU SHOULD DO THE NECESSARY THINGS EACH DAY TO BOOST YOUR POSITIVITY IN ORDER TO BOOST YOUR ENERGY, YOUR PRODUCTIVITY AND YOUR CREATIVITY! Here are some things to increase your happiness.

1. Gratitude

There are HUGE benefits of expressing and receiving gratitude on a daily basis. These benefits are totally underrated- but this could change your entire life. Science tells us that people who are thankful for what they have are happier and reach their goals with greater ease. As published in the Harvard Mental Health Letter:

"Gratitude is a thankful appreciation for what an individual receives, whether tangible or intangible. With gratitude, people acknowledge the goodness in their lives. In the process, people usually recognize that the source of that goodness lies at least partially outside of themselves. As a result, gratitude also helps people connect to something larger than themselves as individuals—whether to other people, nature or a higher power."

Gratitude is also associated with improved health; both physical and emotional. A psychologist at Duke University once stated:

"If thankfulness were a drug, it would be the world's best selling product with a health maintenance indication for every major organ system."

Each day write down 3 things you're grateful for- either- as soon as you wake up- or before you go to bed. This actually RETRAINS YOUR BRAIN to scan for the POSITIVE in your day. Being thankful for your health- every day means that your gratitude means more than being alive- itself. Cultivate gratitude for the little things. This kind of gratitude fosters a sense of deep-seated happiness!

After just 21 days of making this a habit, corporations and individuals have noticed MASSIVE DIFFERENCES IN THEIR POSITIVITY AND PRODUCTIVITY!

Misery is rooted in a perceived sense of lack. But if you have good health and all of your mental faculties intact-you also have the prerequisite basics for improving your situation. Most experts agree that there are no shortcuts to happiness. Even generally happy people do not necessarily experience JOY 24 hours a day. But- a happy person can have a bad day and still find pleasure in the small things of life.

SO- BE THANKFUL FOR WHAT YOU HAVE!

YOUR FUTURE HEALTH AND HAPPINESS DEPENDS LARGELY ON THE THOUGHTS YOU THINK TODAY.

FOR POSITIVITY— START/FINISH YOUR DAY BY THINKING OF 3 THINGS THAT YOU ARE GRATEFUL FOR.

BY FOCUSING ON WHAT'S GOOD RIGHT NOW IN THE PRESENT MOMENT—YOU BECOME OPEN TO RECEIVE GREATER ABUNDANCE IN THE FUTURE!

Remember to say: "**THANK YOU**" –**TO YOURSELF, THE UNIVERSE AND OTHERS**.

2. Fitness

Moving your body through adopting a lifestyle of fitness has a boatload of health benefits. We sit too much these days and can benefit from adopting an identity of someone who moves their body throughout the day.

Exercising at the gym not only releases endorphins which make you feel good but can be a much better energy booster than a late afternoon coffee. However, exercise is only one component of living a "fitness oriented" life. Fitness can be integrated into your day by taking a 2 minute push-up break- or a 3 minute stretching session while on the phone with a client. Research shows that the LITTLE THINGS you do throughout the day are more important than simply getting to the gym 3 times per week. There are lots of options to get more movement into your day—no matter how busy you are. Any incidental exercise can beneficial – so get off your bus one stop earlier or take the stairs…YOUR BRAIN AND YOUR BODY WILL THANK YOU. Perhaps you can squeeze in a TABATA HIIT session.

3. Journaling

Journaling can b a super POWERFUL strategy when incorporated into your daily habits.

WRITING DOWN ONE POSITIVE EXPERIENCE THROUGHOUT THE DAY ACTUALLY TRAINS YOUR BRAIN TO RELIVE THE POSITIVE EXPERIENCE.

Journaling helps improve creativity, strengthen your self-discipline, boost memory and comprehension and **HELPS YOU ACHIEVE YOUR GOALS**.

According to Forbes- Journaling is the **NUMBER ONE PRODUCTIVITY TOOL** that you're not taking advantage of. It's helpful to record wins as well as setbacks- and helps you think about how to get rid of inhibitors blocking your progress.

4. Meditation

Meditation is all the rage in the holistic natural community, Meditation has actually been shown to change the **SIZE AND SHAPE OF YOUR BRAIN!**

It's like resistance training for your muscles leading to more shapely muscles. Meditation actually THICKENS REGIONS OF YOUR BRAIN associated with complex thought, bodily awareness, concentration and problem solving. It also slows down your BRAIN'S NATURAL AGING PROCESS. It also helps to calm your mind, reducing anxiety, and improving your ability to deal with stressful situations. It actually teaches the brain to focus and has been shown to improve YOUR SENSE OF WELL-BEING AND COMPASSION.

Meditation is a super POWERFUL WAY not only to improve your brain function and your body- BUT IT ALSO MAKES YOU HAPPIER!

5. Random acts of Kindness

Random acts of kindness to strangers, colleagues or loved ones makes you and them feel HAPPIER AND MORE POSITIVE. Talking to strangers in public transportation settings (e.g. in buses, subway trains- rather than sitting in silence, has been shown to boost happiness for everyone. Start talking more to strangers. Interacting with others makes people feel happier and has been shown to be good for your immune system. Sending a surprise e-mal to a loved one saying that you are thinking of them has surprise bilateral happiness effects.

When people make a point to conduct 3 to 5 ACTS OF KINDNESS PER WEEK—SOMETHING MAGICAL HAPPENS—

THEY BECOME HAPPIER!

SIMPLE KIND ACTS- a compliment, letting someone ahead of you in line- etc.

THESE SIMPLE ACTS ARE CONTAGIOUS AND TEND TO MAKE ALL OF THOSE INVOLVED FEEL GOOD!

6. EMF (Emotional Freedom Technique)

EMF involves TAPPING WITH YOUR HANDS BEGINNING ON THE TOP OF YOUR HEAD AND CONTINUING DOWN YOUR BODY (TO YOUR HEART TOO!) Just Google it up.

This only takes a few minutes and it produces MARVELOUS RESULTS. Some people call EMF- "Masturbation for the Brain"-☺

7. LOVE HEALS

LOVE is an all -pervasive energy field of love. Listen with your keto-genic LOVING HEART.

NOTHING IS MORE HEALING AND AFFECTS LONGEVITY MORE THAN FEELING LOVED; APPRECIATED AND CARED FOR.

LOVE REALLY DOES CONQUER ALL.

When you are loved and when you are in love- you will be most happy.

FORGIVENESS ENHANCES OUR MENTAL HEALTH.

FORGIVENESS IS A GIFT—NOT JUST FOR YOU—BUT FOR PEOPLE YOU FORGIVE. FORGIVING IS SOMETHING WE ALL CAN DO-IF WE MAKE THAT CONSCIOUS DECISION. AFTER ALL- NO ONE CONTROLS HOW WE FEEL.

EMOTIONS BELONG TO US. THERE IS NO ONE OUTSIDE OF US WHO HAS THE POWER TO PREVENT US FROM EXPERIENCING JOY OR PEACE.

FORGIVENESS HAS TREMENDOUS HEALTH BENEFITS FOR THOSE WHO CONSENT TO FORGIVE.

RECENT RESEARCH SHOWS THAT FORGIVING OTHERS HAS THE FOLLOWING HEALTH BENEFITS:

- Lowered blood pressure

- A stronger immune system

- Decreased stress levels

- decreased back pain, stomach troubles and headaches

Why spend your life playing the "blame game" and losing years wallowing in your anger?

FOCUSING ON YOUR PRESENT BLESSINGS, SKILLS, ABILITIES AND ACCOMPLISHMENTS WILL SET YOU ON THE ROAD TO HEALING— AND RECOVERY.

When we forgive, we don't always forget. When we truly forgive, we may remember…yet we forgive with grace. The person who forgives, can enjoy PEACE, JOY, ENHANCED MENTAL HEALTH AND FREEDOM TO ENJOY ALL THE FUTURE HAS TO OFFER,

There are two kinds of happiness- hedonic (pleasure –oriented) and eudaimonic (fulfilling your life purpose. The term eudaimonic originated with Aristotle and describes the form of happiness that comes from activities that bring you a greater sense of purpose- life meaning or sense of self-actualization. This could be your career or it could be gleaned from volunteering or even taking a cooking class.

What gives you the greatest joy and life satisfaction?

What is your mission on planet Earth? Are you following your JOY? Are you doing what you love to do? What makes you happy and fulfilled?

<u>DON'T WORRY –BE HAPPY BE HEALTHY!</u> <u>BE HAPPY- IT'S A CHOICE!</u>

Self-acceptance is one the most important factors that can produce a more consistent sense of happiness.

<u>BEING HAPPY</u>—is a choice you need to make- much like choosing to eat healthy food or choosing to exercise.

<u>HAPPINESS</u> comes from within—it's not dictated by circumstances alone. This is why if you truly want to be happy—you need to work on <u>YOURSELF FIRST!</u>

<u>In conclusion-</u>

ALL PHYSICAL MANIFESTATIONS OF UNWELLNESS HAVE AN EMOTIONAL COMPONENT (AND VICE VERSA).

LISTEN WITH YOUR KETOGENIC HEART.

LISTENING IS MORE THAN BEING AWARE OF ACHES AND PAINS.

IT INVOLVES MAINTAINING A SUSTAINABLE HEALTHY LIFESTYLE AND HEALTHY DIET.

WELL-BEING IS MORE THAN HEALTHY DIET- IT IS THE COMBINATION OF ALL OF THE HEALING TREATMENTS FROM ALL OF THE "DOCTORS" IN THIS BOOK.

<u>THANK YOU FOR READING THIS BOOK!</u>

MUCH LOVE TO YOU ON YOUR HEALING JOURNEY!

Gary W. Pitts

APPENDIX A
REFERENCES AND SCIENTIFIC STUDIES
152 KETOGENIC Scientific Studies

1. Allen B. et al. "Ketogenic Diets as an adjuvant cancer therapy: History and potential mechanism" Redox Biol. August 7th, (2014) PubMed 25460731.

2. Akram et al. "A focused review of the role of ketone bodies in health and disease" Journal Med. Food (2013) November 16, p. 965-7.

3. Austin GL, et al. "A very-low Carbohydrate Diet Improves Symptoms and Quality of Life in Diarrhea- Predominant Irritable Bowel Syndrome". Clinical Gastroenterology and Hepatology 7.6 (2009): 706-708.

4. Austin GL, et al. "A very-low Carbohydrate Diet Improves Gastroesophageal Reflux and its Symptoms "Digestive Diseases and Sciences 51.8 (2006) 1307-1312.

5. Baranano, K. al. The Ketogenic Diet: Uses in Epilepsy and other neurologic illnesses. Current treatment options in Neurology, 10.6 (2008) 410-19.

6. Bergen. S, Jr. "Hyperketonemia induced in man by medium-chain triglycerides" Diabetes Vol 15 no 10 (1966) 723-725.

7. Bonucelli, G. et al. "Ketones and lactate "fuel" tumor growth and metastasis: evidence that epithelial cancer cells use oxidative mitochondrial metabolism". Cell Cycle (2010), 3506-14.

8. Cahill, G. "Fuel Metabolism in Starvation" Annual Review of Nutrition 26 (2006) p. 1-22.

9. Champ CE, Volek JS et al. "Targeting Metabolism with a Ketogenic Diet during treatment of Glioblastoma Multiforme." J. Neurooncol March (2014) p. 125-131.

10. Champ CE " A Focused Review of the role of Ketone Bodies in Health and Disease" J. Med. Food (2013) Nov. 16th, p.965-7.

11. Chang H et al. Metabolic Profiles of Ketolysis and Glycolysis in malignant Gliomas: Possible predictions of response to Ketogenic diet therapy. J. Clin Oncol 31, (2013) Suppl: abstract e 13048.

12. Clarke K. et al. "Kinetics, safety and tolerability of R-3-Hydroxybuty (R-3 hydroxybutyrate) in healthy adult subjects". Regul Toxicol Pharmacol. August (2012) 63 (3).

13. Cox, Pete J. et al. "Acute Nutritional Ketosis: Implications for exercise performance and metabolism" Extrem Physiol Med (2014) published on line October 29th, 2014, PubMed 212585. DP et al.

14. D'Agostino DP et al. "Therapeutic Ketosis with Ketone Ester delays central nervous system toxicity seizure in rats." Am. J. Physiol Regul. Integr Comp. Physiol. (2013) p. 829-836.

15. Dashti, H. et al. "Ketogenic Diet modifies the Risk Factors of Heart Disease in Obese Patients" Nutrition 19.10 (2003) 901-902.

16. Dashti, H. et al. "Long-term Effects of Ketogenic Diet in Obese Subjects with High Cholesterol Level" Molecular and Cellular Biochemistry 286.1-2 (2006) p. 1-9.

17. Dashti, H. et al. Beneficial effects of Ketogenic diet on obese diabetic subjects. Mol. Cell Biochem 302, (2007) 247-256.

18. Dashti, H. et al. Beneficial effects of Ketogenic diet on obese diabetic subjects with high cholesterol level. Molecular and Cellular Biochemistry (2006) 286 1-9

19. Dresler, A et al. "Type 1 Diabetes and Epilepsy: efficacy and safety of the Ketogenic Diet." Epilepsia 51.6 (2010) 1086-1089.

20. Evangeliou, A et al. " Application of a Ketogenic Diet in Children with Autistic Behaviour" A Pilot Study" Jour-

nal of Neurology 18. 2 (2003) 111-117.

21. Greene A, et al. "Perspectives on the Metabolic Management of Epilepsy through Dietary reduction of glucose and elevation of ketone bodies." Journal of Neurochemistry 36.3 (2003) 529-537

22. Gumbiner B. et al. Effects of composition and ketosis on glycemia during very-low-energy-diet-therapy in obese patients with non-insulin dependent diabetes mellitus. Amer J. Clin Nutr (1996) 63 110-115

23. Feinman, R.D. et al. Metabolic Syndrome and low-carbohydrate Ketogenic diets in the medical school biochemistry curriculum. Metabolic Syndrome and related disorders 1.3 (2003) 189-197

24. Foster GD et al. A randomized trial of a low-carbohydrate diet for obesity. N.Eng J Med 348: (2003) 2082-2090

25. Fine, E. et al. Targeting insulin inhibition as a metabolic therapy in advanced cancer: a pilot safety and feasibility dietary trial. Journal Nutrition (2012) 256

26. Freeman J. et al. The Ketogenic Diet one decade later. Pediatrics 119.3 (2007) p. 535-549.

27. Gano L. et al. "Ketogenic Diets, Mitochondria, and Neurological Diseases" J. Lipid Res (2014) Nov 55 (11) 2211-28.

28. Gasior, M, et al. "Neuroprotective and disease-modifying effects of the Ketogenic Diet" Behav. Pharmacol (2006) Sept. 19th, p. 431-439.

29. Guisado, Joaquin Perez, "Spanish Ketogenic Mediterranean Diet for Weight Loss". Nutrition Journal (2008) October 26, 7:30.

30. Gibson, Alice et al. "Do Ketogenic Diets really suppress appetite? A systematic review and meta-analysis". Obesity Reviews January (2015) 16 (1) 64-76.

31. Gower J. et al. " A lower-carbohydrate, higher-fat diet reduces abdominal and inter muscular fat and increases insulin sensitivity in adults at risk of type 2 Diabetes." J. Nutr. January 14th, (2015) p. 1773-83S.

32. Gumbiner B. et al. "Effects of Diet composition and ketosis on glycemia during very low energy diet therapy in obese patients with non-insulin dependent diabetes mellitus". Amer. J. Clin. Nutr (1996) 63 p.110-115.

33. Guzman M. et al. "Is there an astrocyte-neuron Ketone body Shuttle?"

Trends in Endocrinology and Metabolism, May (2001) p. 167-73.

34. Hartman, AL. et al. The Neuropharmacy of the Keto-
    genic Diet. Piediatric Neurol (2008) 36: 281-2

35. Hartman, AL. et al. Clinical Aspects of the Keto-
    genic Diet, Epilepsia, 48 (1)(2007) 31-4.

36. Hartman, AL "The New Ketone Alphabet Soup: BHB, HCA
    and HDAC" Epilepsy Curr. (2014) Nov-Dec 14(6) p. 355-7.

37. Hashim SA et al. "Ketone Body Therapy: From the Ke-
    togenic Diet to the administration of Ketone Es-
    ter" J. Lipid Res. September (2014) p. 1818-26.

38. Henderson, S. et al. " Ketone Bodies as a Therapeutic for Al-
    zheimer's Disease". Neurotherapeutics 5.3 (2008) p. 470-480.

39. Henderson S. et al. Study of the ketogenic agent Ac-1202 in mild to
    moderate Alzheimer's Disease: a randomized, double-blind, pla-
    cebo-controlled, multicenter trial. Nutr Metab. (Lond) (2009) 6:31.

40. Hoyer S. "Abnormality of Glucose Metabolism in Alzheimer's Dis-
    ease" Annals New York Academy of Sciences Vol. 640, (1991; p 53-58.

41. Hussain D. et al. "Long-term effects of a Ketogenic Diet in
    Obese Patients". Exp. Clin. Cardiol (2004) 9(3) p. 200-205.

42. Hussain A. et al. "Diet Therapy for Narcolep-
    sy" Neurology 62 (2004): 2300-2302.

43. Hussain, T et al. " Effect of Low-calorie versus low-carbohydrate
    Ketogenic Diet in Type 2 Diabetes." Nutrition 28.8 (2013): 1009-14.

44. Huttenlocher PR et al. Medium chain triglycerides as a therapy for
    Intractable childhood epilepsy. Neurology 1971, 21 1097-1103

45. Joo, NS. et al. "Ketonuria after fasting may be related to the
    metabolic superiority." J. Korean Med Sci (2010) 25: 177-179

46. Journavaz FR et al. The role of muscle insulin resistance
    in the pathogenesis of atherogenic dyslipidemia and
    non-alcoholic fatty liver disease associated with meta-
    bolic syndrome. Ann. Rev Nutr (2010) 30, 273-290.

47. Kaghiwaga, Y. et al. " D-b-Hydroxybutyrate protects
    neurons in models of Alzheimer's and Parkinson's Dis-
    eases" PNAS, May 9th, (2000) 97(10) p. 5440-44.

48. Klement et al. "Is there a role for carbohydrate re-

striction in the treatment and prevention of cancer? Nutrition and Metabolism (2011) 1-116

49. Kossoff G. The fat is in the fire: Ketogenic diet for refractory status epilecticus. Epilepsy Curr (2011) 11. 88-89.

50. Kraft et al. "Schizophrenia, gluten and low-carbohydrate, Ketogenic diets, a case report and Review of the Literature." Nutrition and Metabolism 6, (2009) 10.

51. Krajnc N et al. "Management of Epilepsy in patients with Rett Syndrome: Perspectives and Considerations." Ther Clin Risk Manag (2015) June 925-932

52. Kreider RB et al. "A carbohydrate-restricted diet during resistance training promotes more favourable changes in body composition and markers of Health in Obese women with and without Insulin Resistance". Phys Sports May (2011) p .27-40 PubMed 21673483.

53. Krilanovich N.J. "Benefits of Ketogenic Diets" Amer J Clin Nutr (2007) 85 238-9

54. La Gory, Edward et al. A low-carb diet kills tumour cells with a mutant tumor suppressor gene: The Atkins Diet suppresses tumour growth. Cell Cycle (2013);0-1 .

55. Lennox, W.G. "Ketogenic Diet in the treatment of Epilepsy". N. Engl. J. Med (1928) 199 (2): 74-75

56. Liebhaber GM et al. Ketogenic Diet in Rett Syndrome. J. Child Neurol (2003) 74-75

57. Liu, Xin et al. Effects of a low carbohydrate diet on weight loss and cardiometabolic profile in Chinese women: a randomized controlled feeding trial. The British Journal of Nutrition (2013) 1-10.

58. Liu, Y.M. et al. "Medium-Chain Triglyceride (MCT) Ketogenic Therapy". Epilepsia 49 Supp. 8 (2008) p. 33-6.

59. Maalouf, M, et al. " The Neuroprotective properties of calorie restriction, the Ketogenic Diet and Ketone Bodies". Brain Res. Rev. (2009) p. 293-315.

60. Maalouf, M, et al. "Ketones inhibit mitochondrial production of reactive oxygen species production following glutamate excitotoxicity by increasing NADH oxidation". Neuroscience 2007, p. 256-264.

61. Mady, MA et al. The Ketogenic Diet: Adolescents can do it too. Epilepsia, (2003) 847-851 293-315.

62. Manninen AH. Metabolic Effects of the very low carbohydrate diets: Misunderstood villains of Human Metabolism. Journal of the Int'l Society of Sports Nutrition (2004) 1 (2) 7-11.

63. Maroon JC et al. "The Role of Metabolic Therapy in treating Glioblastoma Multiforeme" Surg Neurol Int. April 16th, (2015) PubMed 25949849

64. Martinez-Outselftoom, et al. " Ketone Body utilization drives tumor cell growth and metastasis". Cell Cycle (2012) 3964-71.

65. Masino SA. et al. " Adenosine, Ketogenic Diet and Epilepsy: The Emerging Therapeutic Relationship between Metabolism and Brain Activity." Curr. Neuropharmacol (2009) Sept 7th, (3) p. 257-268.

66. Masino SA, "Mechanisms of Ketogenic Diet Action" (2012) PubMed 22787591.

67. Mattson M. et al. "Beneficial effects of Intermittent Fasting and Calorie Restriction on the Cardiovascular and Cerebrovascular Systems

68. Maurer G. et al. "Differential utilization of ketone bodies by neurons and glioma cell lines: a rational for Ketogenic Diet as experimental glioma therapy. BMC Cancer (2011) 315". J. Nutr Biochem (2005) March 16th; PubMed 15741046.

69. Mavropolous J. al. " The Effects of a Low-Carbohydrate Ketogenic Diet on The Polycystic Ovary Syndrome" A Pilot Study" Nutrition and Metabolism 2 (2005): 35.

70. Mavropolous J. et al. " The Effects of varying dietary carbohydrate and fat content on survival in non-marone incop Prostate Cancer Xenograft Model" Cancer Prevention Research 2 (2009): p. 557-565.

71. McClernon, F. et al. " The effects of a Low-Carbohydrate Ketogenic Diet and a Low-fat diet on mood, hunger and other self-reported symptoms" Obesity (Silver Spring) (2007) 15.1.

72. McDaniel SS et al The ketogenic Diet inhibits the mammalian target of rapamycin (mTOR) pathway. Epilepsia (2011) 52-e7-e-11

73. Maroon JC. Et al. The Role of Metabolic Therapy in treating GlioBlastoma Multiforme. Sur. Neurol Int April 16th (2015) pub med no 25949849.

74. Milder J. "Modulation of Oxidative Stress and Mitochondrial Function by The Ketogenic Diet". Epilepsy Res. (2012) July 100 (3) 295-303.

75. Misra S. et al. "Utility of Ketone Measurement in the prevention, diagnosis and management of Diabetic Ketoacidosis" Diabetes Med. (2015) January p. 14-23.

76. Mitchel G. et al. Medial Aspects of Ketone Body Metabolism. Clin Invest Med (1995) 18(3) 193-216.

77. Mobbs, EV, et al. "Treatment of Diabetes and Diabetic Complications with a Ketogenic Diet". Journal of Child Neurology 28.8 (2013) 1009-14.

78. Morris AA. Et al. "Cerebral Ketone Body Metabolism" J. Inherit Metab Dis (2005) 28 (2) 109-21.

79. Musa, V et al. "Breath acetone is a reliable indicator of ketosis in adults consuming ketogenic meals." Amer J. Clin Nutr (2002) July 6th, 65-70.

80. Newport, Dr. Mary "A new way to produce Hyperketonemia: Use of a Ketone Ester in case of Alzheimer's Disease". Alzheimer's Dement January 11th, (2015) p. 98-103.

81. Noto, H. et al. Low carbohydrate diets and all cause mortality: a Systematic Review and Meta-Analysis of Observational studies. PloS (2013) e 55030.

82. Pacheco, et al. " A Pilot Study of the Ketogenic Diet in Schizophrenia". American Journal of Psychiatry 121 (1965): 1110-1111.

83. Paoli, Antonnio et al. " Ketosis, Ketogenic Diet and Food Intake Control: A Complex Relationship". Front Psychol. (2015) published on line Feb 2, 2015.

84. Paoli, A. et al. " Nutrition and Acne: Therapeutic Potential of Ketogenic Diets. Skin Pharmacology and Physiology 25:3 (2012).

85. Paoli, A. et al. "Ketogenic Diet does not affect Strength Performance in Elite artistic Gymnasts" Journal of the International Society of Sports Nutrition 9.1 (2012) 34.

86. Paoli A. et al. " Ketogenic Diet in Neuromuscular and Neurodegenerative Diseases". Biomed. Res Int (2014) published on line PMC 4101992 July 3, 2014.

87. Paoli, A. et al. "Beyond Weight Loss: A review of the therapeutic uses of very-low carbohydrate (Ketogenic) Diets". European Journal of Clinical Nutrition (2013) published on line on June 26th, 2013.

88. Paoli, A, et al. " Ketogenic Diet for Obesity: Friend or Foe?" Int.

J. Environ. Res. Public Health (2014) Feb 11th (2) 2092-2107.

89. Paganoni S. et al. " High Fat and Ketogenic Diets in Amyotrophic Lateral Sclerosis" J. Child Neurol (2013) Aug. 28th (8) 989-992.

90. Park, S, et al. "A Ketogenic Diet Impairs energy and glucose homeostasis by the attenuation of hypothalamic leptin signalling and hepatic insulin signalling in a rat model of non-obese Type 2 Diabetes." Exp. Biol. Med (Maywood) (2011) Feb 236 (2) p. 194-204.

91. Peloquin Group, "Lose fat by adapting your body to burn fat: Diet and Training strategies to increase Metabolic flexibility for optimum body composition". Published July 7th, 2013.

92. Perez-Guisado J. "Arguments in favour of Ketogenic Diets." Internat. J. Nutr. Wellness (2006) vol. 4:2.

93. Peterman MG. " The Ketogenic Diet in Epilepsy" JAMA 1925; 84(26) 1979-1983.

94. Phelps, J. et al. "The Ketogenic Diet for Type 2 Bipolar Disorder" Neurocase 19-5 (2013): 423-6.

95. Phinney, Stephen, " Ketogenic Diets and Physical Performance" Nutrition and Metabolism (2004) 1:2.

96. Phinney, S. et al. " The Human Metabolic Response to chronic ketosis without caloric restriction: Preservation of submaximal exercise capability with reduced carbohydrate oxidation". Metabolism 32.8 (1983) 769-776.

97. Phinney, S. et al. " Oolichan Grease: A unique marine lipid and dietary staple of the north Pacific coast" Lipids, Jan. (2009) 47-51.

98. Poff, Am, et al. "The Ketogenic Diet an Hyperbaric Oxygen Therapy prolong survival in mice with systemic metastatic cancer" PLoS One (2013) 5522.

99. Poplawski M. et al. "Reversal of Diabetic Nephropathy by a Ketogenic Diet". PLos One 6.4 (2011): e18604.

100. Rho, JM "How does the Ketogenic Diet induce Anti-Seizure Effects?" Neuroscience Lett. (2015) July 26.

101. Rondanelli, M. et al. "Focus on Metabolic and Nutritional Correlates of Polycystic Ovary Syndrome and Updates of Nutritional Management of these critical Phenomena". Arch. Obstet. December 29th, (2014) p. 1079-92.

102. RoseDame R. et al. "Clinical Experience of a Diet Designed to

Reduce Aging." Journal of Applied Research 9 (2009) 159-165.

103. Ruskin, D. et al. " The Nervous System and Metabolic Dys-regulation" Emerging Evidence converges on Ketogenic Diet Therapy" Front Neuroscience (2012) 6:33 PMC 3312079,

104. Schmidt, M. et al. "Effects of a Ketogenic Diet on the Quality of Life in 16 patients with Advanced Cancer: A Pilot Trial" Nutrition and Metabolism 8.1 (2011): 54.

105. Schwartz, Kenneth et al. "Treatment of glioma patients with Ketogenic diets: Report of two cases treated with an IRB-approved energy-restricted Ketogenic diet protocol and review of the literature." Cancer Metab (2015) published on line March 25th, 2015.

106. Seyfried, TN. et al. "Targeting energy metabolism in Brain Cancer through caloric-restriction and the Ketogenic Diet". J. Cancer Res. Ther. (2009) p. 15.

107. Seyfried TN. Et al. " Is the restricted Ketogenic Diet a viable alternative to The Standard of Care for managing malignant brain cancer?" Epilepsy Res (2012) July 100 (3) p.310-26.

108. Seyfried, TN. Dominic D'Agnostino et al. " Cancer as a Metabolic Disease: Implications for novel Therapeutics" J. Carcinogenesis March (2014) p. 515-524"

109. Seyfried, TN. et al. " Metabolic Therapy: a new Paradigm for managing malignant Brain Cancer" Cancer Lett. January 23rd(2015) p. 289-300.

110. Shaffi, et al. " Ketogenic Diet provides neuroprotective effects against ischemic stroke neuronal damages". Adv Pharma Bull December 4th, (2014) p. 479-481. PubMed no. 4312394.

111. Sharman, M. et al. "A Ketogenic Diet favourably affects serum biomarkers for Cardiovascular Disease in normal weight men." Journal of Nutrition (2002): 1879-1885.

112. Sigmore JM. " Ketogenic Diet containing medium-chain triglycerides in Practice". J.Amer. Diet Ass. (1973); 62: 285-290.

113. Stafstrom, C. et al. "The Ketogenic Diet as a Treatment Paradigm for Disease Neurological Disorders" Frontiers in Pharmacology 3 (2012) 59.

114. Strowd R. et al. " Glycemic modulation in neurooncolgy: experience and future directions using a modified Atkins Diet for high-grade brain tumors". Neurooncol Pract. (2015) Sept 2 (3) p. 127-136.

115. Sumithan R. et al. " Ketosis and appetite-mediating Nutrients and Hormones after Weight Loss." European Journal of Clinical Nutrition 67.7 (2013) 759-64.

116. Sussman D. et al. " Gestational Ketogenic Diet Programs Brain Structure and Susceptibility to Depression & Anxiety in the adult mouse offspring". Brain-Behav February 5th, (2015) PubMed no. 4309881

117. Tendler D. et al. " The Effect of a Low-Carbohydrate, Ketogenic Diet on Nonalcoholic Fatty Liver Disease: A Pilot Study." Digestive Diseases and Sciences 52.2 (2007) p. 589-93.

118. Vanitallie T, et al. "Treatment of Parkinson's Disease with Diet Induced Hyperketonemia: A Feasibility Study" Neurology 6.4 (2005) 728-730.

119. Vanitallie TB, et al. "Biomarkers, Ketone Bodies, and the Prevention of Alzheimer's Disease" Metabolism March (2015) 64, S 51-57.

120. Varshneya K. et al. "The Efficacy of the Ketogenic Diet and associated Hypoglycemia as an Adjuvant Therapy for High-grade Gliomas: A Review of the Literature". Cureus (2015) Feb 27, (2) e251.

121. Veech, R.L. "The Therapeutic Implications of Ketone Bodies: the Effects of Ketone Bodies in Pathological Conditions: Ketosis, Ketogenic Diet, Redox States, Insulin Resistance and Mitochondrial Metabolism". Prostaglanding, Leukotriennes and Essential Fatty Acids 70.3 (2004) 309-19.

122. Veech, R .L et al. "Ketone Bodies, Potential Therapeutic Uses" IUMB Life 51 (2001); 241-7.

123. Vidali, S. et al. "Mitochondria: The Ketogenic Diet- A Metabolism Based Therapy" Int. J. Biochem Biol (2015) June 63, p.55-59.

124. Volek, J. Very-low Carbohydrate Diets" in Essentials of Sports Nutrition and Supplements, edited by J. Antonnio et al. N.J. Humana Press (2008).

125. Volek, J.C et al. " The case for not restricting saturated fat on a low-carbohydrate diet" Nutrition and Metabolism 2 (2005): 2

126. Volek J.C. et al. "Very Low Carbohydrate Diets" Essentials of Nutrition and Supplements" edited by J Antonnio et al. NJ. Humana Press 2008.

127. Volek, J. " A Hypocaloric, very-low Carbohydrate diet results in greater reduction in the percent and absolute amount of plasma triglyceride saturated fatty acids compared to a low-fat diet' pa-

per presented on Oct. 20, 2006 at N. Study of Obesity in Boston,

128. Volek J. et al. " An Isoenergetic very-low carbohydrate diet is associated with Improved serum Hgh-Density Lipo-protein in Cholesterol (HDL-C), total cholesterol to HDL-C ratio, triglycerides, and postprandial lipemic responses compared to a low-fat diet in normal weight, normal lipidemic women" Journal of Nutrition, 133.9 (2003) 2756-2761.

129. Volek J. et al. " Modification of Lipoproteins by very low carbohydrate diets" Journal of Nutrition 135.6 (2005) 1339-42.

130. Volek, J. et al. " Dietary Carbohydrate Restriction Induces a Unique Metabolic State Positively Affecting Atherogenic Dyslipidemia, Fatty Acid Partitioning and Metabolic Syndrome" Progress in Lipid Research 47-5 (2008); 212-216.

131. Westman, E. " A Review of very low Carbohydrate Diet for Weight Loss" Journal of Clinical Outcomes Management 6.7. (1999) 36-40.

132. Westman, E. "Is Dietary Carbohydrate Essential for Nutrition? American Journal of Clinical Outcomes 6.7 (1999) 36-40.

133. Westman, E. "Effects of a 6 month adherence to a very low Carbohydrate Program" American Journal of Medicine 113.1 (2002) 30-36.

134. Westman, E. et al. "A Review of Low-carbohydrate Ketogenic Diets" Current Atherosclerosis Reports 5. 6 (2003) 476-483.

135. Westman, E. et al. "Effect of a low-carbohydrate Ketogenic Diet Program compared to a low-fat diet on fasting lipoprotein subclasses" International Journal of Cardiology 114.2 (2006); 212-216.

136. Westman, E. et al. "Carbohydrate Restriction is effective in improving Atherogenic Dyslipidemia even in the presence of weight loss" American Journal of Clinical Nutrition, 84.6 (2006): 1549.

137. Westman E. et al. " Dietary Treatment of Diabetes Mellitus in the Pre-Insulin Era (1914-1922)" Perspectives in Biology and Medicine 49.1 (2006): 77-83.

138. Westman E. et al. "Low-Carbohydrate Nutrition and Metabolism" American Journal of Clinical Nutrition 86 (2007) 276-84.

139. Westman, E. et al. "The Effect of a Low-Carbohydrate, Ketogenic Diet versus a low-glycemic index on glycemic control in Type 2 Diabetes Mellitus" Nutrition and Metabolism 5 (2008): 36.

140. Wheless JW, et al. " The Ketogenic Diet: An effective medical ther-

apy with side effects" J. Child Neurol. (2001): 16(9), p. 633-635.

141. Wilder R et al. " Ketosis and the Ketogenic Diet: Their application to the treatment of Epilepsy and Infections in the Urinary Tract." Int. Clin. (1935), I (45thserv.) 1:12

142. Wood, R. et al. " Carbohydrate Restriction alters Lipoprotein Metabolism by Modifying VLDL, LDL, and HDL Subfraction and distribution and size in Overweight Men" Journal of Nutrition 136.2 (2006) p. 384-389.

143. Wood, r. et al. " Effects of a Carbohydrate Restricted diet on Emerging Plasma Markers for Cardiovascular Disease" Nutrition and Metabolism, 3.1. (2006): 19.

144. Woolf, E. et al. "The Ketogenic Diet for the treatment of malignant Glioma" J. Lipid Res (2015) Jan 56(1) p .5-10.

145. Woodyatt RT, "Objects and method of Diet adjustment in Diabetics" Arch Intern Med. (1921): 28 125-141.

146. Yancy W. et al. " A Pilot trial of a low-carbohydrate Ketogenic Diet in Patientswith Type 2 Diabetes" Metabolic Syndrome and Related Disorders 1.3 (2003): 239-243.

147. Yancy, W. et al. " Effects of two-weight loss diets on health-related Quality of Life" Quality of Life Research 18.3 (2009) 281-289.

148. Yancy, w. et al. "A randomized trial of a low-carbohydrate Diet vs. Orlistat Plus a low-fat diet for weight loss" Archives of Internal Medicine" 170.2 (2010): 136-145.

149. Yancy, W. et al. " A low-carbohydrate, Ketogenic Diet versus a low-fat diet to treat obesity and hyperlipidemia" a randomized controlled trial". Annals of Internal Medicine 140-10 (2004): 769-797.

150. Yang, X, et al. " Neuroprotective and Anti-inflammatory Activities of Ketogenic diet on MPTP Induced Neurotoxicity" Journal of Molecular Neuroscience 42 2 (2010): 143-153.

151. Yin J. et al. " Sirtuin 3 mediates neuroprotection of Ketones against Ischemic Stroke" J. Cereb. Blood Flow Metab. (2015) November 35 (11) 1783-9.

152. Zhao, Z. et al. " A Ketogenic Diet as a Potential Novel Therapeutic Intervention in Amyotrophic Lateral Sclerosis" BMC Neuroscience 7 (2006): 29.

THREE Scientific Studies PROVING THE THERAPEUTIC MAGIC of the Herb "STEVIA"! Zowie!

1. Nabilatul Hani Mohd-Radzman, et al. " Potential Roles of Stevia rebaudiana Bertoni in Abrogating Insulin Resistance and Diabetes: A Review" Published by Hindawi Publishing Corporation, Evidence-based Complementary and Alternative Medicine Volume 2013 October 1st, 2013. Article ID 718049.

2. Ena Gupta et al. "Nutritional and Therapeutic values of Stevia rebaudiana: A Review" published on December 10th, 2013 in the Journal of Medicinal Plants Research, vol 7 (46) pp. 3343-3353.

3. Elena Nikolova, " Development in the Production of Natural Sweetener (Stevia rebaudiana) in Bulgaria." Journal of Environmental and Agricultural Sciences (2015) 3: 61-71.

Selected Scientific studies

1. Mitochondrial Efficiency and Insulin Resistance, Front Physiology (2014)

2. Liver fat, statin use, and incident Diabetes: The Multi-Ethnic Study of Atherosclerosis, Atherosclerosis (2015), July 15th, 242(1) 211-217

3. Diets with High-fat cheese, High-fat meat, or carbohydrate on cardiovascular risk markers in overweight post-menopausal women: A randomized cross-over trial, American Journal of Clinical Nutrition July 15th, (2015).

4. Prospective association of fatty acids in the de novo lipogenesis pathway with risk of Type 2 Diabetes: The Cardiovascular Health Study, American Journal of Clin Nutr. Jan 10th, (2015) 101(1) 153-163.

5. The Lipid Paradox, Critical Care Medicine June (2015) 43(6) p. 1255-64.

6. The relationship between serum low-density lipoprotein cholesterol and in hospital mortality following acute myocardial infarction (the lipid paradox), Amer J. Cardiol March 1st, (2015) 115(5) p. 557-62.

7. Full fat milk and cheese reduce the risk of Diabetes: Study, Published in Telegraph September 16th, (2014), Rebecca Smith.

8. Association between Dairy food consumption and weight change over 9 years in 19,352 perimenopausal women, American J. Clin Nutr Nutr Dec (2006) 84 (6) 1481-1488,

9. High-fat dairy food and conjugated linoleic acid in takes in

relation to colorectal cancer incidence in the Swedish Mammography Cohort, Am J. Clin Nutr (2005) Oct 82(4) 894-900.

10. Association between the consumption of dairy products and incident Type 2 Diabetes-insights from The European Investigation into Cancer Study, Nutrition Review (2015) August 73 (Suppl.1) 15-22 PMC 4502710

11. The relationship between high-fat dairy consumption and obesity, cardiovascular and metabolic disease, European Journal of Nutrition Feb (2013) vol. 52 issue I pp. 1-24.

12. High-fat dairy intake related to less central Obesity: A male cohort study with 12 years' follow up. Scand J. Primary Health Care (2013) June 31 (2) p. 89-94.

13. The relationship between high fat dairy consumption and obesity, cardiovascular, and metabolic disease, European Journal of Nutrition vol 52 Feb. (2013) p. 1-24.

14. Whole fat dairy food intake is inversely associated with obesity prevalence: Findings from the Observation of Cardiovascular Risk Factors in Luxemberg Study, Nutr Res (2014) Nov 34 (11) 936-43.

15. Food sources of fat may classify the inconsistent role of dietary fat intake for incidence of Type 2 diabetes, Am J. Clin Nutr (2015) May 101(5) 1065-80.

16. Yogurt and Dairy Product Consumption to prevent cardio-metabolic Diseases: Epidemiological and experimental studies, Am J. Clin Nutr (2014) May 99 (5) 1235S-42S.

17. A low carbohydrate, whole foods approach to managing Diabetes and Prediabetes, Spectrum Diabetes Journal.org. Nov (2012) no. 4 238-243.

18. Effects of Stepwise increases in dietary carbohydrate on circulating saturated fatty acids and palmitoleic acid in adults with Metabolic Syndrome, Nov. 21st (2014) PloS Journal on line.

19. Higher glucose levels associated with lower memory and reduced hippocampal microstructure, Journal of Neurology, (2013) October p. 1746-1752.

20. Community- based physical activity interventions for Diabetes: a Systematic Review with Meta-Analysis, Front Endrocinol (2013): 4:3.

21. Higher glucose levels may be a factor for dementia, even among persons without Diabetes, N Engl J. Med (2013) 369.

22. Fatty Acids in Energy Metabolism of the Central Nervous System, Journal f BioMed Research International vol. (2014).

23. Medium-chain fatty acids: Functional lipids for the prevention and treatment of the Metabolic Syndrome, Pharmacol Res (2010) 208-212. PubMed 19931617.

24. Mitochondrial Dysfunction in the Elderly: Possible role in Insulin Resistance, Science May 16, (2003) 1140-1142.

25. Glucose-lowering with exogenous insulin monotherapy in type 2 Diabetes dose association with all cause morality, cardiovascular events and cancer, November 14th, (2014) Diabetes, Obes. Metab. PubMed 25399739.

26. Understanding the kidney's role in blood glucose regulation, Am J.Manag Care (2012) Jan 18, 511-16.

27. Lack of suppression of circulating free fatty acids and hypercholesterolemia during weight loss on a high-fat low carbohydrate diet, Amer J. Clin Nutr March 9th, (2010) 91(3) 578-85.

28. Does Food Insufficiency in childhood contribute to dementia in later life? J. Clin Interv Aging (2015): 1049-53.

29. Traditional Chinese Medicine in Treatment of Metabolic Syndrome, Endocrine Metab. Disorder Drug Targets, (2008) June 8(2) 99-111

30. Microb Ecol Health Dis. February 2, (2015) Pubmed 25651995.

31. Oleocantral inhibits proliferation and M1P-1a expression in human multiple myeloma cells, Curr Med Chem (2013) 20:2467-75.

32. Alzheimer's-associated Aboligomers show altered structure, immunoreactivity and synaptotoxicity with low doses of Oleocanthal, Toxicol Appl Pharmacol. (2009) 240:189-97.

33. Docosahaexaenoic acid and adult memory: A systematic review and Meta-Analysis.(1gram and 500mg to 999mg/day of DHA) Journal PloS One, published on line on March 13, (2015), PubMed 4364792.

34. Supplementation with N-3 long-chain polyunsaturated fatty acids or olive oil in men and women with renal disease induces differential changes in the DNA methylation of FADS2 and ELOVLS in peripheral blood mononuclear cells, PLoS One, Oct 17, (2014)

35. Normal Cognitive Aging, Clin Geriatr Med Authority November 29th, (2013) p.737-752.

36. Apoptosis, pyroptosis, and necrosis: mechanisms descriptions of

dead and dying eukaryotic cells, Infect Immun (2005): 73: 1907-16.

37. Gut Microbiota and MA-PI 2 Macrobiotic Diet in the Treatment of Type 2 Diabetes, World J. Diabetes April 15th, (2015) 403-411.

38. Diet Rapidly and Reproducibly alters the Human Gut Microbiome, Nature (2014) Jan: 505 (7484) 559-563, PMC 3957428

39. Gut Dysbiosis is linked to Hypertension, Hypertension June (2015) PubMed 25870193.

40. The clinical significance of the Gut Microbiota in Cystic Fibrosis and the Potential for Dietary Therapies, Clin Nutr August (2014) p. 571-80.

41. The Way to a Man's Heart is through his Gut- Microbiota—Dietary Pro-Prebiotics for the Management of Cardiovascular Risk, Proc Nutr Soc May (2014) PubMed 24767984.

42. Inflammation-associated declines in cerebral vasoreactivity and cognition in Type 2 Diabetes, Neurology July 8th, (2015) PubMed 26156513.

43. Irritable Bowel Syndrome: A Clinical Review JAMA (2014) Mar 313 (9) 949-58. PubMed 25734736.

44. Irritable Bowel Syndrome: A Disease still searching for pathogenesis, diagnosis and Therapy, World J. Gastroenterol (2014) July 20, (27):8807-8820. PMC 4112881.

45. Gut Microbiota as potential orchestrators of Irritable Bowel Syndrome, Gut Liver, May 9th, (2015) 318-331.

46. Diabetes, Obesity and Gut Microbiota, Best Pract Res Clin Gastroenterol Feb 27, (2013) 73-83.

47. Microbial Endocrinology and the Microbiota-Gut-Brain-Axis, Adv Exp Med Biol. (2014) Pub Med24997027.

48. Evidence-based Approach to Fiber Supplements and Clinically meaningful Health Benefits, Part 1 and, Part 2, What to look for and How to recommend an Effective Fiber Therapy, Nutr. Today (2015) Mar: 50 (2) 90-97.

49. Fiber and Functional Gastrointestinal Disorders, Am. J. Gasteroenterol May (2013) 108: 718-27.

50. Fermented foods, Microbiota, and Mental Health, Ancient Practice meets Nutritional Psychiatry, J.Physiol. Antropol Jan. 15th, (2014) PubMed 3904694.

51. Intermingled Klebsiella pneumonia Populations between retail meats and Human urinary tract infections, Clin Infectious Diseases, July 22, (2015) PubMed 26206847.

52. Overweight, obesity and cancer risk, The Lancet Oncology 3, 565-571 (2002).

53. Cancer incidence and morality in relation to body mass index in the MILLION Women Study: cohort study, BMJ 335, 1134 (2007).

54. Cancer attributable to overweight and obesity in the UK in 2010.British Journal of Cancer 105 Suppl. S34-7 (2011).

55. Carcinogencity of tetracholorrinphos, parathion, malathion, diazinon and glyphosate. (organophosphate pesticides) The Lancet Oncology published on line on March 15th, (2015).

56. Thinking the unthinkable: Alzheimeimers, Creutzfedlt-Jacob and Mad Cow Disease: The age-related re-emergence of virulent, foodborne bovine tuberculosis or LOSING YOUR MIND FOR THE SAKE OF A SHAKE OR BURGER, Med. Hypothesis, (2005) 64(4) 699-705.

57. Oleocanthal rapidly and selectively induces cancer cell death via lysosomal membrane permeabilization (LMP) Molecular and Cellular Oncology (2015). Author: O. Legendre.

58. Adrenal Fatigue, Int J. Pharm Compd (2013) Jan-Feb (17) 1 39-44

59. Commitment of human pluripotent stem cells to a neural lineage is induced b pro-estrogenic flavonoid apignenin, J. Advances in Regenerative Biology (2015) 2 (0) dol:10

60. Psychological Stress and the Immune System: a Meta-Analytic Study of 30 years of Inquiry. Psychol Bull. (2004) July 130 (4) 601-30.

APENDIX B
Dr. INTERNET'S 10 RECOMMENDED WEBSITES

- Mercola.com
- Naturalnews.com
- Dr.Jockers.com
- Dr.Perlmutter.com
- AmienClinics.com
- GreenMedinfo.com
- PubMed.com
- AuthorityNutrition.com
- Cronometer.com
- InfoWars.com

CPSIA information can be obtained
at www.ICGtesting.com
Printed in the USA
LVOW13s1038260117

522189LV00004B/11/P

9 781987 985238